347

SAMUEL BELLET, M.D.

Late Professor of Clinical Cardiology and
Visiting Lecturer in Pharmacology,
School of Medicine of the University of Pennsylvania;
Director, Division of Cardiology,
Philadelphia General Hospital

ESSENTIALS OF CARDIAC ARRHYTHMIAS

Diagnosis and Management

1972

W. B. SAUNDERS COMPANY   PHILADELPHIA   LONDON   TORONTO

W. B. Saunders Company: West Washington Square
                       Philadelphia, Pa. 19105

                       12 Dyott Street
                       London, WC1A 1DB

                       833 Oxford Street
                       Toronto 18, Ontario

Essentials of Cardiac Arrhythmias: Diagnosis and Management   ISBN 0-7216-1692-5

© 1972 by W. B. Saunders Company. Copyright under the International Copyright Union. All rights reserved. This book is protected by copyright. No part of it may be reproduced, stored in a retrieval system, or transmitted in any form or by any means, electronic, mechanical, photocopying, recording, or otherwise, without written permission from the publisher. Made in the United States of America. Press of W. B. Saunders Company. Library of Congress Catalog card number 77–183444.

Print No.: 9   8   7   6   5   4   3   2   1

*To my wife, Jean
and
daughter, Joan*

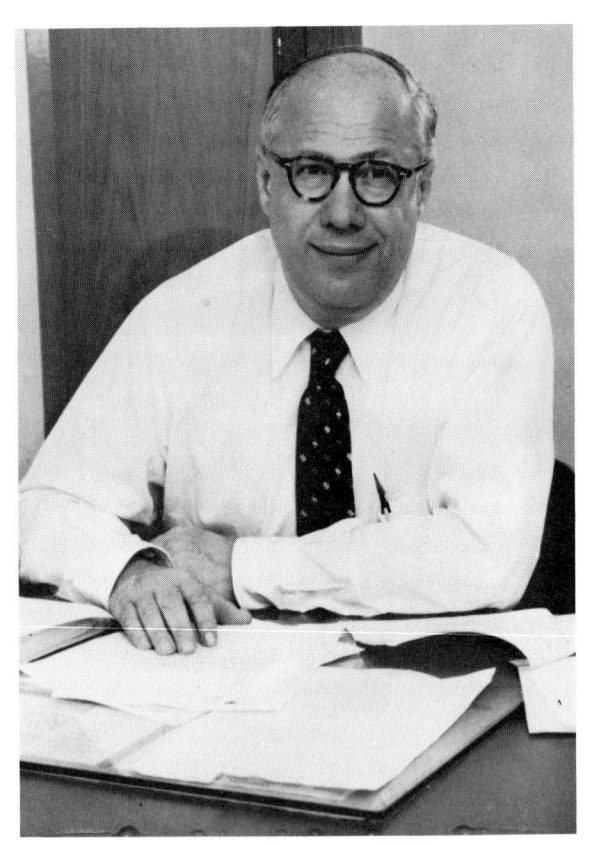

Samuel Bellet, M.D.

Foreword

A certain poignancy attaches itself to a task so close to one's heart that it is completed not only with great effort but even at risk. Just as this is true of the last symphony written by a deaf and ailing Beethoven, so it is true of this book. It represents the final thoughts and distilled clinical wisdom of Dr. Samuel Bellet. He completed it just hours before his untimely death.

In attempting to write the foreword for such a book, published posthumously, it proved difficult to write solely about the book and not about the author, a longtime, cherished friend and associate.

The mid 1920's to 1971, a period that encompassed Dr. Bellet's intensive study of the heart, produced the most startling advances in the field of diagnostic procedures as well as in the prevention and treatment of the real killers: heart block and the serious ventricular disturbances. The responsibility for the recognition of these conditions and for the institution of treatment usually falls upon the intern, resident, nurse, or trained technician on duty in admissions, in the accident wards, or in coronary care units. Realizing that few medical schools can find a place in their curricula for a thorough, comprehensive study of this subject, Dr. Bellet felt that a short, concise text, containing as far as possible just the essentials of cardiac arrhythmias, would be useful to quickly furnish necessary information to students, interns and residents. This book admirably meets these needs.

Those who knew Dr. Samuel Bellet were filled with admiration for his skill in teaching, writing, and research and with affection for his understanding, dedication, and purpose, and will look upon this book as an epitaph worthy of a great scientist and human being.

THOMAS M. MCMILLAN, M.D.
Mobile, Alabama

Preface

The topic of cardiac arrhythmias has been the subject of intense interest in recent years because of the rapid developments that have been made in basic and clinical research. Greater emphasis on arrhythmias has resulted from studies, particularly in coronary care units and situations in which long-term monitoring is available. In addition, the development of additional antiarrhythmic agents has stimulated further study in this area. Advances have also been made in the electrophysiology and mechanisms of production of arrhythmias and in the development of diagnostic methods for their recognition and specific identification, e.g., His bundle recordings.

The object of this volume is to discuss the essential features of cardiac arrhythmias, especially those features pertaining to diagnosis and treatment. It is hoped that this will be of help to physicians engaged in the practice of internal medicine and cardiology, as well as to interns, residents, and medical students. It is in no way intended to displace the larger, more detailed works on this subject. Historical data and physiologic mechanisms are mentioned but briefly; reference is made to sources in which greater detail concerning these aspects of the subject may be found.

The initial chapters include a general discussion of arrhythmias, namely, etiologic factors as related to alterations in physiology and associated clinical states. The subsequent chapters, from 5 to 16, include the discussion of individual arrhythmias: sinus irregularities, atrial flutter and fibrillation, premature beats, paroxysmal atrial tachycardia, A-V heart block, disturbances in the region of the A-V junction, A-V dissociation, paroxysmal ventricular tachycardia, W-P-W syndrome, ventricular flutter and fibrillation, cardiac arrest, and cardiac alternans. A separate chapter is devoted to a discussion of the diagnosis of arrhythmias, including not only the ECG but other modalities, such as esophageal leads, Doppler technique, and His bundle recordings, that are now routinely employed in the diagnosis of specific underlying mechanisms. The next section includes a discussion of those clinical states in which arrhythmias frequently occur, including syncopal attacks, exercise, electrolyte disturbances, and acute myocardial infarction.

The final section, covering therapy, is divided into four main headings, namely, drugs that increase automaticity, drugs that decrease automaticity, mechanical and other procedures employed in therapy, and the various electronic devices used.

Much of the material in this book has been taken from or modified from the 3rd edition of my book *Clinical Disorders of the Heart Beat*, which was published by Lea & Febiger, who have so very kindly granted me permission to use this material.

I particularly wish to thank Leonard N. Horowitz, M.D., for his great effort and devotion in gathering recent material and for his editing and participation in the numerous revisions of the text. I also wish to thank Harriet Beilowitz for her secretarial assistance in preparing the manuscript and illustrations.

I am particularly indebted to Domingo Aviado, M.D., for review of portions of the text.

I also wish to thank the Foundation for Cardiovascular Research for its assistance in the completion of this text.

I wish to extend to the publisher, W. B. Saunders, and their staff my sincere appreciation for their assistance in the preparation of this book.

SAMUEL BELLET, M.D.

Contents

Chapter 1
Anatomy 1

Chapter 2
Physiologic Considerations 11

Chapter 3
Hemodynamics 31

Chapter 4
General Discussion of Arrhythmias 36

Chapter 5
Sinus Irregularities 42

Chapter 6
Atrial Flutter 55

Chapter 7
Atrial Fibrillation 65

Chapter 8
Premature Beats 81

Chapter 9
Paroxysmal Atrial Tachycardia (PAT) 102

Chapter 10
A-V Heart Block 115

Chapter 11
Disturbances in the Region of the A-V Junction 144

Chapter 12
A-V Dissociation 168

Chapter 13
Pre-excitation Syndromes 178

Chapter 14
Paroxysmal Ventricular Tachycardia 189

Chapter 15
Ventricular Flutter and Fibrillation 207

Chapter 16
Cardiac Arrest 214

Chapter 17
Alternation of the Heart 222

Chapter 18
Methods Employed in ECG Diagnosis of an Arrhythmia 229

Chapter 19
Syncopal Attacks 239

Chapter 20
Stress Tests Producing Arrhythmias: Exercise, Emotion, Respiratory Maneuvers, and Atrial Pacing 248

Chapter 21
Pregnancy 257

Chapter 22
Congenital Cardiac Anomalies 261

Chapter 23
Arrhythmias in Infants, Children, and in the Fetus 266

Chapter 24
Endocrine Disturbances 275

Chapter 25
Anesthesia and Surgery 279

Chapter 26
Cardiac Catheterization and Angiocardiography 284

Chapter 27
Brain and Heart Relationships 290

Chapter 28
Coronary Artery Disease and Myocardial Infarction 295

Chapter 29
Disturbances of Electrolyte Balance 312

Chapter 30
Infectious Diseases and Other Disease States 320

Chapter 31
General Methods Available in Therapy 325

Chapter 32
Drugs Which Increase Cardiac Automaticity 329

Chapter 33
Agents Which Decrease Cardiac Automaticity 339

Chapter 34
Digitalis 375

Chapter 35
Electrolytes Employed in Therapy 387

Chapter 36
Other Drugs 394

Chapter 37
Artificial Pacemakers *404*

Chapter 38
Defibrillation and Electric Countershock *426*

Glossary *437*

Index *447*

Chapter 1 *Anatomy*

GENERAL CONSIDERATIONS
NORMAL ANATOMY
  S-A Node
  Atria
  A-V Junction, Bundle of His, Bundle Branches
    and Purkinje Fibers
    Terminology
    Gross Anatomy
    Histology

BLOOD SUPPLY
  S-A Node
  A-V Junction
  Bundle Branches
PATHOLOGIC CONSIDERATIONS
  Relationship to Arrhythmias

In this section we will discuss the anatomic aspects of the heart that pertain directly and indirectly to the origin and normal propagation of the cardiac impulse. Disturbance of function in these structures contributes to the production of cardiac arrhythmias. These structures include particularly the sinoatrial (S-A) node, the atrioventricular (A-V) junction, intra-atrial tracts, bundle branches, and Purkinje fibers.

The heart may be divided into (1) the undifferentiated myocardium, the principal function of which is to pump blood in response to the cardiac impulse; (2) the fibrous tissue, valves, and chorda tendineae, which control the flow of blood; and (3) those tissues of the heart specialized for impulse initiation and propagation (S-A node, intra-atrial tracts, A-V junction, His-Purkinje system, and other specialized fibers).

GENERAL CONSIDERATIONS

Anatomic concepts have been revised in recent years, not only from the standpoint of "anatomy" per se but as a result of studies in histology, electron microscopy, histochemistry, physiology, and pathology. The result of these new correlations has been a clearer understanding of the function of various anatomic structures; this has helped considerably in the study of the propagation of the normal cardiac impulse and the genesis of arrhythmias. Moreover, there is an intimate relationship between the anatomy and the histopathology of pacemaker cells and conduction fibers and the etiology, mechanisms, and manifestations of cardiac arrhythmias.

NORMAL ANATOMY

S-A Node. The S-A node is located in the superior portion of the right atrial wall at the termination of the sulcus terminalis. It is horseshoe-shaped and varies in size from 1.5 to 2.5 cm. in length and 0.4 to 0.7 cm. in width. The "head" of the node is located subepicardially at the junction of the superior vena cava and the right atrium; the "tail" is situated subendocardially at the junction of the auricular appendage and atrium proper. Because of this unique position, the sinus node is affected by those processes which affect the epicardium—notably pericarditis—and also the endocardium, e.g., mural thrombi.

The cells of the sinus node are attached by their basement membranes to an interlacing network of supporting collagen. The arrangement of interweaving bundles contrasts with the more regular pattern of the atrial fibers. The individual cells of the human S-A node may be divided into four groups: (1) P ("pacemaker") cells, located predominantly at the center of the node; (2) undifferentiated myocardial cells, located mostly at the border of the node; (3) transitional cells, with structural properties and often a location intermediate between the previous types; and (4) Purkinje fibers, found at the borders of the node and extending to the atrial muscle and to the specific conduction pathways (James, 1968a).

The P cells are believed to have a pacemaking function. They are small, have little endoplasmic reticulum, and present few connections to adjacent cells, all characteristics which result in slow intercellular conduction and may account for the slow conduction through the S-A node (Hudson, 1960).

Atria. The fibers of the S-A node are in continuity with (1) the transitional cells, discussed previously; and (2) specific pathways that extend from the S-A node to the A-V junction, to the left atrium, and probably to portions of the atrial musculature located at a distance from the sinus node (Fig. 1-1). These tracts have been shown to be composed of Purkinje fibers and apparently undifferentiated myocardial cells. Recent evidence for the existence of these specialized pathways has required revision of the long-held concept that the impulse proceeded from the S-A node by simple radiation over undifferentiated atrial myocardium. Evidence that suggests the presence of specialized conducting fibers within the atria and multiple pathways within the A-V junction includes the following: (1) sinoventricular conduction occurs in potassium intoxication, in which the atrial muscle is electrically bypassed; (2) different forms of the QRS complex can be produced by stimulating different areas of the atria or A-V junction; (3) abnormal A-V conduction can alter the amplitude of the ventricular complex; and (4) in the Wolff-Parkinson-White (W-P-W) syndrome, the change in the pre-excitation ventricular complex sometimes is associated with a change in the location of the atrial pacemaker.

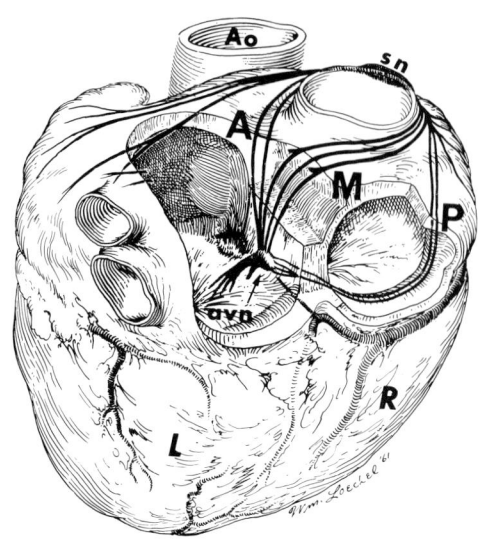

Figure 1-1. This drawing illustrates the three intra-atrial (internodal) pathways. The heart is viewed from above and behind the left atrium. The abbreviations are as follows: A, anterior internodal tract; M, middle internodal tract; P, posterior internodal tract; L, left ventricle; R, right ventricle; Ao, aorta; sn, sinus node; avn, A-V node. The anterior internodal tract leaves the anterior margin of the sinus node and courses forward to enter the anterior interatrial myocardial band; there it divides into two groups, those coursing on into the left atrium (Bachmann's bundle) and those curving back into the interatrial septum and descending to the crest of the A-V node. The middle internodal tract courses from the posterior margin of the sinus node behind the superior vena cava and across the sinus intercavarum to descend along the right atrial side of the septum into the crest of the A-V node. The posterior internodal tract leaves the posterior margin of the sinus node, then courses along the crista terminalis to the eustachian ridge and hence, through the ridge, to the posterior margin of the A-V node. (This latter tract, which is the longest of the three, terminates with most of its fibers *bypassing* the bulk of the A-V node.) (From Sherf, L., and Jones, T. N.: Dis. Chest., 55:128, 1969.)

ANATOMY

Although the concept of internodal pathways is not universally accepted, evidence for their existence is strong. Considerable data have recently been accumulated which indicate that specialized atrial pathways are an integral part of the cardiac conduction system.

A-V Junction, Bundle of His, Bundle Branches, and Purkinje Fibers. The atrioventricular conduction system commences at the A-V junction, situated on the right side of the interatrial septum near the region of the coronary sinus (Fig. 1–2). The specialized atrial conduction pathways terminate at the A-V junction. Most of the fibers enter the upper portion of the A-V junction posteriorly, but some tracts bypass the upper portion of the A-V junction to insert near the origin of the bundle of His. An impulse may travel from the A-V junction and the James bypass fibers by way of the bundle of His to activate the remainder of the atrioventricular conduction system.

Terminology. There has been considerable confusion regarding the application of the terms "A-V node" and "A-V junction." "A-V node" is used loosely to denote all the specialized tissues that constitute the A-V junctional area; however, according to the traditional anatomic definition, the A-V node encompasses a much smaller region. Recent microscopic and physiologic studies make possible a uniform terminology (DeFelice and Challice, 1969): (1) The term "A-V node" should be applied to that area defined structurally by the characteristics of areas b, c, and d in Figure 1–3 and physiologically by the characteristic A-N, N, and N-H potentials. (2) The subdivisions of the A-V node should be labeled in accordance with their physiologic characteristics—the A-N, N, and N-H regions. (3) The term "A-V junction" should be applied to the entire area composed of the A-V node, the specialized tissue of the prenodal atrium, and the tissue from which H potentials are recorded on the atrial side of the fibrous skeleton.

Gross Anatomy. The A-V junction lies on the right side of the interatrial septum, anterior to the coronary sinus, above the base of the septal leaflet of the tricuspid valve (Fig. 1–2). The A-V junction is roughly flask-shaped and measures approximately 8 x 4 x 6 mm. It is continuous with the thinner bundle of His, which passes medially and inferiorly to penetrate the trigonum fibrosum. This "penetrating" part of the bundle of His is continuous with the "branching" part, which runs along the crest of the muscular portion of the interventricular septum. The bundle measures 1 to 4 mm. in width and 15 to 20 mm. in length; in cross section, it is at first triangular, then oval. The bundle passes through the posterior edge of the membranous septum to reach the superior border of the muscular septum (Fig. 1–4). At this point, the bundle of His bifurcates; however, it is now apparent that instead of one bifurcation, as classically taught, there are actually two bifurcation sites (Rosenbaum et al., 1970). The first involves the origin of the posterior division of the left bundle branch, which arises perpendicular to and high in the branching portion of the bundle. More distally, the right bundle branch separates from the anterior division of the left bundle branch. The right bundle branch runs subendocardially in its first and third portions and dips into the septal musculature in its middle third. It courses caudally toward the apex of the heart in the groove between the attachment of the septal and the anterior cusps of the tricuspid valve. At the caudal end of the interventricular septum, it courses through the moderator band to the free wall.

The left branch consists of anterior and posterior hemibranches running toward the anterior and posterior papillary muscles. The posterior branch is broad whereas the anterior is thin and quite delicate. These hemi-

ANATOMY

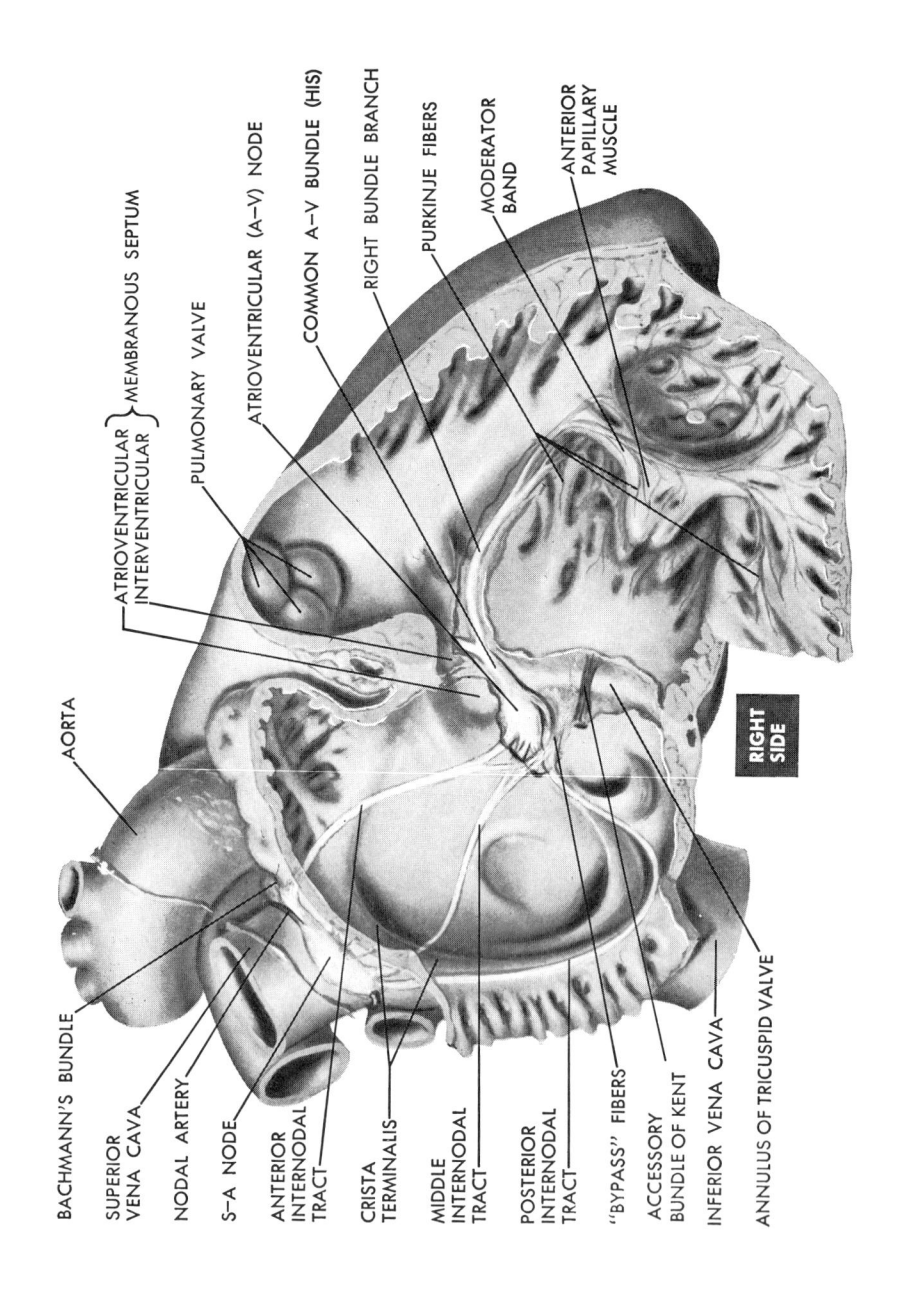

4

ANATOMY

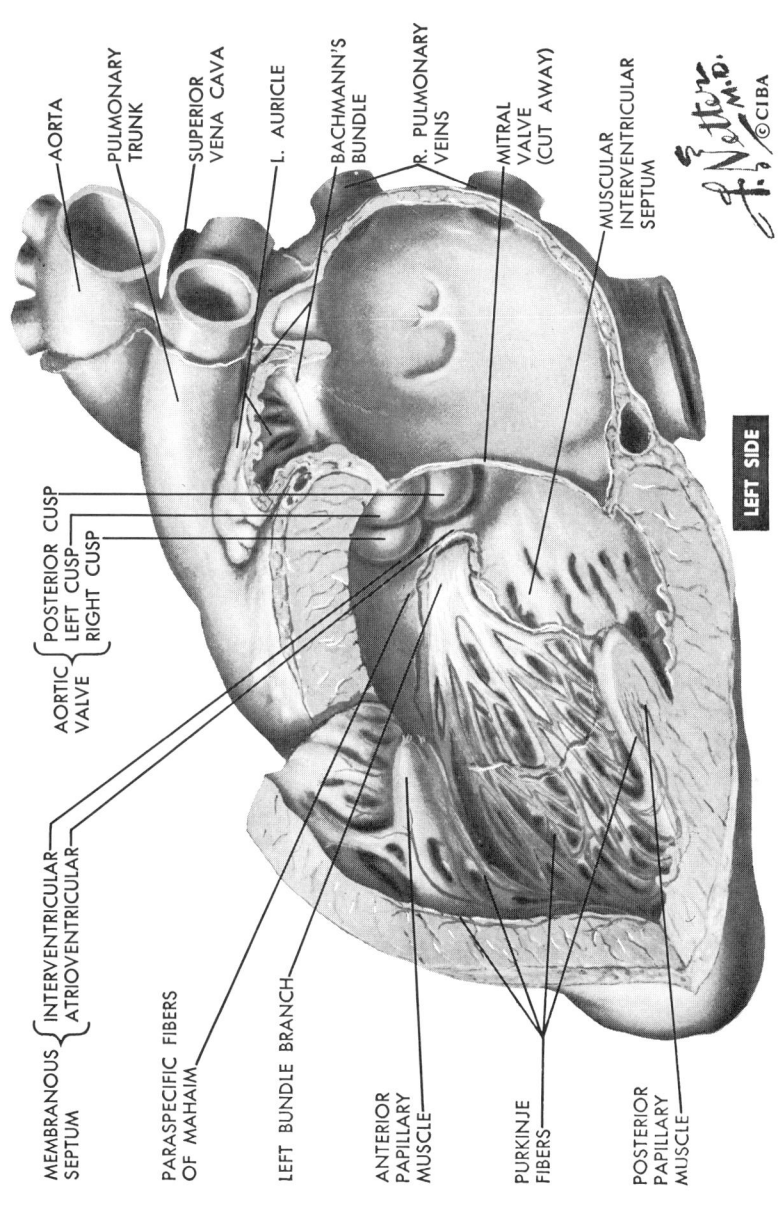

Figure 1-2. Gross anatomy of the heart. (© Copyright 1969 CIBA Pharmaceutical Company, Division of CIBA-GEIGY Corporation. Reproduced, with permission, from THE CIBA COLLECTION OF MEDICAL ILLUSTRATIONS by Frank H. Netter, M.D. All rights reserved.)

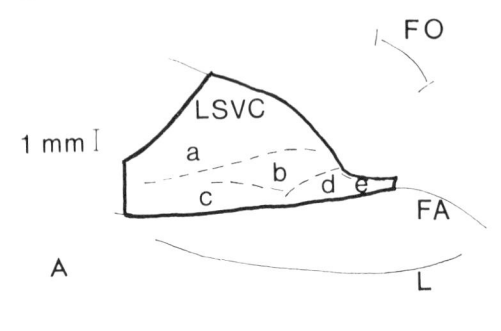

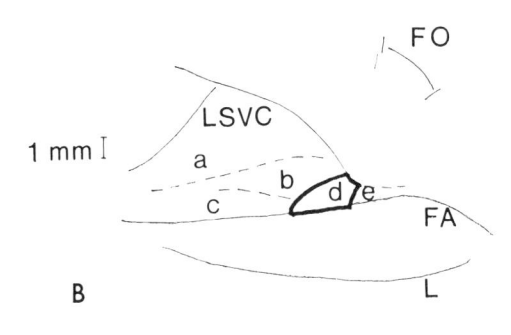

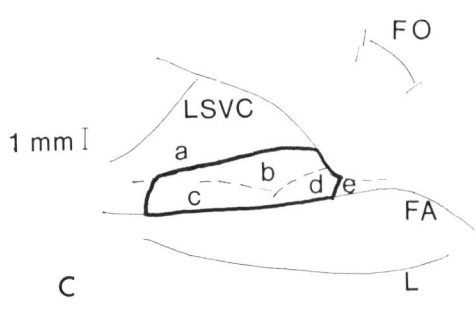

Figure 1-3. Electrophysiologic atrioventricular node of the rabbit. (A) A-V junction; (B) anatomic A-V node; (C) functional A-V node. *LSVC*, Left superior vena cava; *FO*, fossa ovalis; *FA*, fibrous annulus; *L*, septal cusp margin. (Modified from DeFelice, L. J., and Challice, C. E.: Circ. Res., 24:457, 1969.)

branches gradually diverge into numerous fibers descending toward the apex of the heart. They may reach the papillary muscles through the trabeculae carneae or, in the case of the anterior branch, covered only by a thin layer of endocardium, may actually traverse the ventricular cavity.

Histology. The A-V junction consists of delicate fibers ranging from 3 to 11μ in diameter, tightly interwoven into a compact mass. These fibers are less cross-striated than those of the typical myocardium, and they contain fewer myofibrils.

Purkinje cells are observed in the A-V junction, the bundle of His, and bundle branches. They are paler-staining cells than the unspecialized myocardial cells because of their paucity of myofibrils. Nuclei are ovoid in shape and centrally placed, surrounded by a perinuclear clear zone. Their cell boundaries appear smooth with few indentations. This histologic picture of Purkinje cells correlates well with the observed high speed of conduction through them. Three factors are particularly pertinent: (1) the cells are short; (2) the cells have smooth peripheries; and (3) they are joined end to end by intercalated discs. All three factors promote fast conduction (James, 1968a).

BLOOD SUPPLY (Fig. 1-5)

S-A Node. The S-A node is supplied by the terminal branches of the largest artery that nourishes the atria— the ramus ostii cavae superioris. This artery arises from the right coronary artery in 60 per cent of hearts and from the left coronary artery in the remaining 40 per cent. It supplies both the right and left atria and terminates by surrounding the orifice of the superior vena cava. Usually one but in some cases two large branches of the ramus ostii cavae superioris course through the long axis of the sinus node and supply a profuse network of small arterioles and capillaries.

A-V Junction. The A-V junction is nourished by the ramus septi fibrosi, a branch of the right coronary artery in 92 per cent of hearts and of the left circumflex branch in 8 per cent. In the

ANATOMY

Figure 1-4. Photomicrograph (van Gieson stain) of the human common A-V bundle (*B*) and its left branch (*L*). ×50. *M*, ventricular muscle; (*C*) the connective tissue of the membranous portion of septum. (Courtesy of Drs. O. Saphir and M. Lev.) (Katz, L. N., and Pick, A.: Clinical Electrocardiography. Part I. The Arrhythmias. Philadelphia, Lea & Febiger, 1971, p. 20.)

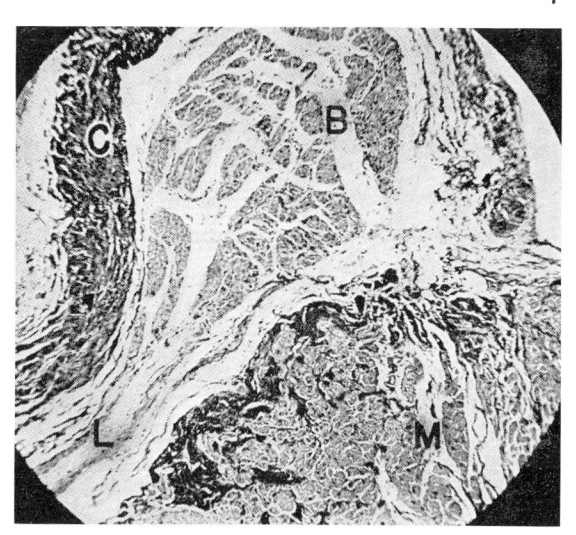

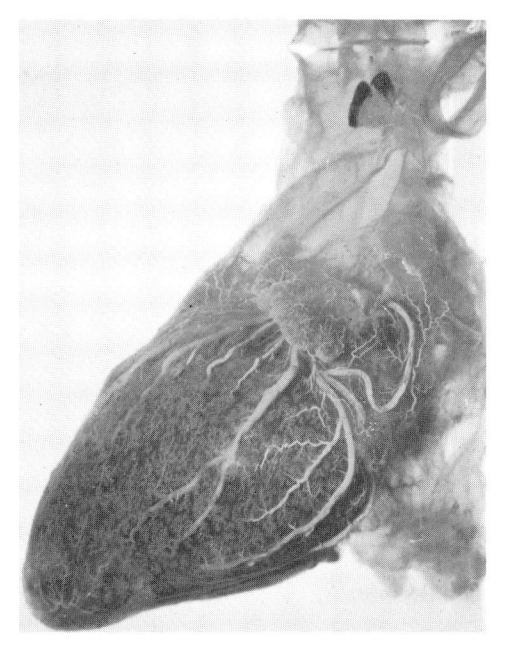

Figure 1-5. The coronary circulation of an adult human heart. The arteries have been injected with vermillion and the specimen rendered transparent (Spalteholz principle). Nothing has been dissected away, yet the vessels can be followed to a considerable depth into the myocardium. The tapering character of the surface coronary arteries of supply contrast with the uniform size of the nutrient arterioles to the myocardium. The viscosity of the mass injected and the pressure used was such that finer arterioles were not injected. Had these vessels been filled with vermillion, it would have appeared that the heart in structure was composed entirely of blood vessels. (Specimen prepared by O. V. Batson, M.D., and S. Bellet, M.D.)

first instance, this branch arises from the posterior descending branch of the right coronary artery at the crus, the point at which it takes an acute downward course to supply the posterior portion of the apex. It then runs anteriorly from the crus following a straight course for 2 to 3 cm. to reach the base of the interatrial septum near the coronary sinus. The ramus septi fibrosi anastomoses grossly with the branches of both the right and left coronary arteries.

Myocardial veins and sinusoids that are intimately related to the A-V junction and the common bundle have also been anatomically demonstrated (Fig. 1-6). The distribution of such venous channels indicates that they may play a significant role in intercoronary circulation in the presence of coronary artery disease. This may also explain the low incidence of bilateral bundle branch block following gradual or acute occlusion of the coronary arteries.

Bundle Branches. The bundle of His and the first part of the right and left bundle branches, contained in the upper portion of the interventricular septum, are also supplied by the ramus septi fibrosi. The conducting tissues immediately distal to this do not have a specific blood supply but are nour-

VENOUS CIRCULATION | ARTERIAL CIRCULATION

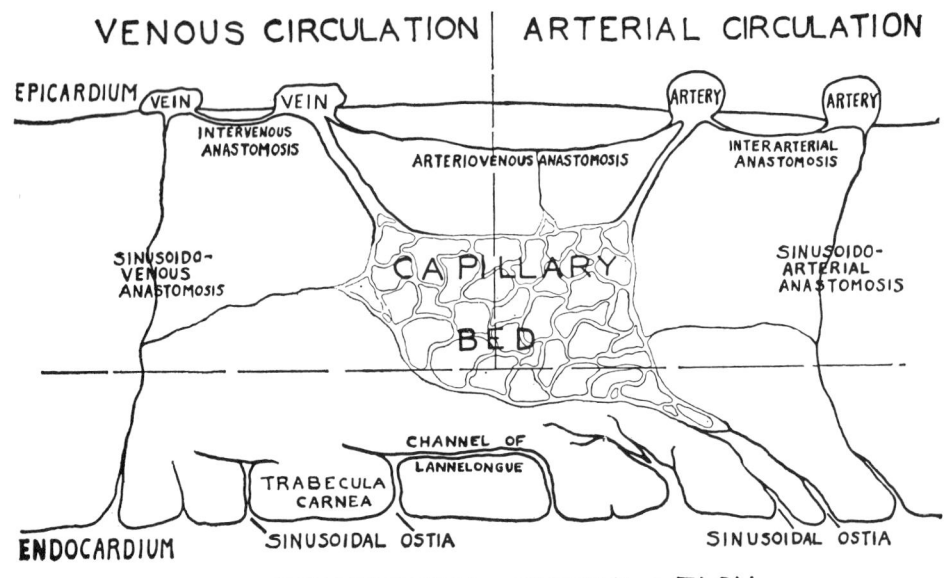

SINUSOIDAL CIRCULATION

Figure 1-6. Diagram of the myocardial circulation. This diagram is based upon the embryologic origin and the adult distribution of the vessels, and the terminology employed is compatible with these points of view and with the terminology generally employed in the vascular system. In development, the endocardial sinusoidal system develops first; the epicardial venous vessels develop next; and, finally, the epicardial arterial vessels develop and join the other two, forming a common capillary bed. The endocardial or epicardial origin of the vessels, as well as their various modes of interconnection, are indicated in the diagram. Sinusoidal ostia are present in all four chambers of the heart. Intervenous anastomoses are obvious with the naked eye. (From Bellet, S.: Nourishment of the Heart by Channels Other Than the Coronary Arteries, *in* the Cyclopedia of Medicine, Vol. III, Philadelphia, F. A. Davis Co., 1933, p. 363.)

ished by vessels that supply the adjacent septal tissues. The anterior portion of the interventricular septum is supplied by penetrating branches of the anterior descending branch of the left coronary artery; the posterior portion of the septum is supplied by the descending branch of the right circumflex; and the middle portion, by both of these branches.

PATHOLOGIC CONSIDERATIONS

Relationship to Arrhythmias. With certain specific exceptions, attempts to correlate pathologic changes observed at necropsy with the arrhythmias present during life have failed to document a consistent association. This is not surprising, since in many instances arrhythmias result from functional derangements rather than from pathologic alterations. On the other hand, quite localized structural changes that can readily be overlooked may be important in the genesis of arrhythmias. A number of recent studies, furthermore, have allowed some correlations to be made between organic disease and electrophysiologic abnormalities.

In an attempt to elucidate the relationship of pathologic findings to arrhythmias, the arrhythmias may be separated into two categories: (1) "ectopic rhythms proper," and (2) "conduction disturbances." Both of these disturbances can occur in hearts presenting no gross or microscopic pathology. An obvious example of an ectopic rhythm frequently occurring in a normal heart is paroxysmal atrial tachycardia. Likewise, it is common to record both atrial and ventricular premature beats in normal subjects. On the other hand, conduction disturbances in normal hearts, which may sometimes occur in normal subjects when they assume the recumbent position, are distinctly less common than "ectopic rhythms." Alterations in the nervous control of the heart may cause some of these phenomena. Alterations in vagal tone may be the mechanism producing transient prolongation of A-V conduction time upon assumption of a recumbent position. Vagal stimulation is often responsible for the genesis of some ectopic rhythms in normal hearts. Thus, not infrequently the A-V junction becomes the cardiac pacemaker as the vagus nerve slows the rate of the sinus node.

Recently, the genesis of several ectopic rhythms has been related to pathologic changes. In subjects with atrial fibrillation, the duration of the arrhythmias and their refractoriness to treatment correlate with the degree of atrial pathology. Various electrophysiologic abnormalities have been demonstrated in biopsy specimens removed from the diseased atria of human subjects with prolonged atrial fibrillation (see Chapter 7).

The incidence of atrial arrhythmias, especially flutter and fibrillation, is markedly increased following atrial infarction. The relationships between the more common type of (ventricular) myocardial infarction and various arrhythmias is a complicated one, involving considerations of altered autonomic tone and varying grades of pump failure; they are discussed in Chapter 28.

Pathologic study and correlated endocardial and epicardial electrophysiologic mapping have documented a circus movement involving both the normal and the accessory A-V pathways in the supraventricular tachycardias associated with the W-P-W syndrome (Cobb, et al., 1968) (see Chapter 13, p. 182). In the W-P-W syndrome, a gross re-entry pathway has been demonstrated, with forward propagation of the impulse over the normal A-V conduction system, then through the ventricular muscle, and in a retrograde direction over an accessory pathway (the Bundle of Kent) to the atrium, which is then activated prematurely (see Chapter 13).

Numerous problems arise when an attempt is made to study the pathology of the conduction elements and then correlate them with the clinical phenomena of ectopic rhythms and conduction disturbances. In the first place, a thorough histologic technique is difficult and time-consuming. Furthermore, lesions of the conducting elements are invariably multiple, thus requiring a careful examination of the entire conduction system (Lev and Unger, 1955). The technique necessary for careful study requires making at least 2000 serial sections which include representative levels of the conduction system. Relatively few such studies have been performed, most of them in relationship to complete A-V heart block (see Chapter 10). Another problem is the reversibility of lesions. Edema and leukocytic infiltration may resolve. Even abnormal collections in elastic tissue may disappear. An ectopic rhythm or conduction disturbance may be related to a pathologic process that is no longer present or has markedly altered when the heart is examined at necropsy.

In summary it may be stated that characteristic pathologic findings have not been demonstrated for most of the arrhythmias. Some advance has been made in correlating pathologic changes, electrophysiologic abnormalities, and some of the arrhythmias. However, most arrhythmias may occur in the absence of any detectable anatomic alteration, and conversely, arrhythmias may be absent in the presence of considerable anatomic change.

In order to understand the cardiac conduction tissues, a correlative study of anatomy, histology, electron microscopy, histochemistry, physiology, and pathology must be undertaken. Simple description of anatomic structures no longer reveals definitive information concerning the significance of these structures in the functioning of the normal heart.

References

Cobb, F. R., Blumenschein, S. D., Sealy, W. C., Boineau, J. P., Wagner, G. S., and Wallace, A. G.: Successful surgical interruption of the bundle of Kent in a patient with W-P-W syndrome. Circulation, 38:1018, 1968.

DeFelice, L. J., and Challice, C. E.: Anatomical and ultrastructural study of the electrophysiological atrioventricular node of the rabbit. Circ. Res., 24:457, 1969.

Eyster, J. A. E., and Meek, W. J.: Experiments on the origin and conduction of the cardiac impulse: VI. Conduction of the excitation from the sino-auricular node to the right auricle and auriculoventricular node. Arch. Intern. Med., 18:775, 1916.

Hering, H. E.: Nachweiss, dass das His'sche Uebergangsbundel Vorhof und Kammer des Saugethierherzens functionell verbindet. Arch. ges. Physiol., 108:267, 1905.

His, W.: Die Thatigkeit des Embryonalen Herzens und deren Bedeutung fur die Lehre von der Herzbewegung beim Erwachsenen. Arb. med. Klin. (Leipzig), 14, 1893.

Hoffman, B. F., and Cranefield, P. F.: Electrophysiology of the Heart. New York, McGraw-Hill, 1960.

Hudson, R. E. B.: The human pacemaker and its pathology. Brit. Heart J., 22:163, 1960.

James, T. N.: Morphology of the human atrioventricular node with remarks pertinent to its electrophysiology. Amer. Heart J., 62:756, 1961a.

James, T. N.: Anatomy of the human sinus node. Anat. Rec., 141:109, 1961b.

James, T. N., and Sherf, L.: Ultrastructure of myocardial cells. Amer. J. Cardiol., 22:389, 1968a.

James, T. N., and Sherf, L.: Ultrastructure of the human atrioventricular node. Circulation, 27:1049, 1968b.

Kent, A. F. S.: Researches on the structure and function of the mammalian heart. J. Physiol., 14:233, 1893.

Lev, M., and Unger, P. N.: The pathology of the conduction system in acquired heart disease. I. Severe atrioventricular block. Arch. Path., 60:502, 1955.

Lewis, T.: Mechanism and Graphic Registration of the Heart Beat. 3rd ed. London, Shaw & Son, 1925.

Paes de Carvalho, A., DeMello, W. C., and Hoffman, B. F.: Electrophysiological evidence for specialized fiber types in rabbit atrium. Amer. J. Physiol., 196:483, 1959.

Purkinje, J. E.: Mikroskopische neurologische beobachtungen. Arch. Anat. Physiol. wissensch. Med., 12:281, 1845.

Rosenbaum, M. B., Elizari, M. V., and Lazzari, J. O.: The Hemiblocks. Tampa Tracings, Oldsmar, Fla., p. 24, 1970.

Rossi, L.: Histopathologic Features of Cardiac Arrhythmia. Milano, Casa Edituce Ambrosiani, 1969.

Truex, R. C., and Smythe, M. Q.: Recent observations of the human cardiac conduction system, with special considerations of the atrioventricular node and bundle. *In:* Taccardi, B., and Marchetti, G. (eds.), Electrophysiology of the Heart. pp. 177–198. Oxford, Pergamon Press, 1964.

Chapter 2 *Physiologic Considerations*

ELECTROPHYSIOLOGY
  Normal Action Potential
  Automaticity and Formation of Cardiac
    Impulse
  S-A Node Initiation of Normal Impulse
PROPAGATION OF CARDIAC IMPULSE
  Methods of Study
    Electrocardiogram
    Electrogram
      Clinical Applications of His Bundle
        Recordings
  Atrial Spread of Impulse
  Atrioventricular Junction
  Ventricular Spread of the Impulse
FACTORS DETERMINING A NORMAL
CARDIAC MECHANISM
PHYSIOLOGIC PROPERTIES OF NORMAL
HEART MUSCLE
  Automaticity
  Excitability
  Conductivity
  Contractility

RELATION OF FUNDAMENTAL
PHYSIOLOGIC MECHANISMS TO
SPECIFIC ARRHYTHMIAS
  Disturbances of Impulse Formation
  Disturbances of Conduction
    Refractory Tissue
    Decremental Conduction
    Inhomogeneous Conduction
    Unidirectional Block and Re-entry
  Combined Disturbances of Impulse
    Formation and Conduction
FACTORS LEADING TO PRODUCTION OF
ARRHYTHMIAS IN HUMAN SUBJECT
  Physical Regulation of Cardiovascular System
  Role of Nervous System
    Autonomic Control
    Sympathetic Effects
    Parasympathetic Effects
  Metabolic Regulation
  Reflex Adjustments
  Endocrine Factors in Cardiac Regulation
  Hemodynamic Alterations
  Pathologic Factors

The study of the etiology, mechanisms, and effect of drugs on arrhythmias involves the integration of knowledge obtained from the experiments upon the single cell, the isolated heart, and the intact animal. In this chapter, the data obtained from these sources are correlated to form a foundation upon which an understanding of the subject of cardiac arrhythmias can be developed. Fundamental to the genesis of their production are the electrophysiologic concepts of impulse initiation and conduction.

ELECTROPHYSIOLOGY

Normal Action Potential. In quiescent cardiac muscle cells, a steady transmembrane potential of about -90 mv is recorded, the inside of the cell being negative with respect to the outside (Fig. 2–1). This is called "resting membrane potential." Electrotonic currents and chemical mediators act on the cell to change its membrane potential. When the membrane potential reaches a critical level termed the "threshold" (usually about -60 mv), a characteristic sequence of self-propagated depolarization and repolarization occurs, which is called the "action potential" or "spike." The spike generates electrotonic currents that spread to adjacent cells, eliciting in them a similar sequence of depolarization followed by an action potential. The impulse spreads as long as it encounters excitable cells in the course of its

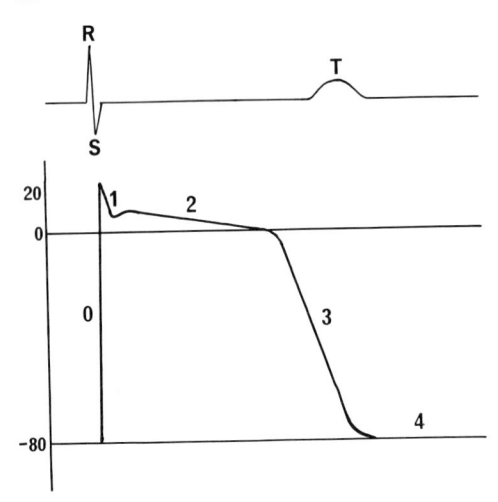

Figure 2-1. Diagrammatic representation of the transmembrane action potential and unipolar electrogram. The zero line is recorded when microelectrode tip is extracellular in position. The transmembrane resting potential (−80) is recorded when the electrode tip penetrates the quiescent fiber. Depolarization and the various phases of repolarization are designated by the symbols 0, 1, 2, and 3; symbol 4 is used to designate the diastolic period. See text for discussion. The top trace shows a unipolar electrogram recorded from the immediate vicinity of the microelectrode tip. Note that the intrinsic deflection of the R wave is synchronous with phase 0 of the transmembrane action potential and that the T wave of the electrogram is inscribed during phase 3.

propagation. Contraction is initiated when a spike potential occurs in cardiac cells containing myofibrils (i.e., unspecialized myocardial fibers).

The normal electrical activity of a cardiac cell is divided into five phases (see Fig. 2-1). Phase 0 denotes the period of rapid depolarization (actually reversal of polarity), which is thought to be due to sodium (Na^+) suddenly entering the cell. The initial rapid return toward the resting potential (repolarization) is called stage 1. There follows a period of slow repolarization — stage 2 and a final rapid repolarization called stage 3, which ends when the resting potential is reached. The repolarization or downsweep of the spike is due to a delayed efflux of potassium (K^+), which brings the cell back to its resting membrane pattern of −90 mv. Stage 4 follows the return of the membrane potential to its resting level and is the period when the cardiac cell restores its ionic composition in preparation for the next spike. The relationship between the transmembrane potential and the unipolar electrogram is illustrated in Figure 2-1.

In the interval during which the cell is refractory to stimulation following phase 0, excitability is gradually recovered. This period, called the "refractory period," is divided into several intervals (see Fig. 2-2).

One of the most fundamental relationships in cardiac electrophysiology is that which exists between the level of the transmembrane potential when excitation is triggered and the characteristics of the ensuing action potential. When excitation occurs at a transmembrane potential near the resting level, the action potential has its most rapid rate of rise and attains its greatest amplitude, thus serving as an excellent stimulus to surrounding cells. However, as the resting potential is reduced, the action potential manifests a lower slope of phase 0 and lower amplitude. This relationship holds whether the impulse is initiated by self-depolarization ("automaticity") or by the arrival of an impulse ("excitability").

Automaticity and the Formation of the Cardiac Impulse. Various cardiac cells are classified by the characteristics of their membrane potential during stage 4. Undifferentiated myocardial cells have a relatively stable potential of −90 mv. Cells in some of the specialized tissues of the heart, however, normally undergo slow depolarization during diastole. Stage 4 depolarization elicits a spike or action potential when the transmembrane potential is reduced to the threshold level, about −60 mv. Cells possessing this property, termed "automaticity," under normal conditions are classified as "automatic cells." These include both the actual

PHYSIOLOGIC CONSIDERATIONS

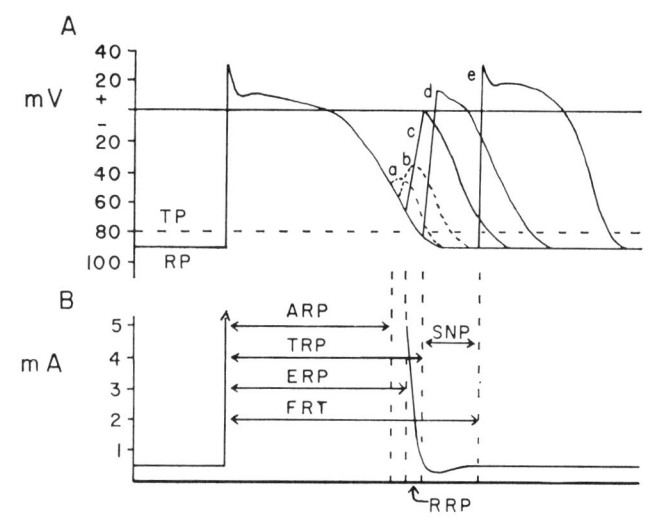

Figure 2–2. (A) Diagrammatic representation of a normal transmembrane action potential and of the responses elicited by stimuli applied at various times during repolarization. The amplitude and rising velocity of the responses are related to the level of membrane potential at the time of stimulation. The earliest responses, (a) and (b), arise at such low levels of membrane potential and are so small and slow rising that they do not propagate (graded or local responses). The first propagated response (c) defines the end of the effective refractory period. Although response (d) arises at a time when the membrane potential approximates the threshold potential (TP), i.e., during the supernormal period of excitability, it is still smaller and more slowly rising than response (e), which occurs after repolarization is complete. The first normal response (e) defines the end of the full recovery time. (B) Schematic representation of the usual relationships between transmembrane potentials and cathodal excitability. The changes in threshold are related to an arbitrary scale of current strength. The fiber becomes inexcitable coincident with the inscription of phase 0 of the action potential. Recovery of excitability, as indicated by changes in threshold, progresses slowly during phase 3. The terminal portion of phase 3 is associated with a period of supernormal excitability. The diagram also illustrates the approximate duration of the absolute refractory period (ARP), the effective refractory period (ERP), relative refractory period (RRP), total refractory period (TRP), full recovery time (FRT), and the period of supernormal excitability (SNP). (From Singer, D. H., and Hoffman, B. F.: Progr. Cardiov. Dis., 7:231, 1964.)

and the potential pacemakers of the heart (see Fig. 2–3).

S-A Node Initiation of the Normal Impulse. The specialized P cells of the S-A node (described in Chapter 1, page 2) possess automaticity both in the isolated preparation and in the intact heart. Of all cells possessing automaticity, those in the sinoatrial node fire at the most rapid rate under normal circumstances. Since the sinus node contains many automatic cells (perhaps 1000 or more), one cell or another is always ready to depolarize and initiate the cardiac impulse 0.6 to 1.0 second after the preceding impulse has discharged all the S-A nodal pacemaker cells. The presence of such a large number of automatic cells normally assures consistent function of the sinus pacemaker despite poor impulse conduction within the node. As a result, the S-A node displays a high degree of "rhythmicity" (i.e., regularity of impulse formation) as well as automaticity.

As long as a normal cardiac mechanism is preserved, the heart rate depends on the degree of automaticity of S-A nodal cells, which in turn reflects the slope of diastolic (stage 4) depolarization and the resting transmembrane potential from which depolarization begins. Any factor that acts (1) to increase the slope of stage 4 depolarization, (2) to decrease the resting potential, or (3) to do both (1) and

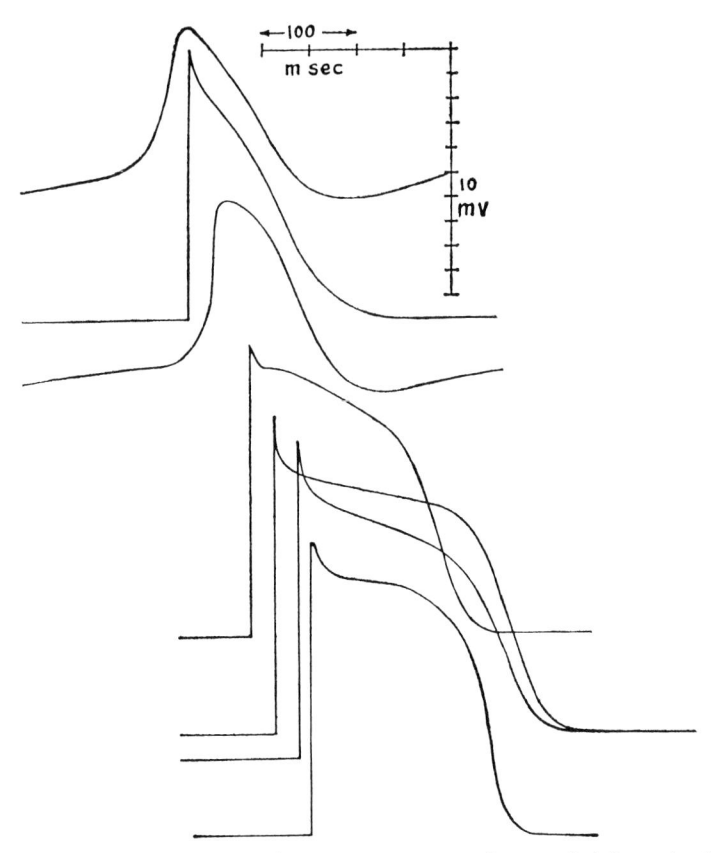

Figure 2–3. Drawings of transmembrane action potentials recorded from the following sites, from above down: sinoatrial node, atrium, N region of the atrioventricular junction, bundle of His, Purkinje fiber in a false tendon, terminal Purkinje fiber, and ventricular muscle fiber. Note the sequence of activation at the various sites as well as the differences in the amplitude, configuration, and duration of the action potentials.

The S-A nodal potential manifests a slow depolarization during phase 4, which is steeper than that of any other automatic tissue, therefore establishing the S-A node as the dominant pacemaker. The action potential of the atrial muscle displays a constant level of potential during phase 4, a rapid rise during phase 0, and a prominent reversal with rapid depolarization. The potential from the N region displays phase 4 depolarization with smooth transition into a slowly rising phase 0. Repolarization is slow and phases 1, 2, and 3 are not well demarcated. In the bundle of His, the transmembrane potential assumes more of the shape of the ventricular muscle transmembrane potential. The phase 0 is rapid and terminates in a sharp spiked reversal followed by a definite plateau. Phases 1, 2, and 3 are clearly demarcated and the duration of the action potential is increased. The Purkinje tracings have a definite spike and phase 1 is very prominent. The slope of phase 2 is lower and the duration longer than in the ventricular fiber. The Purkinje action potential is the longest found in any given heart. The action potential from the ventricular muscle shows a rapid rise during phase 0, a distinct plateau, relatively rapid repolarization, and a steady level of potential between action potentials. (From Hoffman, B. F., and Cranefield, P. F.: Electrophysiology of the Heart. New York, McGraw-Hill, 1960, p. 261.)

PHYSIOLOGIC CONSIDERATIONS

(2) will increase the automaticity of these cells and hence the heart rate (Watanabe and Dreifus, 1968). Any factor that has the reverse effects of (1), (2), or (3) will slow the heart rate. If the rate of impulse formation by the S-A node is enchanced or depressed to an excessive degree, the normal cardiac mechanism is apt to be disrupted, thus producing one of the arrhythmias.

With a normal mechanism, impulses arise in the S-A node quite regularly, usually at a rate between 60 and 140 beats per minute. Automatic fibers other than those of the S-A node ordinarily depolarize less rapidly during stage 4; therefore, they are activated by the impulse propagated from the S-A node before they would reach threshold and initiate a beat themselves (see Fig. 2–3). These automatic fibers thus remain *potential* pacemakers only so long as normal sinus rhythm prevails.

PROPAGATION OF THE CARDIAC IMPULSE

From the S-A node, the cardiac impulse is propagated in sequence through the atrial conduction pathways (activating the atrial muscle), the A-V junction, the His-Purkinje system, and the ventricular myocardium. The impulse proceeds across the atria at a relatively rapid rate (1000 mm./second), slows to 20 mm./second in the A-V junction, and reaches its greatest velocity (4000 mm./second) in ventricular Purkinje fibers, before reaching the ventricular myocardium and causing its contraction. This sequence of events underlies the normal cardiac mechanism, with atrial excitation preceding ventricular excitation by a P-R interval within the usual range.

Methods of Study

The Electrocardiogram. The electrocardiogram is one of the oldest graphic methods of representing cardiac activity and is the graphic method of study most widely employed in human subjects. It yields considerable information concerning: (1) the time required for conduction through various parts of the heart; (2) the course of activation of the heart; and (3) the presence or absence of clinical arrhythmias.

The configuration of the normal electrocardiogram has the following characteristics: (1) Regularity of the formation of sinus impulses is demonstrated by P waves. The P waves are upright and smooth in contour in leads I, II, aVF, and in the precordial leads, except in V_1 and occasionally in V_2; the P wave is normally inverted in aVR. (2) The rate ranges from 60 to 110 per minute and usually decreases with age. (3) Every P wave is followed by a ventricular response. (4) The P-R interval ranges between 0.12 and 0.21 second in duration; it tends to increase with age. Additional characteristics are discussed on page 42 (Fig. 2–4).

THE P-R INTERVAL. The P-R interval represents the period of time between the beginning of atrial and the beginning of ventricular depolarization. The isoelectric period between

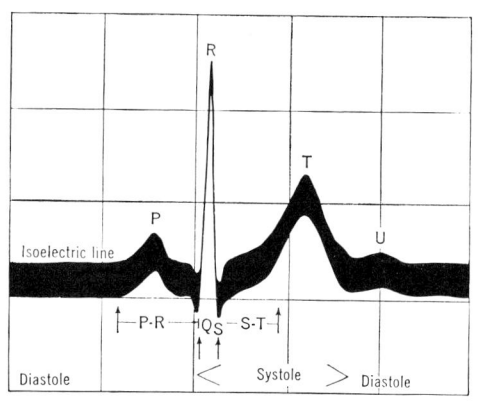

Figure 2–4. Electrocardiogram of a single normal heart cycle. Note the relative shape, size, and direction of the P, Q, R, S, and T waves. A small U wave follows the T wave. The P wave is inscribed by the electrical events that take place during atrial systole; the QRS-T complex is inscribed during ventricular systole; the QRS results from ventricular depolarization while the T wave is the result of repolarization. The U wave is inscribed during the early part of diastole.

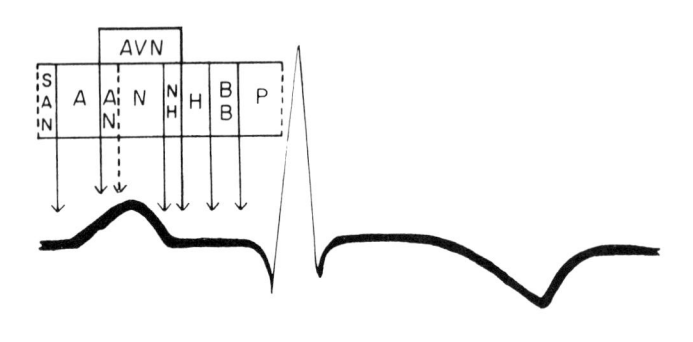

Figure 2-5. Tracing of the lead II electrocardiogram of the canine heart showing the time of activation of the various specialized cardiac tissues. SAN, sino-atrial node; A, atrium; AVN, atrioventricular node; H, His bundle; BB, bundle branches; P, peripheral Purkinje fibers. The subdivisions of the atrioventricular node represent the atrionodal junction (AN), the middle node (N) and the transition from node to His bundle (NH). (From Hoffman, B. F., and Singer, D. H.: Prog. Cardiov. Dis., 7:226, 1964.)

the P waves and the QRS complexes is the seat of electrical activity not shown in the usual electrocardiogram, but which is elucidated by the His bundle electrogram (see Figs. 2-5, 2-6).

Electrogram. Records obtained from cardiac muscle by means of electrodes placed in proximity to the uninjured muscle are called electrograms. These tracings bear a regular relationship to the transmembrane action potential recorded from the same tissue.

The standard 12-lead electrocardiogram provides only indirect information concerning impulse transmission through the A-V junction and the His-Purkinje system. No method existed for studying A-V transmission in the intact human in normal or diseased states until recently, when such a study was made possible by the His bundle electrogram (Damato et al., 1969; Narula et al., 1971, and others).

To record the His bundle electrogram, a bipolar or multipolar catheter electrode is introduced percutaneously into the venous system and under fluoroscopic guidance is advanced through the tricuspid orifice into the right ventricle. It is lodged in proximity to the bundle of His. The catheter sensitivity

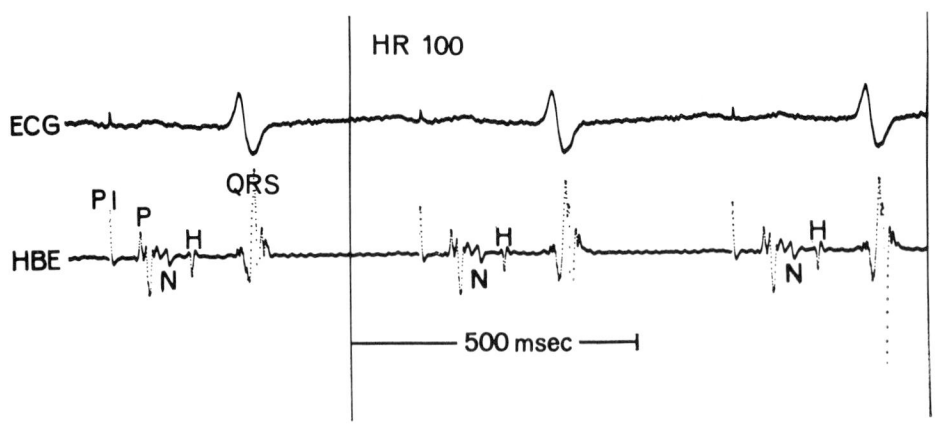

Figure 2-6. Simultaneous ECG and His bundle electrogram (HBE) recordings at a paced atrial rate of 100/minute. PI marks the stimulus artifact; P is the atrial electrogram, N is the nodal potential, H is the His bundle potential, QRS is the ventricular electrogram. The N potential measures 30 msec. and is separated from the H potential by 21 msec. (From Donato, A. N., et al.: Circulation, 39:435, 1969.)

ventricular rate with its adverse hemodynamic consequences. Other homeostatic mechanisms that tend to maintain cardiac function within a normal or relatively normal range include physical regulation (including regulation of venous return and coronary blood flow), neural reflexes, and metabolic and endocrine regulation.

PHYSIOLOGIC PROPERTIES OF NORMAL HEART MUSCLE

The function of the heart muscle depends upon certain inherent properties: automaticity, excitability, conductivity, and contractility. Changes in cardiac function due to an arrhythmia or in response to the treatment instituted may be analyzed in terms of the effect on these properties.

Automaticity. The sinoatrial node ordinarily exhibits the highest degree of automaticity and therefore is responsible for initiating the heart beat. If the function of this primary pacemaker is depressed, either temporarily or permanently, other automatic tissue will take over this function at a lower rate.

In certain abnormal states, the activity of a lower group of automatic cells may be so enhanced as to "usurp" the pacemaker function of the heart from the sinus node. Whenever this occurs, an "ectopic" rhythm is produced. Ectopic rhythms at a slow rate are ordinarily "passive," that is, they result from depression of automaticity in the S-A node rather than enhancement of automaticity anywhere else. An ectopic rhythm that does result from enhanced automaticity of tissue outside the S-A node is called an "active" ectopic rhythm. Active ectopic rhythms usually manifest a rate equal to or above the normal sinus rate of 70 to 100 beats per minute.

The rate of firing of pacemaker cells is influenced by a variety of factors, of which the effects of the nervous system, cardioactive drugs, and the concentration of various metabolites, electrolytes, and hormones in the blood are clinically the most important.

Factors which increase automaticity include: (1) increased sympathetic activity; (2) decreased parasympathetic activity; (2) hypopotassemia; (4) hypercalcemia; (5) hypercapnea; (6) acidosis; (7) hypoxia; (8) hyperthermia; (9) mechanical effects (e.g., increased stretch); and (10) certain drugs, particularly digitalis. The factors which decrease automaticity are (1) decreased sympathetic activity (e.g., effect of beta blocking agents); (2) increased parasympathetic tone (e.g., acetylcholine); (3) hyperpotassemia; (4) hypocalcemia; (5) decreased P_{CO_2}; (6) alkalosis; (7) increased P_{O_2}; (8) hypothermia; (9) decreased stretch; and (10) effect of certain drugs (e.g., quinidine, procaine amide, and diphenylhydantoin).

Excitability. Excitability is that property of living tissue which permits it to respond when stimulated. When a low intensity stimulus elicits a response, excitability is considered to be relatively increased, and when high intensity stimulation fails to elicit a response, the tissue is considered to be relatively inexcitable.

Excitability is increased during (1) the phase of supernormal excitability in the cardiac cycle; (2) increased sympathetic tone; (3) decreased parasympathetic tone; (4) hypopotassemia; (5) hypercalcemia; (6) depression of automaticity; (7) certain arrhythmias; and (8) certain phases of the action of diphenylhydantoin. Excitability is decreased during (1) the absolute and relative refractory periods of the cardiac cycle; and by (2) decreased sympathetic tone; (3) increased parasympathetic tone; (4) hyperpotassemia; (5) ischemia; (6) enhanced automaticity which causes a relative decrease in the resting membrane potential; and (7) effect of certain drugs, e.g., quinidine, procaine amide and digitalis.

tricle, and this may result in a dangerously high ventricular rate—up to 250 or 290 per minute—and, in the presence of a diseased heart, may lead to ventricular tachycardia or ventricular fibrillation.

Ventricular Spread of the Impulse. Having traversed the bundle of His, the impulse enters the bundle branches. The normal sequence of ventricular activation depends on conduction through the three principal subdivisions of the bundle of His: the right bundle branch, the anterior division of the left bundle branch, and the posterior division of the left bundle branch. Since each or several of the branches may conduct normally or demonstrate first, second, or third degree block, at least theoretically many intermediate patterns between unimpaired conduction and complete A-V heart block exist. The anterior and posterior hemibranches, which subdivide into numerous fibers almost immediately reach much of the left ventricle by more direct paths than their counterparts in the right bundle branch. Purkinje fibers ramify in the subendocardial region and supply the interventricular septum and apical midportions of the ventricles richly. The base of the heart is sparsely supplied by Purkinje fibers.

Rapid spread of the impulse occurs over subendocardial Purkinje fibers. From these conducting fibers, the impulse travels more slowly through the myocardium to reach the epicardial surface and the base of the heart. The left ventricular wall is penetrated from endocardial to epicardial surfaces in about 30 msec.; the thinner right ventricle, in about 10 msec.

Conduction by way of the Purkinje fibers occurs at high velocities, in some instances reaching 4000 mm./second. Abnormalities of this conduction tissue alter the timing and sequence of ventricular depolarization. In addition, these fibers under certain conditions possess automaticity, and at slow heart rates may actually function as the pacemaker of the ventricles.

FACTORS DETERMINING A NORMAL CARDIAC MECHANISM

The normal heart beat depends upon the ability of each component of the heart to function within an acceptable range, and on the homeostatic mechanisms to maintain an orderly and regular sequence of activation. Adequate functioning of individual muscle fibers depends on many factors, ranging from their genetic endowment to the provision of sufficient oxygen, hormones, and nutrients. Furthermore, normal myocardial function requires freedom from numerous deleterious factors, such as electrolyte disturbances, inflammation, and degenerative processes. Damage to a small number of cells crucially situated in pacemaker or conduction tissue may cause a significant disruption of impulse formation or conduction. On the other hand, widespread anatomic damage to undifferentiated myocardial cells, as occurs in severe coronary artery insufficiency, might not cause any arrhythmia.

The normal heart efficiently serves the body's demands for oxygen and other nutrients by virtue of various sympathetic and parasympathetic reflexes that adjust the cardiac output to meet its requirements. Sympathetic stimulation enhances the contractility of the myocardium and the automaticity of pacemaker cells, while parasympathetic tone, in general, has the opposite effect. Several mechanisms maintain effective cardiac function over the normal range of rates: (a) at rapid heart rates, the refractory period of the A-V junction, bundle of His, and bundle branches becomes abbreviated, thus allowing conduction of a larger number of impulses; and (b) when the heart rate becomes too high, some of the impulses are blocked in the A-V junction, thus preventing a too rapid

Atrioventricular Junction. In normal hearts the A-V junction is the only pathway over which the impulse from the atria is transmitted across the fibrous skeleton of the heart to the ventricles. From the atrial conduction tracts and musculature, the impulse penetrates the A-V junction. In this area, the transmission of the impulse is delayed and may undergo various modifications which have great importance in a variety of clinical conditions, e.g., A-V heart block, A-V dissociation, and A-V junctional rhythm. If the impulse succeeds in traversing the A-V junction, it reaches the bundle of His and is propagated rapidly to the ventricles.

Many factors cause alterations in the time required for conduction from the atrium to the bundle of His (A-H interval). It is prolonged by rapid atrial rates, carotid sinus stimulation, digitalis, and the presence of certain toxic and degenerative states; it is shortened by atropine and isoproterenol.

Concealed Conduction. Concealed conduction occurs when an impulse partially traverses the A-V junction; however, it fails to be conducted through the entire A-V transmission system and depolarizes only a portion of the A-V junction, thus causing abnormal conduction of the next impulse. Thus, a premature atrial impulse that is blocked in the A-V junction may cause this region to be refractory when the next normal impulse arrives; it may then also be blocked or propagated more slowly than normal. Unless a P wave or some other evidence of the blocked impulse is observed, the diagnosis of "concealed conduction" is made by inference from the altered conduction of subsequent impulses, as observed in the electrocardiogram (Fig. 2-7). Concealed conduction may be demonstrated by His bundle electrography when an impulse preceding altered conduction elicits an H potential but fails to produce a Q wave.

Concealed conduction is considered to be particularly important in producing the "irregular irregularity" characteristic of the ventricular rate in atrial fibrillation.

Effects of Abnormal States. The earlier discussion of the normal electrophysiology of the A-V junction should lead one to conclude that conduction is relatively vulnerable to disturbances in this area. Many clinical disorders caused by degenerative processes, inflammation, ischemia, toxic states, and alterations in autonomic function may result in a decrease of conductivity through this region and produce various degrees of A-V heart block.

Less commonly, conductivity through the A-V junction may be increased. This occurs occasionally with states accompanied by increase in sympathetic tone, and also following therapeutic use of sympathomimetic agents. Enhanced A-V conduction may lead to a dangerously high ventricular rate. This may result in sinus tachycardia. During atrial tachycardia, atrial fibrillation, and atrial flutter, the atrial impulses previously blocked in the A-V junction may be conducted to the ven-

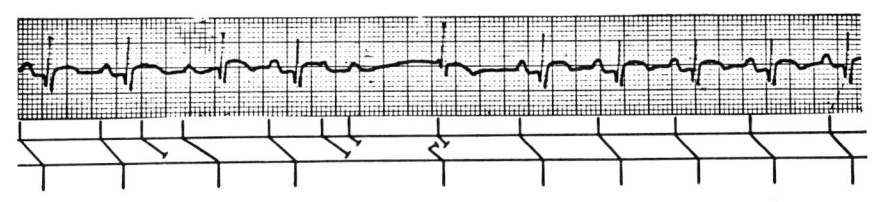

Figure 2-7. Concealed conduction. Atrial premature contractions causing prolongation of the P-R interval as well as apparent Mobitz type II second degree A-V heart block (middle of tracing). (From Moore, E. N., et al.: Amer. J. Cardiol., 28:406, 1971).

PHYSIOLOGIC CONSIDERATIONS

is such that activation of a few cells near the electrode or activation of a larger tissue mass at a distance produces a deflection in the tracing. A characteristic tracing (see Fig. 2–6) thus contains the following deflections: (1) a deflection due to atrial contraction in the prenodal area—presumably the "A wave"; (2) a biphasic deflection due to His bundle activity, called the "H or BH potential"; (3) occasionally, a deflection of low amplitude due to A-V junctional excitation—the "N potential"; and (4) the large, slurred complex due to ventricular contraction—the "Q wave." If the catheter tip is situated over the right bundle branch, the "RB potential" can be recorded. If the catheter electrode is introduced into the arterial system and passed into the left ventricle, a left bundle branch potential can be detected.

The P-A interval, measured from the onset of the P wave in the standard ECG lead and the initial rapid deflection of the A wave, represents the intraatrial conduction time. It is normally 25 to 45 msec. The A-H interval, measured from the first rapid deflection of the A wave to the first rapid deflection of the BH potential, represents the conduction time through the A-V junction. It normally ranges from 50 to 120 msec. The duration of the BH deflection is normally 15 to 20 msec. The H-V interval, or His bundle-to-ventricular muscle conduction time, is measured from the onset of the BH potential to the earliest ventricular depolarization recorded on either intracavitary or surface electrodes. It normally shows the least variation, ranging from 35 to 45 msec. By comparing such tracings with the normal durations of the intervals, one can document and locate the site of the delay, block, or acceleration in conduction in human subjects under various conditions.

CLINICAL APPLICATIONS OF HIS BUNDLE RECORDINGS. The His bundle electrogram allows a precise study of the P-R interval that is not possible with the surface electrocardiogram. Specific electrical events that occur in the A-V junction, the bundle of His, and the bundle branches, which are obscured by the atrial and ventricular electrical activity, are directly available to measurement and observation. For a complete discussion of the clinical applications of His bundle electrography, see Chapter 11.

The QRS complex and T wave are the electrocardiographic representations, respectively, of ventricular depolarization and repolarization. The significance of alterations in their configuration is discussed in this chapter and in Chapters 8 and 10.

Atrial Spread of the Impulse. The impulse initiated in the P cells of the S-A node does not spread radially from cell to cell across the atria as previously hypothesized but actually traverses transitional cells to reach the Purkinje fibers (James and Sherf, 1968). Some of these "Purkinje fibers" terminate in continuity with the atrial myocardium (James and Sherf, 1968), and are thought to underlie sinoatrial (S-A) conduction. Other "Purkinje fibers" join with apparently undifferentiated myocardial cells to form conduction tracts to the left atrium (Bachmann's bundle), and to form the anterior, middle, and posterior internodal tracts to the A-V junction. (See Chapter 1 for a discussion of the anatomy of these tracts.)

S-A conduction and conduction through the specialized tracts usually occur in an orderly sequence, producing (1) activation of the right atrium 0.01 to 0.04 second before activation of the left atrium; and (2) complete atrial contraction, before the impulse can traverse the A-V junction. If the atrial muscle is in a refractory state, conduction over the specialized atrial tracts to the A-V junction may persist. Under these conditions, the sinus impulse is transmitted to the ventricles without inscription of a P wave—so-called "sinoventricular conduction" (Bellet and Jedlicka, 1969).

Conductivity. Conductivity is the ability of a tissue composed of a series of individual cells to propagate an impulse. Conductivity is related to and is a manifestation of excitability. When conductivity is low, the rapid phase of depolarization (phase 0) proceeds much more slowly than usual and the resultant action potential has a subnormal amplitude.

The electrotonic spread of the relatively weak current generated by the action potential of the first fiber causes adjacent fibers to reach their threshold potential more slowly and generate action potentials of subnormal amplitude. The result is propagation of a series of action potentials that are characterized by a slow upstroke, a small amplitude, and low speed of conduction.

Conductivity ordinarily varies considerably among the different tissues of the heart, being greatest in the specialized conduction fibers, less in the myocardium, and least in the N region of the A-V junction.

Factors which tend to enhance conductivity are: (1) certain aspects of cell morphology (i.e., large size, intercalated discs, and nexus structures); (2) the period of supernormal excitability, e.g., the early phase of diastole; (3) increased sympathetic tone and circulating catecholamines; (4) decreased parasympathetic tone; (5) decreased automaticity; (6) shortened refractory period; (7) hypopotassemia; and (8) hypercalcemia. Conductivity is decreased during (1) the cardiac refractory periods; and by (2) decreased sympathetic tone; (3) increased parasympathetic tone; (4) increased automaticity; (5) tachycardia; (6) hypoxia; (7) myocardial disease; and (8) certain drugs, e.g., quinidine, procaine amide, and digitalis (high doses).

Contractility. Alteration in the contractility of the heart, either enhancement or depression, may predispose to the development of arrhythmias. In addition, the physiologic adjustments evoked by clinical arrhythmias and the drugs employed in therapy may all lead to alterations in contractility. Among the many indices that have been employed in evaluating contractility, the most useful are the force of isometric contraction, the velocity of shortening, cardiac output, stroke work, and myocardial efficiency.

Cardiac contraction results from ionic interactions in myocardial cells produced by an action potential; the action potential, in turn, results from an impulse that originates in pacemaker fibers. It is generally believed that the intracellular concentration of free calcium (Ca^{++}) determines the rate of ATP splitting, and hence, of tension development. Marked variation in the amount of intracellular free Ca^{++} occurs during two different phases of the cellular cycle, characterized by a rapid increase at the onset of the action potential and a less rapid decrease during repolarization. Sarcoplasmic reticulum seems to be the specific cellular compartment in which Ca^{++} is stored and from which it is released in response to an action potential.

Factors which are associated with increased contractility include: (1) hypervolemia; (2) increased venous return to the heart; (3) anemia; (4) hypothermia associated with slow rates; (5) exercise; (6) emotion; (7) hyperthyroidism; (8) hypercalcemia; and (9) digitalis, sympathomimetic amines, and bretylium. Contractility is decreased as a result of (1) long periods of bed rest; (2) various types of diffuse myocardial disease; (3) shock-like state; (4) hypothyroidism; (5) hypocalcemia; and (6) certain drugs—quinidine, procaine amide, beta blocking agents, and potassium.

RELATION OF FUNDAMENTAL PHYSIOLOGIC MECHANISMS TO SPECIFIC ARRHYTHMIAS

Disturbances of two processes—impulse formation and conduction—

either singly or in combination, are the main causes of cardiac arrhythmias. In this section, the mechanisms underlying the production of arrhythmias are discussed. Specific details are treated at greater length in individual chapters.

Disturbances of Impulse Formation. Disturbances of impulse formation may occur as a result of altered automaticity. When the automaticity of the S-A node is depressed or when its rhythmicity is interrupted, the normal automatic properties of the potential cardiac pacemakers (i.e., those localized in specialized atrial tracts and the His-Purkinje system) are expressed, resulting in an ectopic rhythm. On the other hand, in the presence of normal sinoatrial automaticity, ectopic rhythms may result from increased automaticity in any region of the heart caused by (1) oscillatory potentials; (2) after-potentials (Brooks et al., 1955); (3) local potential difference between cells; (4) temporal dispersion of repolarization (i.e., inhomogeneous repolarization); and (5) altered conduction.

Disturbances of Conduction. The normal cardiac mechanism depends on conduction of the impulse over the specialized atrial pathways, through the A-V junction, and over the His-Purkinje system to reach the ventricular myocardium. Abnormalities may result if the normal conduction time is increased (first degree A-V heart block), if conduction is not only delayed but also blocked (second and third degree A-V heart block), or if the impulse travels over an abnormal pathway (the pre-excitation syndrome).

Simple conduction delay or block may be caused by (1) the presence of refractory tissue, (2) decremental conduction, or (3) inhomogeneous conduction.

Refractory Tissue. Cells will not conduct impulses which arrive during the absolute refractory period, i.e., during depolarization and the greater period of repolarization.

Decremental Conduction. If an impulse arrives at an excitable cell during its relatively refractory period or when the resting membrane potential has been reduced by phase 4 depolarization or under conditions causing a low resting potential, the resultant spike is characterized by subnormal amplitude and rate of depolarization, which is a normal characteristic of the N region of the A-V junction. This action potential serves as a weaker than normal stimulus to the next fiber and elicits an action potential characterized by even slower depolarization. After progressive decremental passage through a number of cells, the impulse may become too weak to depolarize a distal fiber, even though that fiber is excitable, and conduction is therefore blocked.

Decremental conduction may occur at slow heart rates, because the Purkinje fibers of the ventricles exhibit automatic activity, manifested by diastolic (stage 4) depolarization which lowers the resting potential (Fig. 2–8).

Similarly, low resting potentials that might cause decremental conduction are observed in diseased human atria. In addition, decremental conduction may be caused by stretch, hypoxia, hypopotassemia, antiarrhythmic agents, and digitalis.

Inhomogeneous Conduction. Inhomogeneous conduction of an impulse can result in asynchronous arrival of an impulse and uneven degrees of repolarization when the next impulse arrives. This may disrupt the uniform progression of the depolarization wave and result in decreased conduction or block.

Unidirectional Block and Re-Entry. This may occur (1) at the level of the A-V node and (2) locally within the undifferentiated myocardium. The existence of *parallel conducting pathways in the A-V junction forms the basis for complex arrhythmias resulting from*

PHYSIOLOGIC CONSIDERATIONS

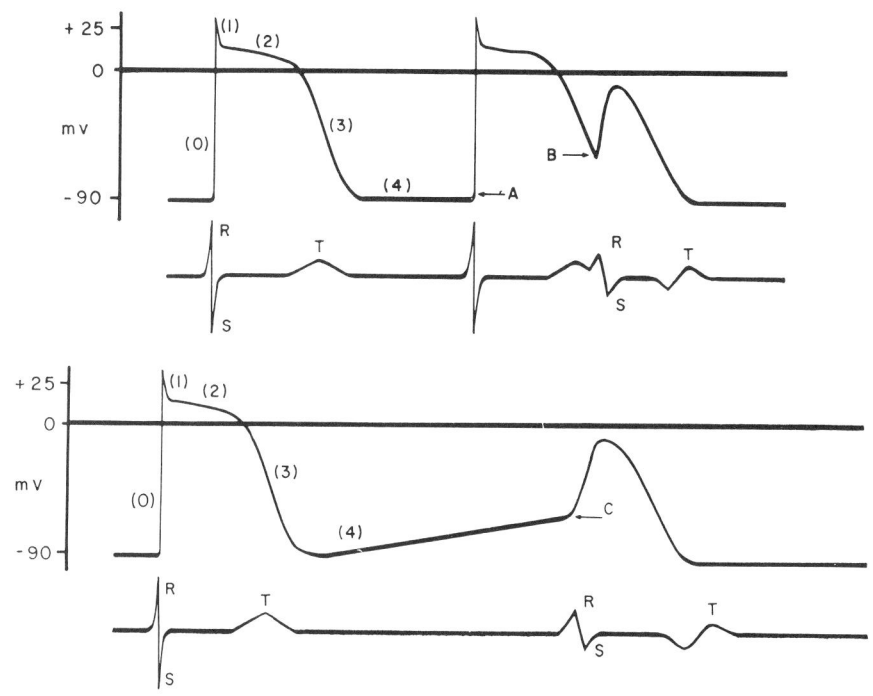

Figure 2–8. Schematic representation of transmembrane potentials and simultaneously recorded surface electrogram from automatic Purkinje cell to illustrate interrelationships between automaticity and conduction. (*Top, left hand side*) Transmembrane action potential recorded during stimulation at a rate sufficiently fast to suppress any tendency for development of phase 4 depolarization. Usual phases of the action potential are designated by numerals in parentheses. (*Right hand side*) Normal action potential initiated at −90 mv resting potential (A) and premature response initiated during repolarization at −60 mv (B). Note decreased amplitude at dV/dt of response and its reduced rate of propagation as indicated by aberration of surface electrogram. (*Bottom, left hand side*) Normal action potential. (*Right hand side*) Action potential initiated in same fiber after development of phase 4 depolarization in response to decrease in frequency of stimulation to a low rate. Since this beat is depicted as being initiated at the same level of membrane potential (C) as the premature response, its amplitude, dV/dt, and speed of propagation are comparably reduced. Note similar aberration in surface electrogram. (From Singer, D. H., Lazzara, R., and Hoffman, B. F.: Circ. Res., 21:537, 1967.)

local unidirectional block and re-entry. Reciprocal rhythm may be due to propagation of an impulse through a healthy portion of the A-V junction and its reflection back to the atrium through another portion of the node, showing a block to forward conduction. Supraventricular tachycardias, A-V heart block, and some cases of the W-P-W syndrome may be explained by unidirectional block at the A-V node.

Local block with gross re-entry has long been postulated to be a conduction disturbance that causes arrhythmias. In this disturbance the same impulse travels over a pathway in a circular fashion.

Combined Disturbances of Impulse Formation and Conduction. It is often difficult to make a clear-cut distinction between disorders of impulse formation and conduction in specific situations. For instance, if conduction through the A-V junction becomes blocked, the rate of diastolic (stage 4) depolarization, and hence the automaticity, becomes enhanced in Purkinje fibers; on the other hand, automaticity of these fibers also affects conduction through them. Many arrhythmias (such as paroxysmal atrial tachycardia with block) require the presence of separate disturbances of both impulse formation and conduction. Combined disorders are characterized by close interaction between disorders of impulse formation and of conduction.

Parasystole. In parasystole, at least one ectopic focus, in addition to the normal pacemaker, fires at a regular and uninterrupted rate. This condition implies that the extra focus is not "captured" by impulses from the normal pacemaker. The focus is protected from incoming impulses (entrance block) by the surrounding ring of tissue, which has low excitability and thus causes decremental conduction of the incoming impulse before it can reach the parasystolic focus. This protection from capture may also lead to exit block as the parasystolic impulse undergoes decrement with subsequent failure of conduction from the focus.

FACTORS LEADING TO THE PRODUCTION OF ARRHYTHMIAS

Any factor that disturbs the fine balance that is normally maintained by the physiologic properties of the single cardiac cell in conjunction with the various homeostatic mechanisms may lead to a clinical disorder of the heart beat. Infection, organic changes, trauma, altered autonomic tone, drugs, and therapeutic procedures may act singly or in concert to derange this balance. We will attempt to describe the effects that some clinical states produce on cardiac cells, the results of these alterations, and their significance. The complexity of this problem is further complicated by the many gaps that exist in our knowledge of this subject.

Under most circumstances, the numerous mechanisms that control and modify cardiovascular function interact to preserve homeostasis. Arrhythmias may result when the normal interrelationship of these mechanisms breaks down; this is most likely to occur in subjects susceptible to functional derangements or in those with organic heart disease. The most important of these regulatory mechanisms are: (1) *physical regulation of blood flow;* (2) *control of autonomic influences on the heart that occur in response to peripheral stimulation (reflexes) and to effects on centers in the central nervous system;* (3) *regulation by metabolites;* and (4) *endocrine factors.*

Physical Regulation of the Cardiovascular System. The cardiovascular system is controlled at least partially by several regional autoregulatory mechanisms which act through physical principles. The heart functions on the Frank-Starling principle, responding intrinsically to alterations of the end-diastolic volume. The arterial system is regulated by distention caused by intraluminal pressure changes. If these mechanisms fail to maintain coronary artery perfusion at a level adequate to support cardiac metabolism, hypoxia and electrolyte and metabolic imbalance, as well as increased stretch of myocardial fibers, may result in the initiation of an arrhythmia.

Role of the Nervous System. The higher centers involved in cardiovascular regulation include those in the cerebral cortex, the hypothalamus, the vasomotor center in the floor of the fourth ventricle, the sympathetic centers of the basal ganglia, and the medullary vagal nuclei (Fig. 2–9). The function of these centers is modified by (1) emotional stimuli; (2) visceral and somatic stimuli; (3) P_{CO_2}; (4) pH; and (5) hypoxia.

Autonomic Control. The limbic system and various nuclei located in the medulla (see also Chapter 27) are strategic in the central control of auto-

PHYSIOLOGIC CONSIDERATIONS 25

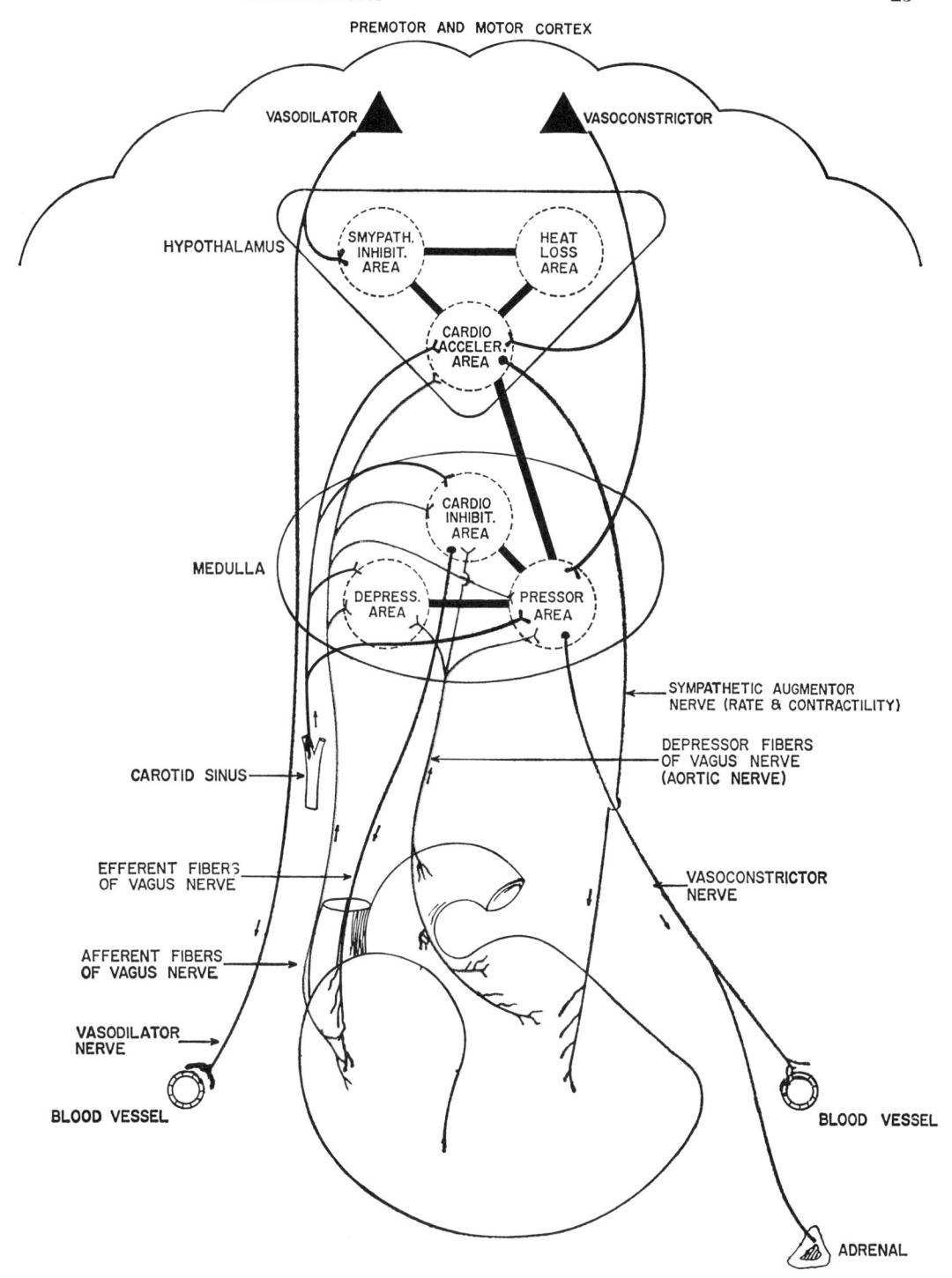

Figure 2-9 Diagrammatic representation of cardiovascular reflex mechanisms. (From Best, C. H., and Taylor, N. B.: Physiological Basis of Medical Practice. Baltimore, Williams and Wilkins, 1966.)

nomic, especially sympathetic, output. Outflow from the limbic system passes over tracts in the midbrain and either continues directly through the spinal posterolateral columns to terminate on the cell bodies of the preganglionic sympathetic neurons or terminates in the nuclei in the medulla. These nuclei give rise to (a) the cardioinhibitory parasympathetic fibers, which course in the vagus, and (b) sympathetic fibers, most of which pass down the spinal cord and a few of which pass via the vagus to the heart; these fibers mediate positive inotropic and chronotropic effects on the heart and the constriction of arterioles and veins. Some fibers terminate at the adrenal medulla where they regulate epinephrine release.

Sympathetic Effects. Sympathetic discharge is influenced by cortical processes and by afferent stimuli from visceral receptors. Impulses from the cerebral cortex are integrated in the limbic system; impulses from visceral and somatic sensory receptors are transmitted through the reticular activating system in the brain stem. These activations cause diffuse discharge to the limbic system and resultant heightening of autonomic tone. Other afferent neurons concerned with the mediation of specific vascular reflexes terminate in the vasomotor and cardioinhibitory centers in the medulla.

Sympathetic stimulation of the heart causing release of epinephrine and norepinephrine from the myocardium (the amount released per discharge is determined by the myocardial concentration) results in (1) an increase in ventricular stroke work and power that is independent of ventricular filling (i.e., represents an increased efficiency of the excitation-contraction linkage); (2) a shortening of the systole and lengthening of the diastole of the ventricle, thus maintaining its "normal" pressure-length curve; (3) the constriction of peripheral veins as part of coordinated control of the circulation, a factor which increases cardiac output; (4) an increase in atrial and ventricular excitability; (5) the prolongation of phase 2 of the action potential, leading to increased contractility independent of changes in end-diastolic volume; (6) alterations in the sequence of ventricular repolarization—alterations which may cause S-T segment and T wave abnormalities in the electrocardiogram; and (7) the production of atrial and occasionally ventricular fibrillation in subjects with underlying disease, or in whom the sympathetic stimulation is exceptionally intense (e.g., following countershock).

Parasympathetic Effects. Although both vagi supply the S-A node and the A-V junction, the S-A node is innervated principally by the right vagus, and the A-V junction is innervated chiefly by the left.

The effects of vagal stimulation upon the atria are generally similar to the effects of acetylcholine, i.e., (1) an increase in the thresholds of excitation, (2) shortening of the action potential, and (3) a decrease in contractility. However, the effects of vagal stimulation have been oversimplified in the past and were considered to result chiefly from its local effects on the S-A and A-V nodes and the atrial muscle. Its effects upon the circulation embody a broader scope and may be summarized as follows: (1) inhibition of the S-A node, tending to decrease the heart rate; (2) nonuniformly distributed decrease in the refractory period of the atrium; (3) decrease in atrial excitability; (4) weakening of atrial contractility; (5) inhibition of the A-V node by prolonging the transmission of atrial impulses to the ventricles; and (6) inhibition of ventricular contractility. In addition, a transient sinus tachycardia occurs at the termination of vagal stimulation; this tachycardia may be due to concurrent stimulation of vagal and sympathetic fibers or to vagal effects on chromaffin cells in the heart.

Metabolic Regulation. Specific metabolic products—hydrogen ion, lactate ion, carbon dioxide, ATP, and histamine—act as vasodilators and partially control regional blood flow. In addition, these products may alter the action of neural and reflex control mechanisms. An example of this is the intensification of effect of arterial chemoreceptor drive upon the bulbar cardiovascular centers by lactate in metabolic acidosis (Folkow et al., 1965). The effects of CO_2, H^+, K^+ and Ca^{++} have been discussed previously.

Reflex Adjustments. The vagal and sympathetic pathways to the heart are functionally altered by reflexes originating from a number of receptors, thus resulting in either cardiac inhibition or acceleration. The reflex adjustments are influenced by: (a) *intrinsic reflexes*, which arise from receptors within the cardiovascular system and are concerned in its homeostatic regulation; and (b) *extrinsic reflexes*, whose afferent limbs originate outside the cardiovascular system, but exert influences on the heart.

Baroreceptors, which monitor intraluminal pressure changes, have been located in the carotid sinus, left ventricle, and right atrium and in pulmonary vessels (Heymans and Neil, 1958). The afferent activity of nerves from these receptors reflexly controls the autonomic tone to the cardiovascular system. The carotid sinus baroreceptors are typical of this group. They are composed of nerve endings that arborize widely in the arterial wall and send both unmyelinated and myelinated sensory fibers to the glossopharyngeal nerve and thence to the medulla (Heymans and Neil, 1958). The endings of these nerves are stimulated by stretching, usually as a result of alterations in blood pressure. A fall in blood pressure within the carotid sinus produces reflexly: (1) increase in peripheral resistance, involving constriction in all types of vessels; (2) increase in pulse rate; (3) increased release of epinephrine; (4) emptying of the blood reservoirs with contraction of the large veins; and (5) increase in cardiac output.

Miscellaneous stimuli perceived by receptors extrinsic to the cardiovascular system may through common afferent or efferent pathways affect the heart and vascular tree. These stimuli include (1) ocular pressure, (2) traction on mesentery, (3) tracheal irritation (e.g., intubation), and (4) pleural irritation.

Endocrine Factors in Cardiac Regulation. (See also Chapter 24.) The adrenal medulla is in effect a ganglion of the sympathetic nervous system, which releases epinephrine and small amounts of norepinephrine in response to nervous impulses. In addition, the adrenal cortex plays an important role in the maintenance of normal cardiovascular function. Mineralocorticoids such as aldosterone maintain intravascular fluid volume by their actions on the kidney. The most important function of adrenocortical hormone is the role of cortisol in maintaining the reactivity of vascular smooth muscle to norepinephrine and epinephrine.

Diseases of the thyroid gland can also cause cardiac dysfunction. In hyperthyroidism, cardiovascular signs constitute an important part of the clinical picture. The heart rate is rapid, the pulse pressure wide, and ectopic rhythms (principally supraventricular) may frequently be seen.

Hemodynamic Alterations. When the heart rate is regular and in the normal range of 60 to 100 beats per minute, each ventricular contraction results in the ejection of a constant stroke volume, and coronary arterial flow is regulated to meet myocardial oxygen demand. With tachycardias or bradycardias, stroke volume and coronary arterial flow may be affected, especially in the presence of myocardial disease in which cardiac function is markedly altered by very slow or very high rates.

These effects may be summarized

as follows: (1) Bradycardia below 20 beats per minute cannot supply the average resting need of 4 to 5 L./minute, since stroke volume cannot be increased beyond 250 ml. (2) Tachycardia results in several deleterious effects: (a) at high rates (150 and over), diastole is so shortened that it infringes on the period of rapid ventricular filling (see Fig. 3-1); (b) blood flow to the left ventricular myocardium, which occurs during diastole, is so reduced that it causes hypoxia; and (c) a shortened diastolic period does not allow the myocardium, which has a low tolerance for oxygen debt, to recover its metabolic balance in preparation for the next beat. (3) Intermittent irregular rhythms can have the same effects as tachycardia, to the extent that one beat closely follows another (Katz and Shaffer, 1966). A protracted decrease may aggravate the pathologic state of the heart by ischemic damage and even the development of infarction.

Hemodynamic disturbances due to organic heart disease or other factors may contribute to the development of arrhythmias, especially by stretch, hypoxia, and reflex alterations in anatomic tone that affect automaticity or conduction in the specialized tissue of the heart.

Pathologic Factors. Organic abnormalities may produce cardiac arrhythmias by various mechanisms. The effect of lesions on the heart depends upon their type and location. As discussed in the previous chapter, circumscribed lesions are most likely to cause arrhythmias if they are situated in the specialized tissues concerned with impulse initiation or conduction; on the other hand, diffuse myocardial disease may produce few signs and symptoms until it is advanced.

Coronary artery disease, with subsequent ischemia and diffuse pathologic changes in the conduction system, is the principal degenerative process involving the heart. Ischemic processes in the heart take two principal forms: (1) developing coronary artery disease with low-grade ischemia leading slowly to diffuse fibrosis and decreased cardiac function; and (2) acute coronary artery thrombosis which is so severe that anaerobic metabolism cannot supply the metabolic needs of the tissue, and consequently localized myocardial infarction occurs, with the production of various arrhythmias.

Acute myocardial infarction results in (1) enhancement of sympathetic tone in response to baroreceptor reflexes and anxiety; (2) depression of contractility with resultant hemodynamic impairment; (3) uneven accumulation of metabolites; (4) efflux of K^+ from infarcted cells, resulting in at least localized hyperpotassemia (see Chapters 15, 16, 28); (5) asynchrony of depolarization and repolarization in the infarcted area on account of the aforementioned factors, with consequent electrophysiologic asynchrony; and (6) a consistent lowering of the fibrillation threshold over the infarcted area.

Inflammatory diseases of the heart include rheumatic fever, bacterial endocarditis, viral and fungal carditis, and myocarditis of various types. These disease processes may cause alterations in automaticity and conductivity and may lead to a decrease of myocardial strength, resulting in serious disturbances in the function of the brain, the kidneys, and the endocrine organs as well as the heart. These disturbances may further affect the heart indirectly. Various arrhythmias may appear as a result of a single factor or of the interaction of several of the factors mentioned above.

Lesions located in the atrium may affect the automaticity of the S-A node or impair conduction of the sinus impulse over the internodal conduction pathways (see Chapter 1). Furthermore, they may cause disturbances in the activation of the atrial myocardium, leading to ectopic beats and fibrillation (see Chapter 7).

The A-V junction may be affected by

pathologic processes in several ways. Inflammation, as in the case of rheumatic fever, may depress conduction through this region, but it also enhances the automaticity of some junctional cells, thus predisposing to ectopic impulse formation. Degeneration and fibrosis may culminate in A-V heart block (see Chapter 10). The presence in this region of abnormal tracts over which impulses can be conducted without delay may underlie the occurence of the W-P-W syndrome (see Chapter 13).

Lesions affecting the ventricles may result in various forms of conduction block (bundle branch block or A-V heart block). When such lesions result in enhanced automaticity, they may cause an idioventricular tachycardia or paroxysms of ventricular tachycardia.

References

Adrian, E. D.: The recovery process of excitable tissues. J. Physiol., 54:1, 1920.

Alanis, J., Lopez, E., Mandoki, J. J., and Pilar, G.: Propagation of impulses through the A-V node. Amer. J. Physiol., 197:1171, 1959.

Bellet, S., and Jedlicka, J.: Sino-ventricular conduction and its relation to sino-atrial conduction. Amer. J. Cardiol., 24:831, 1969.

Bing, R. J., Choudhury, J. D., Michal, G., and Kako, K.: Myocardial metabolism. Ann. Intern. Med., 49:1201, 1958.

Brooks, C. McC., Hoffman, B. F., Suckling, E. E., and Orias, O.: Excitability of the Heart. New York, Grune and Stratton, 1955.

Castellanos, A., Jr., Chapunoff, E., Castillo, C., Maytin, O., and Lemberg, L.: His bundle electrograms in two cases of Wolff-Parkinson-White (preexcitation) syndrome. Circulation, 41:399, 1970.

Damato, A. N., Lau, S. H., Berkowitz, W. D., Rosen, K. M., and Lisi, K. R.: Recording of specialized conducting fibers (A-V nodal, His bundle, and right bundle branch) in man using an electrode catheter technic. Circulation, 39:435, 1969.

Davies, M., and Harris, A.: Pathological basis of primary heart block. Brit. Heart J., 31:219, 1969.

Davis, L., and Hoffman, B. F.: Evidence for specialized pathways in atrial excitation. Fed. Proc., 22:246, 1963.

DeFelice, L. J., and Challice, C. E.: Anatomical and ultrastructural study of the electrophysiological atrioventricular node of the rabbit. Circ. Res., 24:457, 1969.

Durrer, D., van Dam, R. Th., Freud, G. E., Janse, M. J., Meijler, F. L., and Arzbaecher, R. C.: Total excitation of the isolated human heart. Circulation, 41:899, 1970.

Folkow, B., Heymans, C., and Neil, E.: Integrated aspects of cardiovascular regulations. In Dow, P., and Hamilton, W. F. (eds.): Handbook of Physiology, Section 2, Vol. III, p. 1787, Washington, D.C., American Physiological Society, 1965.

Han, J., and Moe, G. K.: Cumulative effects of cycle length on refractory periods of cardiac tissue. Amer. J. Physiol., 217:106, 1969.

Harris, A., Davies, M., Redwood, D., Leatham, A., and Siddons, H.: Aetiology of chronic heart block. A clinico-pathological correlation in 65 cases. Brit. Heart J., 31:206, 1969.

Heymans, C., and Neil, E.: Reflexogenic Areas of the Cardiovascular System. Boston, Little, Brown & Co., 1958.

Hoffman, B. F., Cranefield, P. F., Stuckey, J., and Bagdonas, A. A.: Electrical activity during the P-R interval. Circ. Res., 13:1200, 1960.

James, T. N.: Anatomy of the cardiac conduction system in the rabbit. Circ. Res., 20:638, 1967.

James, T. N., and Sherf, L.: Ultrastructure of myocardial cells. Amer. J. Cardiol., 22:389, 1968.

Katz, L. N., and Shaffer, A. B.: The effect of cardiac arrhythmias on the performance of the heart. In Dreifus, L. S. and Likoff, W. (eds.): Mechanisms and Therapy of Cardiac Arrhythmias. Fourteenth Hahnemann Symposium, New York, Grune & Stratton, 1966.

Lenegre, J.: Etiology and pathology of bilateral bundle branch block in relation to complete heart block. Prog. Cardiovas. Dis., 6:409, 1964.

Lev, M.: Anatomic basis for atrioventricular block. Amer. J. Med., 37:742, 1964.

Mendez, C., and Moe, G. K.: Demonstration of a dual A-V nodal conduction system in the isolated rabbit heart. Circ. Res., 19:378, 1966.

Moe, G. K.: A conceptual model of atrial fibrillation. J. Electrocardiol., 1:145, 1968.

Narula, O. S., and Samet, P.: Wenckebach and Mobitz type II A-V heart block within the His bundle and bundle branches. Circulation, 41:947, 1970.

Narula, O. S., Scherlag, B. J., Samet, P., and Javier, P. P.: Atrioventricular block: Localization and classification by His bundle recording. Amer. J. Med., 50:146, 1971.

Rosenbaum, M. B., Elizari, M. V., and Lazzari, J. O.: Los Hemibloqueos. Buenos Aires, Ed. Paidos, 1968.

Rosenbaum, M. B., Elizari, M. V., Lazzari, J. O., Nau, G. J., Levi, R. J., and Halpern, M. S.:

Intraventricular trifascicular blocks. The syndrome of right bundle branch block with intermittent left anterior and posterior hemiblock. Amer. Heart J., 78:306, 1969.

Sherlag, B. J., Lau, S. H., Helfant, R. H., Berkowitz, W. D., Stein, E., and Damato, A. N.: Catheter technique for recording His bundle activity in man. Circulation, 39:13, 1969.

Singer, D. H., Strauss, H. C., and Hoffman, B. F.: New mode of action of antiarrhythmic agents. Amer. J. Cardiol., 19:151, 1967.

Trautwein, W.: Generation and conduction of impulses in the heart as affected by drugs. Pharmacol. Rev., 15:277, 1963.

Trautwein, W., Kassebaum, D. G., Nelson, R. M., and Hecht, H. H.: Electrophysiological studies of human heart muscle. Circ. Res., 10:306, 1962.

Watanabe, Y., and Dreifus, L. S.: Newer concepts in the genesis of cardiac arrhythmias. Amer. Heart J., 76:114, 1968.

Chapter 3 *Hemodynamics*

GENERAL CONSIDERATIONS
HEMODYNAMIC CONSEQUENCES OF
    ARRHYTHMIAS
    Bradyarrhythmias
    Arrhythmias with Rates in the Normal Range
    Tachyarrhythmias
    Arrhythmias with Variable Rates

EFFECT OF ARRHYTHMIAS ON
    REGIONAL BLOOD FLOW
    Cerebral Circulation
    Coronary Circulation
    Splanchnic and Renal Blood Flow
    Measurement of Phasic Blood Flow in the
        Human Subject

GENERAL CONSIDERATIONS

To assess completely the effect of an abnormal rhythm upon the circulation, it is necessary to measure various parameters of circulatory performance, especially cardiac output, stroke volume, cardiac work, myocardial oxygen consumption, myocardial contractility (dP/dt), and myocardial efficiency.

The ultimate effect of an arrhythmia on the human subject depends on the following factors: (a) the degree of myocardial impairment, especially the presence of atherosclerosis involving the coronary and other regional arteries, and the presence of valvular disease or other abnormalities; (b) slow or rapid heart rates and their duration and effects of the arrhythmia on the cardiac output, which may further affect regional blood flow; and (c) the presence or absence of anxiety, which may exacerbate the clinical situation. The hemodynamic changes caused by an arrhythmia may provoke further disturbance of rhythm, resulting in a vicious circle of decreasing cardiovascular function and efficiency.

Arrhythmias may affect myocardial performance by altering any one or all of the following factors: (1) ventricular end-diastolic volume, which affects myocardial contractility by means of the Frank-Starling mechanism; (2) the intrinsic contractile state of the myocardium; and (3) the synchrony of atrial and ventricular contraction (Fig. 3–1).

During tachyarrhythmias, the rapid phase of ventricular filling is encroached upon and stroke output declines significantly. As the rate becomes markedly elevated, the cardiac output progressively decreases because the stroke volume falls so precipitously that the rate increase cannot maintain an adequate cardiac output. Furthermore, the oxygen requirements of the heart are directly proportional to the heart rate. Hence, rapid heart rates require more oxygen than normal to move the same or even a smaller amount of blood, thus decreasing the mechanical efficiency of the heart. In subjects with myocardial damage or coronary insufficiency, this decrease in mechanical efficiency may utilize the entire cardiac reserve and precipitate symptoms of angina pectoris or congestive heart failure, or both.

Dilatation is the chief compensatory mechanism for bradyarrhythmias. Stroke volume increases so that cardiac output can remain normal. However, the minimal heart rate that can produce a normal cardiac output in patients without heart disease ranges between 20 and 30 beats per minute;

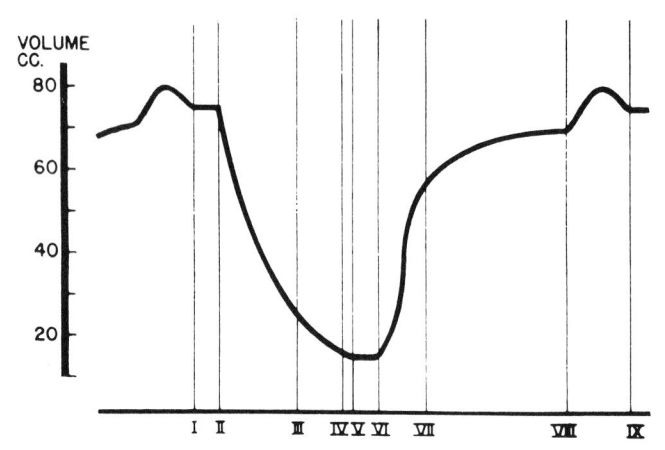

Figure 3–1. Diagrammatic presentation of the volume curve of one ventricle of the human heart at an assumed rate of 80 beats per minute, a stroke volume of 60 cc. and a systolic residue of 15 cc. The curve starts in late diastole. When the impulse in the sinus node spreads to the atria it causes them to contract and relax (between VIII and IX and the homologous portion of the curve ahead of I). The ventricle begins to contract at I, at first isovolumically (between I and II). Then ejection starts. All the blood in the ventricle (except for the systolic residue) is ejected from II to IV; most of it during rapid ejection (II to III), the remainder in the reduced ejection period (III to IV). Diastole begins at IV with a short protodiastole phase (IV to V) and an isovolumic relaxation period (V to VI). Most of the filling of the heart occurs in the rapid inflow phase (VI to VII). After rapid inflow, there is the period of passive filling, diastasis (VII to VIII), due to the *vis a tergo* of the blood coming back to the heart. (From Katz, L. N., and Shaffer, A. B.: *In* Dreifus, L. S., and Likoff, W. (eds.): Mechanisms and Therapy of Cardiac Arrhythmias. New York, Grune & Stratton, 1966.)

most older patients with bradyarrhythmias suffer severe hemodynamic impairment when their heart rate drops below 36 to 30 beats per minute.

The coordination of atrial with ventricular contraction plays an important hemodynamic role in increasing the efficiency of pumping by the heart, and incoordination (e.g., A-V dissociation) or loss of atrial contraction produces unfavorable hemodynamic consequences. Atrial contraction serves two principal hemodynamic roles: (1) it acts as a "booster pump," assisting the passage of the blood from the systemic and pulmonary circulation to the ventricles, and (2) it adds to the efficiency of mitral valve closure, thus preventing regurgitation at the beginning of ventricular systole.

The degree to which atrial contraction contributes to ventricular filling depends on several factors: (1) the time relationship between atrial and ventricular systole; (2) the completeness of ventricular filling at the time of atrial systole; and (3) the strength of atrial contraction, with a resultant increase in cardiac output. Arrhythmias of various types may disrupt one or several of these factors resulting in varying degrees of hemodynamic impairment.

HEMODYNAMIC CONSEQUENCES OF ARRHYTHMIAS

In light of the previous discussion, one can usually predict with a fair degree of accuracy the hemodynamic effect of an arrhythmia in an individual patient on the basis of (1) the heart rate, (2) the type and degree of irregularity, (3) the presence or absence of effective atrial contraction, (4) the effectiveness with which the A-V valves prevent reflux, and (5) the degree of previous myocardial impairment.

The general hemodynamic effects of arrhythmias may conveniently be divided into two general categories: (1) the effects on the heart itself—its rate, its output, and its efficiency, and (2) the hemodynamic alterations that occur in other organs. The effects on the heart are discussed only in general terms in this chapter; more detailed discussion is given in the appropriate chapters. The results in other organs have considerable importance because such alterations may, in turn, further aggravate the hemodynamic state of the heart and circulation. The survival of the patient may often be determined by these extracardiac hemodynamic effects.

Bradyarrhythmias. The most important of the marked bradyarrhythmias (20 to 36 beats per minute) are sinus bradycardia, high-grade partial or complete A-V heart block, and idioventricular rhythm. In these states, the cardiac output is often fixed at a fairly low level, and although certain compensatory mechanisms are operative, such as an increase in oxygen extraction by the peripheral tissues, the circulation often remains in a precarious state.

Because of the low tolerance of the heart, brain, and, to a lesser degree, the kidneys to even slight decreases in cardiac output, a decrease in coronary, cerebral, or renal blood flow may produce marked alteration in their function. These manifestations are more pronounced in the presence of associated disease, especially atherosclerosis and arteriosclerosis. These patients benefit considerably from an increase in the heart rate, accomplished either by the administration of sympathomimetic drugs or by the use of an artificial cardiac pacemaker.

Arrhythmias with Rates in the Normal Range. Arrhythmias with rates of 60 to 110 beats per minute may include partial A-V heart block, A-V dissociation, and A-V junctional rhythm. At these rates slight decreases in the cardiac output and stroke volume may result from the marked asynchrony between the atrial and ventricular beats, but circulatory disturbance due to alterations in rate alone is minimal.

Tachyarrhythmias. Rapid ectopic rhythms (140 to 150 or more beats per minute), if of short duration and occurring in a normal or relatively normal heart, may have little or no effect on cardiac output, especially in the initial stage. However, if the arrhythmia is of long duration in the normal or relatively normal heart or of short duration in the presence of myocardial disease, the blood pressure often falls and the cardiac output may decrease.

Arrhythmias with Variable Rates. Arrhythmias in certain individuals manifest cardiac rates that range between bradyarrhythmias and tachyarrhythmias. Such is the situation of the subject with sinus bradycardia, sick sinus syndrome, sinoatrial block, or complete A-V heart block who tends to develop paroxysms of ventricular tachycardia. This patient suffers in rapid succession the deleterious consequences of both classes of disorders. Such disorders produce profound disturbances in the patient and require special methods for correction which are described elsewhere in this book.

EFFECT OF ARRHYTHMIAS ON REGIONAL BLOOD FLOW

Cerebral Circulation. A decreased cardiac output results in an impairment of the blood flow to the brain, as well as to other organs. The decrease in cerebral blood flow depends primarily upon the type of arrhythmia present. Premature beats, either atrial or ventricular, result in an 8 to 12 per cent reduction. Rapid supraventricular tachycardia causes a reduction of 14 per cent; atrial fibrillation with rapid ventricular rate results in a 23 per cent reduction; and ventricular tachycardia reduces blood supply to the brain approximately 40 to 75 per cent (Corday and Irving, 1961). Furthermore, resistance of the cerebral circulation increases about one-third at the onset and remains increased for the duration of rapid arrhythmias.

Cerebrovascular insufficiency may be observed in patients who manifest significant arrhythmias (bradycardia, below 40/minute; tachycardia, over 150/minute; or a high-grade A-V heart block) (Walter et al., 1970). Specific antiarrhythmic therapy results in significant improvement in most patients.

The Coronary Circulation. Corday and associates (1959) observed in the experimental animal an average reduction in coronary blood flow of 5 per cent during atrial premature beats and 12 per cent in ventricular premature beats. With frequent premature beats, the reduction was 25 per cent; with paroxysmal atrial tachycardia, 35 per cent; with atrial fibrillation and rapid ventricular rate, 40 per cent; and with ventricular tachycardia, 60 per cent. The electrocardiogram may show ischemic changes when the coronary blood flow is reduced by 25 per cent or more.

Splanchnic and Renal Blood Flow. Significant reduction (20 to 40 per cent) in splanchnic and renal blood flow is usually encountered with tachyarrhythmias. In occasional patients ischemic colitis and renal tubular necrosis and their sequelae may result.

Measurement of Phasic Blood Flow in the Human Subject. Recently, instantaneous blood flow velocity has been recorded by the use of the Doppler ultrasonic flowmeter telemetry system (Benchimol and Desser, 1971). In this way, phasic, instantaneous blood flow velocity was measured in cardiac chambers, great vessels, coronary arteries, and regional circulations during ventricular arrhythmias. The velocity patterns closely parallel those of blood flow. Recently, Benchimol and associates (1971) have performed many studies in humans which have given valuable data relative to regional blood flow in various parts of the body. Diminished forward blood flow and stroke output was observed in the presence of ventricular premature beats and ventricular tachycardia (Benchimol and Desser, 1971). Reduced coronary blood flow velocity contributes to impaired ventricular performance during these arrhythmias.

This altered blood flow was closely paralleled by reduced carotid, renal, superior mesenteric, bracheal and dorsal pedis arterial blood velocity during ventricular arrhythmias. The critical factor apparently responsible for reduced ventricular function appeared to be the shortened diastolic filling time due to the prematurity of the ectopic beat or the tachyarrhythmia.

References

Benchimol, A.: Significance of the contribution of atrial systole to cardiac function in man. Amer. J. Cardiol., 23:568, 1969.

Benchimol, A., and Desser, K. B.: Ventricular function in the presence of ventricular arrhythmias. Presented at the 25th Hahnemann Symposium, Cardiac Arrhythmias: Pathophysiology, Pharmacology and Management, Sept. 21–25, 1971, Phila.

Benchimol, A., Ellis, J. G., and Dimond, E. G.: Hemodynamic consequences of atrial and ventricular pacing in patients with normal and abnormal hearts. Amer. J. Med., 39:911, 1965.

Benchimol, A., Stegall, H. F., and Gartlan, J. L.: New method to measure phasic coronary blood velocity in man. Amer. Heart J., 81: 93, 1971.

Corday, E., Gold, H., de Vera, L. B., Williams, J. H., and Fields, J.: Effect of the cardiac arrhythmias on the coronary circulation. Ann. Intern. Med., 50:535, 1959.

Corday, E., and Irving, D. W.: Disturbances of Heart Rate, Rhythm and Conduction. Philadelphia, W. B. Saunders Company, 1961, p. 207.

Janse, M. J., van der Steen, A. B. M., van Dam, R. Th., and Durrer, D.: Refractory period of the dog's ventricular myocardium following sudden changes in frequency. Circ. Res., 24:251, 1969.

Kaplan, M. A., Gray, R. E., Iseri, L. T., and Williams, R. L.: Metabolic and hemodynamic responses to exercise during atrial fibrillation and sinus rhythm. Amer. J. Cardiol., 22:543, 1968.

Katz, L. N., and Shaffer, A. B.: The effect of cardiac arrhythmias on the performance of the heart. In Dreifus, L. S., and Likoff, W. (eds.): Mechanisms and Therapy of Cardiac Arrhythmias. Fourteenth Hahnemann Symposium, New York, Grune & Stratton, 1966, pp. 1–20.

Mitchell, J. H., and Shapiro, W.: Atrial function and the hemodynamic consequences of atrial fibrillation in man. Amer. J. Cardiol., 23:556, 1969.

Shapiro, W., and Chawla, N. P. S.: Observations on the regulation of cerebral blood flow in complete heart block. Circulation, 40:863, 1969.

Skinner, N. S., Jr., Mitchell, J. H., Wallace, A. G., and Sarnoff, S. J.: Hemodynamic effects of altering the timing of atrial systole. Amer. J. Physiol., 205:499, 1963.

Walter, P. F., Reid, S. D., Jr., and Wenger, N. K.: Transient cerebral ischemia due to arrhythmia. Ann. Intern. Med., 72:471, 1970.

Chapter 4 *General Discussion of Arrhythmias*

INTRODUCTION
ETIOLOGY
  Local Cardiac Factors
  Disturbances of Other Organs
  General Factors
INCIDENCE
CLASSIFICATION OF ARRHYTHMIAS
SYMPTOMS AND SIGNS
  Manifestations Associated with Rapid Heart Action
  Manifestations Associated with Slow Heart Action
  Manifestations Associated with Irregular Action of the Heart
  Evaluation of the Symptom of Palpitation
BEDSIDE DIAGNOSIS OF CARDIAC ARRHYTHMIAS
  Guides in Clinical Diagnosis
  Summary of Bedside Diagnosis

INTRODUCTION

In the normally beating heart of a resting human adult, the sinoatrial node discharges 60 to 100 impulses per minute which are conducted through the heart in a well-known sequence, causing contraction of the cardiac chamber and the pumping of blood. Any derangement in the origin of the cardiac impulse, in its rate, or in its conduction results in a "clinical disorder of the heart beat."

The subject of clinical disorders of the heart beat, or the "arrhythmias," as they are usually called, is of considerable interest to the general practitioner, the internist, the cardiologist, the physiologist, the pharmacologist, the anesthesiologist, and the surgeon. The following considerations indicate the importance of these disorders: the diagnosis of an irregularity may be the first evidence of an underlying cardiac abnormality; such disturbances are common and frequently produce intense anxiety in the patient; a rapid rate often precipitates heart failure, especially in the presence of organic heart disease; these disorders can, in most instances, be diagnosed easily, either clinically or by graphic methods; and, finally, in most instances, the result of treatment of these disturbances is extremely gratifying. For example, during an attack of paroxysmal atrial tachycardia, atrial flutter, or atrial fibrillation with a rapid ventricular rate, a patient may manifest intense anxiety, a feeling of impending death, severe precordial pain, heart failure, and in extreme cases, the picture of shock. Proper therapy often results in remarkable improvement within hours.

The following terms have been used synonymously with clinical disorders of the heart beat: (a) *Arrhythmia*—this is the most commonly used term and has been widely accepted, although one of the chief objections to its use is that it implies an irregularity of the heart beat. This frequently is not the case; many of the arrhythmias have an entirely regular rhythm, as for example, paroxysmal atrial tachycardia, atrial flutter, ventricular tachycardia, complete A-V heart block, and others. (b) *Ectopic rhythm*—this term implies

GENERAL DISCUSSION OF ARRHYTHMIAS

an abnormal origin of impulse formation (outside the S-A node) and may thus refer either to a regular or an irregular rhythm. (c) *Dysrhythmia* — this term has enjoyed recent popularity because it is applicable not only to cardiac irregularities but also to disturbances of cardiac rhythm, in which the rhythm is, nonetheless, regular. Because of their wide usage, we shall use the terms "arrhythmia" and "ectopic rhythm" interchangeably with "clinical disorders of the heart beat."

ETIOLOGY

At best, the causes of many clinical disorders of the heart beat are only partly understood. Many instances of ectopic rhythm occur in patients with known organic heart disease, including inflammatory states involving the myocardium (e.g., rheumatic, diphtheric, and other types of myocarditis), degenerative changes (e.g., atherosclerosis, fibrosis), structural abnormalities, and hypertensive heart disease.

Although specific etiologies are characteristic of certain arrhythmias, the possibility of organic heart disease must be suspected initially in every patient with an ectopic rhythm. However, a large number of these disorders, such as sinus arrhythmia, sinoatrial block, and premature beats, are observed in hearts that are clinically normal, especially in children, and are not associated with myocardial abnormality. Atrial tachycardia in about 50 per cent of the cases appears in "clinically" normal hearts. Atrial fibrillation, atrial flutter, and ventricular tachycardia, although occasionally observed in normal hearts, usually occur in association with myocardial damage, often of a severe grade. Some arrhythmias result from obvious disturbances in the heart; the causes underlying the occurrence of others are obscure. Etiologic factors may be divided into the following categories: (a) local cardiac factors, (b) disturbance of other organs, and (3) general factors.

Local Cardiac Factors. These include the effect of cardiac abnormalities associated with hypertensive, rheumatic, viral, or syphilitic origin and other infections that have a special predilection for the heart, congenital anomalies, coronary artery disease with or without acute ischemia, degenerative states, and the presence of congestive failure.

Disturbances of Other Organs. These include functional or organic changes originating in various viscera outside the heart. The central nervous system may be the primary site of origin, owing to psychologic factors, anxiety, varying degrees of sympathetic and vagal stimulation, head trauma, and organic brain disease. Acute and chronic lung disease (pulmonary infarction, pulmonary arteriosclerosis, emphysema, and other states) increases right heart strain and decreases ventilation which in turn leads to hypoxia. Various endocrine disturbances include hypothyroidism or hyperthyroidism, and disturbances in the adrenal glands (hyperaldosteronism) and in the pancreas (diabetes, diabetic acidosis, and hypoglycemia). Gastrointestinal factors include disturbances leading to fluid loss by vomiting, diarrhea, or biliary fistula, the mechanical effect of abdominal distention, and various vagal reflexes. Renal disease may result in hypertension, electrolyte disturbances (hyper- and hypopotassemia, hyponatremia, hypocalcemia), and alterations in fluid balance.

General Factors. These include various infectious and toxic states, anemia, polycythemia, avitaminosis, alterations in electrolyte balance (particularly alkalosis and acidosis with hypo- and hyperpotassemia, hypo- and hypercalcemia, and alterations in magnesium), and the effects of certain drugs, particularly digitalis, diuretics (chlorothiazides, mercurials, and newer agents), quinidine, procaine amide, and other antiarrhythmic agents.

INCIDENCE

The incidence of cardiac arrhythmias varies with the population studied, especially in respect to the age and medical status of the group in question. Another important factor is the method by which arrhythmias are studied, whether by an occasional electrocardiogram or by long-term monitoring; the incidence is higher by the latter method. As would be anticipated, a higher incidence of arrhythmias is encountered in hospital patients. The most complete data concerning the relative incidence of ectopic rhythms in a hospital population have been obtained by Katz and Pick (1956) from the study of 50,000 consecutive patients over a 25-year period. The most frequent arrhythmia was premature beats (14.5 per cent), followed by atrial fibrillation (11.7 per cent), A-V heart block (4.1 per cent), A-V dissociation (1.4 per cent), and atrial flutter (0.5 per cent). Only 35 per cent of the records showed a sinus mechanism with a normal rate; another 20 per cent demonstrated sinus tachycardia, bradycardia, or irregularity of various other types.

Although arrhythmias occur much less frequently in the general, nonhospital population, the incidence is appreciable and is particularly important because of the prognostic significance of certain arrhythmias (see Chapter 28). In a study of electrocardiograms obtained from 5129 adults in a single town, Ostrander et al. (1965) found the following arrhythmias to be relatively frequent: (1) first degree A-V heart block (1.9 per cent); (2) frequent premature beats (1.9 per cent); (3) incomplete left bundle branch block (1.4 per cent); (4) A-V junctional rhythm (0.6 per cent); (5) atrial fibrillation (0.4 per cent); and complete right and left bundle branch block (0.4 per cent).

CLASSIFICATION OF ARRHYTHMIAS

Various classifications of arrhythmias are available. The arrhythmias can be classified according to their mechanisms as: (1) disorders of impulse formation (i.e., those due to abnormal automaticity); (2) disorders of impulse conduction; and (3) disorders due to abnormalities of both impulse formation and impulse conduction. The physiologic concepts underlying these mechanisms have been discussed in detail in Chapter 2; data pertaining to the mechanism of each arrhythmia are found in the appropriate chapter. The arrhythmias may be divided into four groups, according to the portion of the heart in which they arise. Subdivisions of the various categories are discussed in detail under each of the arrhythmias.

A. *Disturbances of rhythm involving the sinoatrial node*
  1. Sinus arrhythmia
  2. Sinus bradycardia
  3. Sinoatrial block
  4. Prolonged sinus pauses (resulting in cardiac standstill or A-V junctional escape)
  5. Wandering pacemaker
  6. Sinus tachycardia
B. *Disturbances involving the atria*
  1. Atrial premature beats
  2. Atrial paroxysmal tachycardia
  3. Atrial flutter
  4. Atrial fibrillation
  5. Intra-atrial block; intra-atrial dissociation
  6. Atrial standstill
  7. Sinoventricular conduction
C. *Disturbances involving the A-V junction*
  1. Atrioventricular heart block (prolonged P-R interval, increasing grades of partial block,

and complete atrioventricular block)
2. A-V junctional rhythm
3. A-V junctional escape, including coronary sinus rhythm
4. A-V junctional premature beats
5. Paroxysmal junctional tachycardia
6. Atrioventricular dissociation (complete or with intermittent capture)
7. Reciprocal rhythm

D. *Disturbances involving the ventricles*
1. Ventricular escape
2. Idioventricular rhythm
3. Ventricular premature beats
4. Ventricular paroxysmal tachycardia
5. Ventricular flutter and ventricular fibrillation
6. Cardiac (ventricular) arrest
7. Heart alternation

SYMPTOMS AND SIGNS

Manifestations Associated with Rapid Heart Action. The response of the patient to a rapid heart rate depends on the ventricular rate, its duration, and the underlying condition of the heart, as well as the mental reaction. In general, palpitation, faintness, dizziness, lightheadedness and at times actual fainting, throbbing in the head or neck, shortness of breath, and discomfort in the precordial region occur. If the rapid rate persists for a sufficiently long period, heart failure may develop in the presence of a previously damaged heart. When the heart has been previously damaged, prolonged tachycardia may precipitate an attack of precordial pain owing to coronary insufficiency and occasionally even myocardial infarction or a shock-like state.

The prognosis is worsened in the presence of an enlarged heart or coronary disease and in older patients. Death may result with 1:1 atrial flutter, the prefibrillatory type of ventricular tachycardia, ventricular flutter, or ventricular fibrillation. The last three arrhythmias may coexist with episodes of cardiac arrest.

Manifestations Associated with Slow Heart Action. The symptoms associated with slow heart action depend on the underlying state of the heart, the age of the patient, the cardiac mechanism (partial or complete A-V heart block, sinus bradycardia), and the ability of the heart to make a circulatory adjustment to the varying requirements of the individual. Moreover, patients with slow heart rates are more susceptible to the development of various other arrhythmias (especially ventricular premature beats) (see p. 96).

Patients with slower heart rates (below 30 per minute) frequently manifest shortness of breath and fatigue on exertion because of the diminished cardiac output and impaired circulatory adjustments following exercise. In addition, many of these subjects have an associated cardiovascular impairment that is aggravated by the slow heart rate. The patient may complain of dizziness and faintness. Symptoms of cerebral insufficiency are observed if the heart rate in these patients is lowered still further for brief periods of time. During periods of ventricular standstill ranging from 3 to 9 seconds, faintness, syncopal attacks, and even convulsive seizures may occur.

Manifestations Associated with Irregular Action of the Heart. Irregular action of the heart usually results from premature beats, sinus arrhythmia, S-A heart block, ventricular escape, varying degrees of A-V heart block, and atrial fibrillation. These irregularities may produce little or no subjective symptoms if the ventricular rate is not unduly rapid. These patients often complain of palpitation, "thumping of the heart," "the heart appears to turn over," and "the heart skips a beat." Generally, the discomfort is moderate, but at times it produces considerable anxiety and is interpreted as "pain around the heart," thus simulating the anginal syndrome.

Irregular heart action associated with rapid ventricular rates above 150 to 160 per minute is usually due to atrial fibrillation, atrial flutter associated with varying degrees of A-V heart block, and repeated short paroxysms of ventricular tachycardia. The clinical manifestations are those described under rapid heart action.

Evaluation of the Symptom of Palpitation. Palpitation, or heart consciousness, is a common symptom which may suggest an ectopic rhythm. To evaluate this symptom more accurately, one should correlate the subjective complaint with objective signs during its presence. Often it is found that "palpitation" is associated with simple acceleration of the heart beat up to 110 per minute, or is a result of a transient increase in blood pressure with change in posture, fear, excitement, exertion, fever, or spontaneous hypoglycemia. Premature beats, A-V heart block, and paroxysmal tachycardia notably evoke the symptom of palpitation. This symptom often occurs in patients with low-grade infections, during convalescence from an acute illness, and is a common manifestation in neurocirculatory asthenia. The psychogenic type of this cardiac disorder is suggested by an anxiety state and the absence of dyspnea or cardiovascular disease.

BEDSIDE DIAGNOSIS OF CARDIAC ARRHYTHMIAS

Guides in Clinical Diagnosis. The following information helps to establish a clinical diagnosis: the patient's description of the type of onset, duration, and frequency of the arrhythmia; whether he is taking drugs with proarrhythmic actions, including digitalis, various diuretics, sympathomimetic amines, or drugs for weight reduction (e.g., thyroid medication, amphetamines) (see p. 400). The patient may or may not give a history of heart disease. If present, it is important to determine whether this is of rheumatic, hypertensive, ischemic, or of other etiology. There may be a history of congestive heart failure or of the anginal syndrome. It should be emphasized that many patients present a history suggestive of cardiac arrhythmia when this is not present. On the other hand, there are often no symptoms with occasional premature beats or other types of irregularities. At times, however, symptoms are perceived in the form of precordial discomfort or precordial pain. The following data are important: the age of the patient, the ventricular rate, the presence or absence of heart disease, the presence or absence of congestive failure, and the type of heart condition or irregularity (if present).

Heart Rate. The heart rate is significant in diagnosis. This may be divided into the following categories: (a) *30 per minute or lower.* This may be due to a complete A-V heart block, sinus bradycardia, or a partial A-V heart block. (b) *40 to 60 per minute.* In the presence of regular or almost regular rhythm, the diagnosis of an arrhythmia is difficult to make on a purely clinical basis. In this group, one may find varying degrees of A-V heart block and A-V junctional rhythm (see Chapter 11). This is an extremely important group because toxic digitalis effects may be a causative factor. (c) If the rhythm is irregular with rates ranging from about *60 to 110 per minute*, one may be dealing with a sinus or other type of vagal arrhythmia, premature beats, A-V heart block and atrial fibrillation, or atrial flutter with varying degrees of A-V response. (d) *Rates 110 to 140 per minute.* This group consists of a gamut of arrhythmias ranging from (c) to (e). These may include vagal arrhythmias, premature beats, various types of A-V heart block occurring alone or in com-

GENERAL DISCUSSION OF ARRHYTHMIAS 41

bination with atrial fibrillation, atrial flutter, atrial tachycardia, or junctional tachycardia. (e) *140 to 180 per minute.* These rates usually result from atrial tachycardia, atrial flutter with 2:1 A-V conduction, or junctional or ventricular tachycardia. A simple tachycardia should be ruled out by having the patient exercise lightly or take deep breaths in order to determine whether the heart rate is labile or fixed. If the rate is fixed, an ectopic focus may be present. An electrocardiogram establishes the diagnosis.

Summary of Bedside Diagnosis. The above data should be available and the clinical state of the patient investigated by the various methods mentioned above. However, in attempting a bedside diagnosis, one should remember that he may sometimes be misled, and consequently the therapy may be inadequate, delayed, or improper. For example, the presence of paroxysmal atrial tachycardia may be an indication for digitalis therapy; however, if paroxysmal atrial tachycardia with block exists, digitalis is usually contraindicated. Therapy based on clinical diagnosis only—except on a temporary basis—should be limited to those instances in which one is acquainted with the patient's history, has knowledge of previous arrhythmias, and does not have an electrocardiograph available.

An integral part of the "bedside" diagnosis of arrhythmias is the electrocardiogram. The information supplied by this test is now increasingly available and is crucial in differentiating between various rhythm disturbances. The diagnostic approach to the electrocardiograph is discussed in Chapter 18.

References

Han, J.: Mechanisms of ventricular arrhythmias associated with myocardial infarction. Amer. J. Cardiol., *24*:800, 1969.

Hinkle, L. E., Jr., Carver, S. T., and Stevens, M.: The frequency of asymptomatic disturbances of cardiac rhythm and conduction in middle-aged men. Amer. J. Cardiol., *24*:629, 1969.

Katz, L. N., and Pick, A.: Clinical Electrocardiography. Part I. The Arrhythmias. Philadelphia, Lea & Febiger, 1956.

Ostrander, L. D., Brandt, R. L., Kjelsberg, M. O., and Epstein, F. H.: Electrocardiographic findings among the adult population of a total natural community, Tecumseh, Michigan. Circulation, *31*:888, 1965.

Singer, D. H., and Ten Eick, R. E.: Pharmacology of cardiac arrhythmias. Prog. Cardiov. Dis., *11*:488, 1969.

Watanabe, Y., and Dreifus, L. S.: Newer concepts in the genesis of cardiac arrhythmias. Amer. Heart J., 76:114, 1968.

Zipes, D. P.: The clinical significance of bradycardiac rhythms in acute myocardial infarction. Amer. J. Cardiol., *24*:814, 1969.

Chapter 5 *Sinus Irregularities*

GENERAL CONSIDERATIONS
CONFIGURATION OF THE NORMAL ELECTROCARDIOGRAM
RELATION OF S-A NODE AND ATRIA TO ARRHYTHMIAS
CONTROL OF THE HEART RATE
SINUS TACHYCARDIA
    Effect of Simple Tachycardia on the ECG
    Symptoms and Signs
    Treatment
    Prognosis
SINUS BRADYCARDIA
    Etiology
    Clinical Features Associated with Bradycardia (Less Than 50 to 60 Beats per Minute)
    Symptoms and Signs
    Diagnosis
    Treatment

SINUS ARRHYTHMIA
    Etiologic Factors
    Symptoms and Signs
    Diagnosis
    Treatment
    Prognosis
WANDERING OF THE PACEMAKER FROM S-A NODE TO A-V JUNCTION
SINOATRIAL HEART BLOCK
    Etiologic Factors (Clinical)
    Symptoms and Signs
    Prolonged Sinus Pauses
    Arrhythmias Associated with S-A Heart Block
    Treatment
    Prognosis
ATRIAL STANDSTILL
    Diagnosis
    Treatment

GENERAL CONSIDERATIONS

Normal sinus rhythm depends upon normal functioning of the S-A node, the dominant pacemaker of the heart. Various clinical disorders of the heart beat arise as a consequence of alterations in function of this structure. These include (a) sinus tachycardia, (b) sinus bradycardia, (c) sinus arrhythmia, (d) wandering atrial pacemaker, (e) sinoatrial block, (f) sinus pauses, and others. However, before discussing sinus irregularities, it is pertinent to discuss certain features of normal sinus rhythm and the control of the heart rate. A detailed discussion of the normal cardiac mechanism is given in Chapter 2.

CONFIGURATION OF THE NORMAL ELECTROCARDIOGRAM

The configuration of the normal electrocardiogram has the following characteristics: (a) Regularity of the formation of sinus impulses, as demonstrated by P waves. The P waves are upright and smooth in contour in leads I, II, aVF, and in the precordial leads, except in V_1 and occasionally in V_2; the P waves are normally inverted in aVR. (b) The rate ranges from 60 to 110 per minute and usually decreases with age. (c) Every P wave is followed by a ventricular response. (d) The P-R interval ranges between 0.12 and 0.21 second in duration and tends to increase with age. The increase is more than half completed by the age of two and one-half years; after ten years of age, there is essentially no further increase. In some apparently normal young adults, the P-R interval may be prolonged to the upper limit of normal.

Departure from any of these features suggests an abnormality. One or more of these abnormalities may result in the production of a clinical disorder of the heart beat. Although the sinus node may dominate the heart rhythm, other pacemakers may also be active in certain cycles. For example, sinus rhythm may be present with sequences of premature beats, with A-V dissociation, or with various degrees of A-V heart block.

RELATION OF S-A NODE AND ATRIA TO ARRHYTHMIAS

Among the automatic tissues of the heart, the sinus node, under normal conditions, possesses the highest spontaneous rate of impulse discharge. However, when the sinus pacemaker slows, when its impulses are carried imperfectly to the remainder of the heart, or when another area of automatic tissue fires more rapidly, an ectopic pacemaker may appear. Other automatic tissues in the region of the atria that might serve as pacemakers are located: (a) at the entrances of the great veins into the atria; (b) around the atrioventricular valve rings; (c) in the A-V conduction pathway; and (d) about the coronary sinus and in the A-N (atrionodal) region of the A-V junction (Hoffman and Cranefield, 1964).

Disease of the S-A node has been observed in various types of sinoatrial block and atrial arrhythmias. However, pathologic alterations have been studied most frequently in the more serious atrial arrhythmias, such as atrial fibrillation and more recently in sinoatrial block and the sick sinus syndrome. Ischemic, sclerotic, and inflammatory changes in the S-A node are observed in most cases of the sick sinus syndrome; however, these alterations are seen in only 25 per cent of cases of other atrial arrhythmias (Hudson, 1960; Schillman et al., 1970).

CONTROL OF THE HEART RATE

The rate of the heart is determined by that of the most rapidly firing pacemaker tissue — normally the S-A node. Its natural tempo is controlled by a balance of antagonistic forces, e.g., the following: (a) *Cardioinhibitory forces (vagal)*, which originate from the nucleus ambiguus in the medulla. This center can be affected reflexly or by higher centers. (b) *Cardioaccelerator forces (sympathetic)* arise in the upper five dorsal segments of the spinal cord and centers in the hypothalamus and cerebral cortex.

The average rate in the adult human subject ranges between 64 and 80 beats per minute. The rate is faster in children and tends to decrease gradually as the individual grows older. At birth, the heart rate ranges from 110 to 150 beats per minute; in patients over the age of 60, the heart rate may range from 50 to 75 beats per minute; also, the rhythm of the S-A node may become somewhat irregular.

In addition to age, several other factors affect the heart rate, viz.: (1) metabolic rate, (2) nutritional state, (3) body temperature, (4) environmental temperatures, (5) body size, (6) posture, (7) exercise, (8) emotional state, and (9) the sleeping state. The adjustments of the heart rate serve an extremely useful purpose in accommodating the heart rate to bodily needs for nutrients, for maintaining adequate cardiac output, and for other functions.

SINUS TACHYCARDIA

The occurrence of a rapid rate arising from the S-A nodal pacemaker is quite common. Rates greater than 110 per minute in adults may be considered a sinus tachycardia; occasionally, rates as high as 180 per minute or even higher may be observed. In children, sinus rates as high as 230 per minute have been recorded.

The tachycardia encroaches mainly upon the "interval of diastasis," with a resultant decrease in ventricular

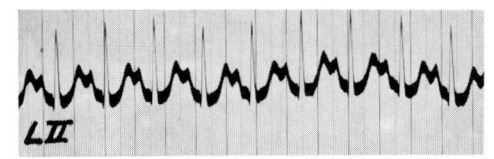

Figure 5-1. Sinus tachycardia with a rate of 186 per minute. (Time intervals measure 0.20 second.) Note the J segment type of ST segment displacement; the P waves follow the peak of the T wave before it has reached the iso-electric line. The P-R interval is relatively short due to the rapid rate.

filling. From the standpoint of work performance, the maximal effective increase in heart rate for the normal adult heart is approximately two and one-half times that of the resting state (i.e., from about 70 beats per minute to a level of 170 to 180 beats per minute). At faster heart rates, the filling period is curtailed and the stroke volume tends to diminish.

Effect of Simple Tachycardia on the Electrocardiogram. The effect of tachycardia on the various deflections of the electrocardiogram depends upon the underlying clinical state and the precipitating cause of the tachycardia. The P waves are increased in amplitude and the P-R interval is usually shortened, but in occasional instances, it is lengthened. The ST-T segments are often depressed; occasionally, they are slightly elevated. ST-T abnormalities may outlast the tachycardia. A previously upright T wave may be flattened and, in rare cases, inverted; occasionally, the amplitude of the T wave may be increased. An inconspicuous U wave may become prominent or even inverted (Fig. 5-1).

Following carotid sinus pressure, sinus tachycardia is usually unaffected; occasionally, it is gradually or partially slowed (Fig. 5-2), particularly in the digitalized patient. In paroxysmal atrial tachycardia, the rate either remains unchanged or slows abruptly to about half the original rate.

Symptoms and Signs. The symptoms and signs depend on the cause and duration of the tachycardia. In the normal heart without associated generalized disease, unless the rate is extremely rapid or of long duration, there may be few or no symptoms due to the tachycardia itself. Frequently, sinus tachycardia is accompanied by an increase in the vigor of contraction, and the symptoms of palpitation, restlessness, agitation, and chest pain may result. The patient often seems apprehensive; vigorous pulsations are observed in the vessels of the neck and a forceful heart beat may be observed in these subjects. Occasionally, a functional systolic murmur may be heard over the apex of the heart.

Treatment. The treatment depends on the underlying cause of the sinus tachycardia: shock, infection, hemorrhage, hyperthyroidism, or other causative agent. Digitalis and diuretics are indicated in the presence of heart failure; however, digitalis in therapeutic doses usually does not slow a sinus tachycardia unless it results from

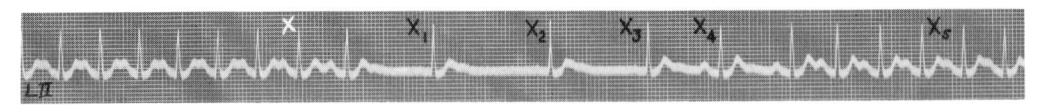

Figure 5-2. Effect of carotid sinus pressure on sinus tachycardia. A sinus tachycardia is present (rate 150 per minute). Carotid sinus pressure applied at X results in marked slowing of the rate. With release of pressure, there is a gradual return to the pre-existing rate. Note the decrease in amplitude and alteration in shape of the P waves and decrease in P-R intervals with the long cycles X_1, X_2, and X_3 (from 0.18 to 0.12 second). This could be the result of shift of the pacemaker within the S-A node as well as improved conduction through the A-V node due to the increased rest period. Note the gradual increase in the P-R interval as the cycle length decreases (X_4) and the return of the P-R interval to 0.18 second as the tachycardia is resumed (X_5).

heart failure. Propranolol has recently been found useful in some cases (see p. 352). Usually no significant effect is observed unless one attacks the underlying cause. Sedatives and psychotherapy are valuable adjuncts in the management of the tachycardia.

Prognosis. The prognosis depends upon the underlying cause of the sinus tachycardia and the response to therapy.

SINUS BRADYCARDIA

Sinus bradycardia is characterized by a slow sinus rate, usually ranging from 35 to 50 beats per minute. Each atrial impulse is followed by a ventricular beat. The slow rate may persist for relatively short periods of time or for hours, days, or years. It may be associated with or occur independently of a sinus arrhythmia. The incidence of sinus bradycardia is greatest between the ages of six and ten and in the older age groups.

Etiology. Sinus bradycardia frequently occurs in athletes and in normal individuals during sleep. It is also common in the older age group. The following are some of the causative factors: (1) Vagal stimulation as a result of Valsalva maneuver, carotid sinus pressure, and ocular pressure result in transient bradycardia; however, vagal reflexes arising from the left ventricle (e.g., as a result of posterior myocardial infarction) may produce sinus bradycardia and hypotension. (2) Factors released by the myocardium following myocardial infarction and retained locally (e.g., glutamic and aspartic acid, potassium) have a negative chronotropic action. (3) Mechanical reflexes, arising in the sinoatrial node, also control the sinus rate. An inverse relationship exists between the degree of distention of the sinus node artery and the rate of the sinus pacemaker. (4) Direct involvement of the sinus node by inflammatory or degenerative processes may cause sinus bradycardia.

Clinical Features Associated with Bradycardia (Less Than 50 to 60 Beats per Minute). Sinus bradycardia is significant not only in itself but also because of its association with a hypotensive state and a low cardiac output in the presence of myocardial disease. The hemodynamic consequences of bradycardia not less than 40 beats per minute are often minimal because the heart can compensate by increasing the stroke volume; however, a diseased heart or one that has sustained a myocardial infarction, with its attendant decrease in ventricular function, may not be able to compensate for this slowing. In addition, the slow rate predisposes to even further slowing and may lead to the production of other types of arrhythmias, such as S-A block, premature beats, and paroxysmal tachycardias.

Several physiologic mechanisms act together to produce these arrhythmias. Temporal dispersion of repolarization enhanced by slow rates generates electrotonic currents, which increase automaticity. Furthermore, slow rates allow the potential pacemaker tissue in the heart to depolarize spontaneously between sinus beats. These changes result in a variety of associated arrhythmias. In addition, slow heart rates, especially in the older age group, may produce manifestations of cerebrovascular insufficiency.

Moreover, patients with sinus bradycardia, particularly older patients (66 to 80 per cent), tend to have disease of the A-V junction and/or of the intraventricular conduction system; symptoms of such disease may be elicited by rapid atrial pacing. Not only does this diffuse involvement of the cardiac conduction increase the probability of occurrence of very slow heart rates but it also affects the site of placement of electrodes if artificial pacing becomes necessary. Evaluation of the A-V junction by His bundle electrography and atrial pacing may be a helpful technique for choosing an appropriate type of pacemaker (see Chapter 37 on pacemakers).

Symptoms and Signs. Relatively few symptoms result from the slow rate itself. Adequate adjustments to increase the cardiac output are made by an increase in stroke volume; in the absence of adequate adjustments, with exercise and emotional stress symptoms such as shortness of breath, easy fatigability, and precordial pain result during the continuance of the slow rate. However, these subjects are prone to syncopal attacks if, as occasionally happens, the rate drops to a still lower figure.

Diagnosis. The diagnosis of sinus bradycardia is suggested by clinical examination but is made definitively with the electrocardiogram (see Fig. 5–3). The differential diagnosis relating to the cause of a slow pulse includes slowing due to S-A and A-V heart block, A-V junctional rhythm, atrial fibrillation, atrial flutter associated with marked grades of A-V heart block, and varying degrees of A-V heart block with sinus rhythm. An electrocardiogram is required to establish a definitive diagnosis.

Treatment. There is no specific treatment for sinus bradycardia. In some patients, however, the persistence of an extremely low rate (e.g., below 36 beats per minute) is not well-tolerated; increasing the ventricular rate by the administration of atropine, isoproterenol, or other sympathomimetic agents may help, but such help is transient. In the presence of syncopal attacks or otherwise symptomatic bradycardia, an artificial pacemaker is indicated (see Chapter 37 on pacemakers).

SINUS ARRHYTHMIA

Sinus arrhythmia is caused by a disturbance in the rhythmic production of the impulse at the S-A node. The ventricles and atria participate equally in this irregularity. Each ventricular contraction is preceded by an atrial systole at the usual intervals. Sinus arrhythmia is most frequently encountered in children and young adults and tends to disappear in adult life, but it may reappear in older patients.

The two types of sinus arrhythmia most commonly observed are: (1) the *respiratory* form, in which the variations in heart rate are cyclic and related to respiration, and (2) the *non-respiratory* form, in which the irregularity occurs without correlation to the phases of respiration.

In the more common form, the irregularity varies with the phases of respiration; the rate tends to increase gradually with inspiration and decrease with expiration. Inspiration tends to diminish vagal tone, while expiration tends to increase it.

In the ventriculophasic type of sinus arrhythmia, the filling of the ventricle mediated through a vagal reflex affects the heart rate. In situations such as partial or higher grades of A-V heart block, the ventricle is filled more during those cycles in which the sinus impulse is blocked, and the sinus rate

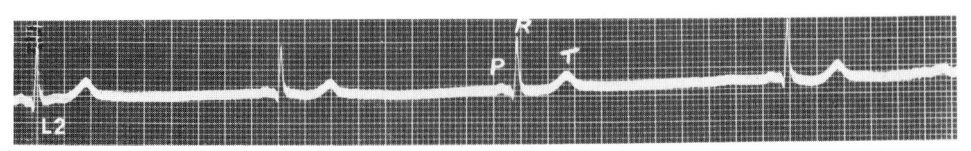

Figure 5–3. Sinus bradycardia, slightly irregular (30 to 34 beats per minute). Both the atrial and ventricular rates are slow (34 per minute) and the P-R interval is normal. With such a slow sinus rate, the possibility of a 2:1 S-A block is to be considered clinically.

SINUS IRREGULARITIES

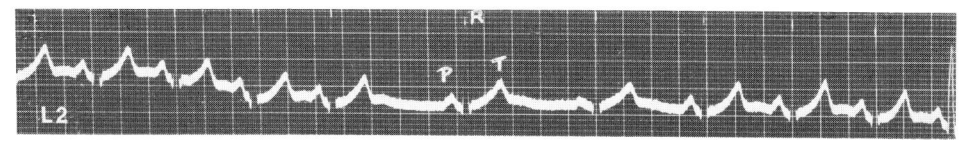

Figure 5-4. Sinus arrhythmia. Note the phasic variation of the R-R interval. The rate increases during inspiration and decreases during expiration. The shorter cycles are associated with a decreased T-P interval. The P-R interval remains constant throughout.

slows (i.e., P-P interval is prolonged) during these periods of increased ventricular filling.

Etiologic Factors. Sinus arrhythmia is observed in normal hearts of children and young adults. By itself, it is not an indication of heart disease; however, its presence does not exclude heart disease, because it often appears in patients with mitral and aortic valvular disease and with various grades of coronary arteriosclerosis in the older age groups.

Other factors include increased intracranial pressure, various types of cerebral dysfunction, and drugs such as digitalis, morphine, and other parasympathomimetic agents.

Symptoms and Signs. In most cases there are no particular symptoms that characterize sinus arrhythmia. In the marked form, the patient may complain of dizziness and faintness. The altered heart action, associated with apnea or Cheyne-Stokes breathing, may give the patient a sense of palpitation.

Diagnosis. Sinus arrhythmias are usually easily diagnosed. A phasic variation in the heart rate, as described above, is quite characteristic (Fig. 5-4).

Treatment. No treatment is required for the common types of sinus arrhythmia. Generally, this arrhythmia may be abolished by any factor that increases the heart rate (e.g., exercise, emotion, atropine, and sympathomimetic drugs).

Prognosis. Sinus arrhythmia *per se* is a normal phenomenon. The prognosis depends on the underlying clinical state. The presence of sinus arrhythmia neither establishes nor rules out the presence or organic heart disease.

WANDERING OF THE PACEMAKER FROM S-A NODE TO A-V JUNCTION

Occasionally, the sinus pacemaker may shift to another portion of the S-A node (the "tail") or to the A-V junction—the so-called "wandering pacemaker." This results in alteration in the configuration of the P waves, the

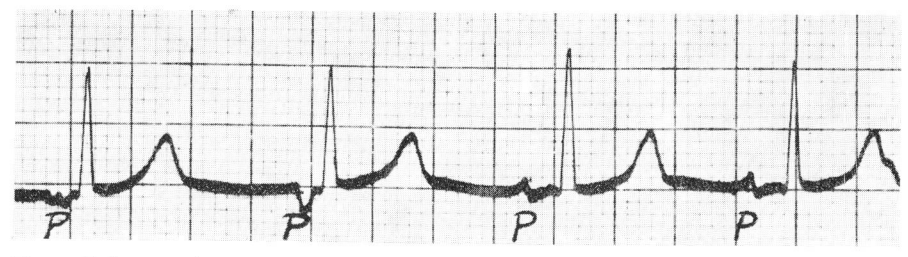

Figure 5-5. Wandering pacemaker. Alteration in configuration of P waves due to a shift in the S-A nodal pacemaker. Note the alterations in configuration of P waves and varying P-R intervals in different cycles. These are due to a shift of the pacemaker to different portions of the A-V node (first two beats) and then to the S-A node (last two beats). The first P wave could be a fusion P (fusion or retrograde and sinus P waves; this is intermediate in type between the second and third P wave).

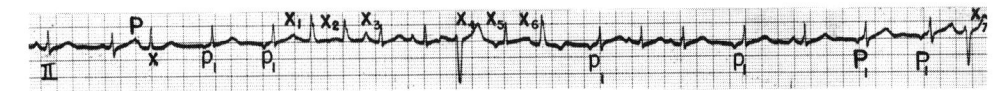

Figure 5-6. Wandering pacemaker with atrial premature beats. (Lead II) Note atrial premature beats at X, X_1, X_2, X_3, X_4, X_6 and X_7; the QRS of X_2, X_4 and X_6 show aberrant conduction. Inverted P waves observed at P_1 are due to a shift of the pacemaker from the S-A toward the A-V node.

length of the P-R interval, and the heart rate (Fig. 5-5). The P wave changes in size, shape, or direction simultaneously with slowing of the rate and changes in the P-R interval. When the pacemaker returns to the sinus node, these changes are reversed.

Vagal stimulation and various parasympathetic drugs have been demonstrated experimentally to cause a shift of the pacemaker from the head, most often to the tail, of the S-A node and occasionally to the A-V junction. Wandering of the pacemaker may be initiated by ectopic premature beats or by a run of such beats that transiently suppresses the sinus node. Shift of the pacemaker may also occur during S-A block (Fig. 5-6).

SINOATRIAL HEART BLOCK

Sinoatrial block is a relatively uncommon condition in which the atria and the ventricles experience a delay or failure of activation by the S-A node for one or more beats. An analogy has been made between the S-A and A-V nodes in grading the degree of block. Theoretically, the block may be divided into first, second, third, or complete S-A block. However, such a differentiation is more difficult to establish with respect to the S-A node.

First degree S-A block may theoretically occur; however, it cannot be recognized because prolongation of S-A node to atrial muscle conduction time cannot be clinically recognized on a human electrocardiogram, although it may be suspected.

Second degree S-A block consists of the following types:

(a) Those manifesting the Wenckebach phenomenon.

(b) Those in which the long cycle is slightly less than twice that of the usual cycle length. Although this may belong in the Mobitz II category, it is more likely a subdivision of the Wenckebach type; this may be more definitely established if sufficient preceding cycles are studied. Also to be ruled out (when the P-P intervals are longer than the normal sequence) is the presence of a non-conducted atrial premature beat (Fig. 5-7).

(c) Those in which the pause is approximately double (or any multiple of) the normal cycle length. Occasionally, the cycle length is less than twice

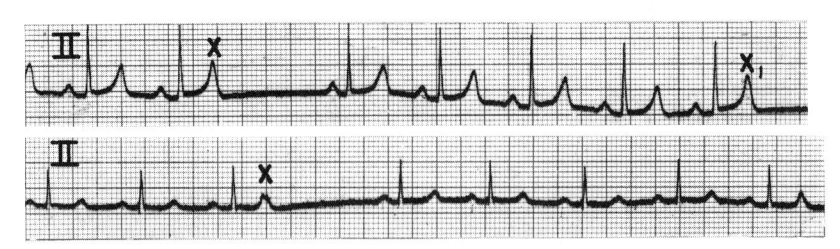

Figure 5-7. Blocked atrial premature beats followed by pauses simulating sinoatrial block. Both tracings represent blocked atrial premature beats occurring superimposed on the T waves marked X and X_1. These represent a superimposition of a P wave on the top of the T wave and are therefore considered as blocked premature atrial beats. The longer cycles are slightly shorter than two P-P intervals. This may be misdiagnosed as S-A heart block.

SINUS IRREGULARITIES

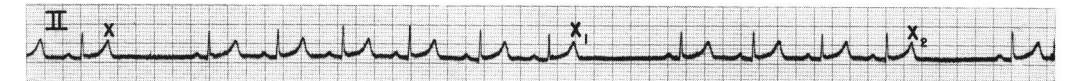

Figure 5–8. S-A Block. Note S-A block in cycle X and cycle X₁. The cycle length is slightly less than that between two normal cycles. The cycles preceding X₂ show a decreasing length, suggesting that this is an example of the Wenckebach type of S-A block.

that of the normal R-R interval. There is no evidence of atrial or ventricular activity (i.e., no P waves or QRST complexes) during the pause except when a junctional escape occurs during a long pause.

The diagnosis of second degree S-A heart block with Wenckebach phenomenon (analogous to Mobitz type I A-V heart block) is made when the following criteria are fulfilled: (1) The P-P interval, including a blocked S-A impulse, is shorter than double the normal P-P interval. (2) The P-P interval after the dropped S-A impulse is longer than the interval preceding the pause. (3) There is a gradual shortening of the P-P interval preceding the long pause. Thus, every third, fourth, or fifth beat may be dropped in a regular or an irregular sequence (see Figs. 5–8, 5–9).

Second degree S-A block without Wenckebach phenomenon (analogous to Mobitz type II A-V heart block) is diagnosed when the pause is nearly an exact multiple (two or more) of the basic P-P interval and preceding cycles are constant. The pauses are equal or multiples of a common divisor (Fig. 5–10). Thus, the beats may be regularly or irregularly dropped. Persistent 3:2 S-A block is another type in which short P-P and R-R intervals alternate with long ones; this simulates a sinus bigeminy.

Third degree S-A block is not detectable clinically, because S-A impulses fail to reach the atrial muscle. This type may be suspected in the presence of atrial standstill.

S-A heart block may be acute, intermittent, or chronic. The irregularity may in fact be observed for a few cycles only; it may progress gradually or the rate may suddenly be halved (e.g., decreased from 75 to 38 beats per minute); this slow rate may persist

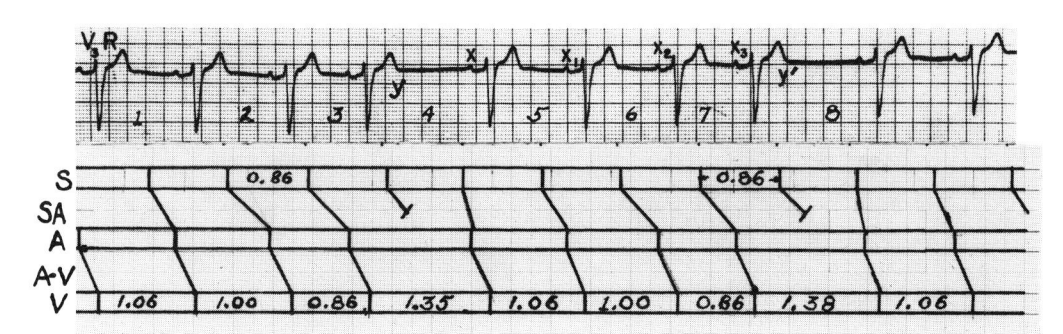

Figure 5–9. Sinoatrial block with Wenckebach phenomenon. A strip of V₃R shows two episodes of 5:4 S-A heart block with Wenckebach phenomenon. The diagram shows theoretical regularly-spaced internal sinus node impulses (occurring 0.86 second apart), which are equal to the length of the shortest R-R cycle in each series. The first of these regular internal sinus node impulses is placed 0.08 second before the P wave that starts the cycle; this is the assumed minimal conduction time from the interior of the sinus node to the atrial muscle (X). S marks the theoretic impulses arising from the S-A node. A denotes the interatrial cycle length, and V denotes the interventricular cycle length. The last internal sinus stimulus, Y, is blocked in cycles 4 and 8 and is not conducted to the atrial muscle. Since the increments in time of the prolonged S-A conduction diminished progressively, the P-P intervals become consequently shorter until the last internal sinus stimulus is blocked, thus producing longer P-P and R-P intervals in cycles 4 and 8.

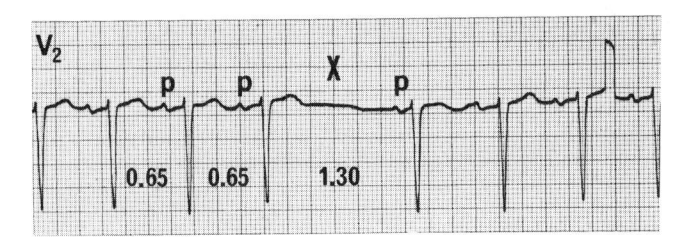

Figure 5–10. Type II second degree S-A heart block. Tracing taken from a 58-year-old woman who manifested a mild grade of digitalis toxicity. Note that the cycle length, X, is exactly twice that of the normal cycle length.

for several minutes or longer. This type, however, is usually transient. The sudden halving of the heart rate is usually preceded by a slight acceleration, followed by longer cycles, which gradually shorten until the usual cycle length is re-established. The disturbance may exist for long periods of time, and it may be the underlying mechanism for long-term bradycardia.

Etiologic Factors (Clinical). S-A block has been observed in subjects with normal hearts (Averill and Lamb, 1960) and in those with disease processes involving the S-A node or the nodal artery (Greenwood and Finkelstein, 1964). The ratio of males to females is 2:1. Of the patients in whom S-A block is found, only 20 per cent are considered to have a normal cardiovascular system; the majority of the subjects had associated atrial disease.

Digitalis is the drug most often implicated in the genesis of S-A block. However, quinidine sulfate and potassium salts may occasionally cause human S-A block. Transient or chronic S-A block has often been associated with the following clinical conditions: (1) inflammation (e.g., acute rheumatic states, other types of myocarditis, and postsurgical trauma); (2) degenerative processes (e.g., post-diphtheric fibrosis and coronary atherosclerosis); and (3) ischemia (i.e., myocardial infarction due to occlusion of the coronary artery that supplies the S-A node).

Symptoms and Signs. Usually, no symptoms are observed with minor grades of S-A heart block. Dizziness and faintness may occur with the sinus pauses, and if they are prolonged, loss of consciousness (syncope) will follow. Ordinarily, the prompt assumption of pacemaker activity by the A-V junction terminates the attack, and this makes the disorder less dangerous than Stokes-Adams attacks in complete A-V heart block. However, many patients with chronic second degree S-A heart block suffer from dizziness; as many as 60 per cent may experience syncopal attacks, and severe brain damage occasionally ensues. There-

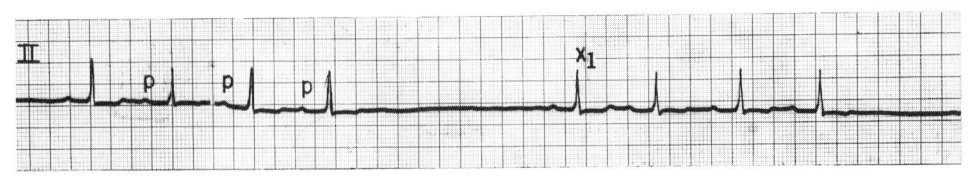

Figure 5–11. Sinoatrial block with prolonged P-R and atrial and ventricular arrest for a duration of three cycles. Following the fourth QRS complex, note the presence of a sinus pause which is equal to that of three cycle lengths. The P-R interval is prolonged; it is shortest after the long pause (0.24 second), and prior to the pause it is 0.28 second. The three complexes following X_1 are similar to those that precede the long pause.

SINUS IRREGULARITIES

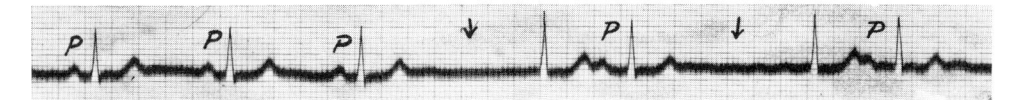

Figure 5–12. Sinoatrial block with junctional escape. At the arrows, a rhythmic atrial beat does not occur, and junctional escape follows. After the escape beat, the P-R interval of the short cycle (fourth and sixth) measures 0.24 second as compared with the normal P-R interval of 0.18 second in the first three beats. This means that the conduction occurred in the relative refractory phase of the preceding beat. Note that the P-P interval occurring between the complex preceding the pause and that following the pause are exactly equal to two normal cycles.

fore, in severe S-A nodal or binodal disease, the manifestations of S-A block may be quite serious.

Prolonged Sinus Pauses. Prolonged sinus pauses may occur during S-A heart block (Fig. 5–11). This is probably caused by the failure of the impulses to leave the S-A node and inability of the S-A node and any other potential atrial pacemaker to generate impulses. Under these conditions, the A-V junction usually escapes and assumes control of the ventricles for one or more beats (Fig. 5–12). If A-V junctional retrograde conduction occurs, each junctional impulse, by retrograde penetration into the sinus node, continues to discharge the sinus node and may contribute to the temporary or permanent elimination of the latter from the control of the heart beat.

Prolonged sinus pauses may be caused by increases in vagal tone, which may occur spontaneously or may follow vagal stimulation produced by carotid sinus or ocular pressure, gagging, vomiting, and other conditions. These pauses may also result from the administration of parasympathetic drugs, particularly acetylcholine; this action has led to the use of acetylcholine in coronary angiography. Quinidine and potassium salts particularly tend to produce sinus pauses by slowing the atrial rate; such pauses may lead to atrial standstill. Such pauses are extremely dangerous because they may produce syncopal attacks, Stokes-Adams seizures, and cardiac arrest.

It is important to note that the absence of P waves in the electrocardiogram does not exclude a sinus origin of ventricular beats. The P wave is representative of atrial, not S-A nodal, activity. Because of the accumulating evidence of the existence

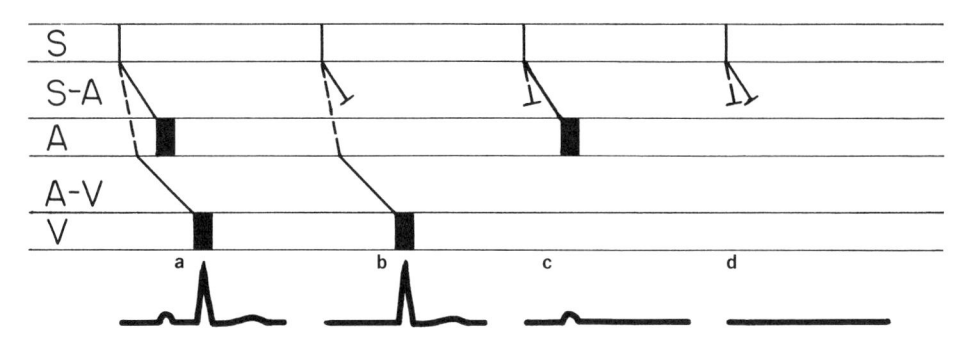

Figure 5–13. (a) Physiologic situation with normal sequence of P-QRS-T. (b) Sinoventricular conduction (without activation of the atrial muscle). Note absence of P wave preceding QRS. (c) Sinoventricular block with atrial activation preserved. Note P wave without ventricular activation. (d) Sinoventricular block together with the block of the sinus impulse conduction of the atrial muscle. Note absence of both atrial and ventricular activity. (From Bellet, S., and Jedlicka, J.: Amer. J. Cardiol., 24:831, 1969.)

of sinoatrial tracts, recent interest has been aroused concerning the existence of sinoventricular (S-V) conduction, which may transmit the sinus impulse to the A-V junction without atrial contraction (Bellet and Jedlicka, 1969). A diagrammatic representation of S-A and S-V conduction is presented in Fig. 5–13. Sinoventricular conduction has been noted during experimental hyperpotassemia (DeMello and Hoffman, 1960; Hoffman and Cranefield, 1964; Vassalle and Hoffman, 1965), digitalis intoxication, and hypothermia. Its presence in clinical situations has been proposed (Fig. 29–1).

Arrhythmias Associated with S-A Heart Block. The pauses observed with S-A block may lead to (a) A-V junctional escape (Fig. 5–12), (b) transient atrial standstill, (c) long periods of bradycardia when 2:1 or higher degrees of S-A conduction occurs, and (d) association with A-V block. In about 70 per cent of patients, S-A block is associated with slight grades of A-V heart block. Atrial pacing tends to bring out latent A-V conduction disturbances.

Sick Sinus Syndrome. In the past few years, the term *sick sinus syndrome* (SSS) has been applied to a group of atrial arrhythmias which occur together. It is associated with (1) severe sinus bradycardia; (2) sinus arrest associated with supraventricular tachyarrhythmias, or, less commonly, periods of cardiac arrest; (3) chronic atrial fibrillation associated with a slow ventricular rate not produced by drugs and with inability of the heart to maintain normal sinus rhythm following countershock; and (4) sinoatrial block unrelated to drugs.

The etiology of the syndrome appears to be ischemic, sclerotic, or inflammatory involvement of the sinus node. Fifty per cent of patients with SSS (average age, 71 years) have coronary artery disease; 20 per cent (average age, 40 years) have cardiomyopathy; 5 per cent have syphilitic heart disease; and in 20 per cent no clear etiologic factor can be determined (Schillman et al., 1970).

The Sluggish Sinus Node Syndrome. In this syndrome, which is closely related to the sick sinus syndrome, the automaticity of the sinus node is depressed. Generalized disease of the sinus node should be suspected when the administration of atropine results in little or no increase in sinus rate or leads to the development of slow A-V junctional rhythms prior to an increase in the sinus rate.

The recovery time of the S-A node following abrupt cessation of suppression of the sinoatrial activity by rapid atrial pacing (at a rate of 130 per minute) provides an objective parameter for evaluating sinoatrial function. In clinically normal hearts the interval between the last pacing impulse and the onset of the first intrinsic P wave ranges from 0.8 to 1.1 second (mean, 0.9 second), whereas in patients with clinical evidence of sinoatrial disease this interval is 1.6 to 7.0 seconds. Sinoatrial function may be assessed also by recording electrograms in the region of the S-A node following pace-induced premature atrial contractions. About two-thirds of subjects with the sick or sluggish sinus syndrome show this abnormal response during right atrial pacing. This group shows manifestations of abnormal A-V junctional conduction in addition to that of the S-A node. In such cases, an atrial pacemaker will not suffice; a ventricular pacemaker is indicated.

Treatment. No treatment is required in the absence of signs or symptoms. If possible, the underlying causes should be determined. When S-A block occurs frequently, and when, in older age groups, the sinus rate drops to a level below 36 beats per minute with resultant syncope, it is advisable to administer drugs that diminish vagal tone (e.g., atropine, isoproterenol for the acute phase). Medications that increase vagal tone, such as digitalis, should be omitted altogether or used with caution. During periods of atrial standstill, because of the danger of severe consequences, vagolytic, sympathomimetic, and alkalinizing agents should be used promptly (see page 329). If episodes are frequent or the sinus pauses prolonged, an artificial pacemaker is usually indicated.

Prognosis. The prognosis of S-A block depends primarily upon the cause (e.g., digitalis), the underlying condition of the heart, the degree of S-A block, the frequency, severity, and length of the episodes, and the type of associated arrhythmias. Except in the most severe types, the prognosis may be considered favorable from the standpoint of the block itself. When S-A block occurs frequently and is associated with prolonged periods of sinus standstill, the prognosis in the past has been more serious. However, with the recent modalities in therapy, especially the use of the artificial pacemaker, the prognosis has improved considerably.

ATRIAL STANDSTILL

Atrial standstill may be *transient,* which is not uncommon, or *persistent,* which is rare. Transient atrial standstill which lasts from several seconds to hours or days is observed under a variety of conditions. The great majority of cases have been associated with drugs or electrolyte imbalance. Two-thirds of cases of temporary standstill are associated with toxic doses of digitalis or the use of quinidine. Transient atrial standstill has been associated with profound sinus bradycardia; S-A block (3:1 or 4:1); responses in A-V junctional rhythm with retrograde conduction to the atria, which render the S-A node refractory; and sinoventricular conduction due to potassium, quinidine, and digitalis.

Persistent atrial standstill may be defined as a condition in which atrial activity is absent for periods of months or years; to date, five authenticated cases have been reported (Allensworth et al., 1969; Bloomfield and Sinclair-Smith, 1965; Lewis et al., 1914).

Atrial standstill may be observed in the terminal phases of many disease states, particularly myocardial infarction. The exact cause of terminal atrial standstill is often difficult to determine; however, in many cases it is the result of hypoxia or hyperpotassemia.

Diagnosis. Transient atrial standstill should not be diagnosed merely

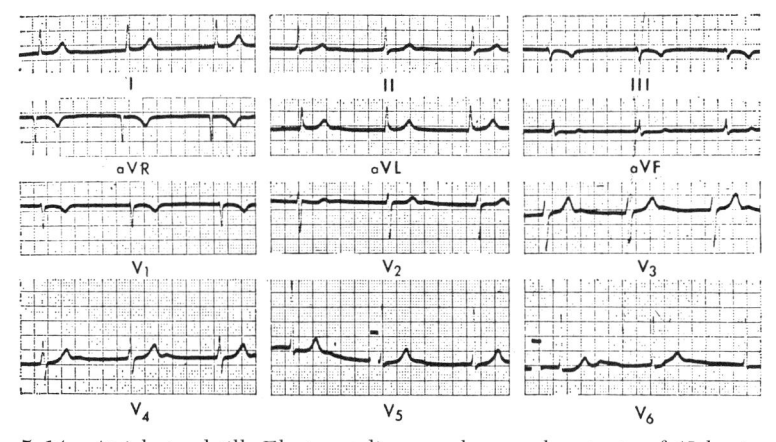

Figure 5-14. Atrial standstill. Electrocardiogram shows a heart rate of 48 beats per minute, QRS duration of 0.08 second and absence of P waves. (From Allensworth, D. C., Rice, G. J., and Lowe, G. W.: Amer. J. Med., 47:775, 1969.)

by the absence of P waves in the routine electrocardiogram but rather by the absence of atrial activity in esophageal or intra-atrial leads (Fig. 5–14) (Bloomfield and Sinclair-Smith, 1965). Transient standstill must be differentiated from mid-A-V junctional rhythm, sinoatrial block, and sinoventricular conduction.

Treatment. The treatment is that of the underlying etiology: to correct drug toxicity or to treat the underlying cardiac disease.

References

Allensworth, D. C., Rice, G. J., and Lowe, G. W.: Persistent atrial standstill in a family with myocardial disease. Amer. J. Med., 47:775, 1969.

Averill, K. H., and Lamb, L. E.: Electrocardiographic findings in 67,375 asymptomatic subjects. Amer. J. Cardiol., 6:76, 1960.

Bellet, S.: Clinical Disorders of the Heart Beat. 3rd Ed. Philadelphia, Lea & Febiger, 1971.

Bellet, S., and Jedlicka, J.: Sino-ventricular conduction and its relation to sinoatrial conduction. Amer. J. Cardiol., 24:831, 1969.

Bloomfield, D. A., and Sinclair-Smith, B. C.: Persistent atrial standstill. Amer. J. Med., 39:335, 1965.

Bouvrain, Y., Slama, R., and Temkins, J.: Sinoatrial block and "sinus disease." Observations on 63 cases. Arch. Mal. Coeur., 60:753, 1967.

Clynes, M.: Respiratory sinus arrhythmias: Laws derived from computer simulation. J. Appl. Physiol., 15:863, 1960.

DeMello, W. C., and Hoffman, B. F.: Potassium ions and electrical activity of specialized cardiac fibers. Amer. J. Physiol., 199:1125, 1960.

Eyster, J. A. E., and Evans, J. S.: Sinoauricular heart block. Arch. Intern. Med., 16:832, 1915.

Eyster, J. A. E., and Meek, W. J.: Experiments on the origin and conduction of the cardiac impulse. VII. Sinoventricular and sinoauricular heart block. Arch. Intern. Med., 19:117, 1917.

Goldreyer, B. N., and Damato, A. N.: A method to evaluate sinoatrial pacemaker function. Circulation, 41–42:III-158, 1970.

Greenwood, R. J., and Finkelstein, D.: Sinoatrial Heart Block. Springfield, Ill., Charles C Thomas, 1964.

Han, J.: Mechanisms of ventricular arrhythmias associated with myocardial infarction. Amer. J. Cardiol., 24:800, 1969.

Han, J., Millet, D., Chizzonitti, B., and Moe, G. K.: Temporal dispersion of recovery of excitability in atrium and ventricle as a function of heart rate. Amer. Heart J., 71:481, 1966.

Higgins, T. G., Phillips, J. H., Jr., and Summner, R. G.: Atrial dissociation. An electrocardiographic artifact produced by the accessory muscles of respiration. Amer. J. Cardiol., 18:132, 1966.

Hoffman, B. F., and Cranefield, P. F.: Electrophysiology of the Heart. New York, McGraw-Hill, 1960.

Hoffman, B. F., and Cranefield, P. F.: Physiological basis of cardiac arrhythmias. Amer. J. Med., 37:670, 1964.

Hudson, R.: The human pacemaker and its pathology. Brit. Med. J., 22:153, 1960.

James, T. N.: Pulse and impulse in the sinus node. Henry Ford Hosp. Med. J., 15:275, 1967.

Lewis, T., White, P. D., and Meakins, J.: The susceptible region in A-V conduction. Heart, 5:289, 1914.

Marriott, H. J. L.: Practical Electrocardiography. 4th Ed. Baltimore, Williams & Wilkins, 1968.

Paes de Carvalho, A.: Cellular electrophysiology of the atrial specialized tissues. *In:* Paes de Carvalho, A., DeMello, W. C., and Hoffman, B. F. (Eds.). The Specialized Tissues of the Heart. Amsterdam, Elsevier, 1962.

Reilley, A., Rosen, K., Loeb, H., Xinno, Z., Rahimtoola, S. H., and Gunnar, R.: Cardiac conduction in the "sluggish sinus node" syndrome. Circulation, 41–42:III-42, 1970.

Sano, T., and Yamagishi, S.: Spread of excitation from the sinus node. Circ. Res., 16:423, 1963.

Schillman, C. L., Rubenstein, J. J., Yurchak, R. M., and DeSanctis, R. W.: The "sick-sinus" syndrome: clinical spectrum. Circulation, 41–42:III-42, 1970.

Vassalle, M., and Hoffman, B. F.: The spread of sinus activation during potassium administration. Circ. Res., 17:285, 1965.

Zipes, D. P.: The clinical significance of bradycardiac rhythms in acute myocardial infarction. Amer. J. Cardiol., 24:814, 1969.

Chapter 6 *Atrial Flutter*

GENERAL CONSIDERATIONS
  Clinical Varieties
ETIOLOGY AND PRECIPITATING
  FACTORS
MECHANISM
SYMPTOMS AND SIGNS
  Relation of the Ventricular Rate and Clinical
    Manifestations
  Auscultatory Phenomenon
HEMODYNAMICS
PATHOLOGY
ELECTROCARDIOGRAM
  The F-R (P-R) Interval in Atrial Flutter
  Ventricular Complexes
  Onsets and Offsets of Atrial Flutter

DISTURBANCES IN RHYTHM
  COMPLICATING FLUTTER
  Atrial Flutter with 1:1 Conduction
  Complete A-V Heart Block
  Ventricular Tachycardia
DIAGNOSIS AND DIFFERENTIAL
  DIAGNOSIS
TREATMENT
  Digitalis
  Quinidine
  Propranolol
  Electric Countershock
  Right Atrial Stimulation
PROGNOSIS

GENERAL CONSIDERATIONS

In spite of the infrequency of atrial flutter, this condition is important because it occurs mainly in diseased hearts, is frequently associated with heart failure, and responds to treatment in most instances.

Atrial flutter is not nearly as common as atrial fibrillation. Nevertheless, the incidence, while still low, is more appreciable in populations in which the presence of heart disease is clinically evident. It is more common in males than in females by a ratio of almost 5:1.

Clinical Varieties. Atrial flutter may be observed either as an established disturbance or as a paroxysmal or transient condition. Chronic atrial flutter is more commonly associated with 2:1 A-V heart block with a ventricular rate of 150 per minute; it may be observed also in conjunction with higher grades of A-V block (i.e., 3:1 and 4:1) and, rarely, with complete A-V heart block. However, because of cardioversion and other recent developments in therapy, particularly the use of propranolol in combination with quinidine, persistent atrial flutter should be quite rare.

ETIOLOGY AND PRECIPITATING FACTORS

Atrial flutter occurs most often in older persons who have moderate to severe grades of chronic heart disease. The etiologic factors are similar to those underlying atrial fibrillation, e.g., *hypertensive, atherosclerotic, rheumatic, and less frequently, congenital heart disease, constrictive pericarditis, and cor pulmonale.* Atrial flutter occurs in approximately 2.5 per cent of patients with chronic cor pulmonale. Atrial flutter has been reported to occur in 1 to 5 per cent of patients with acute myocardial infarction.

Acute conditions may either cause or precipitate it in susceptible persons. Among the factors implicated are *stress* (exercise and emotion), *trauma, infections* (diphtheria, acute rheumatic fever), *hypoxia* (acute myocardial infarction and Stokes-Adams seizures), *hyperthyroidism, drug toxicity* (digitalis, quinidine, epinephrine, and ephedrine), and rarely, *alcoholism* and *diabetic acidosis*.

Atrial flutter develops less commonly as a manifestation of digitalis toxicity than does atrial fibrillation. On the other hand, quinidine administered for the conversion of atrial fibrillation to normal sinus rhythm may precipitate atrial flutter.

MECHANISM

The exact mechanisms underlying all cases of atrial flutter have not as yet been definitely established. No single mechanism has been adduced that will explain the various types of atrial flutter. At present, one is forced to conclude that atrial flutter may be due to either: (1) a circus movement, or (2) a unifocal origin. While the two forms of atrial flutter may be produced by quite distinct experimental methods, the clinical distinction has only recently been studied (Rytand, 1966). The circus movement has been supported by electrograms recorded during thoracotomy in patients with atrial flutter. In a recent case (Wellens et al., 1971), atrial epicardial excitation mapping was performed during open heart surgery in a patient with atrial flutter. The results obtained in this patient excluded a circus movement; the possible mechanisms were an ectopic focus located low in the atrium, or a reciprocal rhythm located in a small area low in the atrium or upper part of the A-V junction.

SYMPTOMS AND SIGNS

The symptoms and signs of atrial flutter depend upon the *degree of heart damage, ventricular rate, duration of the flutter*, and, to some extent, the *emotional state of the patient*. Not infrequently, atrial flutter may be relatively well tolerated and, at times, if the degree of A-V heart block is 3:1 or 4:1, the patient may be entirely unaware of an arrhythmia. In general, the manifestations of atrial flutter resemble those of other types of accelerated heart action (see discussion of paroxysmal atrial tachycardia in Chapter 9); however, since they usually occur in patients with previously damaged hearts, the clinical features are usually more marked.

Relation of the Ventricular Rate and Clinical Manifestations. The symptomatology associated with atrial flutter in the individual patient roughly depends on the ventricular rate. With rates of 150 and higher, the symptoms are usually quite marked; with rates between 100 and 130, they tend to be slight or moderate in severity; and at slower rates, those due to flutter *per se* are minimal. Symptoms when present usually improve notably when the flutter is converted to atrial fibrillation with a concomitant decrease in the ventricular rate, or with a return to normal sinus rhythm. In older persons and in those with associated cardiovascular disease, circulatory collapse may occur when the ventricular rate is rapid, e.g., 1:1 response (Figs. 6–1, 6–2).

A serious drawback to prolonged maintenance with digitalis of patients with chronic atrial flutter and 3:1 or 4:1 A-V heart block is that, although the ventricular rate at rest may be satisfactorily slow, the degree of block may abruptly change to 2:1 or even 1:1 with exercise or emotion. When 1:1 conduction does occur under these conditions, a ventricular rate of 220 to 270 per minute suddenly results; this is often accompanied by alarming symptoms (marked dyspnea, precordial pain, and heart failure). Because of these factors, such cases of flutter should be treated with digitalis given in small doses intravenously or intramuscularly (see p. 377) or converted to

ATRIAL FLUTTER

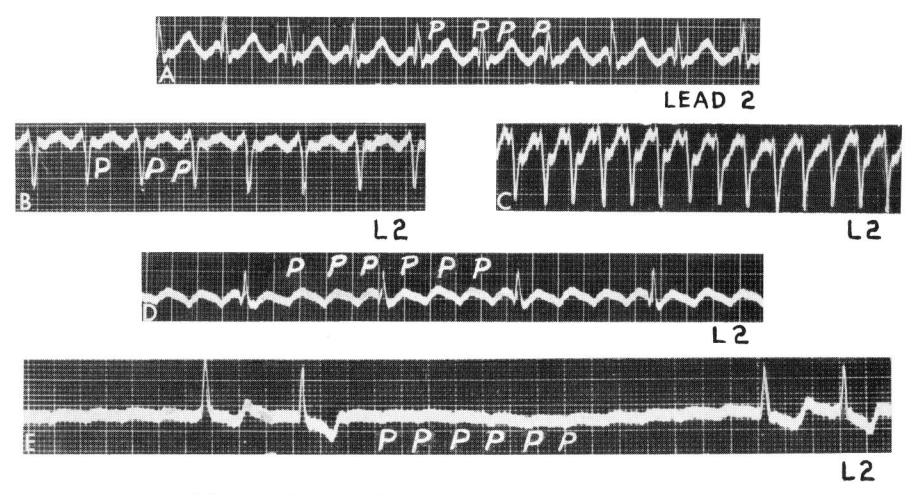

Figure 6–1. Atrial flutter, showing different types of atrial complexes and varying degrees of A-V heart block.

(A) Atrial flutter with a 2:1 heart block. The atrial rate is 250 per minute, the ventricular rate is 125 per minute. Note that the atrial complexes are obscured by the QRS complexes and T waves.

(B) Atrial flutter with a 2:1 heart block.

(C) Atrial flutter with a 1:1 response (atrial and ventricular rate is 250 per minute). The diagnosis of the atrial mechanism was clearly established by other strips that showed higher grades of A-V heart block (Strip B).

(D) Atrial flutter with a 4:1 response.

(E) Atrial flutter with a high degree of A-V heart block and cycle of A-V junctional escapes. Note the short cycle following the escape beat.

Figure 6–2. Atrial flutter with a 1:1 response showing progressive changes following therapy (all leads V₁). (A) Note rapid ectopic rhythm at rate of 264 per minute. This was considered to be atrial flutter with a 1:1 response. (B) Following digitalis the mechanism was converted to atrial fibrillation, thus confirming the original impression of 1:1 flutter. (C) Digitalis was stopped and conversion to normal sinus rhythm was spontaneous. The P-R interval is slightly elevated (0.22 second). Coupled ventricular premature beats are probably due to digitalis toxicity.

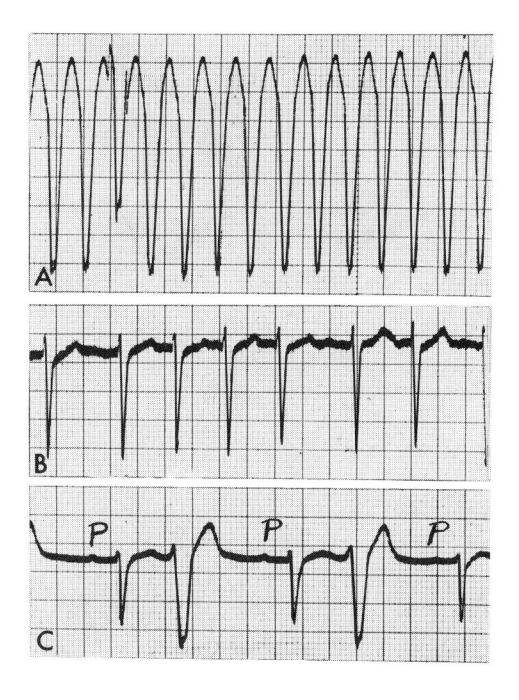

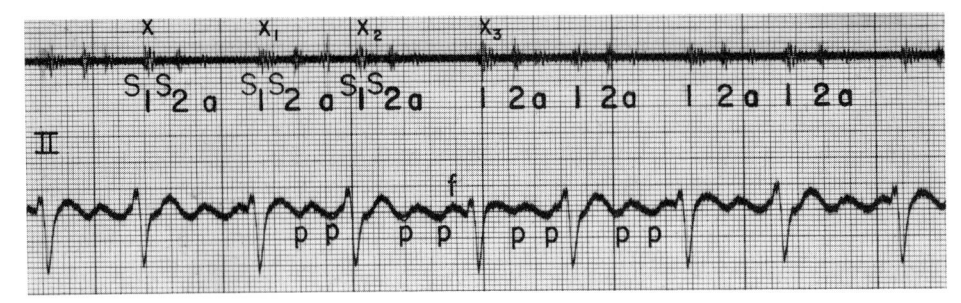

Figure 6-3. Phonocardiogram in atrial flutter with varying degrees of A-V block and varying P-R intervals. Ventricular pseudobigeminy is explainable in two ways: (1) alternating 2:1 and 4:1 conduction with the Wenckebach phenomenon (more probable); and (2) constant 3:1 A-V conduction with alternation of the P-R time. Note the variation in the intensity of the first and second heart sound due to the alteration in the cycle length and varying P-R interval. Note the presence of atrial sounds marked "a."

normal sinus rhythm by electric countershock.

Although not uncommon with atrial fibrillation, embolic phenomena rarely occur as a result of flutter.

Auscultatory Phenomenon. In atrial flutter, the first heart sound may vary in intensity. In contrast to atrial fibrillation, this variation of the first heart sound intensity is not due to the differences in length of the preceding pause but to the variations in the F-R (P-R) interval just preceding the particular ventricular contraction (Fig. 6-3).

Additional heart sounds may be present which are audible during diastole, especially when a high degree of A-V heart block is present. These sounds (S_3 and S_4) are due to atrial contractions or associated movements of the A-V valves.

HEMODYNAMICS

Little change in cardiac output is noted when the ventricular rate is slow (60 to 90 per minute), since there is no distinct alteration in the ventricular diastolic filling period. However, atrial flutter is often associated with a lowered cardiac output when the ventricular rate is rapid (above 150 per minute). Similarly, the blood pressure is higher and cardiac output is greater in atrial flutter with 4:1 and 3:1 than with 2:1 A-V heart block or with 1:1 rhythm in the initial stages. In general, the cardiovascular dynamics approach normal as the ventricular rate approximates the normal range. Therefore, depending upon the ventricular rate during the flutter, conversion to normal sinus rhythm may cause an increase in cardiac output or have no demonstrable influence on hemodynamics.

PATHOLOGY

The pathology associated with atrial flutter is that of the underlying disease states mentioned under etiology (e.g., hypertension, coronary arteriosclerosis, rheumatic heart disease). The heart is usually enlarged and the patients usually have a moderate to severe grade of myocardial damage. The atria are frequently dilated and the atrial muscle is replaced in varying degrees by fibrous tissue.

ELECTROCARDIOGRAM

The diagnosis of atrial flutter is usually clearly established by the electrocardiogram. The distinctive electrocardiographic features are the *characteristic atrial oscillations*. These are rarely seen in lead I, but are more distinct in leads II, III and aVF, and in the precordial leads, V_1, V_2, and V_3R (see Fig. 6–1).

The oscillations are entirely regular at a rate usually ranging between 220 and 370 per minute, the average being 300 per minute. These atrial oscillations are quite evident with slow ventricular rates; they are not always easily recognized with rapid ventricular rates, since the rapidly recurring QRS and T complexes may mask the small atrial waves. Additional help may be obtained by the use of the precordial lead, V_3R, and carotid sinus pressure. Probably the best procedure to determine the atrial mechanism in the doubtful case is the use of the esophageal lead. In such instances, tracings taken at the atrial level will show a sharp positive wave (intrinsicoid deflection), followed by a negative deflection which occurs regularly at a rapid rate (Fig. 6–4). Clear delineation of the atrial waves may also be obtained by Doppler tracings.

Impure atrial flutter represents a transition between flutter and fibrillation. In impure atrial flutter, the F waves vary in contour, amplitude, and duration; the atrial rate is more rapid than that in pure atrial flutter. Transitional forms of electrocardiograms, between atrial tachycardia and flutter or fibrillation, are not uncommon, with the P waves well defined and well isolated in the tracing.

The F-R (P-R) Interval in Atrial Flutter. In many instances the F-R interval is regular and constant, representing a consistent degree of conduction delay in the A-V junction. Such patients usually manifest a consistent degree of A-V heart block (e.g., 2:1, 3:1, or 4:1) with regularly spaced ventricular complexes. The electrocardiogram in many other patients, however, is characterized by an irregular ventricular response; these usually present varied F-R intervals (Fig. 6–5).

Variations in the F-R interval may be due to *concealed conduction* (see p. 18), *A-V dissociation* (this may be associated with junctional tachycardia), *depressed A-V conduction* due to disease of the A-V junction or induced by drugs, *second degree A-V heart block* with Wenckebach phenomenon, or *complete A-V heart block*. In *impure atrial flutter*, the ventricular response is more rapid than in the pure type; the cycle lengths are irregular because of the uneven rate of atrial discharge and variable A-V conduction (Fig. 6–6).

Ventricular Complexes. A rapid rate may cause an increase in intraventricular conduction time due to a relative prolongation of the refractory period of one of the bundle branches, particularly the right. The finding has considerable importance in diagnosis, since simple tachycardia with widened QRS complexes may resemble a ventricular tachycardia; it may be so treated unless one suspects the correct diagnosis and confirms it by the methods outlined elsewhere (see p. 61).

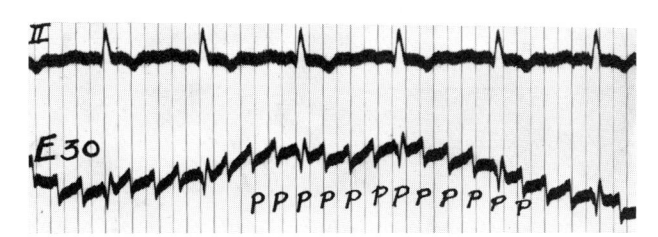

Figure 6–4. Atrial flutter not clearly evident in limb leads, clearly shown by esophageal leads. Limb lead II (*upper strip*) taken simultaneously with esophageal lead (*lower strip*) at atrial level. Upper strip, lead II does not clearly show the atrial complexes. The diagnosis is clearly made by the esophageal lead taken at the atrial level (E_{30}). Note the diphasic atrial complexes occurring at a rate of 310 per minute, which present a characteristic saw-toothed appearance.

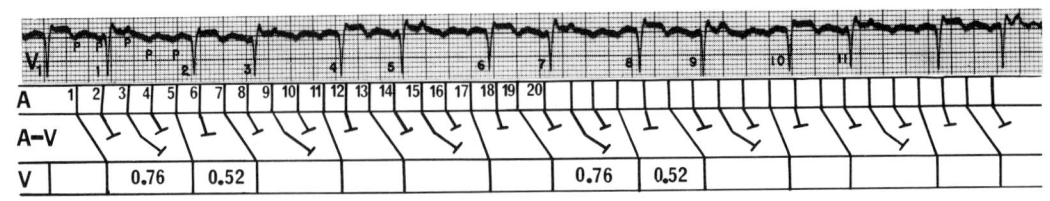

Figure 6–5. Alternating 4:1 and 2:1 flutter, example of "pseudobigeminy." The atrial rate is 280 per minute. Note that *atrial* impulse 5 (see diagram A) is conducted with a short P-R interval. The next impulse (6) is blocked in the A-V node. Impulse 7 is conducted with a longer P-R interval; impulse 8 is again blocked in the A-V node. Impulse 9 has penetrated deeper into the A-V node before being blocked; this shows concealed conduction and represents a dropped beat; impulse 10 is blocked in the node; and 11 is conducted with a short P-R interval. Also note that the longer R-R intervals, measuring 0.76 second, are shorter than four P-P intervals, and the shorter R-R intervals, measuring 0.52 second, are larger than two P-P intervals. This implies that the P-R interval at a 2:1 conduction ratio is longer than the P-R interval at 4:1 conduction ratio, another evidence of Wenckebach phenomenon in this tracing.

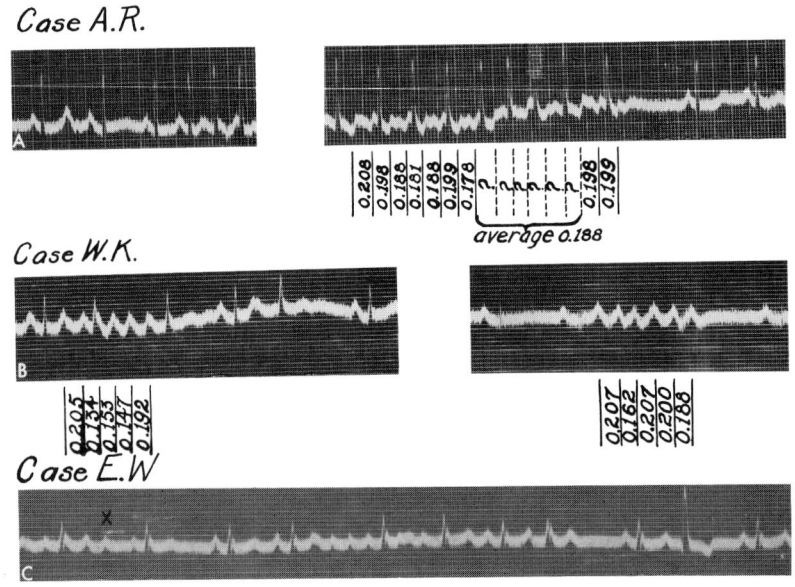

Figure 6–6. Onsets and offsets of atrial flutter (impure). (A) In patient A. R., the onsets invariably were precipitated by exercise or by premature atrial beats. Toward the end of the paroxysm illustrated, the atrial waves are fairly regular in time and also in shape except as the irregularity of the ventricular response modifies them. The last two cycles, 0.198 and 0.199 second in duration, while not longer than some individual cycles, are definitely longer than the immediately preceding ones. The preceding seven cycles are impossible to measure accurately; measured *in toto* and averaged, each has an estimated duration of 0.188 second. Such slight and uncertain changes suggest that the termination of flutter was preceded by slowing of the atria.

(B) In patient W. K., premature atrial beats were also present and at times initiated paroxysms; at other times, onsets were spontaneous. Both types of onsets are illustrated. The behavior of the atrial rate at the time of offsets was inconstant. In the initial strip of B, the last cycle, while not larger than some individual cycles, was longer than the cycle immediately preceding it; in the fourth offset studied the last cycle was definitely shorter than the preceding one. One of each variety of offset is shown.

(C) In patient E. W., the flutter was definitely impure. The flutter waves closely approach in shape the P and T waves, and therefore make it difficult to be certain of the exact point of offset. In the first short paroxysm (marked X), the last atrial wave is definitely faster than the preceding wave. The exact point of the other offset illustrated is uncertain. There are numerous premature beats, but we cannot be certain that any of these impulses actually initiated a period of flutter. (From McMillan, T. M., and Bellet, S.: Amer. J. Med. Sci., *184*:33, 1932.)

Onsets and Offsets of Atrial Flutter. In most instances the paroxysms are initiated by premature atrial beats, but in others no such preliminary disturbances occur. In many of the author's patients, exercise or emotional stress usually precipitated the arrhythmia in susceptible subjects (Fig. 6–6).

The termination of uncomplicated atrial flutter may occur abruptly or it may be preceded by a gradual decrease in the ventricular rate. In the former, the flutter activity ceases and a rather long pause may occur before sinus rhythm resumes (see Fig. 6–6).

DISTURBANCES IN RHYTHM COMPLICATING FLUTTER

Various arrhythmias may be observed in association with atrial flutter; these include different degrees of A-V heart block, ventricular premature beats, and ventricular tachycardia. Except for rare instances of 1:1 conduction, partial A-V heart block is the rule in atrial flutter (Fig. 6–1).

Atrial Flutter with 1:1 Conduction. Atrial flutter with 1:1 conduction occurs when the refractory period of the A-V junction becomes so short that it transmits every atrial impulse. This is accompanied by a rapid ventricular rate (240 to 280 per minute) and usually constitutes a serious cardiac emergency. It merits special consideration because the incidence is probably greater than that suggested by the few cases reported in the literature (Sussman et al., 1966). Indeed, this mechanism, often unrecognized, is probably a cause of acute heart failure and sudden death in patients with atrial flutter (Figs. 6–1, 6–2).

Complete A-V Heart Block. Atrial flutter may occasionally occur with complete A-V heart block (Korst and Wasserberger, 1954). In patients under the age of 55, the etiology is usually rheumatic or congenital, whereas in those over 55 it is less frequently due to these etiologies and is generally due to atherosclerotic or hypertensive heart disease (Rosenbleuth and Garcia Ramos, 1947).

Ventricular Tachycardia. The association of atrial flutter with ventricular tachycardia is relatively rare (Fig. 6–7). This combination is often missed since the nature of the double ectopic rhythm with simultaneous ventricular tachycardia and atrial flutter is not apparent in the routine 12-lead electrocardiogram. It may be due to coronary artery disease or digitalis intoxication (McMillan and Bellet, 1932).

DIAGNOSIS AND DIFFERENTIAL DIAGNOSIS

The diagnosis of atrial flutter is to be considered in any patient with a regular apical rate ranging between

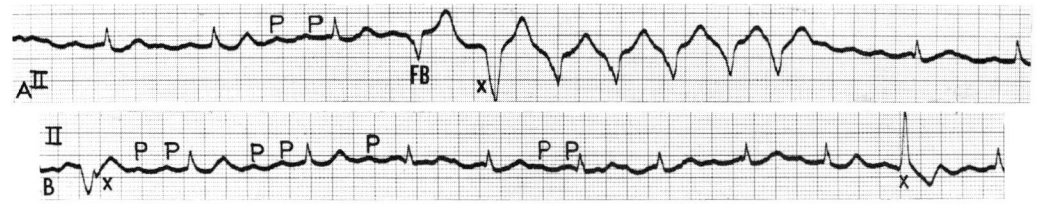

Figure 6–7. Atrial flutter with ventricular tachycardia.
(A) Atrial flutter (rate 216), with 4:1 A-V heart block. Note fusion beat (FB). Starting at X, a 2:1 A-V conduction with aberration of QRS simulating ventricular tachycardia (idioventricular type), 106/minute, is observed.
(B) Note atrial flutter with varying degrees of A-V block. Note aberrant ventricular beats at X. In the middle of the record, there is 3:1 A-V conduction with slight variations of P-R time.

140 and 180 per minute. These patients usually belong to the older age group, show evidence of myocardial abnormality, and often give a history of previous episodes of atrial premature beats, atrial flutter or atrial fibrillation.

In the differential diagnosis, one should consider sinus tachycardia, paroxysmal atrial tachycardia with block, junctional tachycardia, and ventricular tachycardia, when the QRS complexes are widened; occasionally, differentiation from impure flutter is necessary.

The following clinical procedures help in establishing the diagnosis: (1) *Carotid sinus pressure* in atrial flutter results either in no ventricular slowing, or, if slowing occurs, it is usually observed only during the period of carotid sinus pressure. There is no abrupt abolition of the tachyarrhythmia as in paroxysmal atrial tachycardia (Figs. 6-8 and 6-9). (2) The *jugular pulse wave* may be of help, but this is rarely clearly diagnostic. (3) In the *electrocardiogram* the important features in diagnosis are: (a) the *atrial beats are regularly spaced at a rate of 220 to 370 per minute with an average of about 300 per minute;* (b) the flutter waves are usually *most marked in Leads II, III, and aVF;* (c) in the occasional patients with 2:1 and, frequently, with 1:1 response, the diagnosis can be made with certainty only after the *ventricular rate has been slowed by carotid sinus pressure or the P waves identified by esophageal leads;* (d) *the ventricular rate is usually rapid and regular with an average rate of 140 to 150 per minute;* (e) *the ventricular rhythm is often irregular due to the presence of varying degrees of A-V heart block.*

TREATMENT

Treatment should be directed toward the underlying etiologic factor, if this is ascertainable. It may include therapy of acute rheumatic activity and of toxic states, particularly hyperthyroidism. Most patients also require therapy for congestive heart failure. The *therapeutic measures for atrial flutter include the use of certain drugs and electric countershock.*

Digitalis. Digitalis lowers the ventricular rate by increasing the degree

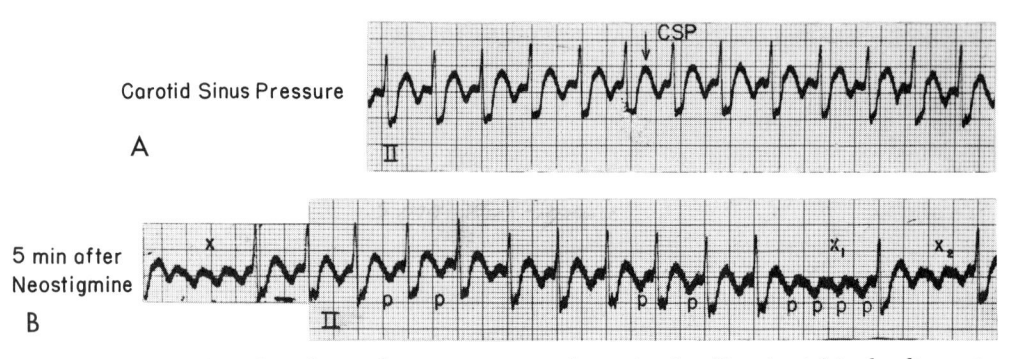

Figure 6-8. The value of carotid sinus pressure and neostigmine (Prostigmin) in the diagnosis of atrial flutter by slowing the ventricular rate.

(A) Shows a regular tachycardia with a rate of 155 per minute. Terminal widening of the QRS complex is due to a right bundle branch block. The exact type of arrhythmia is difficult to establish. Carotid sinus pressure was applied at the arrow; however, no slowing was obtained.

(B) Five minutes after the administration of neostigmine. Note in cycle marked X, the appearance of typical atrial flutter beats with a rate of 300 per minute. Note the resumption of the rapid rate of 150 per minute with 2:1 A-V heart block until cycle marked X_1 where a 5:1 A-V heart block is seen and atrial flutter beats are observed. At X_2 a 4:1 A-V heart block is present. This varying degree of A-V heart block was maintained 11 hours later after the patient had been digitalized.

ATRIAL FLUTTER

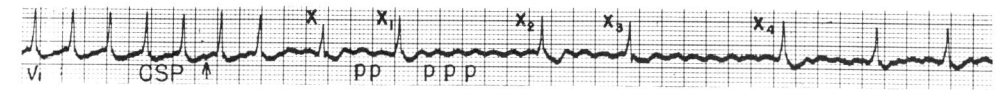

Figure 6–9. Diagnosis of atrial flutter clarified following carotid sinus pressure. The figure shows a rapid arrhythmia, quite regular at a rate of 160 per minute. The exact atrial mechanism cannot be determined at this rapid rate. Following carotid sinus pressure, note that with the slowing of the ventricular rate, the diagnosis of atrial flutter is very clearly made. Note that the P-R interval varies at X, X_3, and X_4.

of A-V heart block; it also manifests an inotropic effect. Usually, its administration is followed by conversion to atrial fibrillation. When the digitalis is discontinued, the fibrillation spontaneously reverts to a normal sinus rhythm in about two-thirds of the patients thus treated. If atrial fibrillation persists after one to two weeks, quinidine or electric countershock may be employed in an effort to convert the atrial fibrillation to a normal sinus rhythm. Occasionally, atrial flutter reverts to a normal sinus rhythm without an observable period of atrial fibrillation.

Patients with paroxysmal attacks of flutter should be digitalized rapidly; even when the atrial flutter persists, the decrease in the ventricular rate improves the cardiac status markedly. For prophylaxis between attacks, digitalis may be given in a maintenance dose; it may not prevent further episodes, but when they recur the ventricular rate will be slower, thus resulting in less severe clinical manifestations. Quinidine sulfate may also be employed for prophylaxis.

Atrial flutter with 1:1 conduction constitutes a medical emergency. Since the ventricular rate of 230 to 265 may gravely compromise cardiovascular dynamics, administration of digitalis by the intramuscular or intravenous route is often warranted.

Quinidine. Because it is successful in converting atrial flutter to a normal sinus rhythm in 30 to 65 per cent of cases, quinidine sulfate is the drug of second choice. When successful, it converts atrial flutter to normal sinus rhythm without an intervening period of atrial fibrillation. The indications and the dosage of quinidine used in converting atrial flutter and fibrillation to normal rhythm are described elsewhere (see p. 349).

Propranolol. Propranolol, a potent beta-adrenergic blocking agent, manifests in addition a quinidine-like effect and has recently been employed in conjunction with quinidine. It has been found useful in the treatment of many cardiac arrhythmias, including atrial flutter. When it is administered in conjunction with quinidine, normal sinus rhythm may result in a greater percentage of cases than with quinidine alone.

Electric Countershock. Electric countershock is often the method of choice for the conversion of atrial flutter to normal sinus rhythm, the conversion rate being between 80 and 100 per cent.

Despite the present high rate of initial success in reversion of atrial flutter, the maintenance of normal sinus rhythm remains a problem. In roughly 20 per cent of the patients, return to flutter or fibrillation occurs in the immediate postconversion period. Three months after conversion, normal sinus rhythm may be observed in as many as 80 per cent of patients; by eight months this figure has dropped to 50 per cent, and at the end of a year, the normal mechanism is manifest in roughly 40 per cent (see p. 427 on countershock).

Right Atrial Stimulation. With resistant cases and those in whom the danger entailed by ventricular depolarization during countershock is considered to be excessive (e.g., digitalis toxicity), conversion may be performed by means of right atrial stimulation. This method has the advantage of not causing ventricular depolarization and does not require anesthesia. The procedure is carried out by means of a unipolar catheter electrode placed in the right atrium by the transvenous route. A stimulus strength of 10 milliamperes is used, and a rate of 180 per minute is effective in most subjects. Occasionally, rates up to 600 per minute must be used.

PROGNOSIS

The prognosis depends upon the severity of underlying disease and the response of the arrhythmia to treatment. When atrial flutter occurs in patients with a severe grade of myocardial damage, the prognosis is that of the basic pathologic condition, plus the effect of the high rate; it is frequently poor unless the arrhythmia is brought under control. However, the prognosis is often quite favorable in uncomplicated cases and in the younger age group.

The prognosis has been substantially improved by the recent use of electric countershock. This method allows almost immediate conversion without undue risk and alleviates the problem of drug toxicity. Episodes of long duration frequently observed prior to the advent of electric countershock are now rarely encountered.

The chief problem at present is the tendency for some subjects to experience recurrent attacks. The problem of maintenance, while a real one, is less than that in atrial fibrillation, perhaps owing to a somewhat lesser degree of underlying atrial disease than in atrial fibrillation. Normal sinus rhythm can usually be maintained by digitalis or quinidine therapy, or both. In some patients, a second trial of cardioversion may be more successful than the first.

References

Bellet, S., and Kostis, J.: Study of the cardiac arrhythmias by the ultrasonic Doppler method. Circulation, 38:721, 1968.

Finkelstein, D., Gold, H., and Bellet, S.: Atrial flutter with 1:1 conduction: Report of six cases. Amer. J. Med., 20:65, 1956.

Korst, D. R., and Wasserberger, R. H.: Atrial flutter associated with complete A-V heart block. Amer. Heart J., 48:383, 1954.

Lown, B.: Cardioversion of arrhythmias, II. Mod. Conc. Cardiovasc. Dis., 33:869, 1964.

Lucchesi, B. R., and Whitsitt, L. S.: The pharmacology of β-adrenergic blocking agents. Prog. Cardiovasc. Dis., 11:410, 1969.

McMillan, T. M., and Bellet, S.: Auricular flutter: Some of its clinical manifestations and its treatment; based on a study of 65 cases. Amer. J. Med. Sci., 184:33, 1932.

Rosenbleuth, A., and Garcia Ramos, J.: Estudios sobre el flutter y la fibrilacion. IV. La Naturaleza del flutter auricular y de la actividas lenta antostenida del musculo auricular aislado. Arch. Inst. Cardiol. Mex., 17:441, 1947.

Rytand, D. A.: The circus movement (entrapped circuit wave) hypothesis and atrial flutter. Ann. Intern. Med., 65:125, 1966.

Semerau, M.: Ueber Ruckbildung der Arrhythmia Perpetua. Deutsch. Arch. Klin. Med., 126:161, 1918.

Sussman, H. F., Duqne, D., and Lesser, M. E.: Atrial flutter with 1:1 conduction. Dis. Chest, 49:99, 1966.

Wellens, H. J. J., Janse, M. J., van Dam, R. T., and Durrer, D.: Epicardial excitation of the atria in a patient with atrial flutter. Brit. Heart J., 33:233, 1971.

Zeft, H. J., Cobb, F. R., Waxman, M. B., Hunt, N. C., and Morris, J. J., Jr.: Right atrial stimulation in the treatment of atrial flutter. Ann. Intern. Med., 70:447, 1969.

Chapter 7 *Atrial Fibrillation*

GENERAL CONSIDERATIONS
INCIDENCE
ETIOLOGY
   Predisposing Factors
   Precipitating Factors
PATHOLOGY AND PATHOPHYSIOLOGY
ELECTROPHYSIOLOGY
HEMODYNAMICS
   Ventricular Function
   Cardiac Output
   Hemodynamic Alterations on Reversion to Normal Sinus Rhythm
SYMPTOMS AND SIGNS
   Relation Between Ventricular Rate and Clinical Manifestations
   Syncopal Attacks
   Cardiac Enlargement
   Heart Failure
   Auscultatory Findings
   Paroxysmal Atrial Fibrillation
ELECTROCARDIOGRAM
   Atrial Deflections
   Ventricular Deflections
   Other Arrhythmias Associated with Atrial Fibrillation
DIAGNOSIS AND DIFFERENTIAL DIAGNOSIS
TREATMENT
   Drug Therapy
   Indications for Conversion to Normal Sinus Rhythm
   Treatment of Paroxysmal Atrial Fibrillation
   Direct Current Countershock
PROGNOSIS

GENERAL CONSIDERATIONS

Atrial fibrillation is probably the most important of the arrhythmias because it is the one most frequently associated with organic heart disease and heart failure. Moreover, it usually responds most satisfactorily to therapy, often with dramatic results.

INCIDENCE

Atrial fibrillation is the second most common of the arrhythmias following premature beats. Of 50,000 consecutive patients, 4316 (8.6 per cent) manifested the chronic variety (Katz and Pick, 1956). Atrial fibrillation occurs most frequently after the age of 40. It is rarely seen in infants, but is not uncommon in older children (predominantly females) in the presence of rheumatic fever or hyperthyroidism. Its incidence later in life is higher in males. Both paroxysmal and the established forms are encountered.

ETIOLOGY

Predisposing Factors. Atrial fibrillation is almost always observed in the presence of myocardial disease, especially the advanced forms. It occurs in about 60 per cent of patients with heart failure. The etiologic factors, however, depend upon the group that is sampled. In a general hospital, rheumatic, atherosclerotic, or hypertensive heart disease constitute the most common etiologies encountered. Much less commonly, there appears to be a tendency in many members of certain families to develop idiopathic atrial fibrillation without evidence of underlying heart disease.

Patients with the underlying processes noted above tend to develop transient attacks of atrial fibrillation which may later develop into the established variety. The established variety is said to be present when atrial fibrillation has been present for months or years; whereas in the paroxysmal variety, attacks occur suddenly and last a few seconds, minutes, or days. The latter type is characterized by a sudden acceleration of ventricular rate, which may range from 140 to 220 beats per minute.

Precipitating Factors. Circumstances that tend to produce both sympathetic and parasympathetic effects apparently lead to the initiation of atrial fibrillation. Precipitating factors include various stress mechanisms including the following: nausea, vomiting, acute gastroenteritis, coughing, heavy ingestion of alcohol, hypoglycemia (spontaneous or post-insulin), severe pain or emotional upset, and, on occasion, digitalis administration. Other less commonly encountered initiating factors include generalized infections, acute exacerbations of carditis, violent exertion, head or chest trauma, subarachnoid hemorrhage, acute coronary occlusion, hyperthyroidism, surgical procedures, electrolyte disturbances, and sympathomimetic drugs.

PATHOLOGY AND PATHOPHYSIOLOGY

The pathology associated with atrial fibrillation is that of the associated disease state. Hearts of patients with atrial fibrillation often show myocardial changes secondary to hypertension and/or coronary arteriosclerosis. In the acute and subacute stages of rheumatic heart disease, the atria show dilatation with a more or less intense grade of inflammatory change which later progresses to fibrosis.

No consistent pathology in the S-A node or atria of hearts with atrial fibrillation is found that could account for the occurrence of the ectopic rhythm. Hudson (1960), however, reported a series of 14 cases in which he was able to correlate the pathologic findings in the S-A node with a clinical history of atrial fibrillation. However, in most of these cases, disease of the atrial muscle was also present. The degree of atrial pathology correlates well with the incidence of atrial fibrillation; this may be the essential factor in the development of this arrhythmia. In patients with mitral stenosis whose atria are essentially normal only rarely does atrial fibrillation occur. However, moderate to severe fibrosis with disruption of atrial architecture almost always results in fibrillation. On the other hand, the incidence of atrial fibrillation does not correlate as well with the degree of mitral valvular damage nor the degree of pulmonary hypertension.

Moreover, patients with prolonged atrial fibrillation frequently manifest an inability to resume normal sinus rhythm following correction of the valvular lesion and attempted conversion; this is probably related to the degree of pathology of the atrium and possibly of the S-A node. Instead of a normal mechanism, chaotic atrial activity is observed, characterized by changing P wave contour, bradycardia, ectopic beats, and runs of atrial and junctional tachycardia. This occurs in 5 per cent of patients with atrial fibrillation of less than one year's duration, and in 45 per cent of patients with the arrhythmia for more than ten years (Lown et al., 1967).

In patients with previous rheumatic activity, Aschoff bodies are frequently present in the left atrial appendage, even in the absence of clinical evidence of active rheumatic disease. In the hearts of patients with atrial fibrillation secondary to hypertensive arteriosclerotic heart disease, there is no definite histologic evidence of a focal change responsible for this arrhythmia. However, distention of the atria, especially the left, is usually found. In patients with atrial fibrillation following myocardial infarction, occlusion of the sinus node artery causing infarction of the S-A node and atrial muscle has been demonstrated. In cases of chaotic atrial activity, coronary atherosclerosis,

ELECTROPHYSIOLOGY

A variety of abnormal mechanisms of impulse formation are operative in atrial fibrillation including oscillatory afterpotentials and alternations in the diastolic resting potential. Automaticity not normally observed in undifferentiated myocardial cells may be seen. These mechanisms may underlie multiple, rapidly firing ectopic foci.

In addition, markedly inhomogenous conduction in atrial tissue taken at surgery from human subjects with atrial fibrillation has been observed. These electrophysiologic abnormalities may cause atrial fibrillation by two mechanisms: (1) rapid ectopic impulse formation, and (2) widespread conduction abnormalities, which give rise to micro-entry circuits (Horan and Kistler, 1961).

HEMODYNAMICS

Atrial fibrillation is associated with marked hemodynamic alterations that contribute to the symptoms and signs observed in this arrhythmia. The hemodynamic consequences of atrial fibrillation result from: (1) failure of the atria to contract; (2) the irregular ventricular rhythm; (3) the short cycle length incident to exercise or emotion; (4) the presence of myocardial changes in rheumatic, arteriosclerotic, or hypertensive heart disease; and (5) associated valvular lesions (i.e., mitral stenosis and insufficiency as an isolated lesion, aortic stenosis or insufficiency, or tricuspid valvular disease).

Ventricular Function. In patients with mitral stenosis and atrial fibrillation, the Starling principle operates on a beat-to-beat basis, and the end-diastolic segment length and diastolic pressure, which are directly related to the length of the cardiac cycle, are the major determinants of the characteristics of the subsequent ventricular contraction, i.e., dP/dt, ejection time (Braunwald et al., 1960). However, the relationship of the preceding cycle length to the stroke volume is not as simple as had been thought. In fact, the influence of a particular change in frequency of contraction on the relationship between cycle length and myocardial contractility appears to extend with diminishing intensity over subsequent cycles. Therefore, the stroke volume of any individual cardiac cycle is altered not only by the cycle immediately preceding it, but in fact by several cycles preceding it.

Cardiac Output. The cardiac output in subjects with atrial fibrillation depends upon many factors. Of considerable importance is the presence or absence of mitral stenosis or other valvular lesions, and the degree of involvement of the heart. However, it may be difficult to determine the extent to which hemodynamic alterations are caused by the arrhythmia in comparison to the underlying disease process. Atrial fibrillation per se may affect the circulation in two ways: (1) by reducing the ventricular filling during diastole because of the absence of atrial contraction, and (2) by the variation in the length of diastole and the frequent occurrence of ineffective ventricular contractions following short cycles. Both of these factors are exaggerated in the presence of rapid ventricular rates and minimized by slow rates. Coronary blood flow is reduced in atrial fibrillation as a result of low cardiac output and the decreased diastolic period. The most marked reduction appears, therefore, with more rapid ventricular rates.

In addition, the cardiac output is usually diminished in mitral stenosis, particularly in the "tight" variety, even with normal sinus rhythm. The increased ventricular rate associated with atrial fibrillation is particularly deleterious in mitral stenosis, because at high rates the diastole is abbreviated, resulting in a subsequent decrease in ventricular filling, which has already been compromised both by the absence of atrial systole and by valvular stenosis.

Atrial fibrillation *per se* results in varying degrees of relative mitral insufficiency, which may be chiefly responsible for the alterations in the arterial pressure pulse contour observed in this arrhythmia.

The response to exercise, as measured by cardiac output and other parameters of cardiac function is impaired during atrial fibrillation. This is due to an abnormally great increase in heart rate in response to physical effort. In addition, this increase in rate exacerbates the other deleterious effects of atrial fibrillation. In such patients, the increase in the cardiac index that occurs in response to exercise is subnormal and is elicited solely by the increased cardiac rate, since the stroke index is relatively fixed.

Hemodynamic Alterations on Reversion to Normal Sinus Rhythm. A large number of studies have been performed to assess the hemodynamic effects of reversion from atrial fibrillation. The reported results suggest that conversion leads to little immediate benefit, but when cardiac output is measured after a delay of hours or days, it is usually increased. The sequence of hemodynamic improvement following conversion is: (a) at three minutes, cardiac output is unchanged, but the heart rate is decreased slightly; (b) after three hours the increase in cardiac output is still not significant, but the decrease in heart rate and the increase in stroke volume are both significant; and (c) after three days, the cardiac output increases (e.g., 5.1 to 6.5 L.) ($p < 0.01$), as does the stroke volume (59 to 93 ml.), and the heart rate decreases from 88 to 70 beats per minute (see Chapter 38).

The hemodynamic response to exercise is also markedly improved following conversion. The following changes after reversion were found to be significant: (a) cardiac output—up 8 per cent; (b) stroke volume—up 30 per cent (c) heart rate—down 24 per cent; (d) arterial pressure—down 8 per cent; (e) peripheral resistance—down 16 per cent; and (f) the time-tension index—up 103 per cent (Benchimol et al., 1965). Clearly, the efficiency of circulatory adaptations to exercise are markedly improved following conversion to normal sinus rhythm.

This delayed return of atrial function has not been investigated in relation to the duration of the arrhythmia, the characteristics of the fibrillatory state, or the underlying pathology. The finding that no hemodynamic benefit results from reversion to normal sinus rhythm in patients classified as "benign fibrillators" (Killip and Baer, 1964) suggests the probable importance of the underlying pathologic state as a cause of the clinical manifestations.

In summary, the benefit of reversion in increasing cardiac output depends on a number of factors: (1) If conversion lowers a rapid ventricular rate to the normal range, the cardiac output will increase. (2) Subjects who have a severe grade of clinical heart disease may benefit more than those with mild grades of organic impairment in whom the heart is relatively well compensated. (3) The return of normal atrial function does not improve hemodynamics immediately, and the full benefit may be realized over a period of several weeks. (4) The maximal cardiac output attainable during exercise may be increased to a greater extent than cardiac output at rest. (5) An improved psychological state and concurrent treatment of associated disorders, such as congestive heart failure, may result in additional improvement in hemodynamics.

SYMPTOMS AND SIGNS

Relation Between the Ventricular Rate and Clinical Manifestations. The clinical manifestations of atrial fibrillation depend largely on two factors: (1) the ventricular rate, and (2) the previous cardiac status. In the average untreated case, the ventricular rate ranges from 110 to 150 per minute. Occasionally, the rate may rise to 160 or even to 200 per minute. Such high rates in older patients with coronary arteriosclerosis may precipitate an attack of severe heart failure and are frequently accompanied by a picture of shock. The symptoms are more marked with a rapid rate in association with mitral stenosis.

On the other hand, one may encounter instances of atrial fibrillation in which the ventricular rate, without digitalis therapy, ranges from 40 to 80 per minute. These instances are usually observed in older patients and are associated with coronary arteriosclerosis and sclerotic changes in the A-V junction.

Syncopal Attacks. Various investigators have observed increased sensitivity to carotid sinus pressure in most patients with atrial fibrillation. The factors that are operative in these cases are: (1) increased parasympathetic activity in the older age group; (2) further increase of the parasympathetic effect with digitalis therapy; (3) the hypoxic state, which affects the central nervous system and which often accompanies mitral or aortic stenosis, enhances parasympathetic effects; and (4) in the presence of mitral stenosis, decreased ventricular filling results in a state of cerebral hypoxia, which by itself, tends to produce syncopal attacks (see Chapter 19, p. 239).

Cardiac Enlargement. Whether or not there is cardiac enlargement depends upon the underlying cardiac lesion, the duration of the fibrillation, and the presence or absence of heart failure. Since atrial fibrillation usually occurs in the presence of pre-existing disease, the heart may already be enlarged due to hypertension or coronary arteriosclerosis. The heart may not be enlarged in the paroxysmal variety, with pure mitral stenosis, in hyperthyroidism, or in instances when atrial fibrillation occurs in so-called "normal" hearts.

Heart Failure. Varying degrees of congestive failure frequently occur with atrial fibrillation, and hepatic congestion is often present. Even when the ventricular rate is fairly well controlled by digitalis, there is usually evidence of dyspnea, breathlessness, and easy fatigability. In the apparently well-compensated patient, the cardiac reserve is rather poor since congestive phenomena readily develop after periods of unusual exertion, excitement, or upper respiratory infection.

Auscultatory Findings. Auscultation reveals a characteristic type of irregularity. This is most pronounced with rates ranging from 90 to 130 per minute. When the ventricular rate is slow or very rapid, the typical type of irregularity is difficult to recognize clinically. At fairly rapid rates during a short cardiac cycle, the ventricular contraction often fails to lift the aortic valve. As a result, only one heart sound is heard and the ventricular contraction is too weak to produce a pulse at the wrist.

Atrial fibrillation must be differentiated from the irregular rhythm of frequent premature beats. This can be done by observing that the long pauses heard frequently with premature beats usually follow a short cycle, while in atrial fibrillation, long pauses may occur which are not associated with such distinct variations. With exercise, premature beats are usually abolished, while in atrial fibrillation, the irregularity frequently becomes more marked.

During atrial fibrillation the phonocardiogram demonstrates a changing intensity of the first heart sound which results from variations in the position of the mitral valve cusps at the time of ventricular systole. If there is a long period of diastole, the blood filling the ventricle will float the valve cusps upwards until they are very nearly closed, and ventricular systole will merely complete the closure, giving a diminished first heart sound. On the other hand, if there is a short cycle, the cusps will be almost wide open and a loud first sound will result.

Systolic murmurs that were audible during normal rhythm are usually preserved during fibrillation. They vary considerably in intensity, depending directly upon the length of the preceding cycle and the consequent variation in ventricular filling—they are louder following the longer cycles and fainter after the shorter cycles. With rapid rates, the murmurs often become inaudible. With the onset of atrial fibrillation and the failure of the atria to contract, the presystolic murmur of mitral stenosis observed with a sinus rhythm disappears; only a diastolic rumble is heard. Its intensity and the phase of diastole when it is heard vary with the cycle length.

Atrial Sounds in Flutter-Fibrillation. Recently, several cases of flutter-fibrillation with audible atrial sounds have been documented (Neporent and da Silva, 1967). In these patients a soft tapping sound was heard at the third left intercostal space parasternally in addition to the usual heart sounds. When a phonocardiogram was obtained at this location, the sounds were shown to be synchronous with atrial contraction. The venous pulse presents no distinct "a" waves, and the peak of the curve occurs during the time interval of ventricular systole. This curve is termed the "ventricular form" of the venous pulse.

Paroxysmal Atrial Fibrillation. The clinical manifestations of paroxysmal atrial fibrillation relate to (a) the sudden onset of the arrhythmia, (b) the elevated ventricular rate, and (c) the previous cardiac status of the patient. The sudden onset results in an abrupt change in cardiovascular dynamics and is frequently accompanied by a marked sense of anxiety, palpitation, shortness of breath, and often precordial discomfort or pain. In patients with myocardial disease, this may precipitate a shock-like state. In such instances, it is mandatory to slow the ventricular rate as rapidly as possible and yet avoid toxic drug effects. On the other hand, in the presence of a relatively normal heart, the symptoms of paroxysmal atrial fibrillation may be relatively slight.

ELECTROCARDIOGRAM

The electrocardiographic manifestations may be divided into: (a) the atrial deflections, and (b) the ventricular deflections.

Atrial Deflections. The atrial oscillations during fibrillation (400 to 700 per minute) are much more rapid than in flutter. The distance between waves is irregular and they vary in size and shape. Sometimes the oscillations are visible in all limb leads, but they are usually more marked in Leads II, III, and aVF. However, they are best seen from surface chest leads, either V_1 or locations on the right precordium, V_3R, or V_4R (Fig. 7–1).

When using Lead I, with the right arm electrode placed over the manubrium of the sternum and with the left arm electrode placed parasternally in the fifth intercostal space, various types of atrial oscillation can be more readily distinguished. This bipolar lead, termed S_5, is influenced mainly by proximity potentials that originate in the atrium.

Esophageal leads taken at atrial levels show rather regular oscillations which resemble those of atrial flutter

ATRIAL FIBRILLATION

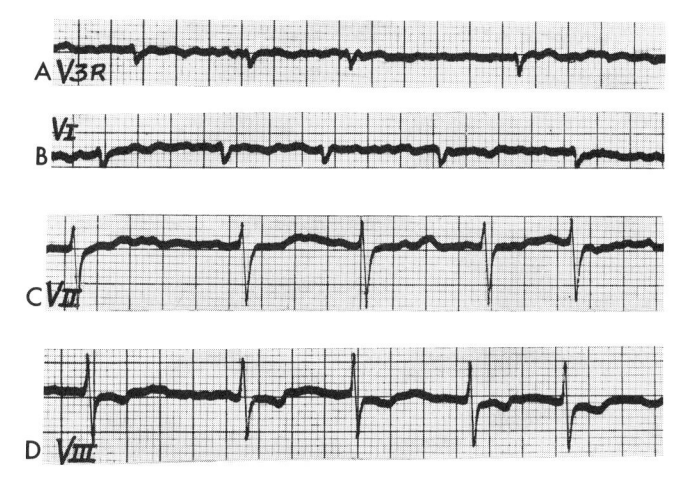

Figure 7-1. Atrial fibrillation showing more marked atrial oscillations in leads from the right side of the precordium. Note that the atrial oscillations are more clearly delineated in the leads V$_3$R and V$_1$ (taken from the right side of the precordium). They are less clearly shown in V$_2$ and V$_3$ and in leads taken from the left side of the precordium.

in the limb leads, but which have a rate that usually ranges from 300 to 350 per minute (Fig. 7-2). Doppler ultrasound tracings and intra-atrial leads may also be used in studying atrial fibrillation (see Fig. 7-3).

The P waves preceding the onset and following the termination of atrial fibrillation may show an increased amplitude or bizarre configurations due to atrial disease and the effects of certain drugs, particularly quinidine.

The P-R interval is often prolonged prior to the onset and following termination of atrial fibrillation. This may be a digitalis effect, but it is also seen in the absence of preceding digitalis therapy. The presence of a prolonged P-R interval apparently increases the susceptibility to the development of atrial fibrillation.

Ventricular Deflections. When the ventricular rate is extremely rapid (140 or more per minute), various degrees of aberration of the QRS complex may occur (simulating bundle branch block); these are probably the result of relative prolongation of the refractory period of the bundle branches, especially the right bundle branch, incident to the high rate. In such cases, the intraventricular conduction time often returns to normal following reduction of the ventricular rate (70 to 100 per minute) (Figs. 7-4, 7-5).

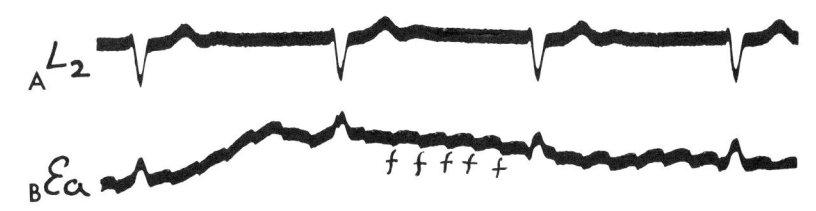

Figure 7-2. The value of esophageal leads in the diagnosis of the atrial mechanism.

(A) Lead II shows a regular ventricular rhythm with a rate of 40 per minute. The atrial mechanism is not clearly shown in this strip. The following possibilities were considered: mid A-V junctional rhythm with hidden P waves, atrial standstill, atrial fibrillation or atrial flutter with a complete A-V heart block.

(B) An esophageal lead taken simultaneously with A shows the characteristic oscillations of atrial fibrillation.

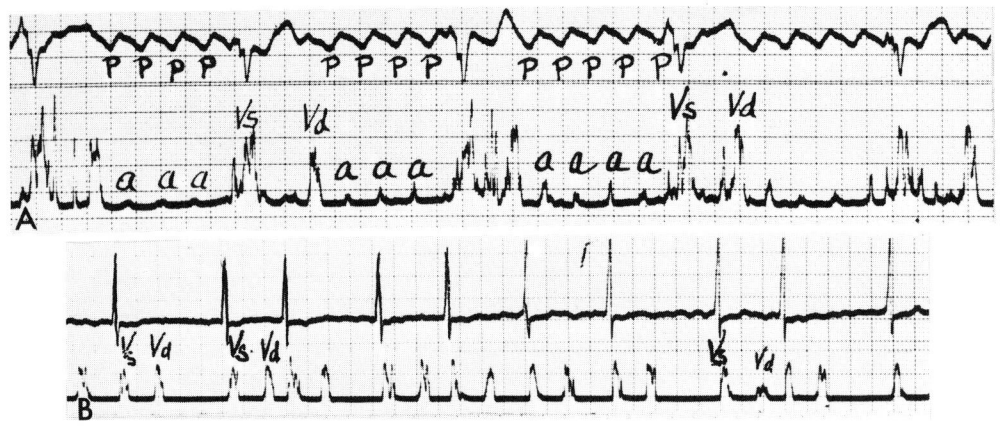

Figure 7-3. (A) Atrial flutter. Tracings from a 70-year-old male with arteriosclerotic heart disease and congestive failure. The distance between the thick time lines represents 0.2 second. The "a" wave on the Doppler tracing corresponds to the P waves of the electrocardiogram. Components "v_s" and "v_d" are also recognized.

(B) Atrial fibrillation. Tracings from patients with hypertensive and arteriosclerotic heart disease and congestive failure. The Doppler tracing consists of deflections "v_s" and "v_d" only. The atrial component ("a") is absent.

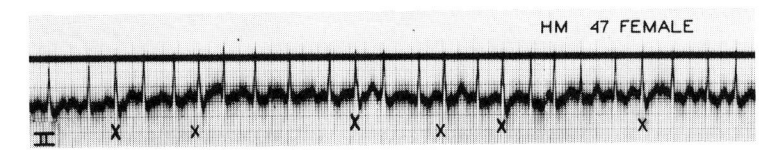

Figure 7-4. Atrial fibrillation with rapid ventricular response (rate 150 per minute) during cardiac catheterization. Note aberrant QRS complexes (at X) terminating the shortest cycles; they represent conducted beats.

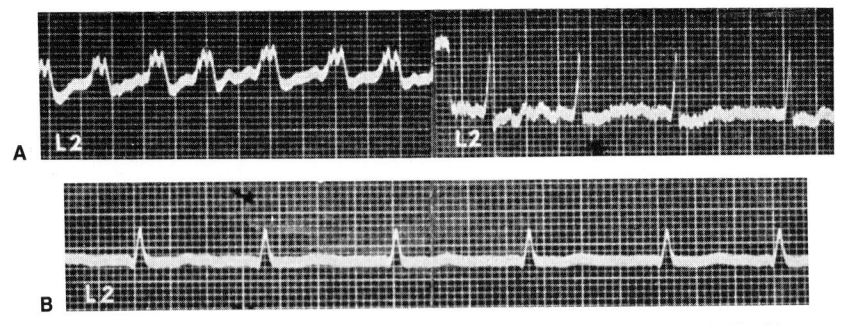

Figure 7-5. Widening of ventricular complexes in association with atrial fibrillation at a rapid ventricular rate. Lead II shows atrial fibrillation with widening of the QRS complexes, with a ventricular rate of 160 per minute. In the second part of A, after digitalization, when the ventricular rate had dropped to 80 per minute, the width of the QRS complexes has returned to normal.

(B) Atrial fibrillation with an almost regular ventricular rhythm. (From Bellet, S., and McMillan, T. M.: *In* Stroud, W. D., and Stroud, M. W. (eds.): Cardiovascular Diseases. Philadelphia, F. A. Davis Co., 1959.)

ATRIAL FIBRILLATION

Figure 7-6. Atrial fibrillation wih varying degrees of A-V heart block.
(A) Atrial fibrillation with rapid ventricular rate, 160 per minute.
(B) Atrial fibrillation with ventricular rate (about 84 per minute), controlled by digitalis.
(C) Atrial fibrillation with probable complete A-V heart block. Note the regular ventricular rate, 38 per minute.
(D) Atrial fibrillation with a slow ventricular rate and coupled ventricular premature beats due to toxic digitalis effect.

The occurrence of conduction block at various levels in the A-V junction can best be explained on the basis of concealed conduction. Following a conducted impulse, the next one reaches the N region during its absolute refractory period and is blocked. Subsequent impulses are blocked upon reaching refractory tissue that is located progressively closer to the atria. Meanwhile, the N region has recovered its excitability. After several impulses have been blocked, one arrives when none of the junctional tissue is refractory, and it is propagated to the ventricles. Thus, in established atrial fibrillation, block occurs primarily between the A-N and N regions.

Other Arrhythmias Associated with Atrial Fibrillation. Atrial fibrillation is often associated with other arrhythmias. Partial A-V heart block is almost always present with atrial fibrillation, although the degree of block usually varies (Fig. 7-6). Complete A-V heart block is occasionally encountered. It may occur as a result of sclerotic changes in the A-V junction and is most often observed in the older age group. Most cases of atrial fibrillation with a slow ventricular rate (40 to 50 beats per minute), however, are due to a high grade of partial A-V heart block and not to complete A-V heart block (see Fig. 7-7). Exercise, the administration of atropine, or sympathomimetic agents usually appreciably increase the ventricular rate in the former group, but they have little effect in the presence of true complete A-V heart block.

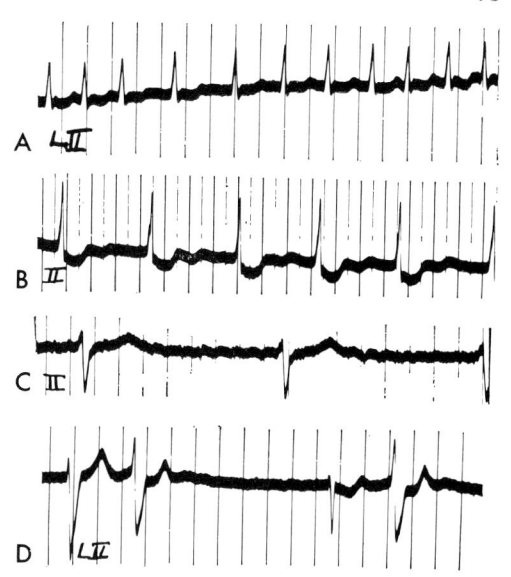

A-V junctional rhythm may be present with atrial fibrillation and may indicate digitalis toxicity or other serious complications. In A-V junctional rhythm, the ventricles are no longer excited by the irregular rhythm from the fibrillating atria but are controlled by a pacemaker in the A-V junction. This diagnosis may be assumed when the ventricular rate is slow and successive R-R intervals are found to be of equal duration; however, the diagnosis may be very difficult to establish due to the absence of P waves and F-R interval characteristics.

Ventricular premature beats are commonly associated with atrial fibrillation occurring occasionally or frequently, coupled or in groups of three or more. Many of these complexes represent the configuration of right bundle branch block suggesting aberrant beats (Fig. 7-8).

74   ATRIAL FIBRILLATION

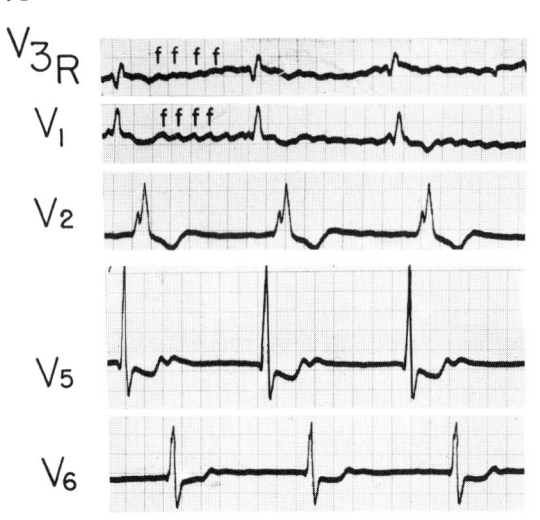

Figure 7-7. Complete A-V heart block with atrial fibrillation. Note the presence of a regular rhythm, rate 40 per minute. The ventricular rate was not altered by moderate exercise or atropine.

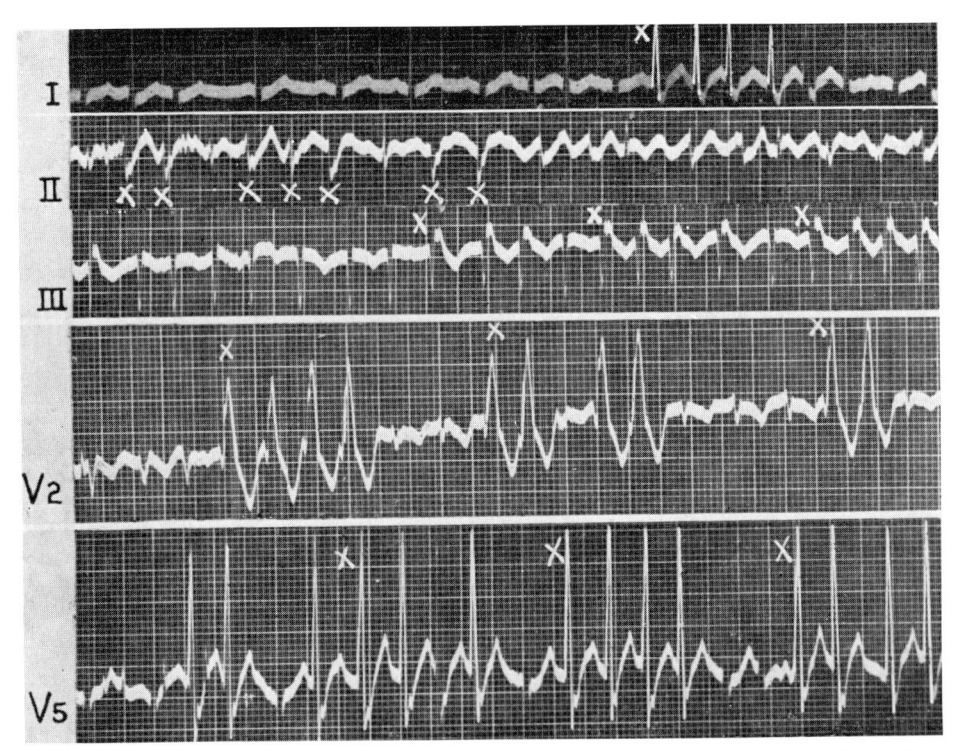

Figure 7-8. Atrial fibrillation accompanied by aberration of the QRS complexes due to delay in the right bundle branch system. These complexes often simulate ventricular beats and ventricular tachycardia. Note the aberration of the ventricular complexes starting at X in lead I. The first beat of the aberrant series is usually following a short pause. The complexes measure 0.10 of a second in width and simulate those of right bundle branch block. Similar episodes are observed at X in leads II, III, V_2, and V_5 (QRS width 0.12 second). Note that the QRS complexes throughout conform to the pattern observed in right bundle branch block.

In a digitalized patient, when the ventricular rate becomes completely and persistently regular in the presence of atrial fibrillation, the following possibilities should be considered: (1) with rapid rates—A-V junctional tachycardia and paroxysmal or nonparoxysmal ventricular tachycardia; (2) with slow rates (40 to 50 beats per minute) —A-V junctional rhythm, A-V junctional tachycardia with exit block, and higher grades of A-V heart block; and (3) with very slow rates (30 to 40 beats per minute)—complete A-V heart block with a pacemaker located in the lower portion of the A-V junction or the His-Purkinje system, depending on the QRS morphology.

The following types of alterations in rhythm in the presence of chronic atrial fibrillation have been observed: (1) conversion of fibrillation to atrial flutter in the absence of quinidine medication; (2) paroxysmal atrial tachycardia with A-V block—these are in most cases due to digitalis; and (3) bidirectional tachycardia.

DIAGNOSIS AND DIFFERENTIAL DIAGNOSIS

Atrial fibrillation may be suspected clinically in patients manifesting an irregular irregularity of cardiac rhythm. It is particularly likely to occur in the presence of myocardial disease, often of an advanced degree and in association with the etiologies mentioned previously. The characteristic symptoms and signs have been discussed. On auscultation, atrial fibrillation must be differentiated from multiple premature beats arising from different foci, atrial flutter associated with varying degrees of A-V heart block, and any type of A-V heart block with an irregular response. In these conditions, exercise may diminish the irregularity, whereas in atrial fibrillation, the rhythm tends to become even more irregular. The electrocardiogram usually establishes the diagnosis.

TREATMENT

Before attempting to treat the atrial fibrillation, one should obtain the following data: (a) the underlying etiology—arteriosclerotic (most common), hypertensive, rheumatic, or thyroid heart disease, etc.; (b) the presence of associated cardiac pathology (i.e., cardiomegaly, valvular lesions); (c) the type of atrial fibrillation, established or paroxysmal form; and (d) the presence or absence of heart failure. In addition to the arrhythmia, treatment should also be directed toward the etiologic and associated factors mentioned previously. The principles of treatment consist of (1) control of the ventricular rate, which is best accomplished by the administration of digitalis; (2) treatment of the congestive failure, which is often present; (3) reversion to normal sinus rhythm in selected cases. Two principal methods are available to obtain reversion: (1) quinidine and (2) electric countershock. These modalities are discussed below.

Drug Therapy

Digitalis. Digitalis is the drug of choice in the treatment of atrial fibrillation. In addition to its efficacy in the therapy of heart failure by its inotropic effect, digitalis slows A-V conduction and thus reduces the ventricular rate. This is accomplished in two ways: (1) by a direct effect on the A-V junction, and (2) by an indirect vagal effect on the A-V junction (see p. 375). The maximal therapeutic effect with respect to the heart rate in atrial fibrillation is said to be obtained when the apical rate drops to about 70 per minute with the elimination of the pulse deficit. Digitalization should be performed rapidly in patients with severe grades of heart failure or a rapid ventricular rate. It may be accomplished gradually in those patients in whom the indications for therapy are not urgent. Caution should be observed in the presence of a rapid, almost regular rate, e.g., a junctional tachycardia or other type of ectopic tachycardia, which may be due to toxic digitalis effects. In such cases digitalis medication increases the toxic effect; omission of this drug tends to abolish it.

The approximate oral digitalizing dose required for a 150-pound person is about 1.2 gm. (18 gr.) of the powdered or whole leaf variety, 1.2 mg. of digitoxin, 2 to 5 mg. of digoxin, or 5 to 10 mg. of lanatoside C (Cedilanid). This dose may be given over a period of four to five days when slow digitalization is desired. When the patient presents a picture of severe congestive failure necessitating rapid digitalization and certainty of absorption, the parenteral route is indicated. Strophanthin, 0.6 mg. ($1/100$ gr.), may be given intravenously, followed in two to three hours by 0.3 mg. ($1/200$ gr.). This dose may be repeated, if necessary, in about six hours.

Others prefer to use lanatoside C (total digitalizing dose, 1.6 mg.) intravenously for rapid digitalization. This should preferably be given in three or four divided doses, several hours apart. The effects of the preceding dose should be carefully noted, preferably by an ECG, before giving additional digitalis.

It should be emphasized that an apical rate of 60 to 70 beats per minute does not necessarily mean that the maximal degree of clinical improvement of congestive heart failure has been achieved. Frequently, peripheral edema and other signs of heart failure may be present even at these reduced rates, and additional digitalis, administered with caution, may be helpful. Digitalis is usually contraindicated in patients with slow ventricular rates (below 50 beats per minute, independent of therapy). In such cases, any further slowing of the ventricular rate may be harmful, inasmuch as the maintenance of the cardiac output at low rates depends upon an increase in stroke volume. This entails further stretching of the myocardial fibers, which may be inadvisable in patients with advanced myocardial disease. In these patients, diuretic therapy often helps in the therapy of the heart failure.

Use of the artificial pacemaker in patients with slow rates offers the following advantages: (1) it prevents excessive slowing of the ventricular rate and the resultant predisposition to syncopal attacks and/or heart failure; and (2) it allows the administration of the full therapeutic dose of digitalis without fear of excessive slowing of the heart rate (Fig. 37–6).

Occasionally, digitalis, even in adequate doses, fails to control the ventricular rate in some patients. Fortunately, such cases are relatively uncommon, but when they occur, the presence of one or more of the following should be suspected: (a) pulmonary embolism (single or multiple), (b) cor pulmonale of severe grade, (c) toxic factors, (d) hypopotassemia; (e) hyperthyroidism, or (f) anemia.

The manifestations of digitalis toxicity in the therapy of atrial fibrillation are qualitatively similar to those generally observed (see p. 380). These include gastrointestinal manifestations —anorexia, nausea, vomiting, and others described in detail in Chapter 34. It should be emphasized that the cardiotoxic effects noted below may occur without these effects. Certain evidences of cardiotoxicity are peculiar to the use of digitalis in atrial fibrillation. The following alterations in the cardiac mechanism may be observed: (1) development of a slow ventricular rate, 30 to 40 per minute, due to high grades of partial or complete A-V heart block; (2) a regular rhythm at a rate of 60 to 70 per minute, due to nonparoxysmal junctional tachycardia; (3) paroxysmal junctional tachycardia at a rate of 140 to 160 per minute; or (4) coupled rhythm or groups of ventricular premature beats. A paroxysmal tachycardia may be truly ventricular in origin or bidirectional (junctional) due to aberration of half the complexes (Fig. 11–

8). The therapy of these dangerous arrhythmias requires a reduction in digitalis dosage, careful electrocardiographic monitoring, and avoidance of electrolyte imbalance. The following drugs are helpful in the treatment of digitalis toxicity: quinidine, diphenylhydantoin, propranolol, and potassium when this electrolyte has been decreased.

Propranolol. Beta blockers, such as propranolol, have proved efficacious in controlling the ventricular rate when digitalis alone has failed to do so (see p. 364). Furthermore, their use may help reduce the required digitalis dosage. They are particularly indicated where a significant anxiety factor is involved. Propranolol should be given with care and in small doses, at least initially, to avoid its negative inotropic effect, which may induce or aggravate heart failure (see p. 367).

Indications for Conversion to Normal Sinus Rhythm. The advisability of converting patients with established atrial fibrillation, particularly the group with obvious heart damage and congestive failure, to normal sinus rhythm is in many instances still a matter of controversy. For therapeutic purposes, cases of atrial fibrillation may be divided into three groups:

Group 1: Patients with recent onset of atrial fibrillation in whom the degree of cardiac damage, cardiac enlargement, and congestive failure may be absent or slight.

Group 2: Patients with a more advanced form of heart disease, moderate degrees of cardiac enlargement, slight to moderate degrees of atrial enlargement, and varying degrees of heart failure.

Group 3: Patients with severe grades of myocardial damage, cardiac enlargement, and heart failure. Of these groups, conversion is most likely to benefit patients in group 1 and, to a lesser degree, those in group 2. However, the treatment of underlying valvular disease may allow subsequent therapy to be beneficial. Patients with a severe grade of heart disease are less likely to revert to normal sinus rhythm or to sustain the reversion, but they may do so in some instances.

The subject of quinidine therapy in arrhythmias is discussed in detail on page 346. Some of the essential features as they relate to atrial fibrillation are discussed below.

Quinidine is the drug most useful in the conversion of atrial fibrillation to normal sinus rhythm, being successful in approximately 60 per cent of patients, although it may vary from 88 per cent (Phillips and Levine, 1949) to 58 per cent (Sandøe et al., 1965), depending upon the observer. However, several difficulties are encountered: hospitalization is required for a period of seven to ten days; there is a risk of quinidine toxicity (see the complete discussion in Chapter 33), and conversion is not realized in 40 per cent of the patients. Quinidine conversion has been indicated less commonly since the advent of electric countershock, which affects reversion in about 80 to 90 per cent of patients within a few minutes and is accompanied by fewer side effects. However, quinidine may still be of use to secure reversion under some circumstances and it is the drug of choice for the maintenance of normal sinus rhythm after conversion.

Several dosage schedules are available which will achieve the therapeutic plasma level of quinidine necessary (4.0–8.0 mg./L) (see page 349). Most patients who revert to normal sinus rhythm will do so with moderate doses of the drug. It must be remembered that in the presence of congestive heart failure or renal insufficiency therapeutic levels of quinidine will be reached with smaller doses of the drug. It has been suggested that reversion to normal sinus rhythm may be obtained with greater certainty and with fewer toxic effects if quinidine is used in combination with propranolol (which has a quinidine-like effect).

Propranolol, 10 to 15 mg. in three to four divided oral doses, may be given for a period of two to four days.

Although many drugs have been recommended for the purpose of converting atrial fibrillation to normal sinus rhythm, none has proved so efficacious as quinidine. Procaine amide, antazoline, potassium, diphenylhydantoin and lidocaine are relatively undependable for this purpose.

Following restoration of normal sinus rhythm, maintenance quinidine (0.2 gm., four times a day, or a long-acting preparation) (see page 351) is given for several months and continued depending upon the tendency for recurrence of atrial fibrillation. Most of the patients who revert to normal sinus rhythm have recurrences of atrial fibrillation. The incidence of recurrence varies in different series. Approximately two-thirds of patients converted to normal sinus rhythm will be back in atrial fibrillation in 12 months. The recurrences of atrial fibrillation are the result of many factors, including long duration of the arrhythmia prior to therapy, degree of myocardial damage (Bailey et al., 1968), dilatation of the heart beyond a volume of 1000 ml., and especially the presence of mitral regurgitation. The maintenance of adequate plasma levels of quinidine over long periods of time may also prove difficult.

The use of propranolol in addition to the quinidine has been efficacious in maintaining normal sinus rhythm for a more prolonged period in many instances (Stern, 1971). This may be due to the decrease in beta-adrenergic effects on the heart.

Treatment of Paroxysmal Atrial Fibrillation. The treatment of paroxysmal atrial fibrillation is a matter of some controversy. In our experience, digitalis is the drug of choice. Its administration will usually have a salutary effect, particularly in patients with pre-existing heart damage, in those in the older age group, and in the presence of congestive failure. It will slow the ventricular rate in paroxysmal atrial fibrillation as effectively as in the established form, and spontaneous reversion to normal sinus rhythm often follows. If this does not occur, other methods of conversion (quinidine and electric countershock) may then be employed. With frequently recurring, troublesome episodes which are unresponsive to drug therapy, the use of an artificial pacemaker with an inherent rate of 60 to 70 per minute with maintenance digitalis therapy has been of considerable help in preventing recurrent episodes (see Fig. 37–6).

Direct Current Countershock. Direct current cardioversion has been found to be effective in causing reversion from atrial fibrillation to normal sinus rhythm in as many as 90 per cent of patients (Aberg and Cullhed, 1968). This method, as compared to reversion by quinidine, has the advantage of a lower incidence of side effects and a briefer period of hospitalization. The indications, technique, and complications of countershock treatment of arrhythmias are discussed in Chapter 38.

The long-term efficacy of direct-current reversion has recently been reviewed (Aberg, 1969; Aberg and Cullhed, 1968; Bjerkelund and Orning, 1969; and Radford and Evans, 1968). Bjerkelund and Orning (1969) report that approximately 30 per cent of reversion last for 12 months or longer and 25 per cent last for 24 months. The problem of maintaining patients in normal rhythm is more difficult in those patients with a severe grade of heart disease, particularly mitral insufficiency. The lack of close control of quinidine plasma levels by quinidine assays compounds this problem.

Complications of Conversion. The chief complications from the use of direct-current countershock to convert atrial fibrillation to normal sinus rhythm include the following: (a) the development of ventricular arrhythmias, which may be of a severe type; (b) the occurrence in occasional instances of cardiac arrest; and (c) the precipitation of an appreciable, although low, incidence of thromboembolic phenomena. Ventricular arrhythmias are more likely to occur if the patient is digitalized at the time of conversion. This subject is discussed in detail in Chapter 38.

PROGNOSIS

The prognosis in atrial fibrillation depends upon the age of the patient, the underlying cardiac condition, the extent of cardiac enlargement or heart failure, and the ease with which the apical rate and heart failure are controlled. In general, persistent atrial fibrillation indicates the presence of a rather serious cardiac condition with impending, if not actual, heart failure. However, with therapy many patients with atrial fibrillation maintain occupations involving moderate physical strain without discomfort.

Those who are required to remain sedentary, because of severe heart damage, obviously have a poor prognosis. The outlook is usually poor in cases in which the ventricular rate is controlled with difficulty by digitalis or where large doses are required to maintain the desired ventricular rate. The sudden appearance of embolic phenomena in the young, or the aged, is usually a serious, and at times, a fatal complication.

The prognosis has been markedly improved in recent years by many advances in therapy; namely, the treatment of heart failure, maintenance of electrolyte balance, certain surgical procedures, and particularly the introduction of cardioversion. Of 290 of these patients followed either until the recurrence of their arrhythmia or for two years, nine died of possible cardiovascular causes. This is a rate of roughly one death per 50 patient years. Considering that the average patient in this series was more than 50 years old, these figures suggest that properly treated atrial fibrillation may reduce life expectancy only moderately in patients without severe organic disease.

References

Aberg, H.: Some aspects on atrial fibrillation. Etiology, treatment, complications, and fibrillatory waves using a new technique. Abst. of Uppsala Dissertations in Medicine, 63, 1969.

Aberg H., and Cullhed, I.: Direct current conversion of atrial fibrillation. Longterm results. Acta Med. Scand., *184:*433, 1968.

Arani, D. T., and Carleton, R. A.: The deleterious role of tachycardia in mitral stenosis. Circulation, 36:511, 1967.

Bailey, G. W. H., Braniff, B. A., Hancock, E. W., and Cohn, K. E.: Relation of left atrial pathology to atrial fibrillation in mitral valvular disease. Ann. Intern. Med., 69:13, 1968.

Bellet, S., Eliakim, M., and Deliyiannis, S.: The electrocardiogram during electro-convulsive therapy as studied by radio-electrocardiography. Amer. J. Cardiol., 25:686, 1962.

Benchimol, A., Lowe, H. M., and Akre, P. R.: Cardiovascular response to exercise during atrial fibrillation and after conversion to sinus rhythm. Amer. J. Cardiol., *16:*31, 1965.

Bjerkelund, C., and Orning, O. M.: The efficacy of anticoagulant therapy in preventing embolism related to DC electrical reversion of atrial fibrillation. Amer. J. Cardiol., 23:208, 1969.

Braunwald, E., Frye, R. L., Aygen, M. M., and Gilbert, J. W., Jr.: Studies on Starling's Law of the heart. III. Observations in patients with mitral stenosis and atrial fibrillation on the relationships between left ventricular end-diastolic segment length, filling pressure and the characteristics of ventricular contraction. J. Clin. Invest., 39:1874, 1960.

Cohen, S. I., Lau, S. H., Berkowitz, W. D., and Damato, A. N.: Concealed conduction during atrial fibrillation. Amer. J. Cardiol., 25:416, 1970.

Corliss, R. J., McKenna, D. H., Crumpton, C. W., and Rowe, G. G.: Hemodynamic effects after conversion of arrhythmias. J. Clin. Invest., 47:1774, 1968.

Friedberg, H. D.: Atrial fibrillation and digitalis toxicity. Amer. Heart J., 77:429, 1969.

Horan, L. G., and Kistler, J. C.: Study of ventricular response in atrial fibrillation. Circ. Res., 9:305, 1961.

Hornstein, T. R., and Bruce, R. A.: Effects of atrial fibrillation on exercise performance in patients with cardiac disease. Circulation, 37:543, 1968.

Hudson, R.: The human pacemaker and its pathology. Brit. Med. J., 22:153, 1960.

Kastor, J. A., and Yurchas, P. M.: Recognition of digitalis intoxication in the presence of atrial fibrillation. Ann. Intern. Med., 67:1045, 1967.

Katz, L. N., and Pick, A.: Clinical Electrocardiography. Part I. The Arrhythmias. Philadelphia, Lea & Febiger, 1956.

Killip, T., and Baer, R. A.: Cardiac function before and after electrical reversion from atrial fibrillation to sinus rhythm. Clin. Res., 12:175, 1964.

Killip, T., and Gault, J. H.: Mode of onset of atrial fibrillation. Amer. Heart J., 70:172, 1965.

Lau, S. H., Damato, A. N., Berkowitz, W. D., and Patton, R. D.: A study of atrioventricular conduction in atrial fibrillation and flutter in man using His bundle recordings. Circulation, 40:71, 1969.

Lown, B., Vassaux, C., Hood, W. B., Jr., Fakhro, A. M., Kaplinsky, E., and Roberge, G.: Unresolved problems in coronary care. Amer. J. Cardiol., 20:494, 1967.

Neporent, L. M., and da Silva, J. A.: Heart sounds in atrial flutter-fibrillation. Amer. J. Cardiol., 19:301, 1967.

Phillips, E., and Levine, S. A.: Auricular fibrillation without other evidence of heart disease. Amer. J. Med., 7:478, 1949.

Radford, M. D., and Evans, D. W.: Long-term results of DC reversion of atrial flutter. Brit. Heart J., 30:91, 1968.

Sandøe, E., Hansen, P. F., Aufred, E., and Oleson, K. H.: Defibrilling av Kronisk Atrieflimren. Resultater og Komplikationer. Ugeskr. Laeg., 127:346, 1965.

Shapiro, W., and Klein, G.: Alterations in cardiac function immediately following electrical conversion of atrial fibrillation to normal sinus rhythm. Circulation, 38:1074, 1968.

Singer, D. H., Harris, P. D., Malin, J. R., and Hoffman, B. F.: Electrophysiological basis of chronic atrial fibrillation. Circulation, 35-36:II-239, 1967.

Stern, S.: Treatment and prevention of cardiac arrhythmias with propranolol and quinidine. Brit. Heart J., 33:522, 1971.

Chapter 8 *Premature Beats*

GENERAL CONSIDERATIONS
INCIDENCE
ETIOLOGY
MECHANISMS PRODUCING PREMATURE BEATS
  Re-entry
  Ectopic Foci
  Parasystole
  Supernormal Recovery of Excitability
EXIT BLOCK
HEMODYNAMICS
  Postextrasystolic Potentiation
  Frequency of Premature Beats
  Effect on Coronary Blood Flow
  Regional Blood Flow
SYMPTOMS AND SIGNS
  Gallops and Murmurs
  Postextrasystolic Auscultatory Effects
ELECTROCARDIOGRAM
  Diagnosis
  Clinical Significance
PREMATURE BEATS WITH COMPLETE A-V HEART BLOCK
PREMATURE BEATS INITIATING ATRIAL FIBRILLATION
TREATMENT
  The Symptomatic Patient
PROGNOSIS
ATRIAL PREMATURE BEATS
  General Considerations
  Etiology
  Pathology
  Mechanism
  Hemodynamics
  Electrocardiogram
  Treatment
  Prognosis
A-V JUNCTIONAL PREMATURE BEATS
VENTRICULAR PREMATURE BEATS
  Electrocardiogram
  Treatment
    The Symptomatic Patient
  Prognosis

GENERAL CONSIDERATIONS

Premature beats are the most common of the arrhythmias. They may be a normal finding, but they may also be the initial evidence of cardiac abnormality. Consciousness of their presence is often the reason for seeking medical aid.

There are several terms referring to premature beats in common usage. However, none is the ideal descriptive term for all situations. "Extrasystole," for example, implies an extra or additional beat and should only be applied to interpolated beats where an extra beat actually occurs. Therefore, in this chapter, the term "premature beat" will be used in most instances; "extrasystole" will be limited to those cases (e.g., interpolated beats) associated with an actual mechanical systole; and "ectopic beats" will be applied to contractions that clearly originate from an ectopic site.

The normal rhythm consists of a regular sequence of beats which arise in the S-A node and are transmitted through the atrial conduction tracts, the A-V junction, and the His-Purkinje system to the ventricles. Each impulse is part of a rhythmic series causing activation of the myocardium in an orderly and regular sequence. Premature or ectopic beats disrupt this normal mechanism. They may arise from any of the automatic tissues of the heart; i.e., the S-A node, various sites in the atria, A-V junction, or cells of the His-Purkinje system (Fig. 8–1). Some premature beats are followed by a compensatory pause, while others are not.

Patients with this ectopic rhythm may be classified into two groups: (1) those who are unaware of the presence of ectopic beats, which are usually diagnosed on routine examination; and (2) those in whom the arrhythmia is associated with the following manifestations: palpitation, a sense of

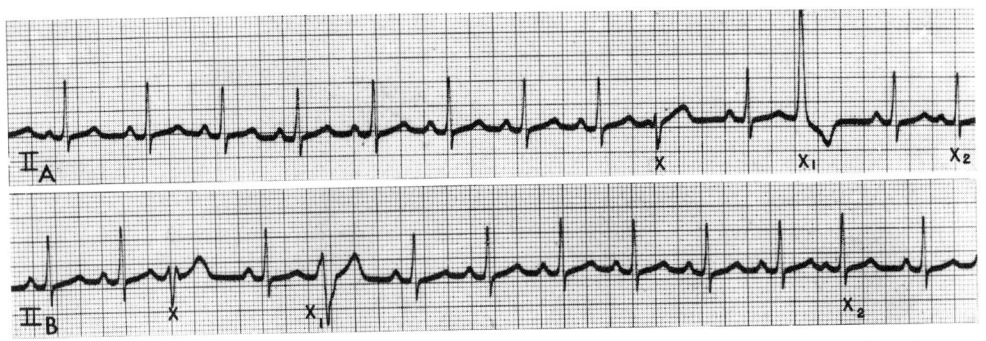

Figure 8-1. Normal sinus rhythm with premature beats of various sites of origin (atrial, junctional, and ventricular).

(A) X and X$_2$ are atrial premature beats. Note the difference in P wave configuration, the shortened P-R interval, and the similarity in QRS configuration in comparison with the other beats. X$_1$ is a premature ventricular beat; note the abnormal configuration and duration, premature onset, and fully compensatory pause.

(B) X is probably a junctional beat (with aberration of QRS) and X$_2$ is atrial; X$_1$ is probably a ventricular premature beat.

oppression in the chest, or even momentary absence of the pulse with a long postectopic pause. Consciousness of the irregularity is often the factor that initially prompts a patient to seek medical care. Since ectopic beats tend to recur over a period of years, they may be associated with or precipitate a variety of other arrhythmias, including atrial tachycardia, flutter or fibrillation, junctional tachycardia, and ventricular tachycardia. In certain instances, premature beats may initiate a tachyarrhythmia, e.g., atrial or ventricular paroxysmal tachycardia.

Premature contractions may occur as isolated beats or in clusters; they may appear infrequently, or they may be recurrent. The usual type occurs at rest and disappears upon effort or excitement; the reverse may be true in certain patients. Premature contractions may occur after each normal beat (bigeminy) (Figs. 8-2, 8-3) or in groups of two (trigeminy) or three (quadrigeminy) or in longer sequences. They may occur in a regular manner, following every second, third, or fourth beat, or they may occur irregularly. Premature beats commonly arise from a single focus but may occasionally originate from multiple foci. The width of the QRS complex may be either normal or increased, depending on the interaction of a number of factors, to be discussed later.

INCIDENCE

Although premature beats have been reported in patients of all ages, they

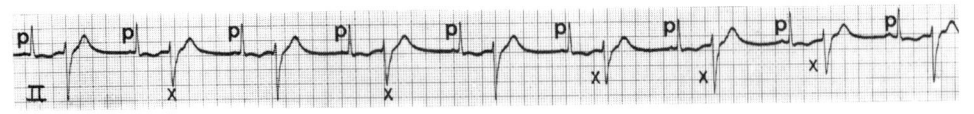

Figure 8-2. Ventricular bigeminy with electrical alternation of premature beats. The beats marked X represent ventricular premature beats and exhibit fixed coupling; i.e., the interval between the onset of the normal QRS and that of the premature beat is the same throughout the tracing (0.44 second). Note the variation in the configuration of the P waves due to a wandering pacemaker. Note that the premature contractions show electrical alternans; i.e., every other premature contraction varies in the size of the S wave as compared to the preceding premature ventricular beat (i.e., fourth X).

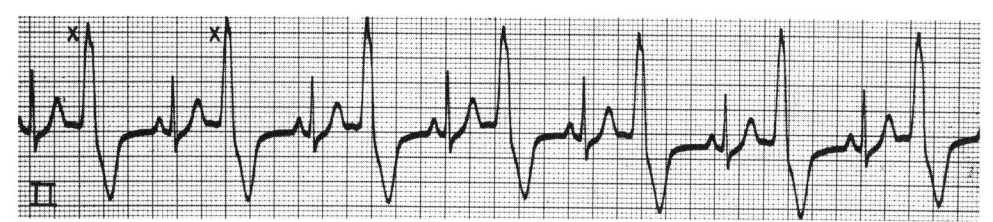

Figure 8–3. Coupled ventricular premature beats (Lead II). The presence of coupled rhythm with a fixed coupling is seen; in the absence of distinct P waves in these pauses, the distinction between fully compensatory pauses and not fully compensatory pauses is impossible.

are rare in the first decade of life; the incidence is greatest between the ages of 50 and 70. At present, data available from continuous magnetic tape and telemetric monitoring reveal that premature beats may be observed in the course of normal everyday activities in subjects with no definite evidence of heart disease, especially in the older age groups (Hinkle et al., 1969). Roughly 5 per cent of an otherwise healthy adult population can be expected to show premature beats on routine electrocardiograms (Chiang et al., 1969). However, the incidence of subsequent coronary artery disease is increased in this group.

The incidence is much higher in a hospital population. Katz and Pick (1956) recorded premature beats in 14 per cent of 50,000 consecutive patients studied by means of the electrocardiogram. Approximately one-half of these originated in the ventricle, one-third in the atria, and one-sixth in the A-V junction.

ETIOLOGY

From the standpoint of the cardiac status, subjects with premature beats may be divided into three groups: (1) those whose cardiac status is normal; (2) a borderline group in whom myocardial disease may be suspected because of age or other factors but cannot be demonstrated clinically, and whose ectopic beats may be due to functional disturbances (particularly overactive sympathetic tone); and (3) those patients with frank myocardial abnormality.

In patients with myocardial abnormality, the most important etiologic factors are: (1) *infectious disease*, especially rheumatic fever, scarlet fever, and other streptococcal infections, diphtheria, and brucellosis; (2) varying *degenerative states* (e.g., coronary artery disease, hypertension, myocardiopathy); (3) *hypoxia*, which often leads to increased myocardial irritability; and (4) *autonomic influences* which may affect premature beats in various ways. Parasympathetic stimuli may abolish, induce, or have no effect on premature beats. Vagolytic agents, however, generally abolish premature beats by increasing the heart rate.

Premature beats may be evoked by a multiplicity of other factors, e.g., (1) *reflexes arising from the gastrointestinal, biliary and genitourinary tracts, or other viscera;* (2) *disturbed psychological states* (discussed in Chapter 27); (3) *various drugs*, including digitalis, quinidine, procaine amide, potassium, sympathomimetic amines, aconitine, acetylcholine, calcium, reserpine, and certain anesthetic agents, particularly cyclopropane; (4) *alterations in certain physiologic states*, particularly alterations in pH and electrolytes, such as hypopotassemia and hypocalcemia (Davidson and Surawicz, 1967); (5) *coffee or tea* which may produce an increase in ectopic beats, due to direct cardiac effects, to electrolyte changes, and to alterations in cardiovascular reflexes; (6) *exercise* which although usually abolishing premature beats, may infrequently elicit ectopic beats in patients with normal hearts and more frequently in subjects with myocardial abnormality; (7) a *sudden increase in blood pressure* which sets into action certain factors that tend to produce premature beats—increased cardiac work and an increase in sympathetic tone and catecholamine release; (8) premature contractions are observed more frequently at *slow heart rates* than at rapid rates (Han et al., 1966).

Clinically detectable myocardial disease is observed in only a minority of the general population with premature beats; 26 of 165 (16 per cent) in one series had evidence of coronary heart disease (Chiang et al., 1969). A higher incidence of myocardial abnormality is found when patients are studied for suspected or known heart disease, as in a hospital population. Such a group may demonstrate an incidence of 75 per cent. When the QRS width of the premature beat exceeds a width of 0.16 sec., myocardial damage, often of a severe grade, is usually present.

MECHANISMS PRODUCING PREMATURE BEATS

Many concepts have been presented regarding the mechanisms that produce premature beats. The following are the important mechanisms involved in the production of premature beats.

Re-entry. The theory of re-entry is premised upon the presence in the heart muscle of one or more areas in which recovery from the refractory state is slower than elsewhere. Following a normally conducted impulse, such tissue remains refractory longer than the adjacent myocardium, so that if the next impulse arrives after a normal interval, this region is unresponsive and the impulse is conducted around the area of block. As this area belatedly becomes responsive, the impulse that initially passed by may return and excite it. This tissue, which is activated late, then serves in effect as an ectopic focus. From it the impulse proceeds throughout the heart as a premature beat, before the next sinus impulse arrives. The re-entry mechanism is particularly valuable in explaining the observed dependence of the ectopic beat on the preceding normal contraction.

A marked difference between the duration of the refractory periods of adjacent tissues occurs under certain conditions in the hearts of experimental animals and in diseased human hearts. The clinically significant circumstances under which this observation has been made include: (a) human atrial tissue characterized by generalized pathologic and electrophysiologic abnormality; (b) artificial stimulation delivered to the dog heart during the refractory period of the right but not the left bundle branch; and (c) marked bradycardia during which the variation in the duration of the refractory periods of adjacent tissue is considerably increased.

Ectopic Foci. An ectopic focus offers an attractive theoretical explanation for premature beats in several respects: (1) the key variable determining the rate of impulse formation in each case (slope of diastolic depolarization, level of resting potential, and characteristics of afterpotentials) may vary in response to virtually any factor that alters cardiac function, thus providing a basis for the frequently observed variations in the frequency, morphology, and coupling interval of ectopic beats; and (2) these variables may, on the other hand, remain relatively constant over an extended period of time. In this respect, it is similar to the normal cardiac mechanism.

Parasystole. Parasystole may be defined as a persistent and regular ectopic focus coexistent with the dominant sinus pacemaker. It may be

PREMATURE BEATS

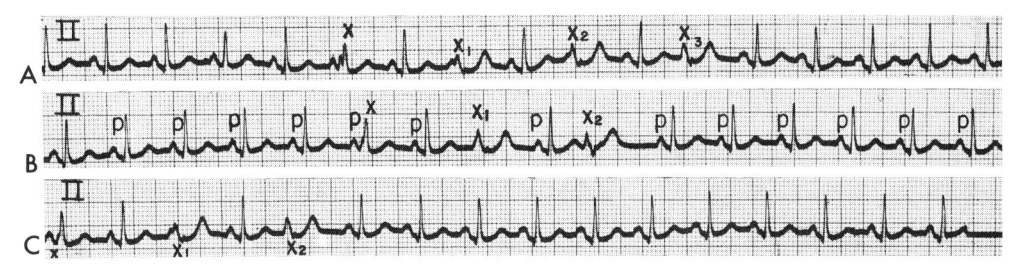

Figure 8-4. Ventricular parasystole. (*A, B,* and *C* represent a continuous strip. The intervals between the ventricular beats are identical.)

(*A*) Note the premature beats at X, X_1, X_2, and X_3.

(*B*) Note fusion beat at X indicating that the premature beats are ventricular in origin. Note also at X_2 that the P wave occurs after the QRS.

(*C*) Note the widened QRS complexes at X, X_1 and X_2. The parasystolic rhythm terminates at the end of X_2.

located in any part of the conduction system except the S-A node, but it is usually located in the deeper parts of the ventricles, rarely in the atria (Fig. 8-4). Long tracings frequently show that parasystole is initiated by a premature beat. The inherent rate of the parasystolic focus may range from 20 to 400 beats per minute. The parasystolic focus is probably constantly active for days, months, or years, and has an almost perfect rhythmicity, rarely varying more than 0.01 second. However, the focus may be only intermittently active.

Normally, the parasystolic focus is not depolarized by impulses from the dominant pacemakers that arrive at a time when discharge would be expected; this situation is described as "*entrance*" or "*protection block*" (see p. 24). Thus, the parasystolic focus may originate impulses, but impulses traversing the surrounding muscle usually do not affect it; occasionally, however, the inherent parasystolic rhythm may be disturbed by impulses from neighboring centers. The dominant pacemaker may or may not be similarly protected. Therefore, either unidirectional or mutual protection may exist. In the latter instance, the two rhythms continue to be totally independent of each other; in the former instance, this does not occur and "capture" of the unprotected pacemaker will occur at times. There is also said to be an "*exit block*," which may inhibit the conduction of the impulse from the parasystolic focus. The nature of these controversial entities is discussed later.

In a long tracing, premature beats of parasystolic origin can be seen to possess a fixed time relationship to each other, although at times beats do not occur when expected. This latter finding is due to the fact that the parasystolic beat falls during the absolute refractory period of the ventricle. However, the interval between these parasystolic beats is an exact multiple of those intervals observed between the regularly recurring beats of the ectopic center.

Attempts have been made to explain all or most coupled beats on the basis of parasystole. This concept may be difficult to disprove in cases of fixed coupling but not in those cases with varying coupling intervals. Fundamental differences exist among the various theoretical mechanisms: reentry involves a passive mode of impulse formation, dependent on the preceding beat, while parasystole represents an independent automatic rhythm. Both are probably operative.

Supernormal Recovery of Excitability. "Supernormal excitability" occurs when an individual cell or the entire heart responds to a stimulus weaker than that considered necessary for excitation during the particular phase in the cardiac cycle. Extensive investigations using artificial pacemakers have demonstrated a brief interval following stage 3 depolarization (for ventricular fibers, this occurs during the downsweep of the T wave in the electrocardiogram) when stimuli 5 to 15 per cent below ordinary threshold values may elicit a response. If stimuli of increasing strength are delivered to the ventricle at this time, one first observes a single premature beat, followed at greater stimulus intensities by a brief run of tachycardia (repetitive responses) and finally by ventricular fibrillation.

EXIT BLOCK

Exit block may be defined as failure of propagation of the impulse from an automatic center to the myocardium. By convention, the poorly understood phenomenon of sinoatrial block is excluded from this definition and the term "exit block" is applied to automatic tissue in the A-V junction and ventricles. The diagnosis of exit block may be made readily in the presence of the following electrocardiographic patterns: (1) ventricular parasystole, in which the impulses obviously fail to be conducted; (2) A-V dissociation or complete A-V heart block, in which the rate of impulse formation from a focus in the A-V junction, His-Purkinje system, or an idioventricular location abruptly doubles or halves (Pick, 1966); and (3) a sudden decrease in rate in a junctional tachycardia.

This conduction depression has been induced experimentally by hypoxia, digitalis, or infusion of potassium with resultant high plasma concentrations of this electrolyte. The occurrence of electrophysiologic evidence of a unidirectional block has been observed in association with ischemia and digitalis toxicity (Greenspan et al., 1971).

Exit block may have considerable clinical significance under certain circumstances. When a patient has been given large doses of digitalis (e.g., to slow the ventricular rate in atrial fibrillation), a slow, regular ventricular rhythm may result, with a pacemaker situated in the A-V junction controlling the ventricles. A digitalis-produced 2:1 exit block may reduce an inherent rate of 100 to 120 beats per minute to an actual ventricular rate of 50 to 60 beats per minute. While such a reduction in the ventricular rate is clearly beneficial, continued administration of digitalis entails the risk of toxicity and the production of more serious arrhythmias. Spontaneous exit block may occur in the absence of a focus of rapid impulse formation. The intersystolic interval may be prolonged to several seconds and result in cardiac standstill if a patient with complete A-V heart block and a relatively slow idioventricular pacemaker develops an exit block; this may lead to loss of consciousness and the development of Stokes-Adams syndrome.

HEMODYNAMICS

The extent of the hemodynamic disturbances depends upon the degree of prematurity, the frequency, and the site of origin of the ectopic impulses, whether in the atria or ventricles.

Postextrasystolic Potentiation. The first beat that follows the pause after a premature beat may show a contractility greater than normal, manifested by (a) a shorter period of isometric contraction and (b) an augmented stroke volume. It has traditionally been held that the degree of this potentiation is directly related to the degree of prematurity of the ectopic beat. The degree of potentiation (a) depends upon the basal frequency of impulse formation; (b) reaches a maximum at a certain interval of prematurity that is related to the basal rate and then decreases with further increases in prematurity; and (c) appears to depend upon the strength of nonpotentiated contractions.

Frequency of Premature Beats. The frequency of ectopic beats is an important factor influencing hemodynamic events. Occasional premature beats do this to only a slight degree; however, the appearance of numerous premature beats or those occurring in couples or groups will materially reduce the cardiac output. The ventricular type may reduce the stroke volume by as much as 25 per cent. Atrial premature beats occurring in couples or groups also reduce the stroke volume and systemic blood pressure, although not to as great an extent as ventricular premature beats.

Atrial premature beats may be associated with various hemodynamic effects: if one occurs very soon after the preceding atrial contraction, it prolongs *atrial repolarization* and is not propagated to the ventricles as a separate beat. The hemodynamic consequences are slight indeed. However, an impulse may occur somewhat later, cause a separate atrial contraction, and fail to be propagated to the ventricles because of refractoriness of the A-V junction. The resultant asynchrony of atrial and ventricular contraction impairs ventricular filling and tends to decrease the cardiac output. If, on the other hand, the atrial premature impulse is conducted normally, its effect will depend upon the prematurity of the beat; the diastolic period of ventricular filling is shortened and the resultant stroke volume is diminished. Such atrial premature beats reduce the stroke volume and are associated with a fall in systemic blood pressure. However, this alteration is less marked than with ventricular premature beats.

The hemodynamic effects of ventricular premature beats depend upon several factors. Most important of these is the degree of prematurity. Frequent premature beats add to the burden of the heart, and their elimination is conducive to more normal heart function. They are much less effective than normal sinus beats because, being premature, they induce contractions before the ventricles are completely filled with blood (Fig. 8–5). The energy expenditure of these beats is not decreased to the same extent as the decrease in work, and their frequent occurrence, therefore, lowers the efficiency of the heart as a pump and may contribute to the development of dyspnea and heart failure. Systemic hemodynamics are relatively less impaired by premature beats arising in the right than in the left ventricle.

Effect on Coronary Blood Flow. Coronary artery and coronary sinus blood flow depends to a considerable degree upon the systolic blood pressure, which in turn depends on the degree of prematurity of the ectopic beat.

Data obtained in dogs indicate that atrial premature beats reduce coronary blood flow by 5 per cent, whereas ventricular premature beats reduce it by 12 per cent. When premature ventricular systoles occur very frequently, a reduction of as much as 25 per cent may occur.

Recently, the instantaneous blood flow velocity has been measured in man by use of the Doppler ultrasonic flowmeter telemetry system. Ventricular premature beats and ventricular tachycardia resulted in diminished flow velocity and stroke output. This was based on decreased ventricular diastolic filling and valvular incompetence. The reduced coronary blood flow velocity contributes to the impaired ventricular performance during these arrhythmias (Benchimol and Desser, 1971; Benchimol et al., 1971).

In considering the effects upon the coronary blood flow produced by ectopic rhythm in the human subject, one should consider (a) the number, frequency, and duration of the ectopic rhythms; (b) their effect on the sys-

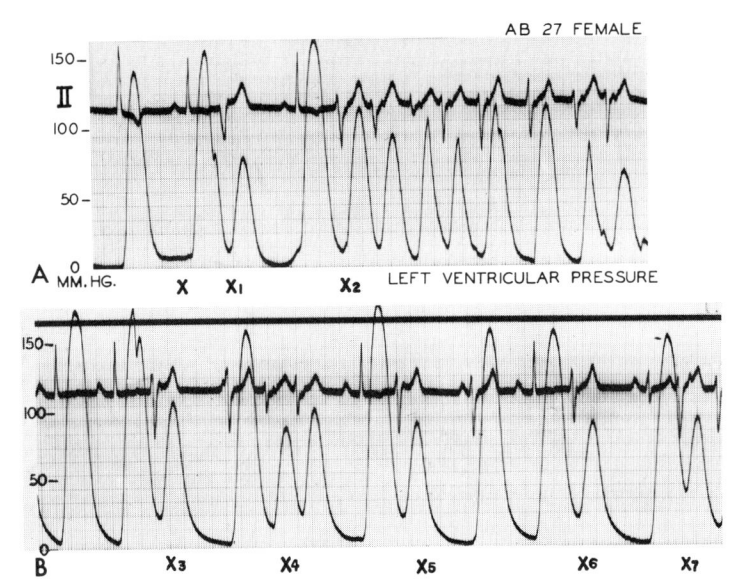

Figure 8–5. Alteration in left ventricular pressure with premature beats (27-year-old female with rheumatic heart disease and aortic stenosis; electrocardiogram recorded during Björck's procedure).

(A) With a normal sinus beat at X, the left ventricular pressure rises to 150 mm. Hg. With a ventricular premature beat at X_1, it is recorded as 80 mm. Hg. A paroxysm of ventricular premature beats at X_2 is accompanied by a marked reduction in ventricular pressure; the systolic pressure rises only to 90 mm. Hg.

(B) Two normal sinus beats at the beginning of the record are followed by a ventricular premature beat. Note the fall in height of pressure curve at X_3. Note that the systolic pressure is lower and the diastolic pressure higher with the ectopic beats at X_4, X_5, X_6, and X_7.

temic blood pressure; (c) their effect on increased stroke output during the compensatory phase; (d) the effect of altered hemodynamics in the presence of diseased coronary arteries and a diseased myocardium; (e) the increase in demand for coronary blood flow that occurs during accelerated cardiac work; and (f) the ability of the diseased coronary arteries to supply this increase in flow.

Regional Blood Flow. The cerebral blood flow is reduced by 8 to 12 per cent during premature atrial and ventricular systole. Ventricular premature systoles decrease the blood flow more than do those of atrial origin. An occasional premature beat may have no adverse effect, whereas if they are frequent, as in coupling, they may have a profound effect in reducing cerebral blood flow (Corday and Irving, 1961).

The renal blood flow is reduced by 8 to 10 per cent when there are frequent atrial or ventricular premature systoles. Occasional premature atrial and ventricular beats have little, if any, effect on the blood supply to the gastrointestinal tract.

Recent studies in man have shown a significant reduction in carotid, renal, superior mesenteric, brachial, and dorsalis pedis arterial blood velocity which mirrors the effects observed in other vascular beds during ventricular arrhythmias (Benchimol and Desser, 1971) (see Chapter 3, p. 33).

SYMPTOMS AND SIGNS

Frequently, the patient is conscious of symptoms which he describes as "palpitation," "the heart turns over," "the heart stops," or "a catch in the throat." If there is a run of premature beats, the subjective sensation may be interpreted as "substernal discomfort," "pressure," or "precordial pain." General symptoms such as anxiety, sweating, weakness, and breathlessness may accompany the short run of beats.

The history frequently relates that the premature beats are not observed while the patient is working or engaged in an absorbing activity, but are more troublesome while resting, particularly lying in bed. While the premature beat in itself may be of little or no consequence, the thought that he might have heart disease causes the patient great anxiety, and he may believe that a serious threat to his life is imminent. When they occur frequently, these symptoms may cause a profound psychological disturbance with a cardiac fixation and fear of sudden death.

The characteristic auscultatory finding consists of an interruption of a normal rhythm by a premature beat or beats, followed by a pause that is usually but not invariably compensatory. However, the characteristics of the heart sounds vary in different cases. The intensity of the first heart sound depends on several factors, which are modified by the altered cardiac dynamics that occur with premature contractions. The first heart sound (S_1) of an atrial premature beat may be similar to that of normal beat or may be louder. The first heart sound of a ventricular premature beat may be fainter or louder than the normal first sound; when it is fainter, the beat usually appears before the end of the rapid inflow phase. Conversely, when it is louder, the beat usually coincides with atrial systole of sinus origin or the end of the phase of rapid inflow, i.e., after a P or T wave. The mechanism which produces these changes in intensity is not fully understood.

The splitting of the second sound has been studied primarily in relation to ventricular asynchrony during premature beats. The majority of ventricular premature beats result in mechanical asynchrony. The auscultatory findings depend on (1) the presence of bundle branch block and other abnormalities during "normal" beats and (2) the site of origin of the ectopic beat. In subjects whose electrocardiograms manifest bundle branch block during normally conducted beats, premature beats may either accentuate or lessen the degree of splitting.

Gallops and Murmurs. When only one heart sound is heard in the presence of a coupled rhythm with a rapid rate, a protodiastolic (S_3) gallop rhythm may be simulated. A short, early systolic murmur of low intensity may be present with ventricular premature contractions which is not heard with normal beats. Systolic murmurs of either the regurgitant or the ejection type are attenuated with the premature beats (Fig. 8–6).

Postextrasystolic Auscultatory Effects. The heart sounds in the cycle after a compensatory pause are different from those in the normal cycle.

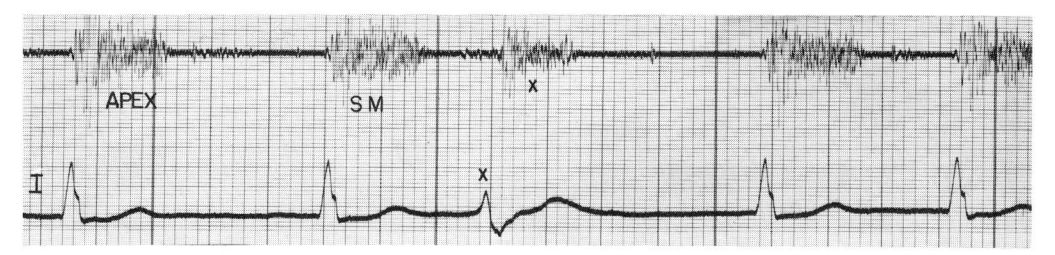

Figure 8–6. Effect of premature beat on character of systolic murmur. Atrial fibrillation. Beat at X represents ventricular premature beat or aberration of a supraventricular beat. The pansystolic murmur recorded at the apex is characteristic of mitral insufficiency. Note that the intensity of the murmur is diminished with the premature ventricular beat at X.

The first sound is accentuated, and the second sound is likely to be accentuated because of the moderately increased pressure in both circuits. Murmurs tend to be exaggerated in the cycle following the pause. Alteration in the intensity of the heart sounds may parallel the variation in pulse pressure which may occur in the several beats after a premature beat.

ELECTROCARDIOGRAM

The cardinal features for recognizing premature beats are (*a*) *prematurity of the beat, and* (*b*) *bizarre deviation from the normal P or QRS configuration*. One may make the following generalization: if these alterations occur in the atrial complexes, they are usually of atrial origin; if they occur in the ventricular complexes they are usually of ventricular origin. When a premature ventricular complex is not preceded by a P wave, then the beat arose in either the A-V junction, the bundle of His, or the ventricles. If the QRS complex is bizarre by comparison with that observed in the normal complexes and if the QRS complex has a duration of 0.12 second or longer, the beat is considered to arise in the ventricle. In this situation, a differential diagnosis must be made between the premature beat and aberration of a supraventricular beat. If the QRS complex resembles that of supraventricular beats and is neither preceded nor followed by a P wave, it is considered to be initiated in the A-V junction. In the presence of persistent intraventricular block, the QRS complex will be prolonged with all beats, and the differentiation between supraventricular and ventricular premature beats is based on the degree of deviation from the QRS of the dominant beats. Special criteria to make this distinction are discussed on page 94.

Diagnosis. The diagnosis may be suspected in the presence of the symptoms enumerated previously and by the characteristic auscultatory findings as well as being confirmed by the ECG. On auscultation, the following clinical states must be considered in the differential diagnosis of premature beats: (1) *Dropped beats in the presence of A-V heart block.* The pause may be confused with the compensatory pause of ventricular premature beats. (2) *Atrial fibrillation* simulating premature beats arising from multiple foci. However, with exercise, the irregularity of atrial fibrillation tends to become more marked, while premature beats usually tend to disappear, although this response is not constant. (3) *Pulsus alternans* simulating coupled beats. However, the marked irregularity observed with coupled beats is absent in pulsus alternans. (4) *Sinus arrhythmia,* which may be differentiated from premature beats by its relation to the phases of respiration. The final diagnosis is made by the electrocardiogram.

Clinical Significance. Once the clinical diagnosis of premature beats has been made, it is important to determine: (1) *the point of origin* (atrial, junctional, or ventricular); (2) *the frequency of the beats;* (3) *whether they are associated with paroxysmal tachycardia;* and (4) *the etiologic factors* (i.e., myocardial abnormality, drugs, psychological disturbances, upper respiratory or other infections, etc.). *It is of primary importance to determine whether or not the premature beats are associated with organic heart disease or are due to functional disturbances. Do they disappear upon exercise? Is there evidence of thyroid dysfunction? Does the electrocardiogram show W-P-W complexes?*

The clinical significance of the various types of premature beats has not been definitely settled. Clear differentiation between those occurring in the normal heart and those occurring in abnormal hearts is often difficult. Although certain patterns of premature beats occur mainly in the presence of myocardial disease, similar types of premature beats may occasionally be observed in hearts that are considered normal. The significance of these beats must be determined by a complete clinical evaluation of the patient.

Although the common variety of premature beats may occur in both normal patients or subjects with myocardial abnormality, the following include the characteristics of premature beats that are suggestive of heart disease: (a) *QRS width.* In the normal group the QRS width varies between 0.06 and 0.16 second, whereas in the abnormal group the QRS varies widely from 0.12 to 0.20 second (Berliner and Huppert, 1955). (b) *Multifocal origin.* (c) *Abnormalities characteristic of myocardial infarction* may be revealed by premature beats. This unmasking may be due to the abnormal sequence of depolarization and repolarization that occurs. (d) *Bizarre depolarization.* A widened and notched summit of the premature ventricular beats is suggestive of underlying heart disease (Gross, 1957; Legrand et al., 1960). (e) *Bizarre repolarization.* The repolarization phase may show a pattern similar to that observed following digitalis or myocardial infarction. (f) Premature beats occurring in groups of two, three, four, or more constitute a repetitive response. They are frequently premonitory to the development of paroxysmal tachycardia (atrial, junctional, or ventricular).

PREMATURE BEATS WITH COMPLETE A-V HEART BLOCK

Premature beats may occur in association with complete A-V heart block, either preceding, during, or following Stokes-Adams seizures. Several features which predispose to ectopic impulse formation in complete A-V heart block have been demonstrated experimentally and may be presumed to operate in human subjects: (1) ectopic beats occur with greater frequency when the heart rate is slow rather than normal (Han et al., 1966); (2) isolated Purkinje fibers display greater automaticity when they are stimulated at slow rates rather than at high rates; and (3) increased excitability, so-called "Wedensky facilitation," may be observed in various tissues beyond a region of block.

PREMATURE BEATS INITIATING ATRIAL FIBRILLATION

It has been shown in human subjects that atrial fibrillation may be initiated by an atrial premature beat. Premature beats occurring early in ventricular diastole during the downstroke of the T wave may lead to ventricular fibrillation. This is particularly apt to occur in the presence of coronary artery disease and especially with acute myocardial infarction. Considerable work has been done on this problem because of its relevance to causes of sudden death and to some of the complications of artificial pacemakers (see Chapter 37). With the widespread use of long-term monitoring of patients in coronary care units, it has become evident that premature beats may have practical importance as an arrhythmia premonitory to the development of ventricular fibrillation. The effect of carotid sinus pressure in suppressing premature beats is discussed in Chapter 33.

ATRIAL PREMATURE BEATS

General Considerations. Atrial premature beats are recognized by the origin of the impulse prematurely from an ectopic focus in the atrial muscle outside the S-A node. It may then be propagated through the A-V junction

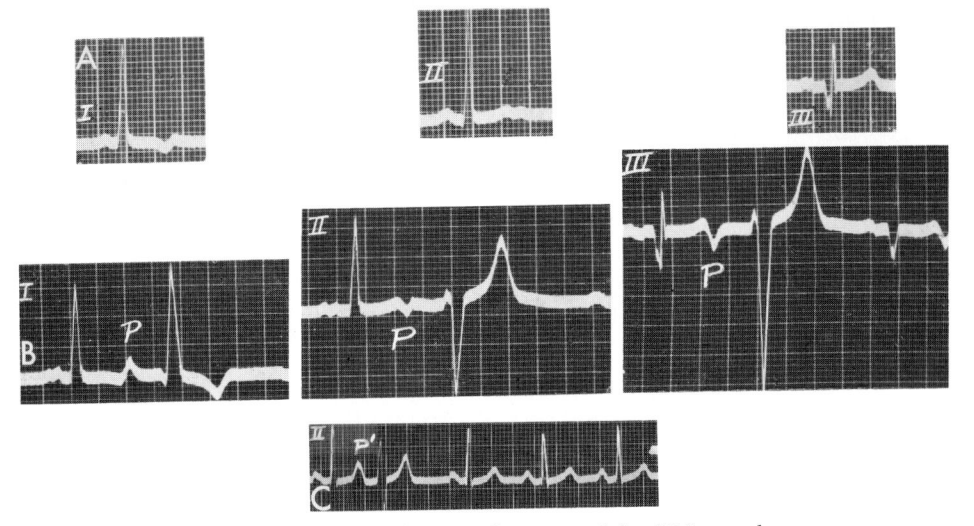

Figure 8–7. Atrial premature beats showing aberration of the QRS complex.
(A) Represents the normal cycles of leads I, II, and III. Note the characteristics of the P wave, QRS complex, and T wave in each lead.
(B) Note the atrial premature beats occurring early in diastole associated with a prolonged P-R interval and aberrant QRS complex in leads I, II, and III. In lead III, after the premature beat, the next sinus beat shows aberrant ventricular conduction.
(C) Note the atrial premature beats (P′) superimposed on the T wave associated with prolonged P-R (0.24 second) followed by aberration of the QRS complex.

and ventricles in a normal manner or may encounter conduction delay and block (Fig. 8–7). The ectopic impulse may discharge the sinus node prematurely with several possible results: (1) A fully "compensatory pause" may occur before the discharge of the next sinus impulse. (2) The ectopic impulse may encounter an unevenly excitable S-A node. It activates the excitable portion, is propagated through the node as the remainder becomes excitable, and finally proceeds to discharge the atrial musculature a second time, resulting in "sinoatrial reciprocation." (3) Premature beats may also temporarily depress S-A nodal automaticity, particularly when several ectopic impulses occur in sequence. This results in a shift of the pacemaker to another portion of the atrium, usually in the vicinity of A-V junction. If the ectopic impulse does not reach the sinus node in time to suppress its regular discharge, a fusion beat will result, without any disruption of the S-A node's regular automaticity.

Etiology. The etiology of atrial premature beats is that of premature beats in general. They tend to occur particularly in subjects with disease (e.g., rheumatic fever) or strain on the lesser circulation or atria (e.g., cor pulmonale, acute myocardial infarction, thyrotoxicosis, hypertension). Atrial premature beats may occur in patients with normal hearts as well as in those who have functional and organic disease. When they occur repetitively, in groups of two or three, they are frequently a precursor of atrial tachycardia, atrial fibrillation, or atrial flutter.

Pathology. The pathology is that of the underlying conditions previously mentioned.

Mechanism. The mechanism of atrial premature contractions is discussed on page 84.

Hemodynamics. As discussed previously, atrial premature beats may or may not have an effect on cardiac output (see p. 87); however, their effects are less marked than those of ventricular premature beats.

Electrocardiogram. The atrial beat occurs prematurely. Since the impulse arises from a point outside the S-A node, it will travel through the atrium in an abnormal direction. It has been traditionally held, therefore, that the P wave will possess an abnormal contour—it may be splintered, notched, diphasic, or inverted. However, recent experimental studies performed on dogs and on human subjects have revealed that stimulation in the atria, near the coronary sinus or in the auricular appendages, does not always yield significantly abnormal P waves in the standard leads (Moore et al., 1967).

If electrocardiograms can be obtained simultaneously from an esophageal and catheter lead in the right atrium, the location of the ectopic focus may be ascertained with greater accuracy by determining the activation sequence of the atria (see p. 107). When, as is frequently the case, the ectopic focus is quite near the S-A node, the premature P wave may closely resemble the normal sinus P wave (Fig. 8-8).

The P-R interval is usually not significantly shortened as compared with normal complexes, since the impulse is propagated in normal sequence over the atrial tracts to the A-V junction and ventricles. However, its length depends to a large degree upon the duration of the P-R interval of the normally conducted beats.

The P-R interval in atrial premature beats may be prolonged under the following conditions: (a) when the impulse occurs early in diastole and reaches the A-V junction during its relative refractory period—this is more commonly observed following a long cycle because the A-V junctional refractory period lengthens with the longer cycle; or (b) as a result of disease of the A-V junction. The P-R interval in most instances is above 0.12 second.

The pause following the atrial premature beat varies in length. It may be that of a normal cycle, it may be longer and compensatory, or it may be intermediate in length between the normal P-R interval and the duration of a fully compensatory pause. The mechanisms of such pauses have already been discussed.

An atrial premature beat is usually followed by a ventricular response. Occasionally, the premature atrial wave may occur so early in the cardiac cycle that the A-V conduction system will not have recovered sufficiently to respond. Under these circumstances, the premature P wave is seen without an accompanying ventricular response (blocked atrial premature beat). One should look for a hidden P wave superimposed on a T wave (it may resemble a U wave because of the altered shape and notched appearance of the T wave (Fig. 8-8).

The QRS complexes immediately following the premature P wave usually have a normal contour, since the ventricles are activated by the normal passage of the atrial impulse through

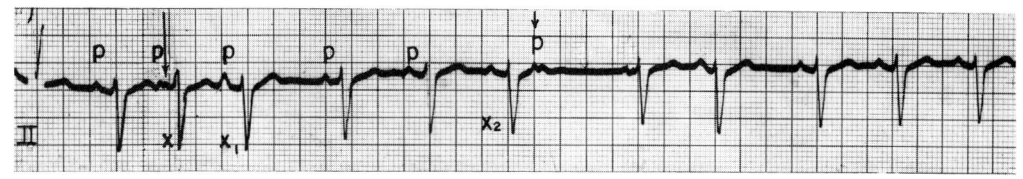

Figure 8-8. Various types of atrial premature beats. Note the presence of an atrial premature beat at X, followed by a P wave of increased amplitude, which is different in configuration from that of the normal P wave and is probably also a premature atrial beat. A blocked atrial premature beat, P, occurs at arrow following X₂. In addition, a slight sinus arrhythmia is present.

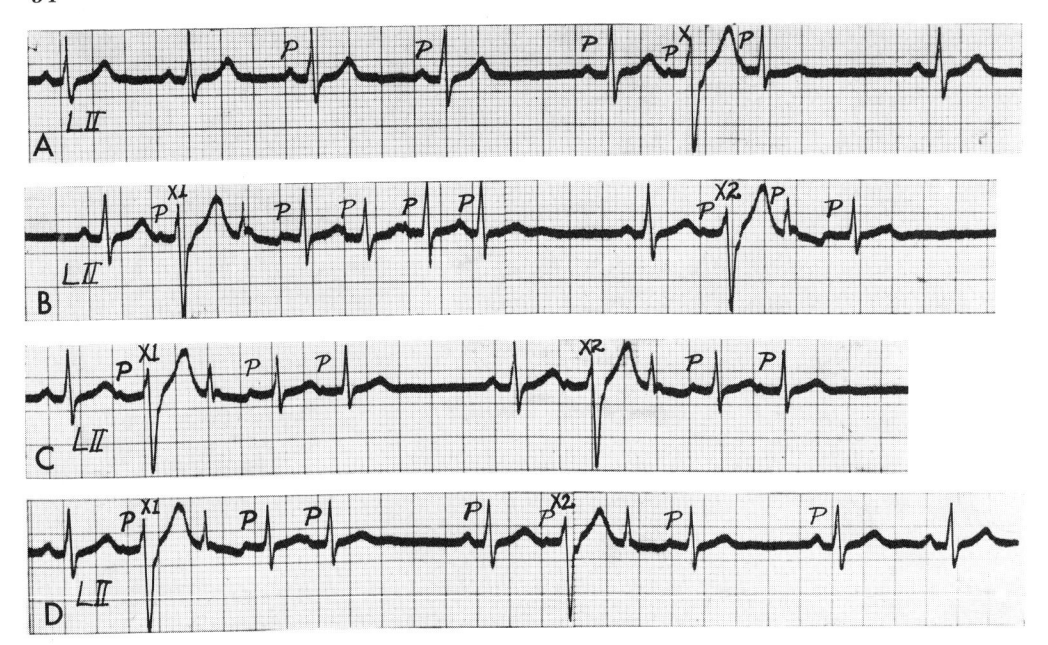

Figure 8-9. Atrial premature beats with aberration of the ventricular complexes. A, B, C, D represent a continuous tracing of lead II.

(A) The complex X following the P wave represents an aberrant ventricular complex; it is supraventricular in origin and is probably an atrial premature beat. This complex is followed by a P wave which is fused with the downstroke of the T wave. X is, therefore, an interpolated atrial beat (with protection block of the S-A node); the next P wave represents another ectopic atrial beat.

(B) Similar aberrant supraventricular complexes are noted at X_1 and X_2. These complexes in B, C, and D initiate other supraventricular beats, which are atrial premature beats in runs (short paroxysms of atrial tachycardia).

(C) Similar aberrant complexes are observed at X_1 and X_2.

(D) Similar supraventricular complexes are observed at X_1 and X_2.

the A-V junction. *If, however, there is some degree of functional impairment in one of the bundle branches, or if the coupling interval between the previous normal impulse and the premature beat is made sufficiently short,* aberrant conduction of the bundle branch will result. The ventricular complex of the atrial premature beat may become widened and notched, similar to that of a ventricular premature beat. This is most apt to occur when the premature beats fall in early diastole, because they then pass into the intraventricular conduction system and the ventricular myocardium while the former are still partially refractory. This causes a delay in the depolarization process of the ventricles and repolarization is abnormal. Thus, the QRS complex will be widened and slurred and the T wave usually will be pointed in a direction opposite to the main QRS deflection. Since it may be difficult to differentiate such a pattern from that of a ventricular premature beat, it is important to evaluate the T wave preceding the premature beat and compare it with T waves not associated with a premature beat. It will often be seen that this T wave is taller, notched, or otherwise deformed by the P wave contained within it (Fig. 8-9).

Aberrant intraventricular conduction of a supraventricular ectopic impulse may take a variety of forms. In one study of atrial premature beats, 18 of 21 subjects showed aberration: 14 manifested right bundle branch block; six, left bundle branch block; and four, "peripheral arborization block" (Rios et al., 1969).

PREMATURE BEATS

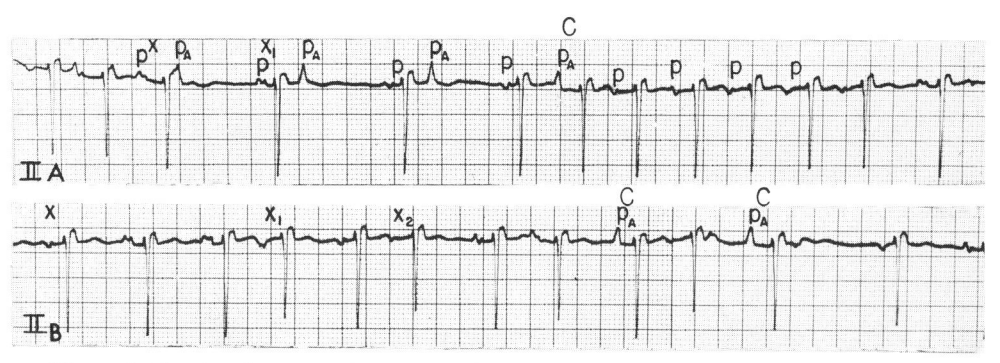

Figure 8–10. Atrial parasystole; parasystolic atrial beats followed by ventricular captures.

(A) Shows the interplay of two atrial rhythms; with the normal atrial beats (marked P), atrial parasystolic beats (marked Pa) are observed. Note the presence of normal bifid P wave in cycle marked X with a prolonged P-R interval (0.24 second). This is followed by a parasystolic P wave that is blocked. The next P wave has a short P-R interval (0.16 second) followed by a second short P wave blocked; the next sinus P has a normal P-R interval. The third parasystolic beat is blocked; however, the fourth parasystolic beat is followed by a capture. This is followed by the restoration of normal atrial beating. It shows increasing length of the P-R interval. The rate of the parasystolic beats is 54 per minute and is perfectly regular.

(B) Shows normal atrial beating with a sinus arrhythmia and wandering of the pacemaker in the presence of premature atrial beats. Note that the P waves at X, X_1, and X_2 are inverted and followed by a prolonged P-R interval. Note the occurrence of parasystolic beats towards the end of the strip.

Note the various patterns of the nonparasystolic P waves: inverted, bifid, diphasic. These indicate different sites of origin. Some occurring after the QRS represent reciprocal beats as shown with simultaneous esophageal leads.

Atrial Parasystole. Atrial parasystole is a disorder manifested by the occurrence of two sets of P waves that are different in configuration. One set of P waves stems from the sinus pacemaker and the other from an ectopic atrial focus. These sets of P waves occur independently of each other (i.e., the protection is mutual), or the ectopic focus may be protected while the S-A node is intermittently or regularly discharged by impulses from it (i.e., the protection is unilateral (Fig. 8–10).

Treatment. Since atrial premature beats do not carry with them so great a risk as ventricular premature beats, either in otherwise asymptomatic patients or in the presence of acute conditions such as recent myocardial infarction, their treatment constitutes, in general, less of an emergency. Therapy should be directed toward the underlying cause if it can be determined. Drugs that are useful in therapy include quinidine, procaine amide, and digitalis if the ectopic beats occur in association with heart failure. Propranolol may prove beneficial when anxiety is a factor.

Prognosis. The prognosis depends upon the underlying cause of the premature beats (e.g., functional derangement, toxic state, mitral valvular disease, coronary atherosclerosis), the frequency and grouping of the ectopic beats, and the response to therapy. Premature beats occurring only occasionally are not of serious import. The condition may become more serious when the premature beats occur frequently and when paroxysmal tachycardia supervenes.

A-V JUNCTIONAL PREMATURE BEATS

An A-V junctional premature beat is one that arises from the A-V junction. The electrocardiographic features depend upon the location of the ectopic focus. As previously described, these foci may originate in either the A-N (atrio-nodal) or the N-H (nodal-His)

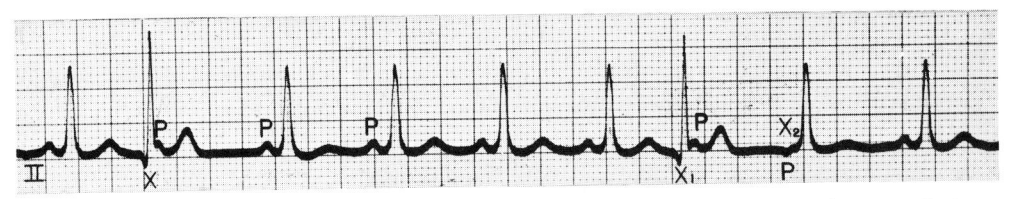

Figure 8–11. Junctional premature beats (Lead II). Note the occurrence of a normal sinus rhythm interrupted by premature beats at X and X₁. These are probably junctional in origin, since the beat resembles the normal beat and is followed by an upright P wave occurring at its normal sequence. Both of these beats are followed by a pause that is fully compensatory. The beat at X₂ is a junctional escape beat following a premature beat and is preceded by an inverted P wave. At X₂, the pause is not fully compensatory.

region. The latter is a more common site of origin. In A-V junctional rhythm, inverted P waves are situated either before or after or are buried in the QRS complex. If situated before the QRS complex, the P-R interval will usually be shortened. Like atrial premature beats, junctional premature beats may also show an aberrant ventricular complex, which may resemble ventricular premature beats. However, they usually resemble normal beats in contour (Fig. 8–11). The occurrence of a premature beat preceded by an inverted P wave with a P-R interval below 0.12 second is an important criterion.

VENTRICULAR PREMATURE BEATS

The etiology of ventricular premature beats is that of premature beats in general. They are due to functional derangement of or damage to the ventricular musculature. The features, symptoms, and signs have been discussed previously (pp. 83–90).

Electrocardiogram. Ventricular premature beats may arise from almost any region of the ventricles or the interventricular septum. The stimulated chamber will be activated before the other with the result that the two ventricles contract asynchronously. This abnormal type of activation produces *ventricular complexes that are slurred, widened, and of considerable voltage.*

The T waves following the premature beats are usually large and opposite in direction to the deflection of the QRS complex. Widening and notching of the premature ventricular complex is not sufficient for diagnosis since this may also result from an aberration or may occur in a patient with an interventricular conduction defect. It must be further shown that these complexes are not a response to preceding P waves. This poses a problem in differential diagnosis, since premature beats arising in the A-V conduction system may give rise to widened ventricular complexes without retrograde activation of the atria.

It has been stated that for the diagnosis of a ventricular premature beat, the *width of the QRS complex should be over 0.12 second;* however, while this is true in the main, it is not always the crucial feature (see page 91). Ventricular premature contractions may appear in the form of isolated beats; they may be numerous; they may arise from one or many foci; or they may occur in pairs or short runs of three or more beats, thereby constituting a potential ventricular tachycardia. When a sequence of six or more of these beats is observed, it constitutes a ventricular tachycardia (Figs. 8–12, 8–13, 8–14).

Ventricular premature beats are usually conducted to the A-V junction and sometimes into the atria. The atrial beats following the ventricular premature beats arise in the S-A node and, therefore, present a normal configura-

PREMATURE BEATS

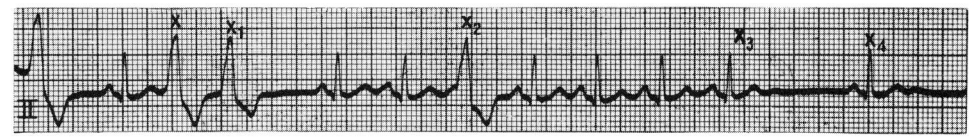

Figure 8-12. Ventricular premature beats, ventricular parasystole with exit block. Note a sequence of two premature beats (X, X₁) followed later by a single premature beat (X₂). Two cycles of S-A block (between X₃ and X₄ and following X₄) is seen after four normal sinus beats.

tion. The premature beats do not disturb the normal sequence of atrial beating and, hence, result in a fully compensatory pause. The P wave that occurs during or just after the premature ventricular beat cannot produce a ventricular response because it occurs during the refractory period of the A-V junction. The first ventricular contraction after the premature beat will be in response to the next rhythmic P wave. The interval between the premature beat and the next ventricular beat is, therefore, longer than the usual R-R interval and is referred to as fully compensatory. In this situation, retrograde conduction of the ventricular impulse to the atria is blocked.

Ventriculoatrial (V-A) conduction is difficult to detect in the surface electrocardiogram. Sinus tachycardia or sinus arrhythmia may either prevent retrograde conduction or make it impossible to detect and analyze. However, A-V conduction may be detected with intra-atrial leads and His bundle electrograms.

Retrograde conduction resulting in a 1:1 response can be obtained using ventricular pacing in a majority of patients with normal A-V conduction time but in only a few patients with prolonged A-V conduction time. Furthermore, the pathways of antegrade and retrograde conduction are not totally independent, as had been postulated. The pathways are interrelated, at least to the extent that transmission in one direction affects the rate of transmission in the other.

If a premature beat occurs sufficiently early enough in the diastolic period at a relatively slow ventricular rate (e.g., 60 per minute), the A-V junction may have recovered sufficiently from its refractory period so that the next sinus impulse is conducted and results in a normal ventricular response. No compensatory pause follows. Such a premature beat is referred to as an *interpolated extrasystole*. The P-R interval following the interpolated beat is often prolonged.

The duration of the intraventricular conduction time of ventricular premature beats depends upon many factors: (a) the QRS width of sinus beats; (b) time of origin (between P and R or T and P) in the cardiac cycle; (c) presence of supernormal recovery; and (d) presence of disease of the ventricular conduction system or myocardium (Fig. 8-15). The QRS duration of premature beats also depends upon the patient's age, as shown in a study of 148 cases in all age groups. In no case of a patient under 21 years was the QRS more than 0.15 sec-

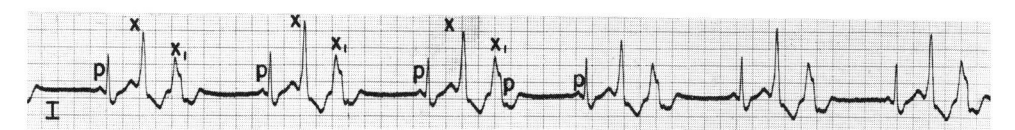

Figure 8-13. Ventricular premature beats occurring in pairs (trigeminy). Note the occurrence of a sinus beat followed by two premature beats at X and X₁. X₁ shows a greater degree of widening than X. Following the pause after X₁, the same sequence is repeated. The premature beats are most probably ventricular in origin. Note nonconducted P waves in the ST segments of X₁; the pauses are fully compensatory.

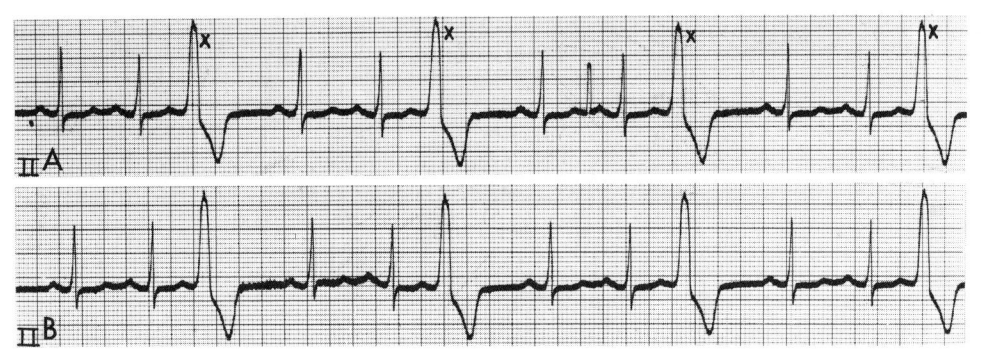

Figure 8-14. Ventricular trigeminy. (A and B) Note the appearance of a ventricular premature beat every third beat (X in strip A). The pauses are fully compensatory.

ond; and in none over 66 years was it shorter than 0.10 second (Huppert and Berliner, 1955).

Fusion Beats

ATRIAL FUSION BEATS. Atrial fusion beats are usually due to a sinus impulse fusing with a retrograde impulse of an A-V junctional or ventricular beat. The latter may be a premature systole or an escape beat occurring during the ventricular pause of marked sinus bradycardia, S-A heart block, or A-V heart block. One rarely finds fusion of the sinus impulse with an atrial premature beat or the fusion of two atrial premature beats, although such fusions are theoretically possible. Atrial fusion beats could also be the result of two impulses of identical origin. For example, in sinus rhythm with a 2:1 A-V heart block and re-entry of the sinus impulse giving rise to reciprocal atrial beats, there could be fusion in the atria of the reciprocal impulse with the next sinus impulse, producing a fusion beat. *Atrial fusion beats manifest a deformed P wave with a short P-R interval.*

VENTRICULAR FUSION BEATS. Ventricular fusion beats result from the *fusion of a supraventricular impulse with a ventricular premature beat, a ventricular escape, or a ventricular complex during idioventricular rhythm.* The supraventricular impulse may have its origin in the sinus node, the atrium, or the A-V junction. These beats may be confused in some instances with premature beats arising from the multiple foci. *Ventricular fusion beats may also result from the simultaneous stimulation of two ventricular foci* or from association of "low junctional" rhythm with reciprocal beats.

Another example would be the *W-P-W syndrome, in which fusion beats are due to the spread of supraventricular impulses along both the normal A-V bundle and an accessory pathway.*

Most fusion beats are premature. In the *most common form of fusion, a ventricular premature impulse fuses with a sinus impulse.* These are usually very late ventricular premature beats, occurring after the P wave of the next beat of the sinus rhythm has started. The ventricular muscle may then be activated in part from the

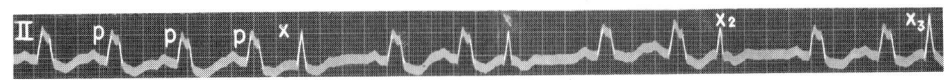

Figure 8-15. Premature beats with narrow QRS complexes occurring in the presence of bundle branch block (Lead II). Normal sinus rhythm (rate 79 per minute) with bundle branch block. Note the occurrence of premature beats at points marked X, X_1, X_2, and X_3. The QRS of the premature beats is quite narrow (0.06 second) as compared to the width of the control (0.14 second).

ectopic focus and in part by the impulse initiated by the sinus node. They can be readily identified by the fact that they fail after a P wave, have a P-R interval shorter than the usual rhythm, and have a configuration between a ventricular and supraventricular complex. On analyzing such a complex, it can be seen that the early part resembles the beginning of a pure ventricular premature beat arising from its usual focus, and the terminal portion resembles the terminal portion of a ventricular complex resulting from a sinus impulse. When these occur regularly in association with a short P-R interval, they closely simulate W-P-W beats.

POSTEXTRASYSTOLIC T WAVE CHANGES. These consist of alterations of the T wave or the duration of the Q-T interval of the sinus beat following the premature beat. There are conflicting opinions regarding the clinical significance of these changes, with the stronger evidence supporting the view that these findings have little importance (Fig. 8–16).

Treatment. The treatment of ventricular premature beats must take into consideration the clinical condition of the patient, particularly in reference to the underlying cardiac status and its etiology, the associated symptoms produced, and the reaction of the patient to the arrhythmia.

In the presence of occasional premature beats, if the patient is not aware of the arrhythmia, it is generally wiser not to bring up the subject since most individuals become quite concerned about changes in cardiac rhythm. The possibility of producing a cardiac neurosis with its deleterious effect should be avoided, if at all possible. In some patients, reduction or elimination of smoking, excessive coffee intake, or certain drugs, such as thyroid hormone or sympathomimetic agents will diminish the frequency of premature beats.

The prophylactic therapy of premature beats is to treat the underlying condition which may cause them. This entails: (1) treating underlying toxic or emotional states; (2) depressing reflexes from the gastrointestinal or genitourinary tract if necessary; (3) treating digitalis toxicity if present; (4) correcting electrolyte imbalance, particularly, potassium deficiency; (5) treating heart failure if present; and (6) curtailing the excessive use of certain stimulants, e.g., coffee, tea, or tobacco.

The Symptomatic Patient. The patient who complains of sensations or symptoms due to premature beats is often considerably relieved by a thorough examination. Definite reassurance in those cases with no abnormal process may be all the therapy needed. If the ectopic beats are due to or associated with an underlying myocardial dysfunction, therapy should be directed towards the underlying clinical state; abolition of the arrhythmia usually has a salutary effect.

The most important antiarrhythmic drugs that may be used to abolish premature beats are (a) *quinidine sulfate*, which may be administered in a dose of 0.2 to 0.3 gm. every four hours, or long-acting quinidine gluconate which

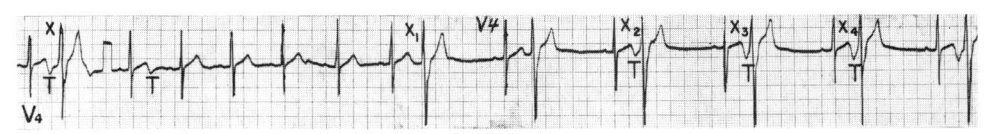

Figure 8–16. The effects of premature beats on the T wave in the beat following the compensatory pause.
(V_4) Note the presence of upright T waves in the normal cycles. Note that, following the premature beat at X, X_2, X_3, and X_4 in the beat following the postextrasystolic pause, the T wave manifests an inversion associated with a terminal downward dip that is usually observed in patients with ischemia.

may be administered in a dose of 0.6 gm. every 12 hours or 0.4 gm. every eight hours; (b) *procaine amide* (Pronestyl), which may be administered in a dose of 0.25 to 0.5 gm. every four hours; (c) *lidocaine*, which has a high degree of priority, may be administered intramuscularly or intravenously when premature beats occur in acute myocardial infarction; (d) *diphenylhydantoin*; (e) *beta blockers*, which may be given orally, especially when an anxiety factor or overactive sympathetic tone is present; and (f) *digitalis*, when the premature beats are associated with congestive failure and are not caused by digitalis toxicity.

When ectopic beats are very frequent, vigorous therapy with one of the aforementioned agents is indicated. The specific choice depends on the underlying clinical state. These drugs are discussed in detail under their specific chapter headings.

Paradoxically, in certain patients, such as those with ventricular ectopic beats superimposed on a bradycardia, those with a definitely prolonged Q-T interval, or those who exhibit a combination of these two features, isoprenaline or orciprenaline (epinephrine derivatives) may be of help (Buchner and Effert, 1968). These drugs increase the ventricular rate while simultaneously increasing the fibrillation threshold and decreasing the tendency towards asynchronous repolarization. When ectopic beats are associated with or occur secondary to a bradycardia, the use of an artificial pacemaker to speed up the rate may have a salutary effect.

The administration of sedatives or tranquilizing agents is indicated in those patients in whom the appearance of premature beats is associated with an anxiety state. Psychotherapy is indicated for those in whom emotional conflicts may be a factor in the production of premature beats.

Prognosis. The prognosis is best determined by the etiology and the underlying condition of the heart, by the frequency of the premature beats, and by their response to therapy. While atrial premature beats ordinarily do not impair the prognosis significantly, ventricular premature beats are associated with a definitely increased risk of sudden death (Chiang et al., 1969). Following acute myocardial infarction, this risk may be accentuated (Baird, 1969).

To aid in determining the prognosis, patients with premature beats have been classified into three groups:

Group 1 consists of patients with clinically normal hearts. If the premature beats are infrequent, the condition is considered to be relatively benign. Patients with premature beats may live for many years without curtailment of physical activity. However, in one study, the likelihood of sudden death occurring over a six-year interval in adults was six times as high in the group with documented premature beats (61 per 1000) as in a group without this arrhythmia (Chiang et al., 1969).

The prognosis is modified in patients in *Group 2*, which consists of those patients who do not have clinically detectable organic heart disease but do have a more severe arrhythmia (i.e., multifocal and/or frequent premature beats, episodes of tachyarrhythmia). In these patients the prognosis depends upon the response to therapy and the incidence of tachyarrhythmia.

Group 3 is comprised of patients with definite myocardial abnormality. The additional occurrence of premature beats in these patients is a cause of concern, especially if the premature beats occur frequently. The appearance of ectopic beats or an increase in their frequency indicates a worsening of the underlying condition. They may forewarn the possible occurrence of ventricular tachycardia, ventricular fibrillation, and Stokes-Adams seizures. In these patients the prognosis depends upon the response to therapy of both the premature beats and the underlying organic disease.

References

Attar, H. J., Gutierrez, M. T., Bellet, S., and Ravens, J. R.: Effect of stimulation of hypothalamus and reticular activating system on production of cardiac arrhythmias. Circ. Res., 12:14, 1963.

Baird, W. M.: Prognostic significance of premature beats in acute myocardial infarction. Clin. Res., 17:288, 1969.

Benchimol, A., and Desser, K. B.: Ventricular function in the presence of ventricular arrhythmias (Abst.). 25th Hahnemann Symposium, Cardiac Arrhythmias: Pathophysiology, Pharmacology and Management, Sept. 21–25, 1971, Philadelphia.

Benchimol, A., Stegall, H. F., and Gartlan, J. L.: New method to measure phasic coronary blood velocity in man. Amer. Heart. J., 81:93, 1971.

Berliner, K., and Huppert, V. F.: Benign ventricular premature systoles. Cardiologia (Basel), 24:184, 1955.

Buchner, M., and Effert, S.: Precipitation of tachycardias by extrasystoles. Germ. Med. Mth., 8:3, 1968.

Bussan, R., Torin, S., and Scherf, D.: Retrograde conduction of ventricular extrasystoles to the atria. Amer. J. Med. Sci., 230:293, 1955.

Chiang, B. N., Perlman, L. V., Ostrander, L. D., Jr., and Epstein, F. H.: Relationship of premature systoles to coronary heart disease and sudden death in the Tecumseh epidemiologic study. Ann. Intern. Med., 70:1159, 1969.

Corday, E., and Irving, D. W.: Disturbances of Heart Rate, Rhythm and Conduction. Philadelphia, W. B. Saunders, 1961.

Davidson, S., and Surawicz, B.: Ectopic beats and atrioventricular conduction disturbances. Arch. Intern. Med., 120:280, 1967.

Dolora, A.: Early premature ventricular beats, repetitive ventricular response, and ventricular fibrillation. Amer. Heart J., 74:332, 1967.

Goldreyer, B. N., and Bigger, J. T., Jr.: Ventriculoatrial conduction in man. Circulation, 41:935, 1970.

Greenspan, K., Anderson, G. J., and Fisch, C.: Electrophysiologic correlate of exit block. Amer. J. Cardiol., 28:197, 1971.

Gross, D.: The apex of ventricular extrasystoles – its diagnostic and clinical significance. Z. Kreislaufforsch, 46:905, 1957.

Han, J., DeTraglia, J., and Moe, G. K.: Incidence of ectopic beats as a function of basic rate in the ventricle. Amer. Heart J., 72:632, 1966.

Hinkle, L. E., Jr., Carver, S. T., and Stevens, M.: The frequency of asymptomatic disturbances of cardiac rhythm and conduction in middle-aged men. Amer. J. Cardiol., 24:629, 1969.

Huppert, V. F., and Berliner, K.: The intraventricular conduction time (QRS duration) of ventricular premature systoles. Cardiologia, 27:87, 1955.

Katz, L. K., and Pick, A.: Clinical Electrocardiography. Part I. The Arrhythmias. Philadelphia, Lea & Febiger, 1956.

Legrand, R., Desruelles, J., Merlen, J. F., and Dubeaux, D. A.: Prognosis of ventricular extrasystoles according to their morphology. Lille Med., 5:461, 1960.

Levine, H. D., Lown, B., and Streeper, R. B.: Clinical significance of postextrasystolic T wave changes. Circulation, 6:538, 1952.

Moe, G. K., Preston, J. B., and Burlington, H.: Physiologic evidence for a dual A-V transmission system. Circ. Res., 4:357, 1956.

Moore, E. N., Jomain, S. L., Stuckey, J. H., Buchanan, J. W., and Hoffman, B. F.: Studies on ectopic atrial rhythms in dogs. Amer. J. Cardiol., 19:676, 1967.

Pick, A.: Electrocardiographic features of exit block. In Dreifus, L. S., and Likoff, W. (eds.): Mechanisms and Therapy of Cardiac Arrhythmias. New York, Grune & Stratton, 1966, pp. 469–476.

Rios, J. C., Sarin, R. K., Pooya, M., and Massumi, R. A.: The various patterns of aberrant intraventricular conduction in induced premature ventricular beats. Amer. J. Cardiol., 23:134, 1969.

Rosenbaum, M.: Classification of ventricular extrasystoles according to form. J. Electrocardiol., 2:289, 1969.

Scherf, D.: The mechanism and treatment of extrasystoles. Prog. Cardiov. Dis., 2:370, 1960.

Smirk, F. H., and Palmer, D. G.: A myocardial syndrome. With particular reference to the occurrence of sudden death and of premature systoles interrupting antecedent T waves. Amer. J. Cardiol., 6:620, 1960.

Chapter 9 Paroxysmal Atrial Tachycardia (PAT)

GENERAL CONSIDERATIONS
ETIOLOGY
MECHANISMS
PATHOLOGY
HEMODYNAMICS
   Comparison of Hemodynamic Effects of Ectopic Tachycardia and Exercise Tachycardia
SYMPTOMS AND SIGNS
ELECTROCARDIOGRAM
VARIANT TYPES OF ATRIAL TACHYCARDIA
   Multifocal Atrial Tachycardia
   Repetitive Atrial Tachycardia
   Persistent Atrial Tachycardia
DIAGNOSIS AND DIFFERENTIAL DIAGNOSIS
   Aids to ECG Diagnosis of the Atrial Mechanism

TREATMENT
   Urgent Treatment
   Procedures Performed by Patients
   Drug Therapy
   Other Procedures
   Prophylaxis Between Attacks
PROGNOSIS
PAROXYSMAL ATRIAL TACHYCARDIA WITH A-V HEART BLOCK (PAT WITH BLOCK)
   General Considerations
   Incidence and Etiology
   Mechanism
   Symptoms and Signs
   Diagnosis
   Treatment
   Prognosis

GENERAL CONSIDERATIONS

Periodic acceleration of the heart beat is a relatively common phenomenon and usually gives rise to the symptoms of palpitation. In only a fraction of the patients with this symptom, however, is the palpitation due to paroxysmal atrial tachycardia (PAT). Frequently, it is due to "pounding" of the heart associated with simple acceleration of the normal heart beat during emotional stress or mild exercise. In some patients, it is due to an ectopic rhythm other than atrial tachycardia, i.e., atrial fibrillation or flutter, or rarely, ventricular tachycardia.

Paroxysms of atrial tachycardia usually start and stop suddenly, lasting a few seconds, hours, or days. The heart rate during a paroxysm ranges from 140 to 220 per minute. Immediately following termination of the paroxysm, the rate is usually approximately one-half of the paroxysmal rate.

Patients with PAT often present a history of isolated atrial premature beats which gradually become more numerous and occur more frequently, ultimately eventuating in paroxysms of PAT. These attacks may occur occasionally, i.e., once per week or month or quite frequently, with many episodes appearing in a single day. At times, they can be related to certain events (see later discussion).

During the paroxysms the ventricular rate is quite regular. The maximal difference between cycles rarely exceeds 0.01 second. This is in contrast with ventricular tachycardia, in which a slight degree of irregularity is usually present. The rate is not influenced by posture or by exercise. Carotid sinus pressure will often stop the paroxysm with resumption of normal sinus rhythm but, if ineffective, it will not even slow the ventricular rate. Relatively few exceptions to this observation have been noted.

ETIOLOGY

Supraventricular tachycardia, of which over half is specifically atrial tachycardia, occurs in approximately 1.1 per cent of hospitalized patients. The underlying etiology in paroxysmal atrial tachycardia is not specifically known; about one-third of cases occur in otherwise normal hearts. The arrhythmia may be observed in association with many conditions: rheumatic heart disease (34 per cent), arteriosclerotic heart disease (14 per cent), hypertensive heart disease (3 per cent), and thyrocardiac disease (5 per cent); and in 10 per cent of the cases, the tachycardia occurs in association with various other clinical states. It is observed in 4 to 8 per cent of those suffering from acute myocardial infarction (Lown et al., 1967; Meltzer and Kitchell, 1966). A variety of conditions may precipitate the paroxysms in a susceptible individual, including: (1) deep inspiration (Montella, 1961), (2) hyperventilation, (3) emotional stress, (4) exercise, (5) changes in position, (6) swallowing, and (7) heavy meals.

MECHANISMS

Recently, the circus movement mechanism or the macro-reentry theory has received substantial support as the electrophysiologic mechanism of PAT (Durrer et al., 1967; Goldreyer et al., 1969). The following findings, characteristic of re-entry, are observed in PAT: (1) the paroxysm can be initiated or terminated by a premature stimulus; (2) there is a regular sequence of cycle lengths that occurs during the establishment of the paroxysm; and (3) once established, the paroxysm has a fixed cycle length (Goldreyer et al., 1969). The macro-reentry pathway may involve the S-A or A-V nodes as well as the atria. The functional dissociation of the proximal A-V junction into α- and β-pathways (see Chapter 2) may facilitate the establishment of the pathway (Mendez and Moe, 1966). A circus movement could be established when a premature atrial beat, encountering a refractory β-pathway, is conducted over the α-pathway and then returned by the now excitable β-pathway to the atrium. Increased refractoriness of both the α- and β-pathways as a result of the action of digitalis, quinidine, or a premature electrical stimulus interrupts the circus movement and terminates the tachycardia.

Recently, it has been proposed that PAT may be due to a sustained reciprocation (circus movement) involving the atrial muscle and the S-A node (Han, 1970).

PATHOLOGY

Infarction of atrial tissue may be present when PAT occurs in a patient with acute myocardial infarction; however, in the majority of cases, in which there are other etiologies, no pathologic alteration is found.

HEMODYNAMICS

The effect of a tachycardia on cardiac hemodynamics depends upon the cause of the arrhythmia, its duration, the previous condition of the heart, and the ventricular rate. In the normal heart, sinus tachycardia usually causes an increase in cardiac output with rates up to 170 to 180 per minute. At faster rates, the period of ventricular filling is shortened, the stroke volume is reduced, and cardiac output falls. In a previously diseased heart this diminution in cardiac output occurs at slower rates. Similarly, supraventricular tachycardia in the absence of organic cardiac abnormality produces little disability initially; however, prolonged paroxysms result in progressive hemodynamic impairment. The systemic systolic, diastolic, and pulse pressures

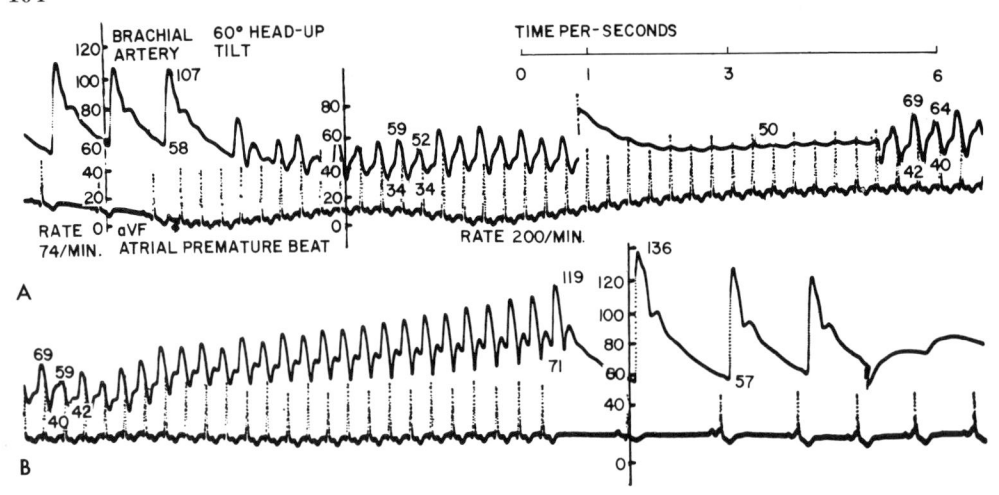

Figure 9-1. Illustrates the drop in brachial artery pressure almost immediately after the onset of paroxysmal atrial tachycardia.

(A) Note the brachial artery pressure, which was 107/58, dropped to as low as 52/34. The hypotensive state is the result of inadequate ventricular filling due to shortening of diastole as a consequence of the tachycardia. As a result, there is a drop in cardiac output.

(B) Note the return of blood pressure to normal with the return of normal sinus rhythm at the end of the strip. (From Saunders, D. E., and Ord, J. W.: Amer. J. Cardiol., 9:223, 1962.)

decrease, particularly in the upright position, and there is a precipitous rise in left atrial mean and pulse pressure with minimal effect upon pulmonary arterial pressures (Fig. 9-1). The most striking alteration is the very low stroke volume (Saunders and Ord, 1962; McIntosh and Morris, 1966; Wright et al., 1970). In the presence of myocardial disease or long duration of the tachycardia, the cardiac output gradually falls.

Comparison of Hemodynamic Effects of Ectopic Tachycardia and Exercise Tachycardia. The effect of rapid heart rates upon the function of the heart as a pump *depends upon whether the tachycardia is secondary to physiologic demands upon the heart or is due to an abnormally rapid discharge from an automatic supraventricular pacemaker or a rapid electronic atrial pacemaker.* In the experimental animal there is a slight to moderate increase in cardiac output following tachycardia produced by electrical stimulation. Similar results have also been observed in the human subject. On the other hand, the stroke volume is either maintained or increased, and consequently the cardiac output goes up during exercise-induced tachycardia (Befeler et al., 1971) as compared with the decrease in stroke volume observed during ectopic supraventricular tachycardia. The exercise-induced increase in stroke volume probably results from the physiologic effects of released catecholamines.

SYMPTOMS AND SIGNS

Paroxysmal atrial tachycardia is characterized by rapid heart action of sudden onset and termination. The symptoms are similar to those observed in the presence of any rapid ectopic rhythm; they depend largely on the state of the heart muscle, its response to an acceleration of the heart beat, the duration of the paroxysm, and the emotional state of the patient. With paroxysms of short duration, the patient may experience relative freedom from symptoms, except for slight palpitation. In the presence of prolonged paroxysms with rapid ventricular rates, especially in patients with organic heart disease, the symptoms may be quite pronounced, including varying degrees of precordial discomfort or pain, weakness, dizziness, or syncope, nausea, and vomiting (which may terminate the paroxysm).

The signs of paroxysmal atrial tachycardia are those of an accelerated and regular heart rate. The pulse is rapid and weak; the heart sounds are usually identical throughout. Minor variations in the intensity of the sounds are noted with the phases of respiration. This constancy in the intensity of the regular rapid sounds is an important feature and may help to differentiate the condition from other types of rapid heart action. The rapid rate may obscure murmurs produced by underlying disease. Gallop rhythm and pulsus alternans are frequently encountered. The blood pressure falls during prolonged paroxysms; circulatory failure, heart failure, or the anginal syndrome may result. In the older age group with arteriosclerosis, the paroxysms may occasionally precipitate a shock-like state resembling that of an acute myocardial infarction. Deaths occurring during paroxysmal atrial tachycardia, although rare, have been observed.

Polyuria, occurring with attacks of all forms of paroxysmal tachycardia is quite typical. Copious diuresis of up to 3 L. begins shortly after the onset of episodes and may last for 30 to 90 minutes in patients with paroxysmal forms of atrial tachycardia, atrial fibrillation, atrial flutter, or junctional rhythms. The mechanism of solute diuresis in these patients is at present believed to be due to inhibition of antidiuretic hormone secretion.

ELECTROCARDIOGRAM

Paroxysmal atrial tachycardia consists of a rapid succession of atrial premature beats that occur at a rate ranging from approximately 140 to 220 per minute. Six atrial premature beats occurring in succession may be considered to be a paroxysm of atrial tachycardia. Because of their ectopic origin, the P waves during the paroxysm vary in configuration to a greater or lesser degree from those observed during normal sinus rhythm. With very rapid rates, the P waves are often superimposed on the T wave of the preceding beat, making it difficult or impossible to recognize them in the ordinary electrocardiogram. When this occurs, the identification of the disturbance can be made only if one ascertains the beginning or the ending of a paroxysm or employs special methods to determine the atrial mechanism (see p. 107).

The ventricular complexes are usually normal in paroxysmal atrial tachycardia; however, widening may occur. This widening is caused by abnormal conduction in the bundle branches as a result of impulses arriving in the conduction system during the relative refractory period which may make a definite diagnosis of atrial tachycardia difficult. In the presence of widened QRS complexes the differential diagnosis between atrial and ventricular tachycardia becomes very important because of the marked difference in prognosis and treatment.

PAT may be associated with the tachycardia-bradycardia syndrome. The interruption period of PAT by periods of cardiac asystole may result in the production of Stokes-Adams seizures.

The following electrocardiographic patterns may be observed during normal sinus rhythm in patients susceptible to the development of paroxysmal atrial tachycardia: (1) atrial premature beats, particularly if they are frequent or in groups of two or more or occur coupled to the preceding normal beat; and (2) preexcitation syndromes (i.e., Lown-Ganong-Levine and W-P-W syndrome).

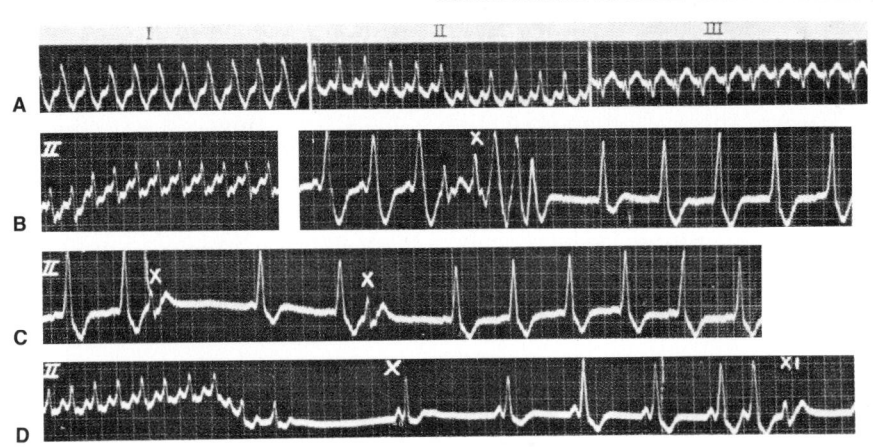

Figure 9–2. Conversion of paroxysmal atrial tachycardia to normal sinus rhythm. Comparison of the effect of methacholine (Mecholyl) and carotid sinus pressure.

(A) Atrial paroxysmal tachycardia with widened ventricular complexes (rate 200 per minute).

(B) Showing effect of methacholine. Note the occurrence of aberrant ventricular complexes resembling those of ventricular tachycardia or flutter at X, prior to restoration of normal sinus rhythm.

(C) Continuous with end of strip B. Note the presence of W-P-W beats at a relatively slow rate with atrial premature beats at X. Note that these premature beats resemble the ventricular complexes of lead II during the paroxysm.

(D) Attack of paroxysmal atrial tachycardia in the same patient, showing effect of carotid sinus pressure. Note the restoration of normal sinus rhythm (with W-P-W) at X without the occurrence of the bizarre ventricular complexes noted in B. Note the atrial premature beat at X_1.

The transitional period between PAT and normal sinus rhythm may be critical because asystole or ventricular tachyarrhythmias may transiently occur. The type of transitional arrhythmias observed depends upon the methods of conversion (e.g., carotid sinus pressure, drugs, countershock) (Fig. 9–2).

Conversion to normal sinus rhythm occurs in five general patterns: (a) asystole lasting up to six seconds, followed by normal sinus rhythm; (b) slight slowing of the ventricles, followed by sudden conversion; (c) precipitous conversion (most common); (d) slowing, asystole, and then conversion; and (e) ventricular tachycardia, a prefibrillatory ventricular arrhythmia, and premature beats followed by normal sinus rhythm (Hellerstein et al., 1951). I have encountered occasional episodes of ventricular tachycardia and ventricular flutter during this transition period.

VARIANT TYPES OF ATRIAL TACHYCARDIA

Several variants of the typical types of PAT have been described:

Multifocal Atrial Tachycardia. Multifocal atrial tachycardia (chaotic atrial tachycardia) is a relatively uncommon arrhythmia; it may be confused with several other atrial arrhythmias (e.g., atrial flutter, wandering atrial pacemaker). It is distinguished by the following electrocardiographic features: (1) an atrial rate of over 100 beats per minute; (2) discrete P waves of distinctly varying morphology representing at least three different foci; and (3) most common occurrence is in elderly patients who, with few exceptions, are quite ill and often have coexisting cardiovascular and pulmonary disease. Multifocal atrial tachycardia often evolves into atrial fibrillation or flutter.

Repetitive Atrial Tachycardia. The repetitive type of atrial tachycardia consists of brief paroxysms of atrial tachycardia (e.g., 3 to 8 beats), frequently separated by only one or two sinus beats. It is somewhat more resistant to therapy than the continuous type.

Persistent Atrial Tachycardia. Occasional instances of atrial tachycardia have been documented in which the arrhythmia has lasted for months or years (Dolara and Possi, 1965). With the advent of newer methods of therapy, such cases must now be rare indeed.

DIAGNOSIS AND DIFFERENTIAL DIAGNOSIS

The diagnosis of paroxysmal atrial tachycardia should be suspected in a patient who gives a history of a sudden acceleration of the heart beat that lasts for varying periods of time and stops suddenly. A history of atrial premature beats and the presence of a regular rhythm with a rate ranging from 140 to 220 per minute during the paroxysm should lead one to suspect atrial paroxysmal tachycardia. The ECG criteria for the diagnosis of paroxysmal atrial tachycardia are: (1) the P waves usually differ from those of sinus beats or merge with the preceding T waves; (2) the rhythm during the paroxysm is quite regular; (3) the QRS complexes are usually normal in shape but may show aberration; and (4) the first normal beat at the end of a paroxysm is usually followed by a postparoxysmal pause (Figs. 9–3, 9–4).

Aids to Electrocardiographic Diagnosis of the Atrial Mechanism. Not infrequently it is quite difficult to determine the type of atrial mechanism in the electrocardiogram because of the rapid rate and consequent poor delineation of the atrial complexes and widened QRS complexes. Under these conditions, the following procedures may be utilized:

Carotid sinus pressure may help in the following ways: *It will terminate an atrial and occasionally a junctional tachycardia;* occasional atrial premature beats during the transition period suggest paroxysmal atrial tachycardia.

The best method is the use of the esophageal lead (Fig. 9–5). With this procedure, the atrial complexes are quite prominent and the nature of the atrial mechanism can be ascertained easily, even at rapid rates.

Characteristic alterations may also

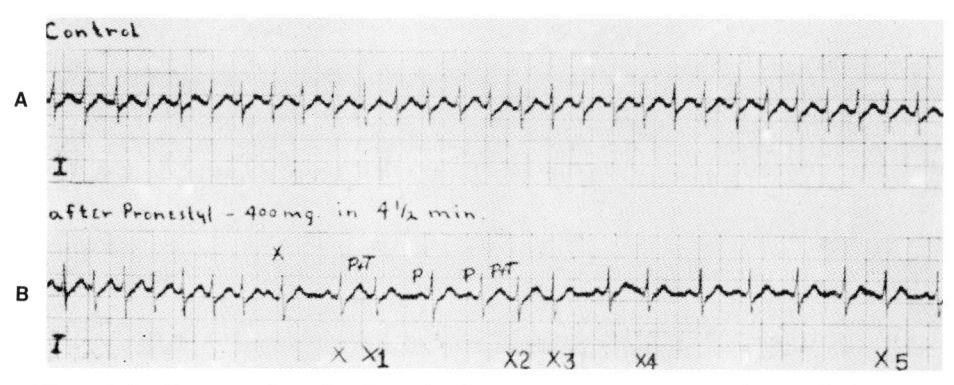

Figure 9–3. Paroxysmal atrial tachycardia showing conversion to normal sinus rhythm.
(A) Atrial paroxysmal tachycardia with a rate of 200 per minute is shown. The P wave is superimposed on the preceding T wave. There is no widening of the QRS complex.
(B) Note end of paroxysm at X following the intravenous administration of 400 mg. of procaine amide (Pronestyl). The return to a normal sinus rhythm is accompanied by atrial premature beats (P + T) at X_1, X_2, X_3, X_4, and X_5.

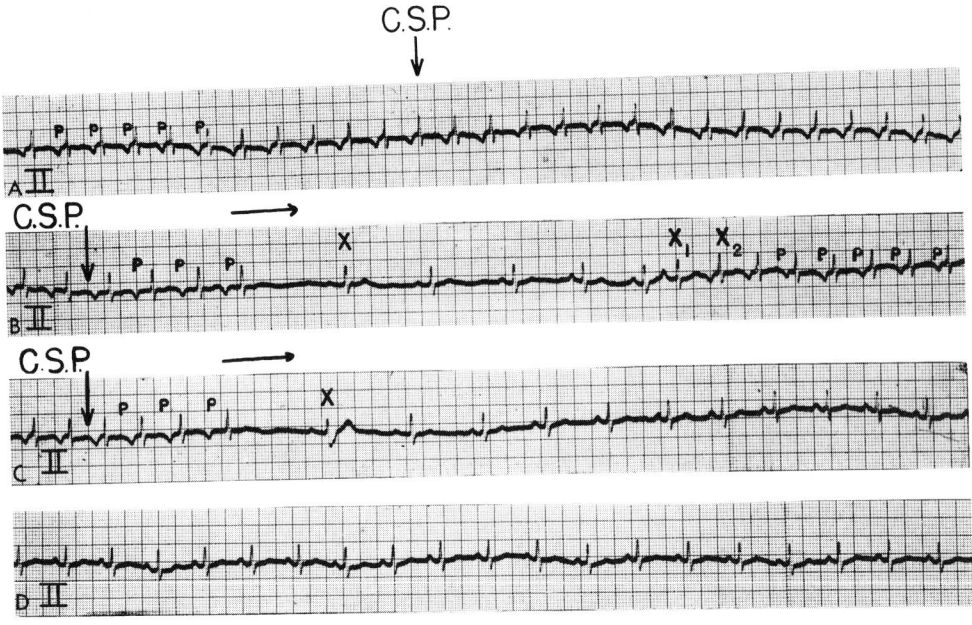

Figure 9-4. Supraventricular tachycardia (probably atrial).

(A) Note the presence of supraventricular tachycardia (atrial?) with a ventricular rate of 150 per minute. The P waves are inverted. The P-R interval measures 0.12 sec.

(B) Ventricular rate 150 per minute; P-R, 0.20 second. Following carotid sinus pressure, note the return to a normal sinus rhythm at X, a premature atrial beat at X_1, followed by a return of the paroxysm at X_2.

(C) Following carotid sinus pressure during another episode, note the return to a normal sinus rhythm at X.

(D) Sinus tachycardia.

be observed in the Doppler tracing and intra-atrial leads. Recently, the His bundle electrogram has been employed to distinguish between a ventricular and atrial origin of the paroxysm.

The differential diagnosis involves *PAT with block, sinus tachycardia, junctional tachycardia, atrial flutter,* and *ventricular tachycardia.*

TREATMENT

The principles of therapy of paroxysmal atrial tachycardia involve the use of (a) parasympathetic stimulation (the treatment of choice), by mechanical means, drugs, or a combination of both; (b) antiarrhythmic drugs; (c) electric countershock in selected cases; and (d) right atrial pacing. All of these methods are based on the principle of increasing parasympathetic discharge to the heart or inhibiting atrial ectopic pacemaker activity.

Urgent Treatment. This is important to those patients who manifest acute distress which at times may approach a shock-like state. Rapid abolition of the episode is desirable and at times mandatory. Conversion may be effected by carotid sinus pressure (technique is described on p. 342), which is successful in about 80 per cent of cases. If unsuccessful, the subject should be given neostigmine, 2 cc. of 1:4000 solution intramuscularly. The maximal effect occurs in about 20 minutes. Carotid sinus pressure, if initially ineffective, will often be successful in reversion after this drug has been given.

The following drugs and procedures may be employed cautiously in the therapy of PAT: (1) Edrophonium (Tensilon), intravenously, has been used recently with considerable success. (2) Vomiting, induced by ipecac, may also cause parasympathetic stimulation and restore the rhythm to normal. (3) Digitalis in the form of digoxin or Cedilanid (intravenously or intramuscularly) is often successful and a preferred method for immediate conversion. (4) Electric countershock is indicated when some of the previous measures have failed in conversion (details are given in Chapter 38). (5) Atrial pacing in refractory cases will frequently revert the atrial tachycardia directly to a normal sinus rhythm; occasionally, atrial fibrillation may occur as a transient mechanism (see p. 75).

Procedures Performed by Patients. Some procedures may be performed by patients and are relatively safe and often successful in the abolition of the paroxysm: (1) Extending the head backward as far as possible may produce some degree of carotid sinus stimulation. (2) With the patient in the semirecumbent position, pressure is applied in the upper region of the neck, in the area of the carotid sinus, with the thumb pressed backward toward the vertebral column. Although many patients cannot perform this maneuver correctly, a knowledgeable member of the family is often able to do so. (3) Blowing into a balloon, particularly one that is difficult to inflate, may produce a sufficient parasympathetic effect to abolish the ectopic rhythm. (4) Other procedures include breath holding, performing a Valsalva maneuver (forced expiration with the glottis closed after deep inspiration), or the Müller procedure (forced inspiration made against the closed glottis after deep expiration). (5) The patient may put his finger down his throat and attempt to retch. This may produce a sufficient parasympathetic effect to stop the attack. (6) The use of an ice collar around the neck is often effective in terminating a paroxysm in a few minutes. (This should be kept in the refrigerator in between attacks.)

Drug Therapy. Drugs which increase the parasympathetic stimulation to the heart are effective in controlling PAT either alone or in conjunction with carotid sinus pressure. Neostigmine (Prostigmin) and edrophonium (Tensilon), both anticholinesterase agents, are the most commonly used drugs of this type.

Digitalis preparations are extremely useful in therapy. They are effective during attacks and act prophylactically between attacks. Digitalis helps to stop the attacks by the following mechanisms: (a) sensitizing the carotid sinus so that carotid sinus pressure will be more effective; (b) increasing, in some hearts, the refractory period of the atrial muscle owing to a preponderance of the direct muscular effect (if this actually occurs); and (c) increasing A-V conduction time. Full digitalization followed by a daily maintenance dose may prevent the recurrence of the ectopic rhythm. Patients with this arrhythmia may be maintained on digitalis for a period of three to four months or longer. It is the drug of choice in the therapy of the recurrent episodes occurring in patients with the W-P-W syndrome.

Quinidine is an important drug in the treatment of supraventricular tachycardia. It terminates an attack by increasing the refractory period of the atrial muscle and by decreasing the automaticity of ectopic pacemakers. For therapy during an attack, quinidine gluconate may be given in a dosage of 0.4 gm. intramuscularly every two hours for a total of five doses. For prophylactic therapy, oral quinidine (0.2–0.3 gm., three times daily) is preferable.

Procaine amide is one of the preferred methods of treatment and, in our opinion, should be used if carotid sinus pressure and neostigmine or digitalis fail to terminate the attack.

Its administration will stop the attack in about 80 per cent of the cases (Bellet et al., 1952; Berry et al., 1951). This is accomplished through a mechanism quite similar to that of quinidine.

Sympathomimetic drugs, especially phenylephrine (Neo-Synephrine), have been used successfully in the treatment of supraventricular tachycardia. The vasoconstriction and hypertension produced by this drug result in the simultaneous stimulation of cardioinhibitory centers via the carotid sinus and aortic arch.

Alprenolol, propranolol, and other sympathetic blocking agents may be efficacious in the therapy of acute episodes or for the prophylactic treatment of PAT, especially in that group of patients resistant to other drugs or those in whom anxiety is a significant factor. Serious side effects, however, have been observed in approximately 5 per cent of patients using these drugs. Beta-blocking agents should not be used in the presence of congestive heart failure or severe myocardial damage, except in selected instances (see Chapter 33).

Other Procedures. The following procedures have occasionally been employed but do not constitute a preferred method of therapy: (1) *Electric countershock.* (2) *Electrical stimulation delivered to the atria by an artificial pacemaker electrode* has terminated the paroxysm in 50 to 70 per cent of patients (Barold et al., 1969). Most subjects revert to normal sinus rhythm, but some develop atrial fibrillation, generally with a reduced ventricular rate. (3) In refractory cases, cardiosuppression may be affected by a pacemaker inserted into the atria or ventricles (usually more efficacious).

Prophylaxis Between Attacks. If the paroxysms tend to recur frequently, the following drug regimen often helps to prevent attacks: (1) digitalization may be induced and followed by a maintenance dose, which may be continued for months; (2) procaine amide, 0.25 to 0.5 gm., four times daily; or (3) quinidine sulfate, 0.2 gm., four to five times daily. In some subjects, such therapy may not suffice to stop recurrent attacks.

In patients in whom overactive sympathetic tone is considered to be a factor in precipitating attacks, propranolol is indicated in an initial dose of 10 mg., three to four times daily, and may be increased to 20 mg., four times daily. In refractory patients, particularly in the group of hyperreactors, we have been able to stop repeated episodes by the use of methimazole (Tapazole).

Psychotherapy. The life situations and emotional state of the patient are significant factors in the precipitation of episodes of paroxysmal atrial tachycardia. These are important aspects to be considered in therapy.

PROGNOSIS

The prognosis of paroxysmal atrial tachycardia is usually good insofar as individual attacks are concerned. The prognosis is less favorable in the following situations: (a) in a long continued paroxysm; (b) when severe myocardial damage is present; (c) in those infrequent instances in which the attacks recur repeatedly in spite of therapy, e.g., those associated with the W-P-W syndrome; and (d) when the attacks are accompanied by precordial pain or cardiac collapse and in association with acute or chronic myocardial infarction.

PAROXYSMAL ATRIAL TACHYCARDIA WITH A-V HEART BLOCK (PAT WITH BLOCK)

General Considerations. Paroxysmal atrial tachycardia with A-V block (PAT with block) is an important arrhythmia. Prompt diagnosis is essential because of its therapeutic and prognostic implications.

Incidence and Etiology. Atrial tachycardia with block is generally considered uncommon, occurring only one-sixth to one-third as frequently as the common type of PAT (El-Sharif, 1970; Freiermuth and Jick, 1958).

The following etiologic factors are observed: (1) digitalis intoxication; (b) digitalis administration in nontoxic doses; (3) hypopotassemia; (4) coronary artery disease, hypertension, or myocardial infarction (Mark and Shaw, 1969); (5) cor pulmonale; and (6) occasionally, certain drugs other than digitalis (e.g., quinidine and isoproterenol).

Mechanism. PAT with block is due to a unifocal atrial pacemaker beating at a rapid rate. Intracardiac records have shown that the site of stimulation, at least in some cases, is located in the right atrium near the sinus node and spreads from above downward. The A-V block has been attributed to the following factors: (a) *the rapid atrial rate;* and (b) *the direct and vagal effect of digitalis on the A-V node, resulting in the conduction delay.* Hypopotassemia would tend to increase A-V block. The first factor may be the more important, since even in the normal heart, an increase in the atrial rate by electrical stimulation predisposes (in the absence of digitalis effects) to the development of A-V heart block (Fig. 9–5).

Symptoms and Signs. PAT with block is usually observed in relatively ill patients. An aggravation of the clinical state characterized by the appearance or worsening of congestive failure and by cardiac or gastrointestinal evidence of digitalis toxicity usually occurs following the occurrence of PAT with block. Often, its occurrence may be precipitated by conditions leading to potassium depletion, e.g., anorexia, vomiting, diarrhea, or administration of powerful potassium-wasting diuretics.

The ventricular rate in PAT usually ranges from 140 to 180 per minute; however, rates of 100 to 120 per minute have been observed. The rhythm may be regular; however, a regular rhythm may be interrupted by varying periods of irregularity due to an increase in or a variation in A-V conduction (Fig. 9–6).

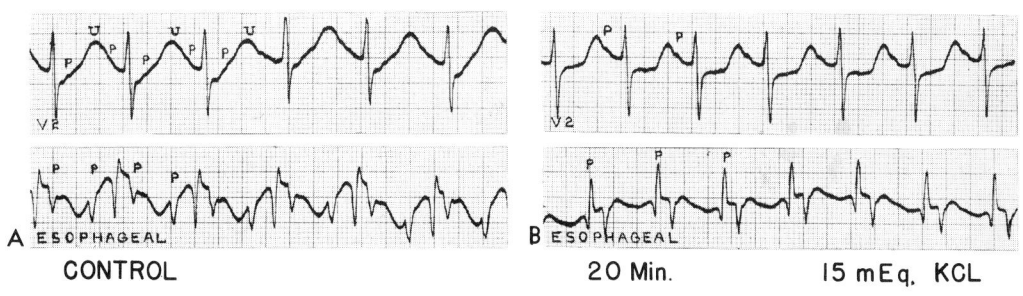

Figure 9–5. Paroxysmal atrial tachycardia with 2:1 A-V heart block due to hypopotassemia (no digitalis medication). Electrocardiogram of a 34-year-old woman with a clinical diagnosis of epilepsy. There was no underlying heart disease or history of digitalis medication, but the patient had intractable vomiting and the serum potassium level was 1.0 mEq./L.

(A) The upper strip of the control tracing shows a hypopotassemic pattern and barely visible P waves. In the esophageal lead, the P waves established the diagnosis of an atrial tachycardia with 2:1 A-V block.

(B) Following 15 mEq. of potassium, the atrial tachycardia with block has disappeared, although with this amount of potassium the hypopotassemic pattern remains. The administration of a total of 11 gm. of potassium chloride in 48 hours resulted in a return of the electrocardiogram to a normal pattern. (From Bettinger, Surawicz, Bryfogle, Anderson, and Bellet: Amer. J. Med., 21:521, 1956.)

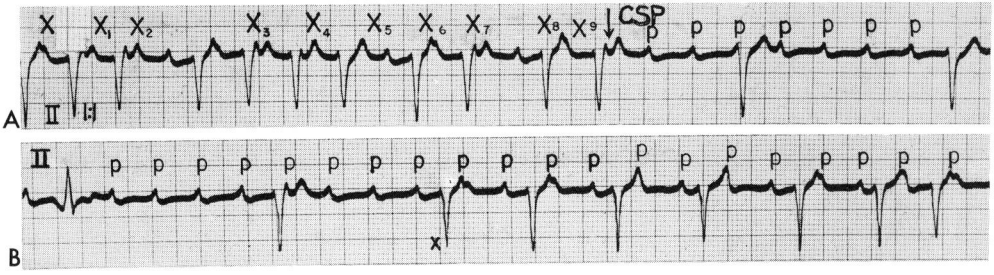

Figure 9-6. Paroxysmal atrial tachycardia with varying degrees of A-V heart block. Complete A-V heart block occurs transiently following carotid sinus pressure.

(A) Paroxysmal atrial tachycardia. The atrial rate is 167 per minute; the ventricular rate varies depending upon the degree of A-V heart block. In cycles X and X_1, the ventricular rate is 167 per minute (i.e., 1:1 response); in cycle X_2, 2:1 A-V block is present; cycles X_3, X_4, and X_6 manifest a 1:1 response; X_5 is 2:1; X_7 is 2:1; X_8 is 1:1; and X_9 is 1:1. Following carotid sinus pressure (at arrow), a transient complete A-V heart block can be observed; the atrial rate is unaffected.

(B) Shows paroxysmal atrial tachycardia with varying degrees of A-V block. The first QRS in the record is probably an escape beat.

Diagnosis. The diagnosis may be suggested by the presence of the aforementioned symptoms and signs; however, the final diagnosis depends upon the electrocardiogram; in the presence of 1:1 conduction, carotid sinus pressure may occasionally aid in establishing the diagnosis.

This arrhythmia manifests the following characteristics: (1) The P complexes resemble those of normal S-A origin since the ectopic site is usually located close to the S-A node; however, it occasionally originates close to the A-V junction, in which case the P waves may be abnormal in morphology. (2) An isoelectric baseline is present between the P waves. (3) The atrial rate is regular and ranges from 150 to 250 per minute; however, in 75 per cent of the episodes it is less than 190 per minute. The lowest reported atrial rate in PAT with block is 106 per minute (Lown et al., 1960). (4) Occasionally, the atrial rhythm may be irregular and an analysis may demonstrate cycle lengths that are multiples of a basic interval suggesting the presence of an exit block. (5) The degree of block may vary from 2:1 with occasional periods of 1:1 response to a Wenckebach type. (6) The degree of A-V block usually can be increased by carotid sinus pressure (Fig. 9-7).

The differential diagnosis includes the following: (1) *Sinus tachycardia* may be simulated when the ectopic pacemaker rate is slow (110 to 140 per minute) or in the presence of a 2:1 A-V heart block when the non-conducted P wave is superimposed on the succeeding T wave. (2) *Paroxysmal atrial tachycardia* of the common type may be diagnosed when the P-R intervals are prolonged. However, the heart rate in PAT usually exceeds 140 per minute; carotid sinus pressure, if successful, converts the tachycardia to a normal sinus rhythm. (3) *Junctional tachycardia* may be suggested in the absence of discernible P waves or when P waves are conducted retrograde from the A-V junction. (4) *Atrial flutter* is frequently diagnosed in the presence of 2:1 A-V heart block, particularly when the atrial rate ranges from 200 to 250 per minute.

The diagnosis in a puzzling case may often be clarified by the use of the following procedures: carotid sinus pressure, V_3R leads in the third and fourth interspaces, and the esophageal lead.

Treatment. The treatment depends upon the underlying clinical state and, in particular, the underlying cause of the PAT with block. In the presence of digitalis toxicity, administration of

PAROXYSMAL ATRIAL TACHYCARDIA (PAT)

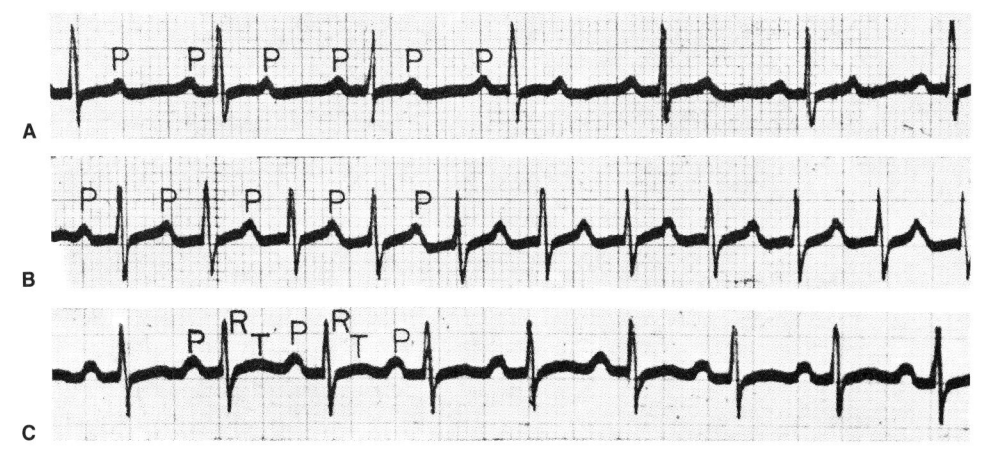

Figure 9-7. Paroxysmal atrial tachycardia with 2:1 A-V block, conversion to normal sinus rhythm with potassium.

(*A*) Shows an atrial rate of 184 per minute and a ventricular rate of 92 per minute (2:1 A-V heart block).

(*B*) Note that the ventricular rate has increased to 160 per minute. The response is now 1:1 with a prolonged P-R interval, 0.21 second (effect of administration of potassium chloride).

(*C*) Note the return to sinus rhythm with a ventricular rate of 130 per minute; the P-R interval now measures 0.18 second (after 22 mEq. of potassium has been infused in 36 minutes). (From Bettinger, Surawicz, Bryfogle, Anderson, and Bellet: Amer. J. Med., *21*:521, 1956.)

the drug should be stopped. Since diuretic therapy may be an additional factor, this should also be discontinued. Before giving potassium, one should obtain the serum potassium level, since the value may be either low, normal, or elevated. Elevation could be the result of acidosis, dehydration, and a shock-like state. If the serum potassium is low, potassium may be cautiously infused, preferably intravenously under continuous electrocardiographic monitoring. If toxic effects do occur with this procedure, the potassium infusion may be stopped immediately, or one may administer 50 per cent glucose or molar sodium lactate to reverse the cardiotoxicity (Fig. 34-8). If digitalis toxicity is not the cause of the arrhythmia and hypopotassemia is not present, digitalis may be given as a therapeutic measure (Morgan and Breneman, 1962).

Other drugs, such as procaine amide and quinidine, may be used. Combined use of potassium with procaine amide often facilitates the reversion, and smaller amounts of each drug are required when the two are used together. Magnesium sulfate has been used and has been instrumental in stopping the episodes in occasional cases.

Electric countershock has been employed successfully in patients suffering PAT with block (Mark and Shaw, 1969). Care should be taken in using this procedure with patients who manifest digitalis toxicity (see p. 385).

Prognosis. The prognosis generally depends on the etiology, rapid recognition of the arrhythmia, and prompt therapy. Because PAT with block is usually accompanied by a serious form of heart disease, the prognosis is often poor. The outlook is more favorable in those cases that are associated with transient and correctable types of electrolyte disturbances (e.g., hypopotassemia precipitated by vomiting or diarrhea) and when digitalis toxicity is the chief factor, if these conditions are recognized and the appropriate therapy instituted promptly. The mortality ranges from 28 per cent (Freiermuth and Jick, 1958; Lown et al., 1960) to 58 per cent (Lown et al., 1960).

References

Barker, P. S., Wilson, F. N., Johnston, F. D., and Wishart, S. W.: Auricular paroxysmal tachycardia with auriculoventricular block. Amer. Heart J., 25:765, 1943.

Barold, S. S., Linhart, J. W., Samet, P., and Lister, J. W.: Supraventricular tachycardia initiated and terminated by a single electrical stimulus. Amer. J. Cardiol., 24:37, 1969.

Barrow, J. G.: Treatment of paroxysmal supraventricular tachycardia with lanatoside C. Ann. Intern. Med., 32:116, 1950.

Befeler, B., Hildner, F. J., Javier, R. P., Cohen, L. S., and Samet, P.: Cardiovascular dynamics during coronary sinus right atrial and right ventricular pacing. Amer. Heart J., 81:372, 1971.

Bellet, S., Zeeman, S. E., and Hirsch, S. A.: Intramuscular use of Pronestyl. Amer. J. Med., 13:145, 1952.

Berry, K., Garlett, E. L., Bellet, S., and Gefter, W. I.: Use of Pronestyl in treatment of ectopic rhythms. Amer. J. Med., 11:431, 1951.

Bjerkelund, C., and Orning, O. M.: An evaluation of DC shock treatment of atrial arrhythmias. Acta Med. Scand., 184:481, 1968.

Bouveret, L.: De la Tachycardie Essentielle Paroxystique. Rev. Med. (Paris), 9:755, 837, 1889.

Dolara, A., and Possi, L.: Persistent supraventricular tachycardia. Amer. J. Cardiol., 16:449, 1965.

Durrer, D., Schoo, L., Schuilenburg, R. M., and Wellens, H. J. J.: Role of premature beats in the initiation and termination of supraventricular tachycardia in the Wolff-Parkinson-White syndrome. Circulation, 36:644, 1967.

El-Sharif, N.: Supraventricular tachycardia with A-V block. Brit. Heart J., 32:46, 1970.

Freiermuth, L. J., and Jick, S.: Paroxysmal tachycardia with atrioventricular block. Amer. J. Cardiol., 1:584, 1958.

Furman, R. H., and Geigen, A. J.: Use of cholinergic drugs in supraventricular tachycardia. JAMA, 149:269, 1952.

Goldreyer, B. N., Bigger, J. T., Jr., and Heissenbuttel, R.: Reentrant supraventricular tachycardia. Clin. Res., 17:243, 1969.

Han, J.: The mechanism of paroxysmal atrial tachycardia. Amer. J. Cardiol., 26:329, 1970.

Hellerstein, H. K., Levine, B., and Feil, H.: Electrocardiographic changes following carotid sinus stimulation in paroxysmal ventricular tachycardia. J. Lab. Clin. Med., 38:820, 1951.

Lister, J. W., et al.: Rapid atrial stimulation for treatment of supraventricular tachycardias. Circulation, 37–38:VI-130, 1968.

Lown, B., Vassaux, C., Hood, W. B., Jr., Fakhro, A. M., Kaplinsky, E., and Roberge, G.: Unresolved problems in coronary care. Amer. J. Cardiol., 20:494, 1967.

Lown, B., Wyatt, N. F., and Levine, H. D.: Paroxysmal atrial tachycardia with block. Circulation, 21:129, 1960.

McIntosh, H. D., and Morris, J. J., Jr.: The hemodynamic consequences of arrhythmias. Prog. Cardiov. Dis., 8:330, 1966.

Mark, H., and Shaw, R.: Non-digitalis-induced paroxysmal atrial tachycardia with block. I. Management with cardioversion. J. Electrocardiol., 2:171, 1969.

Meltzer, L. E., and Kitchell, J.: The incidence of arrhythmias associated with acute myocardial infarction. Prog. Cardiov. Dis., 9:50, 1966.

Mendez, C., and Moe, G. K.: Demonstration of a dual A-V nodal conduction system in the isolated rabbit heart. Circ. Res., 19:378, 1966.

Montella, S.: Phasic respiratory paroxysmal atrial tachycardia. Amer. J. Cardiol., 7:613, 1961.

Morgan, W., and Breneman, G.: Atrial tachycardia with block treated with digitalis. Circulation, 25:787, 1962.

Saunders, D. E., Jr., and Ord, J. W.: The hemodynamic effects of paroxysmal supraventricular tachycardia in patients with the Wolff-Parkinson-White syndrome. Amer. J. Cardiol., 9:223, 1962.

Sowton, E., et al.: Long-term control of intractable supraventricular tachycardia by ventricular pacing. Brit. Heart J., 31:700, 1969.

Vassaux, C., and Lown, B.: Cardioversion of supraventricular tachycardias. Circulation, 39:791, 1969.

Wright, J. S., Fabian, J., and Epstein, E. J.: Immediate effect on cardiac output of reversion to sinus rhythm from rapid arrhythmias. Brit. Med. J., 3:315, 1970.

Chapter 10 A-V Heart Block

GENERAL CONSIDERATIONS
TYPES OF A-V HEART BLOCK
  First Degree A-V Heart Block (Partial)
  Second Degree A-V Heart Block
  Third Degree Heart Block (Complete)
PHYSIOLOGIC AND ELECTROPHYSIO-
  LOGIC ASPECTS
  His Bundle Recordings
    First Degree A-V Block
    Second Degree A-V Block
      Wenckebach or Mobitz Type I
      Mobitz Type II
    Third Degree A-V Block
    Value of His Bundle Recordings
  Summary

PARTIAL A-V HEART BLOCK

ETIOLOGY
PATHOLOGY
PHYSIOLOGIC EFFECTS
SYMPTOMS AND SIGNS
ELECTROCARDIOGRAM
  First Degree A-V Heart Block
  Second Degree A-V Heart Block
    Wenckebach Type (Mobitz Type I)
    Mobitz Type II
TREATMENT
PROGNOSIS

COMPLETE A-V HEART BLOCK

ETIOLOGY
HEMODYNAMICS
  Congenital Complete A-V Heart Block
  Acquired Complete A-V Heart Block
CLINICAL FEATURES OF ACQUIRED
  COMPLETE A-V HEART BLOCK
TYPES OF COMPLETE A-V HEART
  BLOCK
ELECTROCARDIOGRAM
  Retrograde Conduction
  The P-P Intervals
  Types of Ventricular Complexes
  Ventricular Rate and Rhythm
  Association with Other Arrhythmias
PATTERNS OF COMPLETE A-V HEART
  BLOCK (UNIFASCICULAR, BIFASCICU-
  LAR, AND TRIFASCICULAR)
  Anatomy
  Classification of Fascicular Blocks
DIAGNOSIS AND DIFFERENTIAL
  DIAGNOSIS
TREATMENT
  Drugs
  Artificial Pacemakers
PROGNOSIS

STOKES-ADAMS SEIZURES

CLINICAL FEATURES
THERAPY
PROGNOSIS

GENERAL CONSIDERATIONS

There have been important recent developments in our knowledge of the physiology of the A-V conduction system and in the pathogenesis, hemodynamics, and therapy of complete A-V heart block and Stokes-Adams seizures. The term "A-V heart block" refers to disturbances occurring in the A-V conduction system which includes the A-V junction, the bundle of His, or the region even lower in the ventricular ramifications of the Purkinje fibers.

Normally, the impulse is conducted from the atria to the ventricles through a narrow neuromuscular structure, the A-V junction. The period required for the cardiac impulse to pass from the S-A node to the ventricles (the P-R interval of the electrocardiogram) usually ranges from 0.12 to 0.21 second. The P-R interval, to some degree, depends upon the cardiac rate. A formula has been presented for predicting this interval for various cycle lengths in normal hearts (Bazett, 1920). Most of this interval is occupied not by propagation through the atrial pathways, where conduction is relatively rapid, but through the A-V junction, where the transmission is much slower. The term "A-V heart block" is applied to the abnormal mechanism whereby the atrial impulse is delayed or completely fails to reach the ventricle.

TYPES OF A-V HEART BLOCK

A-V heart block may be divided into two main types — partial and complete — and may be temporary, intermittent, or permanent. Usually, the degree of block increases with age.

First Degree A-V Heart Block (Partial A-V Heart Block). In adults with a normal heart rate, the first stage of A-V heart block is said to occur when the conduction time (the P-R interval) exceeds 0.21 second (Fig. 10–1). Normal conduction time may vary in children and at high rates. As the block becomes progressively more severe, the conduction time is further prolonged; however, no dropped beats occur at this stage.

Second Degree A-V Heart Block. Second degree A-V heart block is characterized by failure of some, but not all, atrial impulses to reach the ventricles in a heart in which the ventricles are ordinarily controlled by the sinus pacemaker. Two types are observed to occur: (1) *Wenckebach type, Mobitz Type I*, the common type, with progressive prolongation of the P-R interval preceding the dropped ventricular beat; and (2) *Mobitz Type II*, a less common type in which the "dropped" ventricular systole occurs without any previous prolongation of the P-R interval. In its more advanced form, several consecutive atrial impulses are blocked, giving rise to a high degree of partial block and to intermittent periods of prolonged ventricular asystole, which must be differentiated from sinus arrest and other conditions that also give rise to the same effect. Progressive prolongation of the P-R interval followed by a dropped ventricular beat is known as the "Wenckebach phenomenon" or "Mobitz Type I" heart block. The form with constant P-R intervals but sudden dropped beats is known as the "Mobitz Type II" type of A-V heart block.

Third Degree Heart Block (Complete A-V Heart Block). In complete A-V heart block, the atria beat regularly at a rate of 70 to 80 beats per minute in response to the sinus pacemaker. However, the ventricles also beat regularly, usually at 20 to 40 beats per minute in response to their pacemaker situated in the lower portion of the A-V junction, the bundle of His, or the upper portion of the interventricular septum. These two pacemakers function entirely independently of

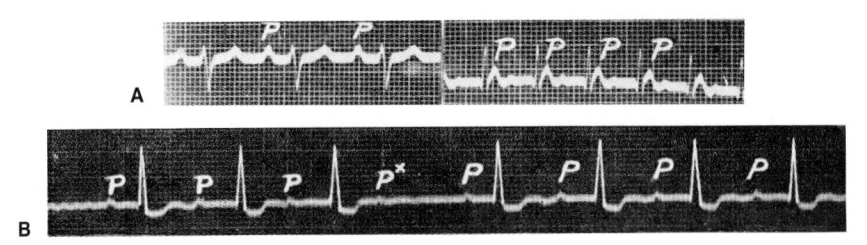

Figure 10–1. Various types of partial A-V heart block.
(A) Initial strip shows prolongation of the P-R interval, which measures 0.22 second. Second strip: note the P-R interval prolongation with the tachycardia (ventricular rate, 150 per minute). Note that the P wave of the prolonged P-R interval is situated immediately following the preceding QRS complex between the QRS and T wave. This P wave controls the following QRS complex.
(B) Shows progressive prolongation of P-R interval until a dropped beat is observed at Px (Wenckebach phenomenon). The same sequence is repeated in the latter part of the tracing.

each other. During the evolution of complete A-V block, occasional atrial impulses may be transmitted through the A-V junction to produce an effective ventricular beat (incomplete form of complete heart block). In complete A-V heart block, the atrial rate is subject to normal autonomic regulation, while the ventricular rate (except for the congenital type) is either totally unaffected or occasionally accelerated only by profound sympathetic discharge.

The association of atrial flutter and atrial fibrillation with complete A-V heart block is discussed on page 129.

PHYSIOLOGIC AND ELECTROPHYSIOLOGIC ASPECTS

His Bundle Recordings. (See also Chapter 2.) Recent studies including the micro-electrode technique and particularly His bundle recordings obtained in the human subject have been instrumental in changing many of our concepts relative to the sites of origin and disease states involved in the various types of A-V heart block, partial or complete (Damato et al., 1969; Narula et al., 1971; Rosen, 1971).

The P-R interval in standard leads represents the total transmission time from the S-A node, through the atria, A-V node, bundle of His to the onset of ventricular activation (Fig. 2–5). However, the standard electrocardiogram fails to give information relative to the exact site of the region or regions involved, i.e., the P-H and H-Q sectors.

His bundle recordings enable division of the P-R into two main subdivisions: (1) *P-H (80–140 msec.)*, from the beginning of atrial depolarization (P wave) to His bundle depolarization. It measures intra-atrial and A-V conduction time; and (2) *H-Q (35–55 msec.)*, from His depolarization to the onset of ventricular activation (initial deflection of QRS) and is a measure from the distal His and bundle branches (Figs. 10–2, 10–3). Data obtained from the His bundle electrogram help to establish the site of block and may have a bearing on the prognosis and treatment.

First Degree A-V Block. In the absence of bundle branch block, first degree A-V heart block signifies an increase in the P-H interval. First degree A-V block with bundle branch block usually signifies prolongation of the P-H and H-Q intervals.

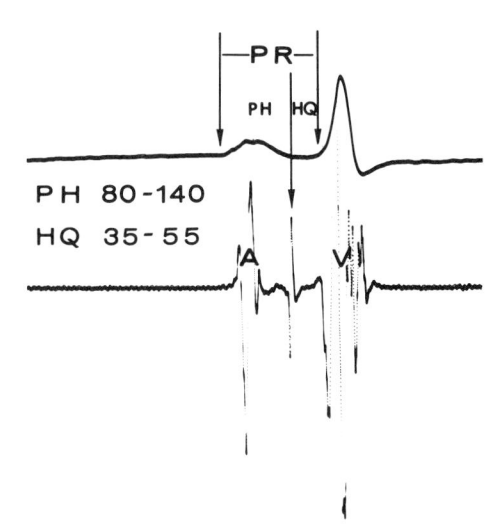

Figure 10–2. Measurement of intervals in the His bundle electrogram. Simultaneous electrocardiogram (top tracing) and His bundle electrogram (bottom tracing) are shown. The P-R interval is from the onset of the P wave (first arrow) to the onset of the QRS (third arrow). The His bundle electrogram (second arrow) occurs between the atrial (A) and ventricular (V) electrograms. The P-R interval can thus be subdivided into P-H and H-Q subintervals. The normal ranges of P-H and H-Q are given in msec. (From Rosen, K. M.: Circulation, 43:961, 1971.)

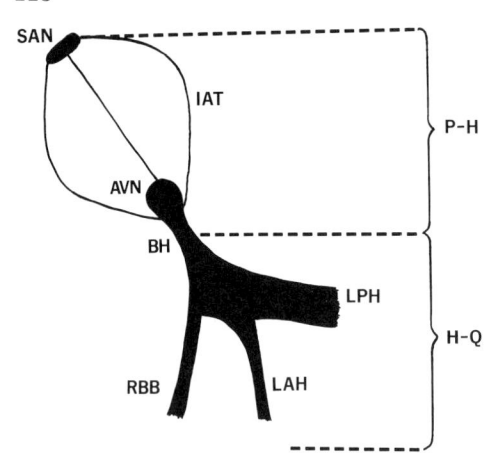

Figure 10-3. Diagrammatic representation of the cardiac conduction system illustrating the intervals which are measured in the His bundle electrogram (compare with Fig. 10-2). SAN: sinoatrial node; IAT: intra-atrial tracts; AVN: atrioventricular node; BH: bundle of His; LPH: left posterior hemibranch; LAH: left anterior hemibranch; RBB: right bundle branch.

Second Degree A-V Block

WENCKEBACH OR MOBITZ TYPE I HEART BLOCK. This type of second degree heart block may manifest several different and distinct alterations in the His bundle electrogram depending upon the site of delay: (1) Progressive prolongation of the A-H interval until a beat is dropped between the A and B-H deflections indicates delay in the A-V node. In dropped beats the A wave is not followed by either a B-H or V deflection. (2) Block occurring in the distal bundle of His is recorded as a dropped beat between the B-H and V deflections following progressive prolongation of the H-V interval with a normal QRS complex.

MOBITZ TYPE II A-V HEART BLOCK. In this type of A-V heart block, the His bundle electrogram shows that the block is represented by a dropped beat (usually) distal to the B-H deflection (the A-H and H-V intervals remain constant).

Third Degree A-V Heart Block. Third degree A-V heart block may be due to block proximal to, involving, or distal to the bundle of His. Each type represents different electrocardiographic patterns depending on the site of A-V disturbance or block.

Value of Atrial Pacing in Studying Suspected A-V Block. Atrial pacing stresses A-V conduction, thereby eliciting A-V conduction disturbances at increased pacing rates in patients with incipient disturbances of the A-V conduction system which are not demonstrable at normal rates. It increases the A-H and usually manifests no effect on the H-Q interval. With premature atrial stimulation, there is prolongation of the A-H and to a lesser degree the H-Q, the segment which may result in QRS widening (aberration). In the development of second degree block proximal to the His bundle, at a pacing rate of 130 per minute or lower, A-V nodal dysfunction is suggested. Development of second degree A-V block distal to the bundle of His at any heart rate below 200 per minute suggests disease of the His-Purkinje system.

Value of His Bundle Recordings. As a result of clinical experience and correlation with surface electrocardiograms, His bundle recordings have been found of value in the following situations: (1) By use of atrial pacing, it helps in the evaluation of patients who are suspected of having Stokes-Adams attacks but have normal sinus rhythm. (2) In second degree A-V block, it helps to determine the site of block—proximal or distal to the Bundle of His Type I proximal to the His-Purkinje system, and Type II distal to the bundle of His (some exceptions are noted); the latter, which is of more serious prognostic importance, merits close observation and has a bearing on the prognosis and treatment. (3) In complete A-V heart block, it helps to determine the site of block: (a) block distal to the B-H (Bundle of His) is most common; (b) block in the B-H; and (c) block proximal to the B-H is noted especially in the congenital type. In acute coronary occlusion with inferior infarction, block normally occurs proximal to the B-H, suggesting A-V nodal dysfunction. In anterior infarction, block often appears distal to the B-H and indicates involvement of the interventricular septum or bundle branches. (4) This method often demonstrates the mechanism responsible for the W-P-W. (With atrial pacing there is failure of prolongation of the P-R while the P-H lengthens and the H potential is often noted in the QRS.) (5) It is useful in the interpretation of complex arrhythmias; recording of the H potential is of help in the differential diagnosis of supra- and ventricular tachyarrhythmias. (6) It shows the presence of increased His bundle depolarizations because of antegrade and retrograde block.

The preceding data is quite helpful in understanding cardiac conduction in health and disease.

Summary. The precise localization of the site of delay in the various types of A-V heart block is of considerable interest not only insofar as it represents electrophysiologic data obtained from the human subject, but also because of its therapeutic and prognostic implications. However, at present, the method is limited by its availability to those clinics in which it is commonly employed. The percentage of cases in which the findings would significantly affect the therapy of a given patient (although important in the individual case) would appear to be somewhat limited.

PARTIAL A-V HEART BLOCK

In a study of 6732 electrocardiograms taken on 4264 patients, Logue and Hanson (1944) observed 100 instances (1.5 per cent) of first degree heart block, with P-R intervals of 0.22 second or longer.

ETIOLOGY

In children, A-V heart block is due most often to congenital defects or infection, particularly rheumatic fever and diphtheria. In older patients and adults, infections, digitalis toxicity, and degenerative states (coronary artery disease and primary fibrosis of the conducting system) become the predominant causes. The etiology of complete (third degree) heart block is discussed later (p. 124). Clinical, partial (first and second degree) heart block has been observed to result from the following conditions: (a) *Infections:* in the acute phase of rheumatic fever or diphtheria, heart block may occur or may be postponed until later in life; infections accompanied by myocarditis (e.g., measles, mumps, typhus, acute infectious mononucleosis, and upper respiratory and various other viral infections). These infections usually result in low grades of A-V heart block with a return to normal rhythm after the infection subsides. (b) *Congenital cardiac anomalies* (see under *complete heart block,* p. 262); (c) *Vagal stimulation* as a result of carotid sinus pressure, and vagal reflexes originating in the gastrointestinal tract or other viscera. These may be enhanced in certain disease states, e.g., influenza, and with the use of certain drugs, particularly digitalis. (d) *Degenerative conditions:* Degenerative states, particularly coronary artery disease and changes localized to the A-V conduction system resulting in isolated fibrotic changes, are the most common causes of the A-V heart block in older patients. A-V heart block, partial or complete, occurs not infrequently in acute myocardial infarction. (e) *Hypoxia* may produce heart block by a depressant effect on the A-V junction, which is extremely sensitive to a lack of oxygen, or by increasing vagal sensitivity. (f) *Certain drugs:* Digitalis (see p. 383). Quinidine and procaine amide produce slight P-R interval prolongation as a result of a direct effect on the A-V junction. Propranolol and other beta-blocking agents depress A-V conduction (see p. 365) and (g) *P-R prolongation in presumably normal subjects:* Occasionally, P-R prolongation occurs in the absence of any clinically demonstrable heart disease or other conditions known to produce heart block. In a survey of 67,375 apparently healthy male pilots whose ages ranged from 17 to 54 years, 350 cases of first degree A-V heart block were observed (P-R, 0.21 to 0.39 sec.), an incidence of 5.2 per thousand (Johnsson et al., 1959). A significant relationship between age and the duration of the P-R interval was noted in this study.

PATHOLOGY

The pathology of partial A-V heart block has not been adequately investigated since most studies have been performed in complete A-V heart block. It is probable that less severe stages of the same pathologic processes that underlie complete A-V block may also cause partial A-V heart block. These include: (a) *degenerative states,* including ischemic coronary artery disease and the so-called "isolated fibrosis" of the conduction system; (b) *inflammatory conditions,* including rheumatic fever, acute infections, and all forms of myocarditis; and (c) *congenital anomalies.*

PHYSIOLOGIC EFFECTS

An increase in sympathetic tone and a reciprocal decrease of vagal tone appear to be responsible for the decrease in the P-R interval which occurs when both normal subjects and patients with A-V heart block stand up.

In partial A-V heart block, the P-R interval is usually decreased immediately after exercise; however, exercise may lead to a higher degree of block in certain patients with partial A-V heart block. These findings suggest that the transient vagal effects that occur in the postexercise period may reveal a latent disturbance in A-V conduction (Fig. 10–4).

SYMPTOMS AND SIGNS

The symptoms of partial A-V heart block are largely influenced by the underlying clinical state; however, unless the heart rate is slow, there are few symptoms due to the heart block itself. The important symptoms in higher grades of partial and complete

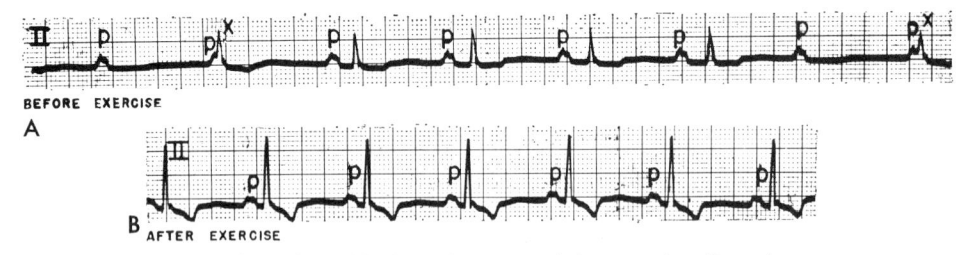

Figure 10–4. Partial A-V heart block (Mobitz type II) showing the effect of exercise in restoring normal sinus rhythm with normal P-R.

(A) Shows normal sinus rhythm with prolonged P-R (0.26 second) and second degree A-V heart block (Mobitz type II). Junctional escapes are present in the first and last QRS complexes, marked X. Note constant P-R of 0.26 second and the sudden pause in the first cycle and the last cycle without alteration in the preceding P-R.

(B) After exercise, the P-R interval is back to normal (0.18 second) and all evidence of A-V heart block has disappeared.

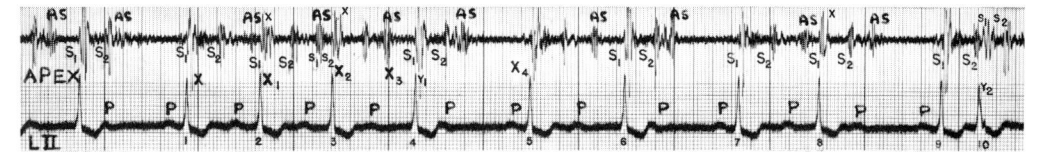

Figure 10–5. Variations in the intensity of the first heart sound occurring in the presence of partial A-V heart block with Wenckebach phenomenon. The first heart sound following QRS_1 with a relatively normal P-R interval shows a moderate amplitude; QRS_2, with a slightly prolonged P-R interval, shows a diminished amplitude; QRS_3, with an increased P-R interval, shows a diminution in S_1. However, QRS_4 with a long P-R interval shows considerable amplitude of the first heart sound. QRS_5, with a normal P-R interval following a long pause, shows a moderate amplitude of S_1; however, QRS_6, with a longer P-R interval, also shows an increased amplitude of S_1. QRS_7 shows a moderate amplitude at S_1. A longer P-R interval with QRS_8 shows a diminished amplitude at S_1. QRS_9, following a long pause and a short P-R interval, shows an increased amplitude of S_1. The premature beats of QRS_{10} (Y_2) is followed by a moderate amplitude of S_1 and S_2.

In summary, therefore, it would appear that the amplitude of S_1 bears a general relationship to the preceding P-R interval length; this relationship is not absolute and depends also, to some degree, on the preceding cycle length.

A-V heart block are giddiness, fainting, and temporary loss of consciousness, with or without convulsive seizures. These manifestations of cerebral hypoxia occur when the brain fails to receive blood for a period of three to nine seconds or longer because of ventricular fibrillation or ventricular asystole.

Auscultation. It is well known that the intensity of the first heart sound varies with the relationship of atrial to ventricular contraction: with a short P-R interval, the first heart sounds tend to be loud, and with a moderately prolonged P-R interval, the first heart sound is characteristically diminished in intensity (Fig. 10–5).

Partial A-V heart block is always present with atrial fibrillation and almost always with atrial flutter and not infrequently with paroxysmal atrial tachycardia. It is often present in association with sinoatrial block and following digitalis therapy of various arrhythmias.

The auscultatory phenomena in A-V heart block are to be differentiated from those of premature beats, S-A block, sinus arrhythmia, sinus bradycardia, and A-V junctional rhythm. A 3:2 A-V heart block may simulate bigeminal rhythm. The diagnosis is clearly established by the electrocardiogram.

ELECTROCARDIOGRAM

First Degree A-V Heart Block. The electrocardiogram clearly shows regularly recurring, normally shaped P waves with P-R intervals which are prolonged beyond 0.21 second in adults and beyond 0.18 second in children. Although the P-R interval may vary considerably in length, at times it may be almost as long as a normal cycle length (0.8 second or longer with conducted beats). First degree A-V heart block is usually associated with a regular rhythm; dropped beats are not encountered.

Second Degree A-V Heart Block

Wenckebach Type (Mobitz Type I). This pattern of A-V heart block is characterized by progressive lengthening of the P-R interval until a point is reached at which no ventricular complex follows the P wave. There is, therefore, the appearance of progressively shorter cycles (despite the lengthening P-R interval) separated by a long cycle; the long cycle is less than the sum of the two short cycles preceding it. (If this process is pro-

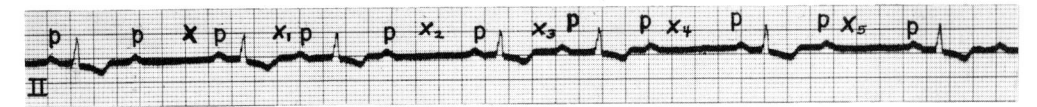

Figure 10-6. Partial A-V heart block with Wenckebach periods (3:2 alternating with 2:1 A-V block). Note the presence of 2:1 A-V heart block in the first cycle (X), followed by a period of 1:1 response with a prolonged P-R interval (X_1), followed again by 2:1 A-V heart block in the third cycle (X_2), followed by a period of 1:1 response in the fourth cycle (X_3). In the last two cycles 2:1 A-V heart block persists (X_4 and X_5). Note the relatively shorter P-R interval preceding the QRS complex with a long cycle as compared to the more prolonged P-R interval preceding the QRS with a short cycle (see text).

nounced enough, it may cause 2:1 A-V heart block) (Fig. 10-6).

Mobitz Type II. In this situation the P-R interval is fixed, although it may be less than, equal to, or greater than 0.20 second. At intervals, a single ventricular beat is dropped, possibly resulting in a variety of ratios of atrial to ventricular beats (e.g., 3:2, 6:5, 9:8) (Fig. 10-7). Frequently associated with Mobitz Type II A-V heart block is a widening of the QRS complex to 0.12 second or longer. This widening is indicative of the conduction disturbance, discussed previously, in which the sinus impulse is permanently blocked in one bundle branch and intermittently blocked in the other. Furthermore, varying ratios of ventricular response to supraventricular stimuli, such as 3:1 or higher, may in fact result from blockade of the impulse alternately in the A-V junction and the lower conducting system (Watanabe and Dreifus, 1967).

CONCEALED CONDUCTION. Concealed conduction is defined as an incomplete penetration through the A-V junction of a sinus impulse and is recognizable by an unexpected delay or block in the subsequent impulse or the displacement of an ectopic impulse. The concept of concealed conduction was introduced into electrocardiography to explain a lengthening of or change in the refractory period of the atrioventricular conduction system caused either by atrial activity that fails to propagate to the ventricles or by ventricular activity that fails to reach the atria (see Chapter 2).

Langendorf and Pick (1960) have shown that a local conduction delay or complete failure of propagation can occur at the junction of two fibers whose action potentials are different

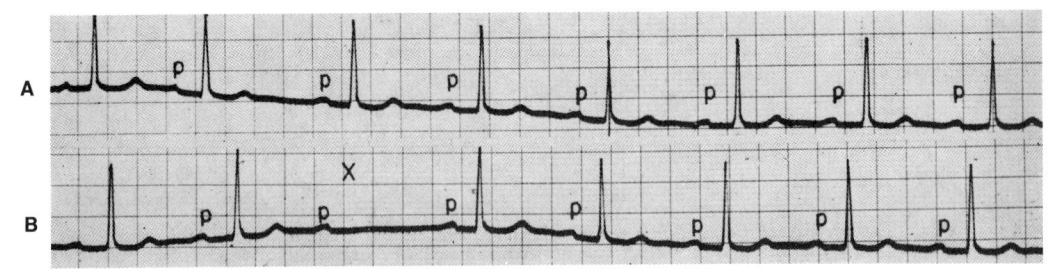

Figure 10-7. Partial A-V heart block: Mobitz type II. *A* and *B* represent a continuous record. Note the presence of a partial A-V heart block with a constant degree of P-R interval prolongation measuring 0.28 second. Slight irregularity in the ventricular rate is due to a sinus arrhythmia. Note the sudden appearance of a 2:1 A-V heart block in cycle X of strip B, without any change in the length of the preceding P-R intervals. The P-R after the A-V block is slightly shorter (0.24 second) than that observed in previous short cycles and this is followed by cycles of P-R prolongation similar to those that preceded the 2:1 A-V heart block. Note narrow QRS width.

in duration. Such disturbances of conduction are observed whenever the propagation of excitation in one fiber precedes complete repolarization of an adjacent fiber. This situation is possible because the cells of the conduction system show a progressively longer refractory period from that of the sinus node to the ventricular terminations of the His-Purkinje system.

TREATMENT

No specific treatment is usually required for minor grades of A-V heart block; the treatment is that of the underlying cause, if ascertained (e.g., rheumatic heart disease or other infections, acute myocardial infarction, and digitalis intoxication). When the A-V heart block follows an acute myocardial infarction, the patient should be monitored and carefully observed in a coronary care unit to note whether further progression occurs.

Drugs Employed in the Therapy of Partial A-V Heart Block. Drugs are usually not indicated in minor grades of A-V heart block. They may be employed in higher grades or when the block is progressive. Attention should initially be focused on the underlying etiology.

The effects of atropine depend upon the dose administered. In full doses (1.0 mg., intravenously), A-V block is notably diminished; however, its use in these cases is limited because the effect is transient. Atropine should therefore be used only when the heart rate is quite slow (20 to 36 per minute).

By increasing cardiac automaticity, isoproterenol will increase the ventricular rate and decrease the degree of A-V block. Like atropine, it is ordinarily not indicated in partial A-V heart block except in cases with very slow rates.

Alkalinizing agents will also increase the heart rate and shorten the P-R interval in A-V heart block. These effects are transient, however. These agents are of particular efficacy in the presence of hypoxia, acidosis, and hyperpotassemia.

In A-V heart block due to digitalis intoxication, therapy consists of discontinuing digitalis medication which usually suffices (see Chapter 34). Since propranolol in full doses may induce or exaggerate A-V heart block as a result of its β-adrenergic blocking action, its administration is usually contraindicated.

PROGNOSIS

The prognosis of partial A-V heart block depends on the degree and underlying etiology and can best be determined by evaluating the heart as a whole. Minor grades of heart block are in themselves not serious; some subjects live for years without notable evidence of cardiac impairment.

Mobitz Type II A-V block is usually associated with serious organic heart disease. This type is particularly dangerous because: (a) it may lead to Stokes-Adams seizures by producing cardiac arrest; and (b) the underlying pathologic process, located relatively low in the A-V conduction system may prevent the occurrence of a junctional escape or an idioventricular rhythm. If and when complete heart block supervenes, even transiently, the resultant ventricular rate is likely to be quite slow (in the range of 25 to 34 beats per minute), unstable, and susceptible to the occurrence of episodes of cardiac arrest.

The prognosis in higher grades of A-V heart block depends on the etiology, symptomatology, degree of progression, and the development of syncopal episodes. The previously unfavorable prognosis of patients with high grades of A-V heart block and syncopal episodes has been improved by the use of artificial pacemakers; the effect of pacemaker therapy on this group is discussed on page 417.

COMPLETE A-V HEART BLOCK

ETIOLOGY

In the general hospital population complete A-V heart block is seen in about 0.5 per cent of the electrocardiograms; however, complete heart block is observed to occur in approximately 7 per cent of patients with myocardial infarction who are studied by continuous electrocardiographic monitoring (Stock and Macken, 1968).

The underlying conditions producing complete A-V heart block may be divided into congenital or acquired. Congenital factors are rare, underlying only 3 to 8 per cent of cases that come to necropsy.

The age of patients when complete A-V heart block was first observed by Penton et al. (1956) varied from 10 to 85 years (averaging 59.2 years), with 85 per cent occurring between 40 and 80 years. The average age at death in 126 fatal cases was 63.2 years.

The pathologic processes responsible for the acquired type of complete heart block may be divided into four categories: (1) degenerative (most common), (2) inflammatory, (3) infiltrative, and (4) traumatic. Both congenital and acquired A-V heart block produce a similar histologic picture—discontinuity of the conducting tissue with replacement by fibrosis and/or calcification (Figs. 10–8, 10–9, 10–10).

Degenerative Processes. This group may be divided into those due to: (a) vascular insufficiency, (b) degeneration of unknown etiology limited to the conduction system, and (c) pressure of an expanding lesion.

Recent evidence suggests that complete A-V heart block is commonly due to fibrosis of the conduction system, either alone or in association with diffuse myocardial fibrosis. "Isolated fibrosis of the conduction system" or "primary heart block" is the most important cause of heart block. Lev (1964) has described "sclerosis of the left side of the cardiac skeleton" due to aging and calcification of the fibrous cardiac skeleton, a pathologic process which appears similar to "primary heart block" (described previously).

Degenerative processes in the con-

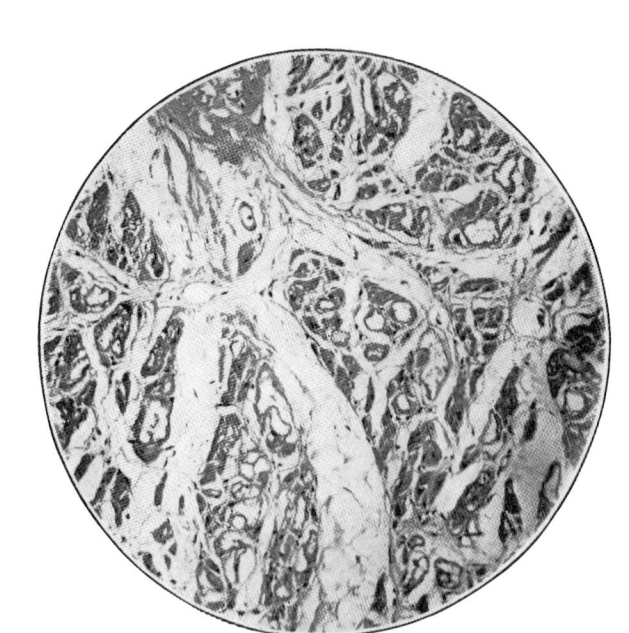

Figure 10–8. Section of A-V junction (×400). This section is representative of those taken throughout the entire A-V junction. Note vacuolization of muscle bundles, probably the result of lipoid degeneration.

A-V HEART BLOCK 125

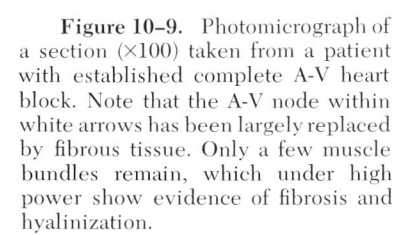

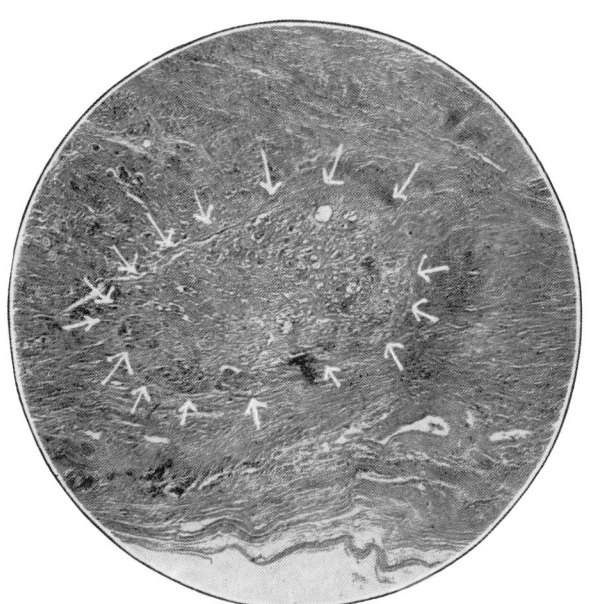

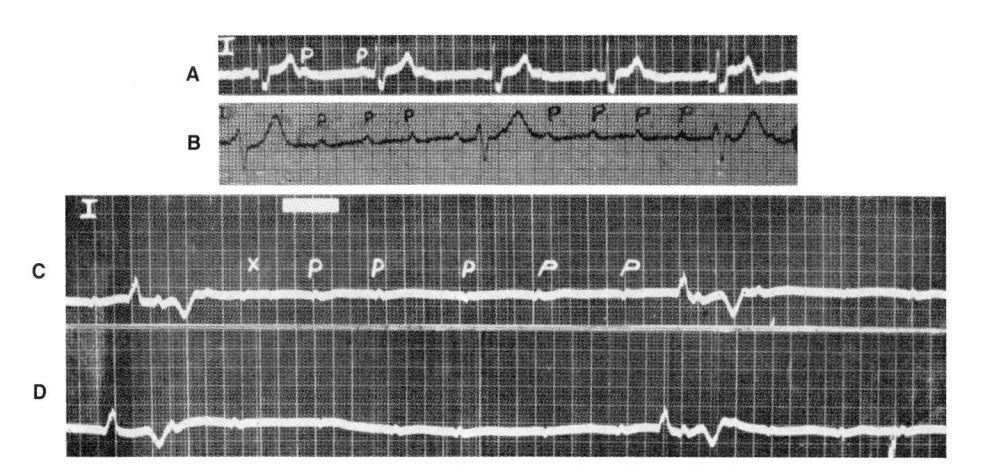

Figure 10-9. Photomicrograph of a section (×100) taken from a patient with established complete A-V heart block. Note that the A-V node within white arrows has been largely replaced by fibrous tissue. Only a few muscle bundles remain, which under high power show evidence of fibrosis and hyalinization.

Figure 10-10. Illustrates progression in the degree of A-V heart block.
(A) 2:1 A-V heart block. The atrial rate is 96 and the ventricular rate is 48 per minute.
(B) Taken one week later, shows a complete A-V heart block. The atria are beating at a rate of 120; the ventricles, at a rate of 23 per minute.
(C) Taken one week after B, shows that the complete A-V heart block is associated with an extremely slow ventricular rate (10 beats per minute) suggesting so-called *block in block*, 2:1 (as compared with the rate of 23 beats per minute in B). Note the varying P-P intervals and varying configuration of P waves, indicating different sites of origin; the two occurring together at X represent atrial premature beats. The patient experienced numerous Stokes-Adams attacks during this period, and eventually succumbed in one of them.
(D) Similar to C. Necropsy revealed a tuberculoma infiltrating the A-V node and the bundle of His.

ducting elements secondary to an expanding lesion may result from: (a) inflammatory expansion of the collagenous extension of the fibrous skeleton of the heart, as in acute rheumatic fever and other less clearly defined disease states; (b) calcific deposits in the interventricular septum, frequently extending out from diseased mitral and aortic rings; (c) calcification of valves; and (d) primary or secondary neoplasm of the heart.

HEMODYNAMICS

Congenital Complete A-V Heart Block. The hemodynamic consequences of most cases of congenital complete heart block are quite different from those of the acquired type. The most significant physiologic consequences of the slow cardiac rate are the increased stroke volume and the increased end-disastolic heart volume. During exercise, the ventricular rate may rise to nearly 100 beats per minute as the atrial rate reaches 180. The increase in rate is determined by the oxygen-transporting capacity of the blood, the stroke volume, the ability to increase the ventricular rate, and the adaptation of the peripheral circulation. Physical working capacity is normal or only slightly reduced in most instances. Furthermore, the hemodynamics at rest show essentially normal features. The pressures in the right heart, the lesser, and the systemic circulations are within the normal range. The end-diastolic pressure for both ventricles, judged from the right ventricular end-diastolic pressure and the pulmonary capillary venous pressure, are normal owing to the ejection of a large stroke volume through the semilunar valves.

Acquired Complete A-V Heart Block. The chief differences between the hemodynamics in acquired and congenital complete A-V heart block are as follows: in the acquired form, the heart rate is usually slower; the cardiac output is less and shows a greater tendency to be fixed, being augmented only slightly with increased work or excitement.

At rest, the slow heart rate is compensated for largely by the prolonged diastolic period of ventricular filling and myocardial recovery, resulting in an increased stroke volume up to 250 ml. At rates below 20 and at higher rates (20 to 30 per minute) in patients with a diseased myocardium that cannot produce a maximal stroke volume, even the resting output may be subnormal, thus resulting in congestive heart failure, salt and water retention, and manifestations of cerebrovascular insufficiency. When slow heart rates result from causes other than complete heart block, variation in cardiac output, stroke output, blood pressure, and pulse pressure are observed, whereas in complete A-V heart block these are practically fixed at a subnormal level. In the normal subject, the responses to exercise and emotion are rapid and adequate; however, in the presence of complete A-V heart block, such responses are usually insufficient to meet increased demands. Therefore, in the presence of a slow ventricular rate, the patient may present no symptoms at rest, but the inadequate increase in cardiac output may cause him to demonstrate easy fatigability, dyspnea, or giddiness during exercise (see discussion under pacemakers, Chapter 37).

The hemodynamic consequences of complete A-V heart block can be markedly altered by therapy. Cardiac output is most significantly increased by isoproterenol, digitalis, or an artificial pacemaker. Isoproterenol often increases pacemaker activity; in some cases, it enhances passage of the sinus impulse across the A-V junction and may transiently restore sinus rhythm.

Digitalis may be helpful as a result of its inotropic effects and its prevention of certain tachyarrhythmias. However, its usefulness is limited unless it is employed with an artificial pacemaker because digitalis can adversely affect the idioventricular pacemaker.

The use of an artificial pacemaker frequently enables a patient with complete A-V heart block to engage in his normal activities without precordial pain, shortness of breath, or notable fatigability. There is an optimal rate of pacing for each patient, which yields the maximal increase in cardiac output; beyond this rate, cardiac output falls (Benchimol et al., 1965c; McNally and Benchimol, 1968). During exercise, stroke volume may remain maximal up to a rate of 100 beats per minute; thereafter, cardiac output falls despite higher rates, owing to a decreased stroke volume (Bevegard et al., 1967). This effect is most marked in severely diseased hearts; it is not seen in normal hearts until ventricular rates over 150 are reached (McNally and Benchimol, 1968).

CLINICAL FEATURES OF ACQUIRED COMPLETE A-V HEART BLOCK

The symptoms depend on the age of the patient, the severity of cardiac involvement, and the underlying clinical state. Palpitation is common and is observed in about 20 per cent of patients, particularly those with a heart rate of 30 beats per minute or less. Symptoms associated with myocardial dysfunction are common; the patient may be practically bedridden as a result. He usually experiences easy fatigability, shortness of breath, occasional episodes of precordial or substernal pain, and dizzy spells. In the more serious variety, the fatigue and shortness of breath are quite marked, the pain is often severe, and dizzy spells and syncopal attacks are frequent. The cerebral blood flow, which in the presence of varying degrees of cerebral atherosclerosis may be in a precarious state at 30 to 36 beats per minute, drops to the level of cerebrovascular insufficiency with a further reduction in the heart rate and decrease in the cardiac output.

The signs of complete heart block result from the slow heart rate and the adjustments made by the heart to compensate for it. The ventricular rate is usually unaffected by carotid sinus pressure. In following a patient who goes in and out of complete A-V heart block, it is observed that, as the heart rate slows, the systolic pressure usually rises and the diastolic pressure falls. In this way, the heart may be able to

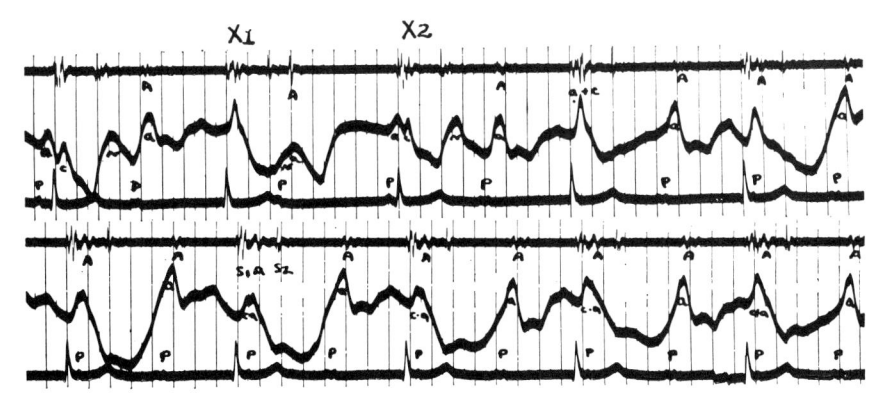

Figure 10–11. Simultaneous phonocardiograms, jugular pulse and lead II in a patient with complete A-V heart block. Note the variations in the intensity of the first heart sound due to varying lengths of the P-R interval. The intensity of the first heart sound is diminished at X_1 when the P-R interval is long, and is increased at X_2 where the P-R interval is relatively short. Note the atrial sounds marked A which follow the "a" wave of the jugular pulse and the P wave in the electrocardiogram.

increase the stroke volume and thus maintain a minimal output, even at a rate of 30 beats per minute.

The most pathognomonic sign of complete heart block (aside from the slow heart rate) is the change of intensity of the first heart sound, which is best heard at the apex. This is due to the variation in the relationship between the atrial contraction and the first heart sound.

Frequently, faint atrial sounds may be heard during the long diastolic intervals. A systolic murmur is often heard in the third interspace to the left of the sternum, probably due to relative valvular insufficiency (Fig. 10-11).

The venous pressure is elevated and cervical venous pulsation is unrelated to ventricular contractions. Venous cannon waves are observed in the neck and occur when the P wave falls between the QRS and T waves (i.e., when the right atrium contracts against a close tricuspid valve). The heart is enlarged in most cases of complete A-V heart block.

Urine formation and other renal functions are decreased at low ventricular rates. The low cardiac output may result in symptoms and signs of renal and cerebrovascular insufficiency.

TYPES OF COMPLETE A-V HEART BLOCK

Complete A-V heart block may be (1) established or permanent, or (2) transient. In one series, 176 patients had permanent and 19 additional patients had repeated transient complete heart block (Penton, et al., 1956). The established form is the type most frequently encountered, and once observed, it usually persists throughout the life of the patient. This form is generally considered to be due to irreversible changes, involving the A-V junction, bundle of His, or bundle branches. Sometimes, for reasons that are difficult to determine, occasional periods of sinus control with A-V transmission of impulses may be observed even after a documented period of complete A-V heart block which lasts many years. However, such occurrences are rare. It is not unusual to encounter instances of complete A-V heart block, thought to be of the established variety, in which normal rhythm is temporarily restored by the administration of isoproterenol, epinephrine, or molar sodium lactate (Bellet and Wasserman, 1957; Bellet et al., 1955, 1956).

When the ventricular rate is 50 to 60 beats per minute or higher and the ventricles appear to beat independently of the atria, there may be complete A-V dissociation, but not necessarily a complete A-V heart block. Digitalis and potassium commonly cause A-V dissociation but only rarely cause even transient complete A-V heart block.

ELECTROCARDIOGRAM

A positive diagnosis of A-V heart block can be made from an electrocardiogram. Although an electrocardiographic diagnosis is usually easily made, in some cases it may prove difficult. Every case of complete A-V heart block also manifests complete A-V dissociation, but only a portion of cases of A-V dissociation are associated with complete A-V heart block. In the latter condition, a lesion of the A-V conduction system prevents transmission of the atrial impulses to the ventricles; no such lesion necessarily exists in simple A-V dissociation. The distinction between the two is very important. In the acquired form of complete A-V heart block, the ventricular rate is usually unaffected by atropine or exercise, which usually increase the rate in A-V dissociation.

Complete A-V heart block is characterized by ventricular complexes that occur regularly and evenly at a rate of 20 to 40 beats per minute, while the

A-V HEART BLOCK

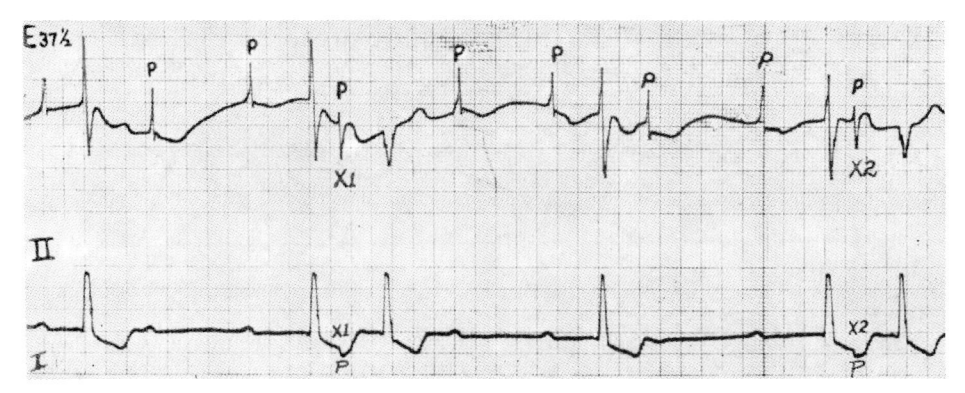

Figure 10–12. (Lead II) Complete A-V heart block with ventricular reciprocal beats. Taken simultaneously with esophageal lead at atrial level (upper strip).

At X_1 and X_2, the atrial beats (which are delineated clearly in the esophageal leads) occur earlier than their anticipated time. They both occur early in diastole at the same period following the end of the preceding QRS (0.16 second). Note that these P waves (X_1 and X_2) show negative deflections. Note that in lead II the P waves at X_1 and X_2, representing retrograde conduction, are of extremely low amplitude. However, they are clearly displayed in the esophageal leads. Both of these P waves are followed by ventricular beats at the same time interval. The P waves during short ventricular cycles are clearly negative and occur only after longer preceding P-R intervals. These negative P waves represent retrograde activation of the atria and are followed after a fixed P-R interval by ventricular complexes (reciprocal beats). The fully compensatory pause is shorter by 0.08 second than other interectopic ventricular intervals; this time represents the delay in conduction of the reciprocal beat below the site of origin of the ventricular rhythm. *Note difference of shape of QRS in the reciprocal beat as compared with basic QRS in the esophageal lead only; this is not seen in lead II.* This difference may be due to aberration of the coupled beat or to conduction through a different A-V pathway during reciprocal beating.

atria usually beat at a normal rate. The ventricular rate may be higher under some circumstances, especially following emergence from a Stokes-Adams attack, when the rate may transiently reach 100 beats per minute.

Complete A-V heart block may exist in the presence of an abnormal atrial mechanism. Occasionally, one may observe complete A-V heart block with atrial fibrillation, atrial flutter, or paroxysmal atrial tachycardia. At times, complete A-V heart block may be associated with atrial standstill. This situation has been observed with potassium and quinidine intoxication. Under these conditions, the slow rate may be due to a slow idioventricular rhythm.

Retrograde Conduction. It has been known for some time that the A-V junction has a bidirectional conduction capacity (see p. 18) and that its conduction fibers can be excited by impulses arising below as well as by those arising above the bundle of His. Retrograde conduction or the transmission of an impulse across the A-V junction from ventricles to atria may occur during ventricular tachycardia, premature beats, and complete A-V heart block. In the presence of complete A-V heart block and ventriculoatrial (V-A) conduction, the atrial component is usually represented by distorted and inverted P waves (Fig. 10–12).

To date, the most accepted theory of the mechanism underlying retrograde conduction is decremental conduction involving a unitary conduction pathway. The greatest barrier to transmission is at the ventricular end so that orthograde impulses, having undergone decrement throughout the A-V junction, are unable to penetrate for any distance through this structure. On the other hand, the ventricular

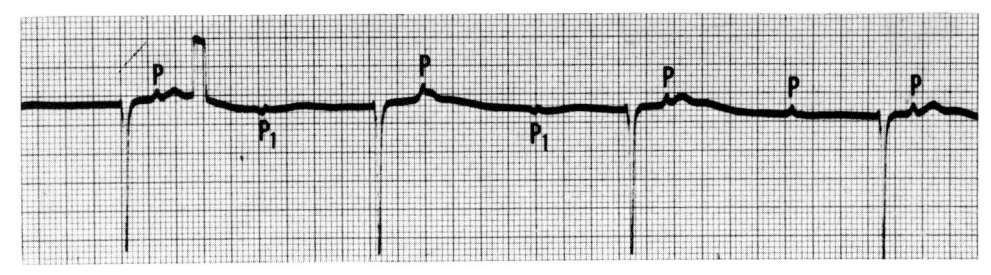

Figure 10–13. Complete A-V heart block with narrow QRS complexes (0.08 second) in an 80-year-old male with arteriosclerotic heart disease. The ventricular rate is 33 per minute; the atrial rate is 75 per minute; there is no relationship between the atrial and ventricular contractions. The atrial beats vary in configuration; the beats marked P_1 probably have an ectopic atrial origin. The narrow QRS complexes suggest that the ventricular pacemaker is located in the lower part of the A-V junction or bundle of His. This origin of the pacemaker is infrequently observed in older subjects.

impulses pass this barrier at full strength and are propagated in a retrograde direction.

Artificial pacemaker stimulation of the ventricles in complete A-V heart block may result in retrograde conduction. The incidence of this observation varies with the method employed in pacing (Kastor et al., 1969).

The P-P Intervals. It has been frequently observed that in cases of A-V heart block (partial or complete), the P-P intervals which contain a ventricular complex are shorter than those which do not contain one. The best explanation for this effect is that the ventricular contraction produces traction on the right atrium, and this mechanical stretch increases the automaticity of the sinus node (Rosenbaum and Lepeschkin, 1955).

Types of Ventricular Complexes. Ventricular complexes in complete A-V heart block are of two main types. The first type, of normal width and duration, is most commonly seen in the congenital variety, but it may occasionally occur in acquired A-V heart block (Fig. 10–13). In the second type, the ventricular complexes display prolonged intraventricular conduction, with notched and slurred QRS complexes; this group is associated with 85 per cent of adult cases of complete A-V heart block.

Widened ventricular complexes in complete heart block may be due to unusual pacemaker location as well as different combinations of bundle branch block. Not infrequently, widened ventricular complexes may occur only intermittently, owing to presumed shifts in the location of the ventricular pacemaker.

Ventricular Rate and Rhythm. The ventricular rhythm is usually quite regular. However, the characteristics of pacemakers in the A-V junction and below the bifurcation of the bundle of His differ in that rhythms originating from the former tend to be quite regular, averaging 45 to 50 beats per minute; the latter are slower, with characteristic rates of 24 to 44 beats per minute, and tend to be irregular and prone to develop episodes of unexplained cardiac arrest. In addition, the ventricular rhythm in complete A-V heart block may be slightly irregular under the following circumstances: (a) most commonly, when the rhythm of the idioventricular pacemaker is slightly irregular; (b) when the idioventricular pacemaker shifts from one focus to another for one or two beats or a longer period; (c) when ventricular premature beats are present; (d) when occasional normally conducted beats occur; (e) when, occasionally, a high grade of partial A-V heart block merges

A-V HEART BLOCK

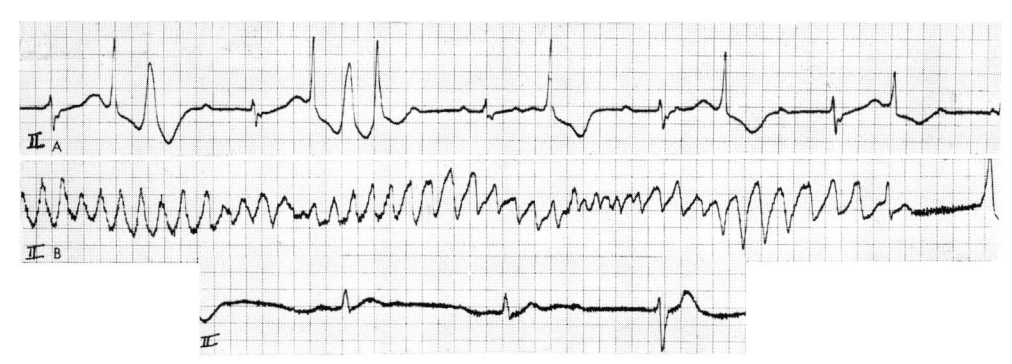

Figure 10–14. Patient with complete A-V heart block showing numerous ventricular premature beats and an episode of ventricular fibrillation leading to Stokes-Adams seizure. Treatment by molar sodium lactate.

(A) Control tracing showing complete A-V heart block and frequent premature beats, some of which occur in groups of two and three. The compensatory pause is constant regardless of how many premature beats (one, two, three) occurred. This means that all premature beats discharged the idioventricular focus.

(B) Continuous record, four minutes after infusion of 100 ml. of molar sodium lactate in ten minutes, shows transient ventricular flutter and fibrillation prior to restoration of a slow ventricular rhythm. (From Bellet, S., and Wasserman, F.: Circulation, 15:591, 1957.)

into varying periods of complete A-V heart block; (f) when two or more lower pacemakers compete; (g) often when atrial fibrillation accompanies complete A-V heart block, though the irregularity in this instance is usually slight; and (h) after emergence from a Stokes-Adams seizure, when the ventricular rate may be initially rapid (100 or more per minute), then gradually slows to the original control rate of 30 to 40 per minute (Fig. 10–14).

Association with Other Arrhythmias. Atrial flutter and fibrillation are only rarely associated with complete A-V heart block. Korst and Wasserberger (1954) collected a series of 71 cases of atrial flutter associated with complete A-V heart block. The occurrence of premature beats, especially ventricular, is not uncommon. These may be observed as isolated beats, or they may occur frequently; they may appear in sequences of two, three, or more and constitute a ventricular tachycardia. Such episodes are often premonitory of the development of Stokes-Adams attacks.

PATTERNS OF COMPLETE A-V HEART BLOCK (UNIFASCICULAR, BIFASCICULAR, AND TRIFASCICULAR)

The concept that progressive lesions in the bundle branches may be related to the evolution of partial and complete A-V heart block has recently assumed added importance. A consideration of the normal anatomy of the A-V and interventricular conduction system is necessary before discussing the individual patterns in the evolution of complete A-V heart block.

Anatomy. The A-V bundle emerges from the membranous septum at its anterior end and divides into two branches, the left and right (see Fig. 1–2). The anatomy and distribution of these two branches are quite different. The right bundle continues undivided as a cylindrical fascicle to the right anterior papillary muscle and then branches at this point into numerous, small, interlaced ramifications. The left bundle, upon emerging from the septum divides almost immediately into: (1) a short, thick, posterior branch,

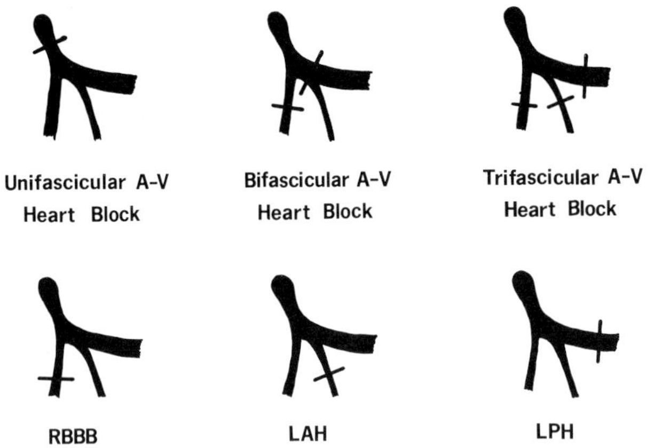

Figure 10–15. Diagrammatic representations of the A-V conduction system illustrating the various types of complete A-V heart block (top row) and the individual fascicular blocks (bottom row). RBBB: right bundle branch block; LAH: left anterior hemiblock; LPH: left posterior hemiblock.

which runs to the posterior papillary muscle; and (2) a long, thin, anterior branch which, covered with endocardium, crosses the ventricular cavity to the anterior papillary muscle. The origin of the left anterior branch and the second segment of the right bundle run in close proximity in the anterosuperior portion of the septum and share a common blood supply (see p. 7). Therefore, lesions in this area would be expected to affect both fascicles (Fig. 10–15). Furthermore, the left anterior branch, being situated along the subendocardial portion of the intraventricular septum and partially traversing the ventricular cavity as a false tendon, is more vulnerable to damage. Conduction delay and block, either intermittent or permanent, may occur in each of the fascicles or any combination of two or three of them. The following discussion includes the electrocardiographic patterns of disturbances in each of a combination of the three main branches.

Inasmuch as the A-V conduction system is anatomically as well as functionally divided into three fascicles, it is obvious that complete A-V heart block may arise from interruption of the main bundle (unifascicular block), interruption of the two main bundle branches (bifascicular block), or interruption of the three individual fascicles (trifascicular block).

Classification of Fascicular Blocks. In approximately 85 per cent of patients with the acquired form of complete A-V heart block, there is involvement of both bundle branches of varying degrees of severity, accompanied by disease of the A-V junction. The electrocardiographic characteristics of block of each of the fascicles (right bundle branch block, left anterior hemiblock, and left posterior hemiblock) and of block of combinations of these fascicles (left bundle branch block, right bundle branch block with left anterior or posterior hemiblock) are discussed in the following sections.

Right Bundle Branch Block (RBBB) (Block of the Right Bundle Branch). Right bundle branch block may be the result of disease or functional alterations which interrupt this conduction pathway. The electrocardiographic criteria for the diagnosis of RBBB are: (1) QRS prolongation to more than 0.12 second; (2) delayed onset of the intrinsicoid deflection (R′) in the right ventricular leads; (3) increased amplitude of the R′ deflection in the right precordial leads; (4) secondary S-T and T wave changes; and (5) often a QR or SR′ pattern in lead aVR (Fig. 10–16). The electrocardiographic manifestations of right ventricular hypertrophy and cor pulmonale must be differentiated from those of right bundle branch block. Clinically,

A-V HEART BLOCK

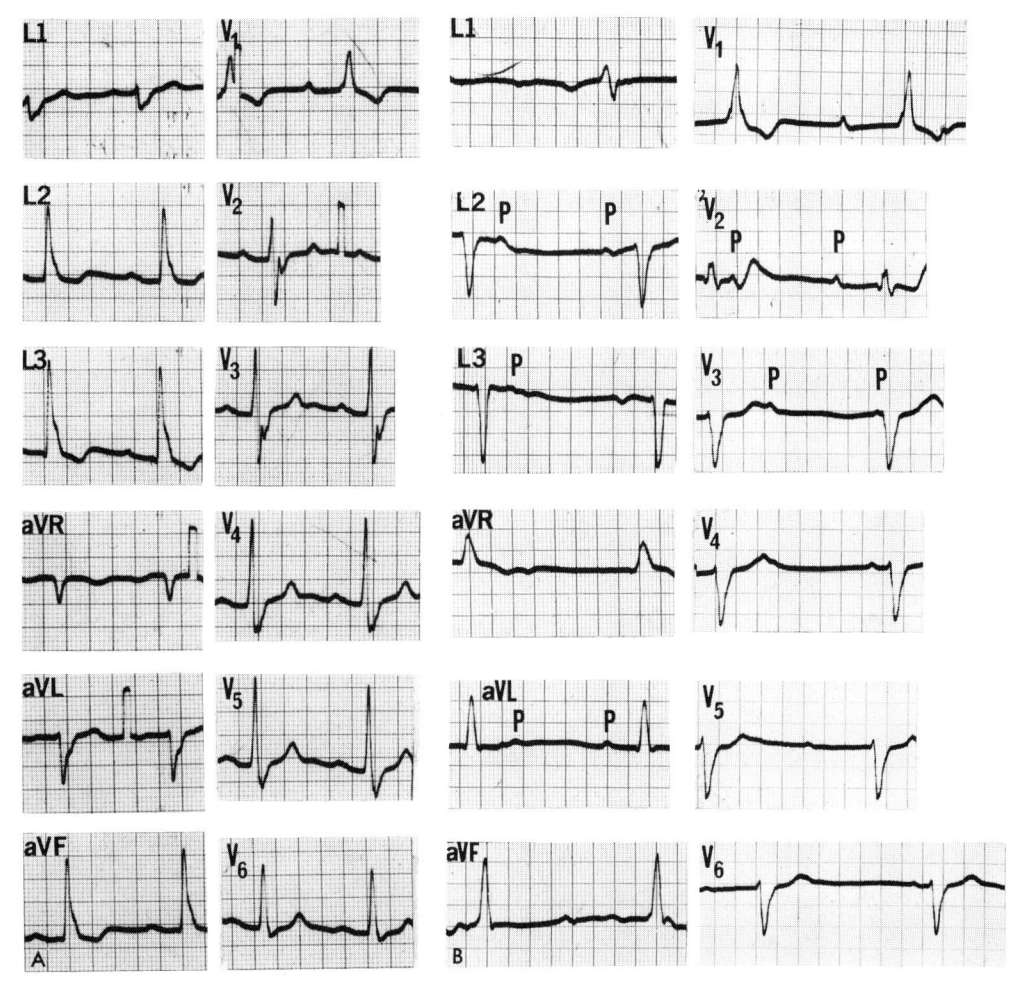

Figure 10–16. (A) Right bundle branch block with left posterior hemiblock. Note the right axis deviation, widened QRS and prolonged P-R interval (0.28 second). Tall R waves are observed in the right precordial leads.

(B) One year later, patient has developed complete A-V heart block. Note the presence of a left axis deviation in the limb leads and tall R waves in the right precordial leads.

RBBB is associated with coronary artery, hypertensive and valvular heart disease, myocarditis, congenital heart disease, emphysema, and other types of pulmonary disease, and it is associated transiently with pulmonary embolism.

Left Anterior Hemiblock (LAH) (Block of the Antero-Superior Division of the Left Bundle Branch) (Fig. 10–17). The electrocardiographic criteria for pure left anterior hemiblock (LAH) are: (1) electrical axis about −60°; (2) main QRS forces oriented superiorly and to the left; (3) a QI/SIII pattern or an apparent counterclockwise rotation of the heart on the longitudinal axis; and (4) a QRS complex of normal width or not prolonged by more than 0.02 second. LAH is often associated with varying degrees of A-V heart block.

Left Posterior Hemiblock (LPH) (Block of the Posterior Inferior Division of the Left Bundle Branch)(Fig. 10–16). The electrocardiographic cri-

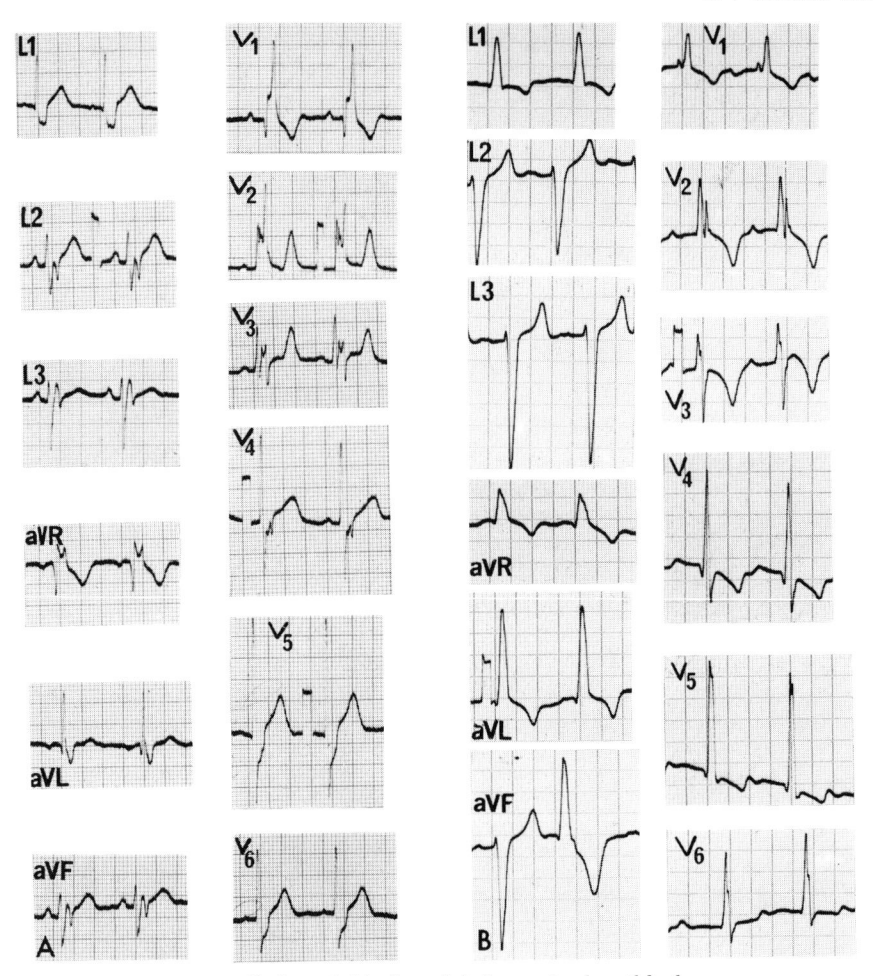

Figure 10-17. Right bundle branch block with left anterior hemiblock.
(A) Shows right bundle branch block with left-axis deviation. Note the terminal widening of the QRS complexes in leads I, II, and III and the tall R waves in the right precordial leads. This is due to the combination of right bundle branch block and left anterior hemiblock.
(B) Note the marked left-axis deviation in the limb leads, the presence of right bundle branch block in the right precordial leads, and partial A-V heart block (P-R measuring 0.28 second). This represents a left anterior hemiblock plus right bundle branch block.

teria are: (1) electrical axis between +80° and +120°; (2) SI/QIII pattern in vectorcardiogram; and (3) prolongation of QRS complex. A simple vertical heart and right ventricular hypertrophy due to emphysema must be ruled out. Clinically, pure left posterior hemiblock is very uncommon since the posterior branch is anatomically the least vulnerable fascicle. In fact, it is almost never seen unless diffuse damage to the conduction system has occurred, in which case it is accompanied by RBBB or LAH (Rosenbaum et al., 1969).

Various Combinations of Fascicular Block

RIGHT BUNDLE BRANCH BLOCK (RBBB) WITH LEFT AXIS DEVIATION (LAD) (Fig. 10–17). The most commonly observed electrocardiographic pattern seen during the evolution of complete A-V heart block is that described by Wilson et al. (1934), Rosenbaum et al. (1967, 1969) and others as characteristic of right bundle branch block (RBBB) with marked left deviation of the cardiac axis. During its developmental stages when complete block occurs intermittently, this pattern may be discerned from the morphology of the QRS complexes of the conducted beats. The underlying pathology is thought to consist of: (a) a lesion of the right bundle branch, and (b) damage of the anterior division of the left bundle branch (Lasser et al., 1968). Permanent or transient lesions in the remainder of the left bundle branch cause progression to clinical complete A-V heart block.

Lopez (1968) has recently investigated the evolution of complete A-V heart block in 31 patients for whom serial electrocardiograms were available. Twenty-four had manifested right bundle branch block prior to the development of complete A-V heart block; all showed left axis deviation, ranging from slight to marked. On the basis of these serial electrocardiograms, Lopez proposed that several stages occur in the development of acquired complete A-V heart block: (1) either the right or the left bundle branch is blocked, with normal conduction to the opposite side; (2) the initial bundle branch block persists while a conduction delay develops in the opposite side, resulting in a partial A-V heart block; and (3) in the third stage, both bundle branches become blocked, and the ventricles are driven by a subsidiary pacemaker (Lopez, 1968). The congenital type and the uncommon cases of acquired complete A-V heart block with the pacemaker in the A-V junction (unifascicular block) do not fit into this scheme.

RIGHT BUNDLE BRANCH BLOCK (RBBB) WITH LEFT AXIS DEVIATION (LAD) AND QV$_1$ (RBBBQV$_1$). In the presence of anterior infarction, the transition to complete A-V heart block is by way of bilateral bundle branch block in contrast to that of inferior infarction, which is usually by way of first or second degree A-V heart block. Recently, Stock and Macken (1968) found that right bundle branch block (RBBB) with a significant Q wave in V$_1$ (RBBBQV$_1$) was the usual form of BBB observed in patients who developed complete A-V heart block with anterior infarction (Fig. 10–18).

Degrees of Bundle Branch Block. Varying degrees of bundle branch block, analogous to the degrees of A-V heart block, have been observed experimentally and clinically (Katz and Pick, 1956; Friedberg and Schamroth, 1969). The concept of progressive

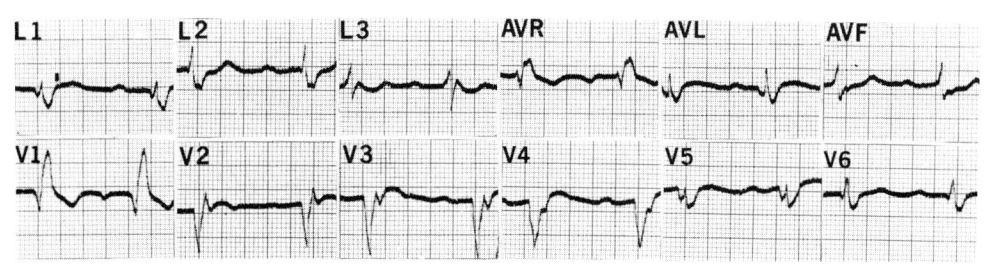

Figure 10–18. Right bundle branch block with left anterior hemiblock and first degree A-V heart block. This pattern has been designated "RBBBQV$_1$."

This electrocardiogram is taken from a patient who had an extensive anterior myocardial infarction which progressed into the healed stage. Note the presence of right bundle branch block in the limb leads; the significant Q waves in V$_1$ and V$_2$; QS in V$_3$, V$_4$, and V$_5$; and the prolonged P-R interval (0.28 second). This patient therefore has a complete right bundle branch block and a left anterior hemiblock, probably the result of an extensive anteroseptal infarction and a partial A-V heart block. The right bundle branch block and Q waves in the right precordial leads have been classified as the type of RBBBQV$_1$ that is very susceptible to the development of complete A-V heart block since the right bundle and the anterior branch of the left bundle are blocked and the ability to maintain a normal sinus rhythm is due to the remaining (posterior) fascicle of the left bundle branch (see text).

stages of bundle branch block is important in understanding the evolution of complete A-V heart block, since minor degrees of bundle branch block may progress to complete bundle branch block. Furthermore, this concept is important for the recognition of those instances of partial A-V heart block in which one bundle is permanently and completely blocked and the other branch exhibits only intermittent block. Under these conditions, in addition to the pattern of bundle branch block, varying degrees of A-V heart block will be present, depending upon the facility with which the supraventricular impulses can pass through the A-V junction and the bundle branches to the ventricular myocardium.

Partial (incomplete) RBBB has essentially the same pattern as complete RBBB. However, several differences exist: the electrocardiographic characteristics of partial RBBB are: (1) a prolonged QRS complex ranging from 0.08 to 0.12 second; (2) relatively broad S wave in leads I and V_6; and (3) early R and late R' waves over the right precordium (V, V_2, V_3R, and V_E). The differentiation between right ventricular hypertrophy and partial RBBB may be difficult; the latter may be diagnosed if a tall R' wave is also seen in lead V_3 and V_4, and if the initial notching (r wave) in lead V_1 is 0.02 second or longer.

First degree LBBB is characterized by: (1) decreased or absent Q wave and initial slurring of the R wave in the leads over the left ventricle (II, aVL, V_5, V_6); (2) prolonged QRS complex ranging from 0.07 to 0.12 second; (3) late onset of intrinsicoid deflection in lead V_6; (4) small QRS complexes in leads V_1 and V_2; and (5) counterclockwise rotation of horizontal vectorcardiographic loop. Second degree LBBB is characterized by: (1) increased

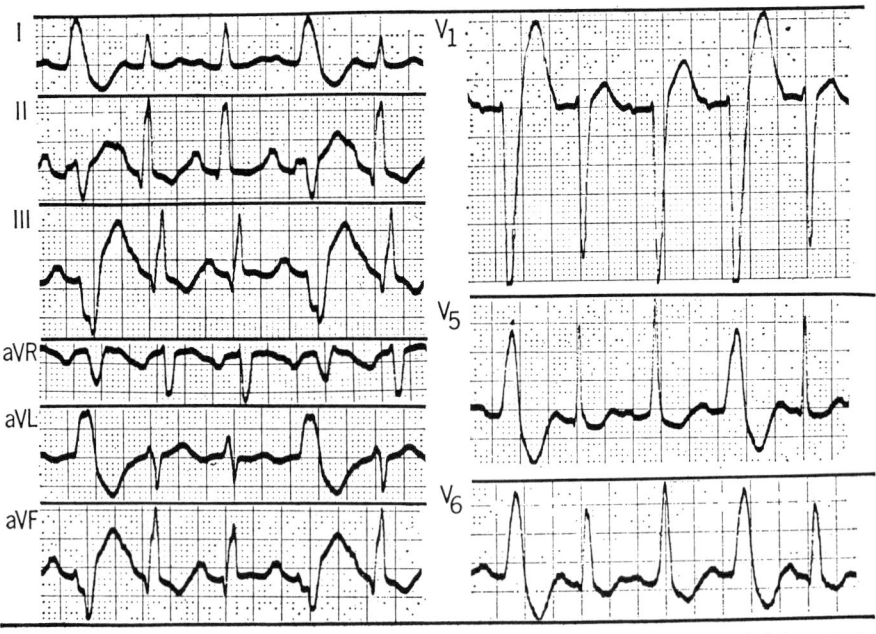

Figure 10-19. Electrocardiogram showing the Wenckebach phenomenon in left bundle branch block. Note the following sequences: The second and fifth beats show normal intraventricular conduction. The beats following this show increasing QRS width; the second beat of the sequence reflects the pattern of incomplete bundle branch block; the third beat shows a typical pattern of complete left bundle branch block. (From Friedberg, H. D., and Schamroth, L.: Amer. J. Cardiol., 24:591, 1969.)

slurring of the R wave in left ventricular leads; (2) absent Q wave in leads V_5 and V_6; (3) inverted and asymmetrical T waves in leads I, aVL, V_5, and V_6; (4) QRS prolongation ranging from 0.11 to 0.15 second; (5) absent r wave in leads V_1 and V_2; (6) beginning of reversal of vectorcardiographic loop to clockwise; and (7) shift toward left axis deviation.

Wenckebach Phenomena in Bundle Branch Block. The bundle branches, like the A-V junction, display types of partial block. Wenckebach phenomenon has been observed in bundle branch block (Katz and Pick, 1956; Friedberg and Schamroth, 1969), and it is recognized by those characteristics of Wenckebach phenomenon that are applicable to other parts of the conduction system via a regular sequence of prolonged conduction culminating in complete block of an impulse. However, when the bundle branches are involved in this phenomenon, one must be careful to differentiate rate-dependent aberration (Fig. 10–19).

DIAGNOSIS AND DIFFERENTIAL DIAGNOSIS

The diagnosis of complete A-V heart block should be suspected in any subject with a regular rhythm at a heart rate below 36 per minute; it should be distinguished from sinus bradycardia, S-A block, idioventricular rhythm, A-V junctional rhythm, and A-V dissociation. Furthermore, the possibility of A-V heart block should be suspected in the presence of a slow ventricular rate and in those patients who suffer from attacks of vertigo, unconsciousness, or convulsions. In the last group, a complete A-V heart block may be transiently observed during these episodes. Exercise, emotion, and atropine will not appreciably increase the ventricular rate in complete A-V heart block (except for the congenital type) but will do so in sinus bradycardia, partial A-V heart block, and other conditions under vagal control. Other manifestations, mentioned under Clinical Features, should be looked for, particularly the alteration in the intensity of the first heart sound and variations in the jugular pulse (see p. 127). A slow idioventricular rhythm may occur in conjunction with an A-V block or may occur independently of it (e.g., in the advanced stage of hyperpotassemia and following emergence from a period of cardiac arrest). In atrial tachycardia and atrial flutter, the diagnosis of complete A-V heart block is usually made by the slow ventricular rate (30 to 40 per minute) and the absence of a fixed relation between the regularly spaced QRST complexes and the P or F waves, respectively. The effect of exercise and atropine may help to exclude an A-V nodal from an idioventricular pacemaker.

The diagnosis of complete A-V heart block should be made with caution in the presence of atrial fibrillation. The presence of a slow ventricular rate, ranging from 20 to 40 per minute with an almost regular rhythm, may be due to complete A-V heart block or may result from a high grade of partial block. This may be caused by the effects of digitalis or by hypoxia, or it may occur spontaneously in older patients owing to sclerotic changes of the A-V junction.

To meet the criteria of a true complete A-V heart block, the same criteria (relative to the ventricular pacemaker) must be met as in patients with atrial complexes arising from the S-A node. These are: (1) little or no effect on ventricular rate following exercise and emotion; (2) failure of the ventricular rate to respond to carotid sinus pressure; and (3) little or no effect on the ventricular rate following the use of atropine and sympathomimetic drugs. Exceptions are found in cases of congenital complete A-V heart block.

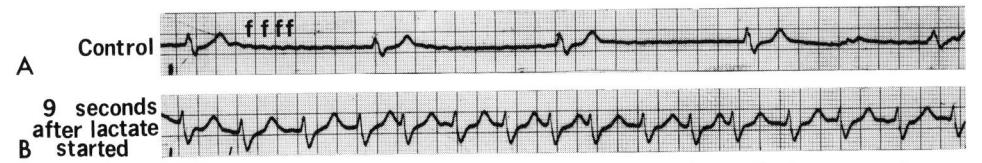

Figure 10-20. The effect of molar sodium lactate in increasing cardiac rhythmicity in the presence of atrial fibrillation with an apparently complete A-V heart block due to digitalis.

(A) Shows the presence of atrial fibrillation with a regular ventricular rhythm with a rate of 32 per minute; this is suggestive of a complete A-V heart block. The patient was in a state of shock and the blood pressure was 70/40.

(B) Nine seconds after 20 ml. of molar sodium lactate had been administered intravenously. Note that the ventricular rate has increased to about 115 per minute, and the rhythm is slightly irregular.

The slow heart rate in A was probably due to transient depression of A-V conduction in the A-V node and not due to complete A-V heart block.

We find that very few cases of atrial fibrillation with slow heart rates meet these criteria. Indeed, the ventricular rate often responds rather easily to the above procedures with increases in rate of from 30 to 110 beats per minute (Fig. 10–20). A definite diagnosis of complete A-V heart block should be made prior to implantation of an artificial pacemaker.

Occasionally, simple complete A-V dissociation may be confused with complete A-V heart block. This point is important when one plans to implant an artificial pacemaker in the mistaken diagnosis of complete A-V heart block. This problem of diagnosis may arise when both the atria and ventricles are beating at a very slow but almost identical rate. Under these circumstances, in A-V dissociation, there are almost as many QRS complexes as there are P waves, and there is no primary impairment in A-V conduction. Exercise or atropine will cause an increase in the ventricular rate and a transient restoration of the normal relationship between the P waves and the QRS complexes.

Occasionally, complete A-V heart block may be present with an atrial rate that is almost exactly twice that of the ventricular, thus suggesting the presence of a 2:1 A-V heart block. The use of exercise or atropine in this instance will accelerate the atria but not the ventricles, thus clarifying the diagnosis.

TREATMENT

The treatment of complete A-V heart block depends to some degree upon the etiology and the clinical manifestations. The therapy of the established type of heart block includes the use of drugs and artificial pacemakers. Even in asymptomatic individuals with established complete block, it is questionable whether to permit a patient to be treated by drug therapy alone, since it is only of partial efficacy and at best transient and undependable. The treatment of choice is the insertion of an artificial pacemaker, whether or not the patient has previously had a Stokes-Adams attack.

Effects of Drugs. Drugs are rarely effective in abolishing established complete A-V heart block and restoring A-V conduction; moreover, their action in improving A-V conduction is transient. These preparations act in one of several ways: (1) by improving A-V transmission and returning the control of the ventricles to a higher pacemaker; and (2) by removing factors that tend to depress A-V transmission (e.g., acidosis and potassium effects).

Atropine. Atropine is currently in favor as the agent for drug therapy in complete A-V heart block because of its low incidence of serious side effects. By reducing vagal tone it accelerates the ventricular rate in the presence of certain types of complete A-V heart block. Thus, in doses of 2 mg. intravenously, atropine is effective in increasing the ventricular rate in the congenital type of complete A-V heart block and in those varieties of acquired complete A-V heart block with a narrow QRS arising from a focus high in the A-V conducting system. It has little effect in the acquired type with a ventricular pacemaker situated below the bifurcation of the bundle of His.

Sympathomimetic Amines. Isoproterenol is useful in increasing the automaticity of cardiac pacemakers and it may cause an increase in cardiac output due to increased ventricular rate in complete A-V heart block. At a fixed cardiac rate (as in the paced subject), isoproterenol results in increased stroke volume (Benchimol et al., 1965c). It may transiently abolish complete A-V heart block by improving A-V conduction and by stimulating higher pacemakers.

Epinephrine is not commonly used in the treatment of complete A-V heart block, except when Stokes-Adams attacks occur as a result of ventricular standstill. In those instances, 0.5 mg. diluted, 1:10,000 in 5 ml. of saline, every three to five minutes is recommended. Epinephrine increases the ventricular rate through its sympathomimetic effect. It is often efficacious in the arousal of ventricular or supraventricular pacemakers. Zoll et al. (1958) found that epinephrine and isoproterenol were equally effective in arousing ventricular pacemakers in patients without intrinsic ventricular activity who were kept alive at the same time by prolonged, external electrical cardiac stimulation. However, particularly in nonemergency situations, epinephrine should be used with caution, since its stimulatory effect on the heart muscle may result in the production of dangerous types of ectopic rhythms, even ventricular fibrillation.

Sodium Bicarbonate and other Alkalinizing Agents. Sodium bicarbonate has tended to supplant the use of molar sodium lactate in counteracting the adverse effects of acidosis on the heart, especially those associated with slow heart rates. When the slow ventricular rate is associated with hypoxia or acidosis, molar sodium lactate or sodium bicarbonate will increase the rate in more than 25 per cent of patients.

Artificial Pacemakers. The application of artificial pacemakers in the therapy of human subjects with complete heart block is a relatively recent development. The use of an artificial pacemaker is indicated to improve cardiac output in symptomatic complete A-V heart block and for prophylaxis in patients who suffer from Stokes-Adams attacks (see pp. 141 and 418).

PROGNOSIS

The true prognosis for complete A-V heart block in asymptomatic patients is unknown, since the condition is discovered only in those from whom an electrocardiogram is obtained. Prior to the initiation of long-term pacing on a large scale, 50 to 60 per cent of subjects who suffered a first Stokes-Adams attack died within a year, most often from a subsequent attack (Johansson, 1966). In many series, artificial pacing has been found to markedly improve long-term survival rates. The life expectancy of patients with pacemakers is now within 10 per cent of that of a normal population comparable in age and sex (see p. 418).

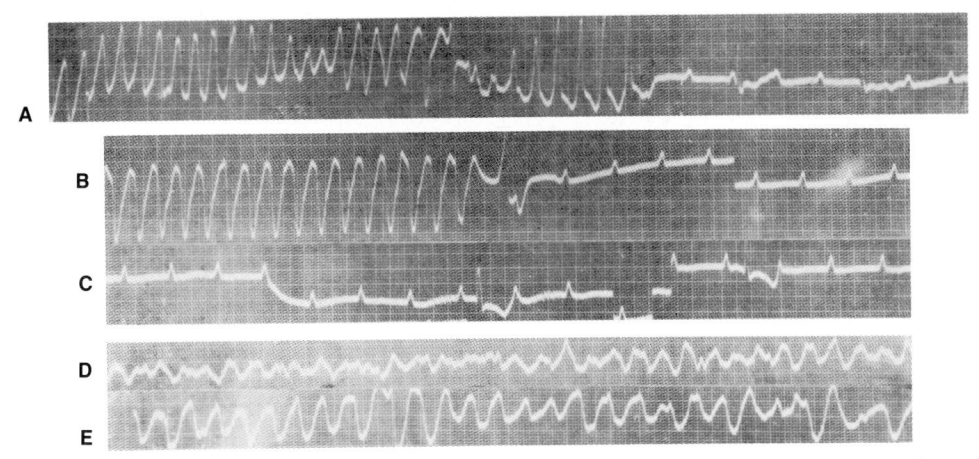

Figure 10–21. Cardiac mechanisms during a Stokes-Adams attack. Strips A, B, C, D, and E are taken from the same patient who had a complete A-V heart block (lead II), and sustained many Stokes-Adams attacks over a period of 24 hours.

(A) Paroxysm of ventricular flutter with a ventricular rate which averages about 200/minute. Note the markedly aberrant type of ventricular complexes. The end of the strip shows the spontaneous resumption of complete A-V heart block.

(B) Ventricular flutter with a rate of about 200 per minute terminating in ventricular standstill; atrial beating is maintained at a rate of 100 per minute.

(C) Emergence from an attack of ventricular standstill, with the appearance of occasional idioventricular beats.

(D and E) Ventricular fibrillation. Note the markedly aberrant type of ventricular response. The patient recovered from this paroxysm, but succumbed during a subsequent attack.

STOKES-ADAMS SEIZURES

Stokes-Adams disease is a condition characterized by sudden attacks of unconsciousness, with or without convulsions, and frequently accompanies heart block. In a broad sense, these seizures may result from any alteration in cardiac mechanism that results in a sudden drastic reduction in the cardiac output and, consequently, in the cerebral blood flow, e.g., following the sudden onset of a very slow heart rate or marked acceleration of the heart beat (Fig. 10–21). Essentially, the syncopal attacks and convulsive seizures which typify this syndrome are due to failure of the brain to receive an adequate blood supply for a period of three to nine seconds or longer.

CLINICAL FEATURES

The clinical manifestation of the Stokes-Adams seizure depends not only upon the type and duration of cardiac disturbance but also upon the state of the cerebral circulation of the patient. The manifestations of cerebral origin may range from light-headedness to loss of consciousness, with or without actual convulsive episodes.

In general, only occasional feeble heart sounds are audible and respirations are very slow or absent. The electrocardiogram may show ventricular standstill with some atrial activity, atrial standstill with maintenance of a very slow ventricular rate, ventricular fibrillation, or complete cardiac asystole. These arrhythmias may occur singly or in various combinations.

THERAPY

The therapy of Stokes-Adams seizures may be divided into treatment during the attack and prophylaxis between the attacks. Both medical and pacemaker therapy have a place in the treatment of this disorder.

The immediate aim in treatment during a Stokes-Adams attack is to institute artificial respiration and restore adequate blood flow to the vital organs. *A vigorous blow over the lower sternum may restore cardiac beating, at least temporarily.* External cardiac massage should be performed. When the circulation has been restored in this manner, one should infuse isoproterenol (0.1 mg. in 10 mg. saline) by intravenous drip (in combination with a peripheral vasoconstrictor such as phenylephrine).

Ventricular fibrillation may be terminated by means of a direct-current cardioversion (see p. 427); however, pacing by external electrodes may be necessary with prolonged asystole. As soon as feasible, a transvenous pacemaker should be installed. Until this is effected, sustained external cardiac massage is performed by means of rhythmic pressure applied over the sternum approximately 60 times per minute to maintain blood flow. At the same time, artificial respiration should be maintained throughout the resuscitation procedure until spontaneous respirations have returned.

Following a single Stokes-Adams attack, a temporary pacemaker should be immediately inserted followed by a permanent device. Because of their far greater effectiveness and reliability, pacemakers have largely replaced drugs in the prophylaxis of recurrent Stokes-Adams attacks.

Additional measures beyond the use of a pacemaker depend upon the adequacy of cardiac output. In subjects with myocardial disease that limits the response to pacing, tolerance of exercise and emotional stress may be limited. Isoproterenol has been shown to further increase cardiac output in paced subjects (Benchimol et al., 1965a). When acidosis and hyperkalemia complicate the picture, the use of a thiazide diuretic or sodium bicarbonate is often efficacious.

PROGNOSIS

Death frequently occurs during a Stokes-Adams seizure; indeed, this is the most common cause of death in untreated complete A-V heart block. It has been estimated (Johansson, 1966) that 50 to 60 per cent of patients without a pacemaker die within the first year after their initial Stokes-Adams attack. In the series of Penton et al. (1956) the average duration of life after the first sign of complete A-V block was 26.2 months. With the advent of reliable pacemaker therapy the prognosis of patients with Stokes-Adams seizures has become much better. With the devices presently in use, the prognosis of subjects with Stokes-Adams attacks is within 10 per cent of that for a group of similar age (70 at onset) and sex (largely male). In a series of his own patients, Chardack (1969) found that 25 of 48 (52 per cent) were alive 5 to 8 years after surgical implantation of myocardial electrodes. Other authors have reported similar results (Johansson, 1966; Siddons and Sowton, 1967). At present, the principal limitations on longevity are (1) the age of the patient; (2) the severity of the underlying disorder; (3) the occurrence of a rhythm in competition with the pacemaker, leading to ventricular fibrillation; and (4) the various forms of failure and other complicating factors of the pacemaking device. Hopefully, the reliability of pacemakers can be further improved.

References

Adolph, R. J.: Diagnosis and medical management of complete atrioventricular block. Heart Bull., 17:16, 1968.
Alanis, J., and Benitez, D.: Transitional potentials and the prolongation of impulses through different cardiac cells. *In* Santo, T., Mizukira, V., and Matsuda, K. (eds.): Electrophysiology and Ultrastructure of the Heart. New York, Grune and Stratton, 1967, pp. 153–175.
Bazett, H. C.: Analysis of time relations of electrocardiogram. Heart, 7:353, 1920.

Bellet, S., and Wasserman, F.: Indications and contraindications for the use of molar sodium lactate. Circulation, 15:591, 1957.

Bellet, S., Wasserman, F., and Brody, J. I.: Molar sodium lactate; its effect in complete A-V heart block and cardiac arrest occurring during Stokes-Adams seizures and in terminal state. New Eng. J. Med., 253:891, 1955.

Bellet, S., Wasserman, F., and Brody, J. I.: Effect of molar sodium lactate in increasing cardiac rhythmicity: Clinical and experimental study of its use in the treatment of patients with slow heart rates, Stokes-Adams syndrome and episodes of cardiac arrest. JAMA, 160:1293, 1956.

Benchimol, A., Evandro, E. G., and Dimond, E. G.: Stroke volume and peripheral resistance during infusion of isoproterenol at a constant fixed heart rate. Circulation, 31:417, 1965a.

Benchimol, A., Palmero, H. A., Liggett, M. S., and Dimond, E. G.: Influence of digitalization on the contribution of atrial systole to the cardiac dynamics at a fixed ventricular rate. Circulation, 31:417, 1965b.

Benchimol, A., Wu, T., and Liggett, M. S.: Effect of exercise and isoproterenol on the cardiovascular dynamics in complete heart block at various heart rates. Amer. Heart J., 70:337, 1965c.

Bevegard, S., et al.: Effect of changes in ventricular rate on cardiac output and central venous pressure at rest and during exercise in patients with artificial pacemakers. Cardiovas. Res., 1:21, 1967.

Chardack, W. M.: Cardiac pacemakers and heart block. *In* Gibbon, J. H., Sabiston, D. C., and Spencer, F. C. (eds.): Surgery of the Chest. Philadelphia, W. B. Saunders, 1969, pp. 824–865.

Chatterjee, K., et al.: The electrocardiogram in chronic heart block. A histological correlation with ECG changes in 42 patients. Amer. Heart J., 80:47, 1970.

Damato, A. N., Lau, S. H., Helfant, R. H., Stein, E., Berkowitz, W. D., and Cohen, S. I.: Study of atrioventricular conduction in man using electrode catheter recordings of His bundle activity. Circulation, 39:287, 1969.

DeLeon, A. C., Bellet, S., and Muller, O. F.: The effect of acidosis and of hyperpotassemia on the idioventricular rate in complete A-V heart block (unpublished data, 1961).

Fisch, C., and Knoebel, S. B.: Junctional rhythms. Prog. Cardiov. Dis., 13:141, 1970.

Friedberg, H. D., and Schamroth, L.: The Wenckebach phenomenon in left bundle branch block. Amer. J. Cardiol., 24:591, 1969.

Hanssen, P.: Incidence of auricular flutter and auricular fibrillation associated with complete auriculoventricular dissociation. Acta Med. Scand., 136:113, 1949.

Johansson, B. W.: Complete heart block. A clinical, hemodynamic and pharmacological study in patients with or without an artificial pacemaker. Acta Med. Scand., 180, Suppl. 451, 1966.

Johnsson, R. A., Averill, K. H., and Lamb, L. E.: Non-specific T wave changes. *In* Lamb, L. E. (ed.): First International Symposium in Cardiology in Aviation. Texas, Brooks Air Force Base, 1959.

Kastor, J. A., Sanders, C. A., Leinbach, R. C., and Hawthorne, J. W.: Factors influencing retrograde conduction. A study of 30 patients during cardiac catheterization. Brit. Heart J., 31:580, 1969.

Katz, L. N., and Pick, A.: Clinical Electrocardiography, Part I. The Arrhythmias. Philadelphia, Lea & Febiger, 1956.

Kaufman, J. G., Wachtel, F. W., Rothfield, E., and Bernstein, A.: The association of complete heart block and Adams-Stokes syndrome in two cases of Mobitz type II block: case reports. Circulation, 23:253, 1961.

Korst, D. R., and Wasserberger, R. H.: Atrial flutter associated with complete A-V heart block. Amer. Heart J., 48:383, 1954.

Langendorf, R., and Pick, A.: Approach to the interpretation of complex arrhythmias. Prog. Cardiov. Dis., 2:706, 1960.

Langendorf, R., Pick, A., Edelist, A., and Katz, L. N.: Experimental demonstration of concealed A-V conduction in the human heart. Circulation, 32:386, 1965.

Lasser, R. P., Haft, J. I., and Friedberg, C. K.: Relationship of right bundle branch block and marked left axis deviation to complete heart block and syncope. Circulation, 37:429, 1968.

Lev, M.: Anatomic basis for atrioventricular block. Amer. J. Med., 37:742, 1964.

Lev, M., Kinare, S. G., and Pick, A.: The pathogenesis of atrioventricular block in coronary disease. Circulation, 42:409, 1970.

Lev, M., and McMillan, J. B.: A semi-quantitative histopathologic method for the study of the entire heart for clinical and electrocardiographic correlations. Amer. Heart J., 58:140, 1959.

Logue, R. B., and Hanson, J. F.: Heart block. Amer. J. Med. Sci., 207:765, 1944.

Lopez, J. F.: Electrocardiographic findings in patients with complete atrioventricular block. Brit. Heart J., 30:20, 1968.

McNally, E. M., and Benchimol, A.: Medical and physiological considerations in the use of artificial cardiac pacing. Parts I and II. Amer. Heart J., 75:380, 864, 1968.

Moe, G. K., Childers, R. W., and Merideth, J.: An appraisal of "supernormal" A-V conduction. Circulation, 38:5, 1968.

Narula, O. S., and Samet, P.: Wenckebach and

Mobitz type II A-V heart block within the His bundle and bundle branches. Circulation, 41:947, 1970.

Narula, O. S., Scherlag, B. J., Samet, P., and Javier, R. P.: Atrioventricular block: Localization and classification by His bundle recordings. Amer. J. Med., 50:146, 1971.

Penton, G. B., Miller, H., and Levine, S.: Some clinical features of complete heart block. Circulation, 13:801, 1956.

Rosen, K. M.: The contribution of His bundle recordings to the understanding of cardiac conduction in man. Circulation, 43:961, 1971.

Rosenbaum, M. B., Elizari, M. V., and Lazzari, J.: Los Hemibloqueos, Ed. Paidos, Buenos Aires, 1967.

Rosenbaum, M. B., et al.: Intraventricular trifascicular blocks. The syndrome of right bundle branch block with intermittent left anterior and posterior hemiblock. Amer. Heart J., 78:306, 1969.

Rosenbaum, M. B., and Lepeschkin, E.: The effect of ventricular systole on auricular rhythm in atrioventricular block. Circulation, 11:240, 1955.

Siddons, H., and Sowton, E.: Cardiac Pacemakers. Springfield, Ill., Charles C Thomas, 1967.

Stock, R. J., and Macken, D. L.: Observations on heart block during continuous electrocardiographic monitoring in myocardial infarction. Circulation, 38:993, 1968.

Watanabe, Y., and Dreifus, L. S.: Second degree atrioventricular block. Cardiovas. Res., 1:150, 1967.

Watanabe, Y., and Dreifus, L. S.: Newer concepts in the genesis of cardiac arrhythmias. Amer. Heart J., 76:114, 1968.

Watt, T. B., Murao, S., and Pruitt, R. D.: Left axis deviation induced experimentally in a primate heart. Amer. Heart J., 70:381, 1965.

Wenckebach, K. F., and Winterburg, H.: Irregular Heart Action. Leipzig, Wilhelm Engelmann, 1927.

Wilson, F. N., Johnston, F. D., and Barker, P. S.: Electrocardiogram of an unusual type in right bundle branch block. Amer. Heart J., 9:472, 1934.

Zoll, P. M., et al.: Intravenous drug therapy of Stokes-Adams disease: Effect of sympathomimetic amines on ventricular rhythmicity and atrioventricular conduction. Circulation, 17:325, 1958.

Chapter 11 Disturbances in the Region of the A-V Junction

A-V JUNCTIONAL RHYTHM
  General Considerations
  Incidence and Etiology
  Pathology
  Symptoms and Signs
  Electrocardiogram
    QRS in A-V Junctional Rhythm
  Diagnosis
  Treatment
  Prognosis
CORONARY SINUS RHYTHM
  Incidence and Etiology
LEFT ATRIAL RHYTHM
A-V JUNCTIONAL TACHYCARDIA
  Paroxysmal Form
    Electrocardiogram
    Therapy
    Bidirectional Tachycardia
  Nonparoxysmal Form
    Etiology and Treatment
A-V JUNCTIONAL ESCAPE
  Etiology
  Electrocardiogram
  Treatment

RECIPROCAL RHYTHM
  General Considerations
  Terminology
  Etiology
  Diagnosis
  Treatment
WIDENING OF QRS COMPLEXES
  Types of QRS Widening
    QRS Prolongation with Acceleration of Heart Rate
    Mechanisms
    QRS Prolongation at Slow Rates
    QRS Prolongation Independent of Rate
  Etiology and Clinical Significance

ABERRATION

GENERAL CONSIDERATIONS
ECG CHARACTERISTICS
DIFFERENTIAL DIAGNOSIS
SIGNIFICANCE
THERAPY OF ABERRATION

A-V JUNCTIONAL RHYTHM

General Considerations. The major part of the A-V junction is located in the lower portion of the interatrial septum near the fibrous skeleton of the heart, anterior to the ostium of the coronary sinus. The distal portion of the A-V junction includes that portion of the bundle of His proximal to its bifurcation, which extends through the membranous interventricular septum. The term "A-V node" was originally applied by Tawara (1906) to the initial portion of this system; however, the physiology of the A-V junction has recently been reinvestigated. These recent studies have indicated that some of the older concepts are no longer valid; nevertheless, the traditional interpretations can still, in a general way, be utilized clinically.

Until recently, it was held that the "A-V node" possessed a high degree of automaticity and, hence, was considered to be a pacemaker site. Many anatomic and physiologic investigations have modified this view (see Chapters 1 and 2 for a detailed review of this work). Present concepts may be briefly summarized as follows: the traditional "A-V node" of the light microscopist (as most commonly described) corresponds to the N-H region of the electrophysiologist; the "functional A-V node" of other anatomists, e.g., Truex and Smythe (1964), also includes the electrophysiologic A-N and N regions; the "A-V junction" includes the three regions of the A-V node, in addition to specialized prenodal atrial tissue and the bundle of His (DeFelice and Challice, 1969). Automatic fibers have been observed in the A-N and N-H regions, in the coronary sinus region, situated just proximal to the A-V junction, and in the His-Purkinje system (DeFelice and Challice, 1969). If the traditional "A-V node" lacks automaticity, then the A-V rhythms may be explained as originating either somewhat lower down in the nodal-His junction or a little higher up in the coronary sinus area, rather than in the A-V node proper. The possibility that some of the upper nodal beats may have an origin in the left atrium or in the coronary sinus area has also been considered (DeFelice and Challice, 1969), but this has not been definitely established.

Normally the A-V junction serves as a bridge for the transmission of impulses from the atria to the ventricles. This structure may be the site of impulse formation in the following circumstances: (1) when the sinus pacemaker fails; (2) when the automaticity of the S-A node falls below that of the A-V junction; (3) when the rate of impulse formation in the A-V junction is so enhanced that its rate exceeds that of the sinus node; and (4) when conduction fails in the N region due to Wenckebach-type second degree A-V heart block or in certain types of complete A-V heart block.

When, under these conditions, the A-V junction assumes the pacemaker function, an A-V junctional rhythm results, with its various manifestations and modifications. Failure or depression of the S-A node results in unmasking of the natural rate of the A-V junction (approximately 40 to 50 beats per minute); this is termed the *slow* or *passive* type of A-V junctional rhythm. Under certain conditions, the automaticity of the A-V junctional cells may be much greater, producing an A-V junctional tachycardia. Neither type is very common, but the slow form is seen much more often than the rapid. Both forms of A-V junctional rhythm are almost always temporary disturbances; in only a few instances have these disturbances approached permanency.

An impulse originating in the A-V junction is usually conducted in both directions: in a forward (antegrade) direction, thus activating the ventricles, and in a retrograde direction, activating the atria. The impulse, however, may be blocked in either one or both directions (Pick and Langendorf, 1968).

For the purpose of this chapter, we will continue to employ the terms "upper," "middle," and "lower" nodal (junctional) rhythms, which have been used and well understood for years. However, one should recognize that these terms represent only rough approximations, and indeed, this classification may not be applicable under certain circumstances (Waldo et al., 1968).

Incidence and Etiology. A-V junctional rhythm is rare in children; it is noted most frequently in the middle and later decades of life. In a hospital population, 1 per cent (502 of 50,000) manifested A-V junctional rhythm (Katz and Pick, 1956).

A-V junctional rhythm is a disorder which usually occurs secondary to disturbances of function in the S-A node, to disease of that structure, to parasympathetic effects, or to the effects of certain drugs. Often, this state is associated with incomplete A-V dissociation. The precipitating factors include: (1) vagal stimulation of various types (e.g., during the phases of respiration or following electric countershock), which may depress S-A nodal function; (2) injury to the S-A node by toxic or infectious processes, myocarditis (especially rheumatic), and degenerative states; (3) digitalis intoxication; (4) the effect of certain drugs (e.g., potassium, quinidine); (5) atropine during the initial state of its effect; and (6) episodes of sinus bradycardia accompanying acute myocardial infarction; under these circumstances, 7 to 10 per cent of patients manifest A-V junctional rhythm.

Pathology. Relatively few cases present characteristic pathologic findings: the pathology observed is that of the conditions described under etiology. In the persistent type of A-V junctional rhythm, the sinus node may be extensively damaged or entirely destroyed by the disease process. Destruction of the sinus node has been demonstrated by careful pathologic study in several series of patients with chronic atrial fibrillation in whom normal sinus rhythm could not be restored because of damage to this structure. Episodes of A-V junctional rhythm frequently result following countershock in these patients.

Symptoms and Signs. No symptoms or signs are produced by the common type of A-V junctional rhythm itself unless it is associated with an extremely slow or rapid heart rate or unless it occurs in subjects with underlying disturbances in circulatory function. Only slight hemodynamic impairment is produced in otherwise healthy individuals by the disruption of the relationship between atrial and ventricular systole in A-V junctional rhythms. The significant physical signs are a persistently slow pulse often accompanied by some degree of irregularity. Following exercise or emotion, owing to alterations in vagal or sympathetic tone, the rhythm may transiently revert to normal or periods of A-V dissociation may develop. When this occurs, the auscultatory phenomena are similar to those described under A-V dissociation (see p. 175).

Electrocardiogram. There is one common feature in A-V junctional rhythm: the P waves, if present, often differ in shape from P waves originating in the sinus node. This occurs because an impulse arising in the A-V junction follows a course through the atria roughly opposite to that of a sinus impulse. The P waves are often inverted in human A-V junctional rhythms, including those instances when the pacemaker is situated in the coronary sinus or bundle of His. However, some instances of A-V junctional rhythms may produce positive P waves. These may include "isorhythmic" A-V dissociation and junctional rhythms in patients with altered cardiac position or derangement of the atrial conduction pathways.

Patients manifesting the "lower nodal" electrocardiographic pattern studied by the His bundle electrogram (see Chapter 2) demonstrate that the activation of the bundle of His precedes that of both the A-V junction and the ventricles (see Figs. 11–1, 11–2).

An A-V rhythm with no visible P wave may occur in the following instances: (a) if the P wave is buried in the QRS or, rarely, in the T wave (Figs. 11–3, 11–4); (b) in the presence of atrial fibrillation; (c) in failure of retrograde conduction to the atrium; or (d) in atrial standstill. This pattern of A-V rhythm may be simulated by sinoventricular rhythm during hyperpotassemia and quinidine intoxication. The diagnosis may be established by careful inspection of a long tracing, since A-V junctional rhythm is generally unstable, and may go in and out of periods of A-V dissociation. In those tracings in which the P waves are continuously buried in the QRS complexes, the atrial mechanism may be difficult to establish.

DISTURBANCES IN THE REGION OF THE A-V JUNCTION

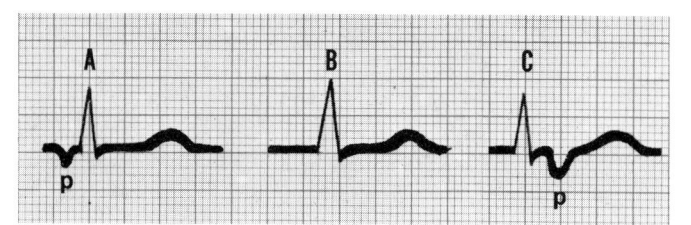

Figure 11–1. Diagrammatic representation of various types of A-V nodal rhythm.

(A) Denotes lower nodal A-V rhythm. Note the inverted P wave and the P-R interval measuring 0.12 second.

(B) No P wave is discernible; this is a mid A-V nodal rhythm with a P wave probably hidden in QRS.

(C) Lower nodal rhythm shows an inverted P wave following the QRS.

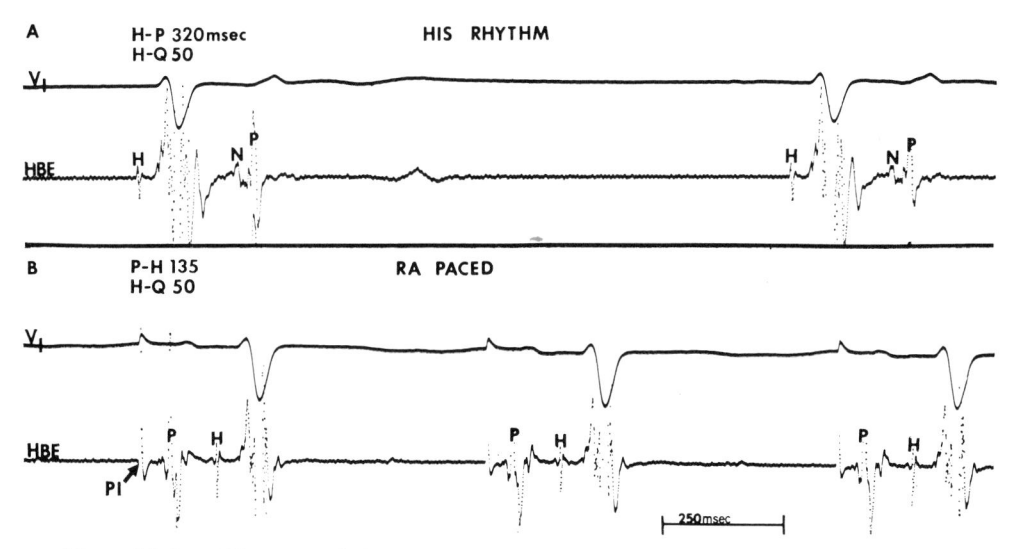

Figure 11–2. A-V junctional rhythm. His bundle recordings. (*Panel A*) His rhythm with retrograde conduction to the atria. Each QRS complex is preceded by a single His deflection (H). The retrogradely conducted P wave is preceded by an A-V nodal potential (N). (*Panel B*) Antegrade conduction during right atrial pacing. H-Q time same as in panel A. (From Damato, A. N., and Lau, S. H.: Circulation, 40:527, 1969.)

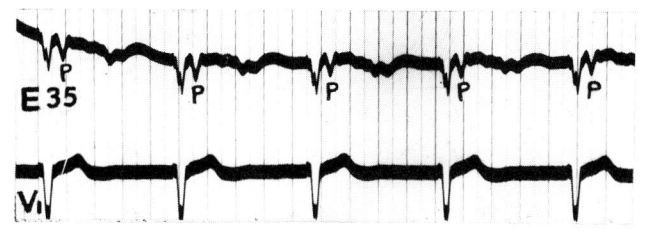

Figure 11–3. A-V junctional rhythm. V_1 taken simultaneously with esophageal lead at atrial level. Note presence of inverted P waves in esophageal lead which follow the QRS complex. This indicates a junctional ("lower nodal") origin. These P waves are not discernible in V_1.

However, the following procedures may be helpful to demonstrate P waves and the atrial mechanism: (1) Atropine may be administered or the patient exercised; both of these procedures tend to decrease vagal tone, often affecting the two pacemakers unequally and separating the atrial and ventricular rhythms by producing a transient A-V dissociation or a return to normal sinus rhythm. (2) A jugular pulse tracing taken simultaneously with the electrocardiogram will record an "a" wave occurring synchronously with the wave of the carotid pulse. (3) Use of the Doppler tracing (Fig. 11–5). (4) A recording from the esophageal lead taken with the electrode at the atrial level is one of the best methods of establishing the type and sequence of atrial activity. (5) Tracings from a right intra-atrial lead will establish the diagnosis.

Also, transition from sinus to A-V junctional rhythm and back again to sinus rhythm is not infrequent. It may be noted by a gradual change in the P-R interval or the shape of the P wave. This shift in the origin of the impulse may be observed with the "wandering pacemaker" and transient periods of A-V dissociation (Fig. 11–4).

QRS in A-V Junctional Rhythm. Irrespective of the P wave pattern or morphology, the QRS complexes are usually supraventricular in form. They

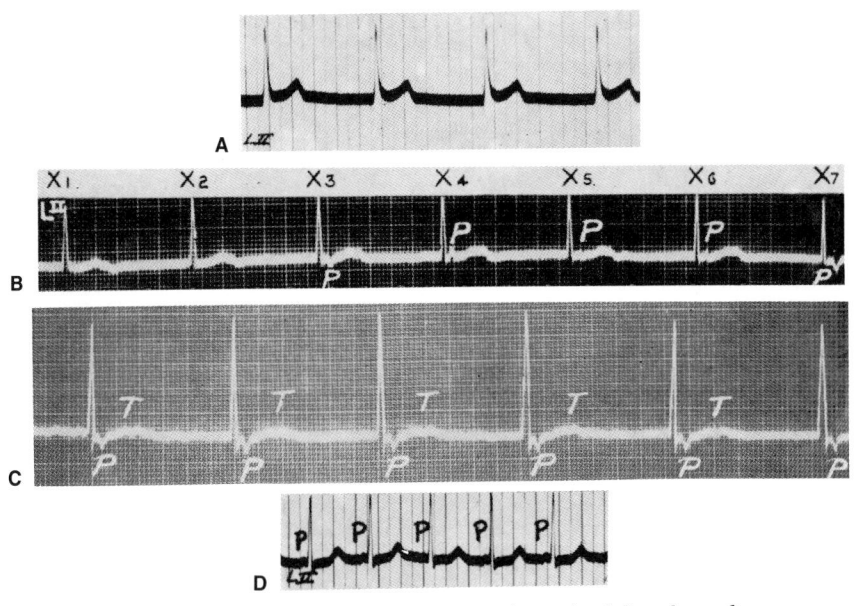

Figure 11–4. A-V nodal rhythm, A-V dissociation, and A-V (nodal) tachycardia.

(A) "Mid A-V nodal" rhythm. No P waves are observed; they either are buried in the QRS complexes or may be absent (atrial standstill).

(B) Incomplete and partial A-V dissociation in the presence of sinus bradycardia and "lower nodal" rhythm. Regular sequence of ventricular complexes at a rate of 50 per minute. Small positive P waves are buried in the QRS at X_1 (downstroke) and X_2 (upstroke), or follow the QRS complex with practically the same R-P interval but changing amplitude of P at X_4, X_5, and X_6. Negative P waves follow the QRS complex at X_3 and X_7; the latter is deeper than the former. Atrial fusion of sinus and retrograde activation occurred at X_3, X_5, and X_6. P wave at X_4 may be totally of sinus origin, and, at X_7, is probably of nodal origin without fusion.

(C) "Lower nodal" rhythm. The ventricular rate and atrial rate are both regular at 50 per minute. Note that the P wave follows the QRS at a regular R-P interval of about 0.12 second.

(D) "Upper nodal" tachycardia (rate 115 per minute). The P waves precede the QRS complexes, are diphasic, and the P-R interval is very short (0.08 second).

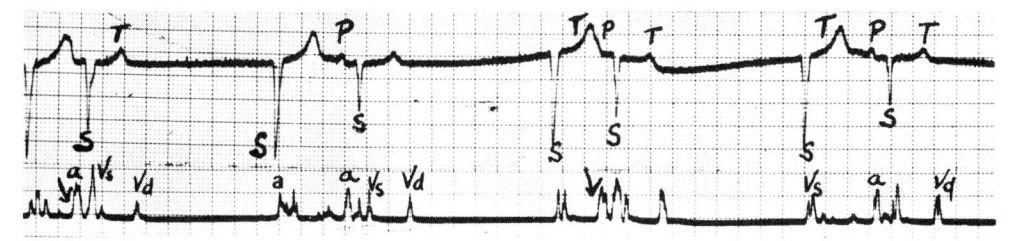

Figure 11-5. A-V nodal escape beats. Tracing from a 43-year-old woman with rheumatic heart disease, mitral insufficiency, and digitalis toxicity. Interval between thick time lines is 0.2 second. Note the relationship of the components of the Doppler tracing to the deflections of the electrocardiogram. The arrow points at a sequence where the P wave is hidden in the T, but the "a" wave is easily recognized in the Doppler tracing.

are of normal width and shape, although occasionally one may observe aberration.

Diagnosis. Although an A-V junctional rhythm may be suspected when the apical rate ranges from 40 to 50 beats per minute, the diagnosis is made only by the electrocardiogram. When the P wave is situated before the QRS complex, the P-R interval is usually short, less than 0.12 second. With a slow (or "passive") A-V junctional rhythm (40 to 50 beats per minute), this can be recognized unmistakably. If the P wave follows the QRS complex, the R-P interval may measure 0.16 to 0.20 second with normal conduction (Scherf and Cohen, 1966). Conduction disturbances may, of course, alter all of these relationships.

Inversion of the P wave and variation in the P-R interval should take into consideration variation in antegrade and retrograde conduction times. For example, prolongation of antegrade conduction may result in the P wave preceding the QRS even though the site of impulse may be "low nodal" (Fisch and Knoebel, 1970). In a similar manner, depression of retrograde conduction might result in the QRS preceding the P wave even if the rhythm were "upper nodal" (Fisch and Knoebel, 1970).

The conditions to be differentiated are atrial fibrillation with an almost regular slow ventricular response (A-V junctional rhythm), A-V dissociation, atrial standstill, sinoventricular conduction, and idioventricular rhythm.

Treatment. There is no specific treatment for this condition; therapy should be directed toward the underlying clinical state.

Prognosis. The prognosis in A-V junctional rhythm depends on the underlying clinical state. Persistent A-V junctional rhythm is usually a sign of widespread myocardial damage; however, it may occasionally be the result of a small isolated lesion. The occurrence in the postinfarction period of A-V junctional rhythm (not tachycardia) by itself is not usually associated with a poor prognosis.

CORONARY SINUS RHYTHM

Coronary sinus rhythm is probably a subdivision of A-V junctional rhythm. The pacemaker arises in the A-V junction close to the coronary sinus in the proximal portion of the A-V junction. The following electrocardiographic criteria characterize coronary sinus rhythm: (a) the P-R interval may range from 0.10 to 0.17 second; (b) the P wave is of low voltage or indiscernible in lead I; (c) the P wave is negative in leads II and III and is frequently peaked (occasionally, it may show an intrinsicoid deflection); and (d) the

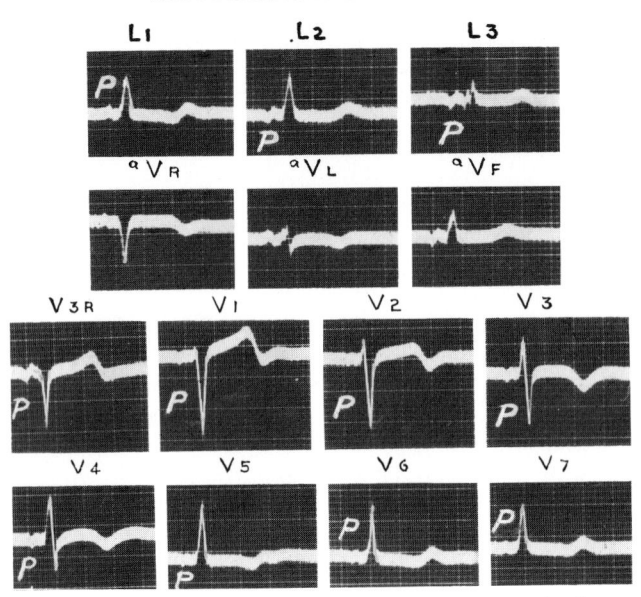

Figure 11-6. Coronary sinus (supranodal) rhythm. The P wave in lead I is upright but of low amplitude. Note inverted P waves in leads II, III, aVF, and V₃R and inverted P waves in the precordial leads V₁ to V₅. In V₆ and V₇, the P waves are diphasic. The P-R interval measures 0.14 second. (See text.)

electrical axis of the P wave is deviated to the left (Fig. 11-6).

Incidence and Etiology. Scherf and Harris (1946) collected 31 instances in 23,610 consecutive tracings (1.3 per thousand); Katz and Pick (1956) found 172 instances in 50,000 electrocardiograms (3.4 per thousand). Coronary sinus rhythm probably results from disease or transient functional depression of the sinus node. It is most frequently observed in patients with arteriosclerotic or hypertensive heart disease; it is occasionally encountered in rheumatic heart disease or as the result of the effects of digitalis.

LEFT ATRIAL RHYTHM

Experimental and clinical evidence suggests that in certain instances the pacemaker may arise in the left atrium. To a large degree, this rests on electrocardiographic and vectorcardiographic evidence. This electrocardiographic diagnosis depends on one or both of the following features: (1) inverted P waves in V₆ with upright, isoelectric, or inverted P waves in lead I; and (2) negative P waves in lead I and V₆ with "dome-and-dart" waves in V₁; (3) the presence of these findings in atrial flutter with which it is commonly associated. On the basis of vectorial analysis, it has been pointed out that the P wave inversion in V₆ is the most sensitive specific sign of this arrhythmia.

The proposed theory concerning the origin of left atrial rhythm may be correct; however, it is difficult to establish from the available evidence. To be ruled out are all ectopic rhythms arising in the lower portion of the right atrium and A-V junctional rhythm with retrograde conduction. Until these points are settled, the electrocardiographic patterns previously mentioned should be considered as originating from one of the several possible foci until more definitive evidence is obtained. It has been suggested that since the ectopic focus cannot be definitely placed in the left atrium, a general term such as "ectopic rhythm" might be used to refer to this rhythm.

A-V JUNCTIONAL TACHYCARDIA

When a sustained junctional rhythm ranges in rate between 80 and 110 beats per minute (the inherent rate, which is unmasked during bradycardia, is 40 to 50 beats per minute), it may be due to what is called "nonparoxysmal junctional tachycardia." This form must be distinguished from "paroxysmal junctional tachycardia," which usually has a faster rate (between 140 and 220 beats per minute). The etiologic factors and treatment of paroxysmal A-V junctional tachycardia are similar to those of paroxysmal atrial tachycardia (see Chapter 9).

Paroxysmal Form

Electrocardiogram. The QRS complexes and position of the P waves are similar to those of premature beats of similar origin (Fig. 11-7). Four electrocardiographic patterns of A-V junctional tachycardia, with features similar to the corresponding junctional rhythm, may be recognized. These are (1) P wave preceding the ventricular complex (old classification: "upper nodal"); (2) P wave concealed by the QRS ("midnodal") (in this case, atrial standstill should be excluded); (3) P wave succeeding the QRS ("lower nodal"); and (4) coronary sinus tachycardia (Scherf and Cohen, 1966).

Therapy. The therapy is that required by the underlying cause. Carotid sinus pressure or other methods for increasing vagal tone result in transient abolition of the complexes of junctional origin, in most cases. If vagal stimulation is not effective, digitalis may be administered, except in those patients in whom the arrhythmia is a manifestation of digitalis intoxication.

Bidirectional Tachycardia. A bidirectional type of junctional tachycardia (formerly thought to arise from the ventricles) is not uncommon and usually results from toxic digitalis effects (Fig. 11-8).

Rosenbaum et al. (1969) have suggested that bidirectional tachycardia may be explained by the differing electrophysiologic properties of the individual fascicles. The right bundle branch has the longest recovery time of the three fascicles and it is not unexpected that conduction delay and block due to a rapid supraventricular rate causes the pattern of RBBB. The anterior division of the left branch, possessing the next longest recovery time, also may be blocked. Furthermore, the sinus impulse, conducted normally in the left posterior hemibranch to activate the ventricles, arrives too early to activate the left anterior branch retrogradely. The second impulse from the rapid supraventricular focus reaches the left posterior branch in a refractory state, but the left anterior branch is now recovered and conducts the beat, resulting in the second type of QRS complex. This

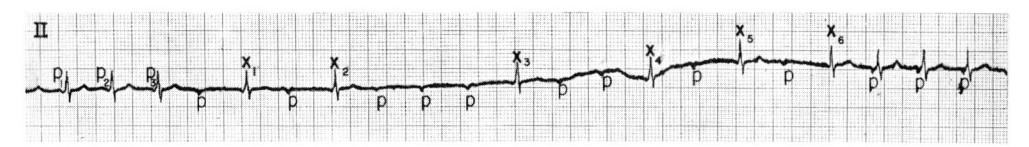

Figure 11-7. A-V junctional tachycardia with varying degrees of A-V heart block. Shows a junctional tachycardia, rate 117 per minute; this is maintained during periods of ventricular standstill. Note the inverted P waves and the short P-R interval at P_2 and P_3. During the ventricular pauses, note the continuance of the inverted atrial beats, which maintain the retrograde conduction and the same heart rate. Note the resumption of the 1:1 response after X_6.

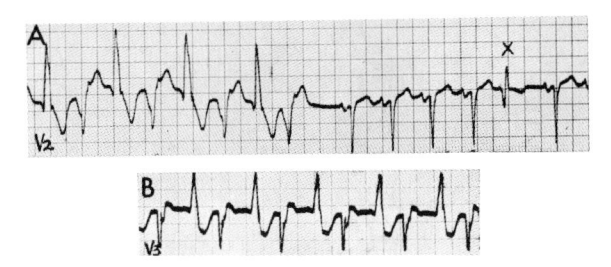

Figure 11-8. Bidirectional type of junctional tachycardia. (See junctional tachycardia, p. ,,,.)

(A) Shows termination of tachycardia with return to normal sinus rhythm. Note that the ventricular complexes after conversion are downward in direction and are similar to, but narrower than, the downward-directed complexes of the paroxysm. Note ventricular premature beat at X.

(B) Simulates bidirectional junctional tachycardia due to digitalis. The basic rhythm (ventricular or A-V junctional with aberration) is represented by upward-directed QRS complexes. Downward-directed complexes are ventricular premature beats with fixed coupling (which is *shorter* than the interval between the premature beat and the following QRS).

repetitive cycling produces the pattern of bidirectional tachycardia.

The supraventricular QRS complexes may be abolished with carotid sinus pressure (CSP) (Fig. 11-8). This observation has led to the theory that this arrhythmia may be due to two independent foci, one supraventricular and one ventricular.

Inasmuch as this arrhythmia occurs in patients with severe myocardial damage of various etiologies, the prognosis is usually poor and is associated with a high mortality.

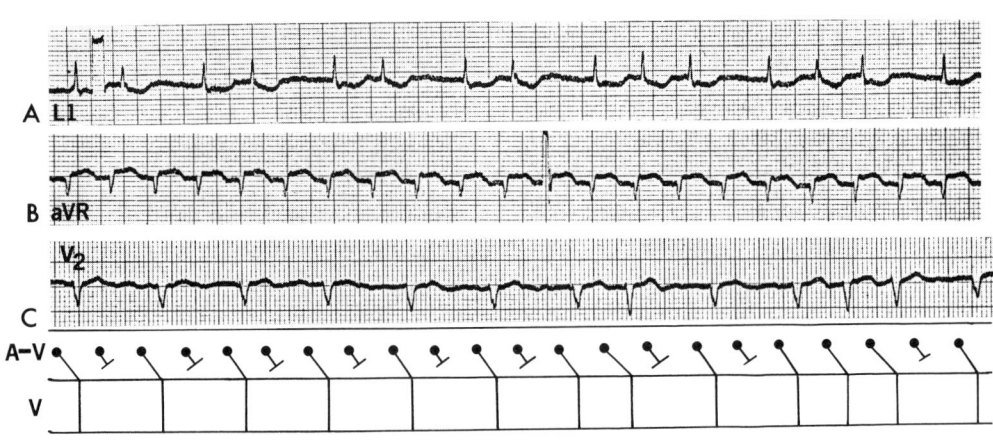

Figure 11-9. A-V junctional tachycardia with exit block and pseudobigeminy. These tracings were obtained on a 65-year-old female with chronic atrial fibrillation who was in digitalis toxicity. Intermittent second degree A-V block of A-V junctional impulses results in intermittent irregularity or pseudobigeminy of the ventricles.

(A) (Lead I) Atrial fibrillation. At the beginning of this strip, notice regular 3:2 periodicity (pseudobigeminy); at the end of this strip there are 4:3 Wenckebach periods.

(B) (aVR) A-V junctional tachycardia with a rate of 160 per minute, probably due to digitalis toxicity. No exit block is present. This pattern could be misinterpreted as atrial tachycardia.

(C) (V$_2$) In lead V$_2$, repeated 2:1 exit block is manifested as a regular ventricular rate of 80 beats per minute. In the left half of the strip, 2:1 exit block of the A-V junctional tachycardia mimics "A-V junctional tachycardia" with a rate of 80 beats per minute. In the right half of the strip, the following ratios of conduction are present: 3:2, 2:1, 4:3 block (Wenckebach periodicity).

Nonparoxysmal Form

Etiology and Treatment. In nonparoxysmal junctional tachycardia, the ventricular rate ranges from 80 to 110 beats per minute in contrast to the more rapid paroxysmal form. The nonparoxysmal type may be produced by excessive digitalis given for the treatment of atrial fibrillation; this may simulate conversion to normal sinus rhythm because of the regularity of the ventricular complexes. Such a mechanism may occur as a result of exit block (Fig. 11–9). These episodes may be observed in up to 30 per cent of patients with atrial fibrillation who are receiving digitalis (Urbach et al., 1969).

A-V JUNCTIONAL ESCAPE

Following parasympathetic stimulation, the excessive slowing of the S-A node is often interrupted by an A-V junctional impulse or A-V junctional escape beat. This is a very important homeostatic mechanism, since sudden death from heart disease would be much more frequent than it actually is if this mechanism were not operative. If escape of the A-V junction does not occur under these conditions, automatic tissue in the region of the bundle of His or below its bifurcation may take over control of the ventricular rhythm. If the latter mechanism also fails, death may result from prolonged cardiac arrest (standstill), or the development of ventricular flutter or fibrillation. Junctional and ventricular escape are often responses to relatively mild hypoxia; on the other hand, severe hypoxia, as may result from anesthesia, occasionally from Stokes-Adams seizures, and from the effects of certain drugs (e.g., quinidine and potassium), may actually depress these lower pacemakers to such a degree that complete cardiac standstill or ventricular fibrillation and death may result.

Etiology. A-V junctional escape occurs: (1) with spontaneous sinus slowing; (2) with S-A block (see Fig. 5–12); (3) as a result of partial A-V heart block with failure of an atrial impulse to discharge the lower pacemaker; (4) following a premature beat that temporarily suppresses the S-A pacemaker; (5) following carotid sinus pressure during normal sinus rhythm or in the postparoxysmal pause after termination of a supraventricular tachycardia (Figs. 11–10, 11–11); and (6) when the S-A node is depressed by excessive vagal tone, occurring in a variety of conditions, such as hyperactive carotid sinus reflexes, digitalis intoxication, rheumatic carditis, coronary artery disease, and certain other disease states (see Chapter 5). It is frequently observed in the older age group in association with sinus bradycardia.

Electrocardiogram. A-V junctional escape is easily recognized in the electrocardiogram by the slow rate (40 to 50 beats per minute). The essential feature of an escaped beat is that it occurs after a long pause. It is often not preceded by P waves; frequently, the P-R interval may be short and the P waves may be inverted (Fig. 11–11). The QRS may simulate those of normal beats or aberration may be present. If a series of escape beats appears at a rate slightly in excess of the sinus bradycardia, A-V dissociation may result.

Escape beats may occur singly or in brief runs. Rarely, this same mechanism may initiate persistent junctional rhythm or even junctional tachycardia. If the A-V junctional pacemaker continues to function and does so at a rate greater than that of the re-activated S-A node, the resultant rhythm may be: (a) A-V dissociation, (b) the nonparoxysmal form of junctional tachycardia, or (c) a combination of "a" and "b." This first type has been called "passive junctional rhythm" or the assumption of pacemaker activity by default. The

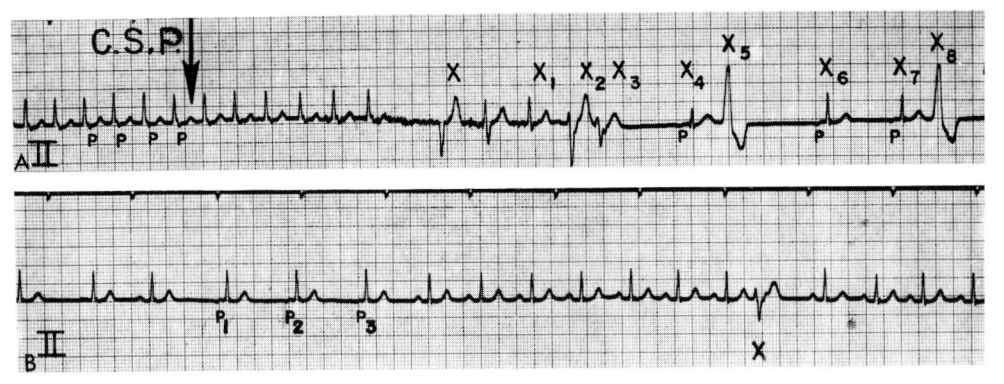

Figure 11-10. Paroxysmal junctional tachycardia.

(A) The paroxysm manifests a regular rhythm with a rate of 180 per minute. Note that the P waves are inverted and immediately follow the QRS complex (lower nodal rhythm). Following carotid sinus pressure, note the presence of a postparoxysmal pause and a junctional escape beat at X, a normally appearing QRS at X_1, followed by premature beats or aberrantly conducted beats at X_2 and X_3. Note the occurrence of a junctional escape beat at X_4 preceded by an inverted P wave and followed by a premature beat, probably ventricular in origin, at X_5. This is followed by a compensatory pause and junctional beats at X_6 and at X_7.

(B) Note the restoration of normal sinus rhythm with a wandering pacemaker from the S-A to the A-V node (inverted P waves at P_1, P_2, and P_3) and the restoration to normal sinus rhythm thereafter, except for a premature beat at X.

second type occurs when the junctional pacemaker manifests greater automaticity than the sinus node (e.g., due to digitalis effects); this has been regarded as the assumption of pacemaker activity by "usurpation."

Treatment. If A-V junctional escape is observed only occasionally, treatment is not necessary. However, in the presence of prolonged periods of junctional escape, the underlying condition, as previously noted, must be determined and treated. If recurrent episodes of escape occur, prophylactic measures may be employed. These may include management of a rheumatic carditis, discontinuance of digitalis, and the use of sympathomimetic amines or atropine. Treatment is especially urgent if the junctional escape rate is so slow that syncopal attacks occur. Under these conditions, an artificial pacemaker is indicated.

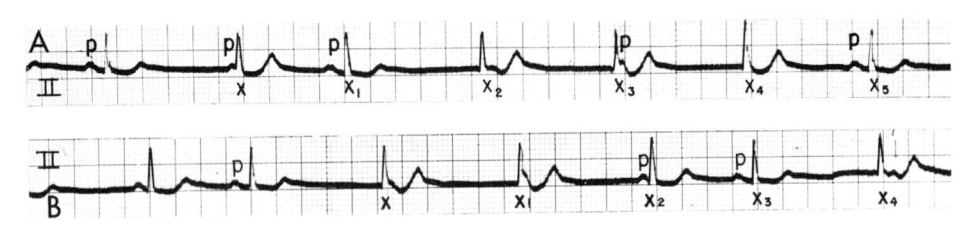

Figure 11-11. Normal sinus beats with a wandering pacemaker, periods of A-V junctional escape, and intermittent A-V dissociation.

(A) Note the normal P-R interval, followed by a junctional escape beat at X, the normally conducted beat at X_1, another escape beat at X_2, X_3, and X_4, with a conducted beat at X_5. The sinus rate is 68 per minute with the conducted beats and 58 per minute with the escape beats. Intermittent A-V dissociation occurs at X_2, X_3 and X_4.

(B) Shows periods of A-V junctional escape at cycles marked X, X_1, and X_4. Intermittent A-V dissociation is present at X, X_1, X_2, and X_4.

RECIPROCAL RHYTHM

General Considerations. Reciprocal rhythm is a relatively rare type of arrhythmia. It may be defined as a disturbance of rhythm whereby an impulse arising in the sinus node, atria, A-V junction, or ventricles activates the atrial or ventricular chamber and, during its passage through the A-V junction, enters another A-V pathway, which permits the impulse to return to activate the same chamber once again. Reciprocal rhythm, as it occurs in man, has been associated chiefly with an A-V junctional pacemaker. Two additional types of reciprocal rhythm have been described: reciprocal rhythm with impulses of atrial origin, and reciprocal rhythm with impulses of ventricular origin (Kistin, 1963).

Clinical and experimental evidence suggests that one mechanism for reciprocal rhythm may be the existence of multiple and separate pathways for atrioventricular and ventriculoatrial conduction. The extensive literature on this subject has been discussed recently (Kistin, 1963; Moe, 1966; Schamroth and Dubb, 1965; Schamroth and Yoshonis, 1969).

The existence of two or more longitudinally dissociated pathways in part or all of the A-V junction has been proposed on indirect physiologic evidence and suggestive anatomic findings (see Chapter 2). Clinical findings have been described which are consistent with the presence of two or more pathways in the upper and middle portions of the A-V junction; these may form a common pathway in the remainder of the junction, or they may be completely separate throughout the length of the A-V junction (Schamroth and Yoshonis, 1969).

Reciprocal rhythm thus represents a form of re-entry. For example, propagation of a junctional impulse proceeds in a forward direction through one portion of the A-V junction to stimulate the ventricles and in a retrograde direction to activate the atria. The impulse from the atria then re-enters another portion of the A-V junction, which is now excitable and is conducted to activate the ventricles for a second time.

Less commonly, reciprocal beats may arise in the atria or ventricles. Reciprocal rhythm of atrial origin occurs when the sinus or atrial impulse, somewhere in its course toward the ventricles, turns back to activate the atria, thus producing both a QRS complex and a retrograde or reciprocal P wave (Schamroth and Yoshonis, 1969) (see Fig. 11–12). In reciprocal rhythm of ventricular origin, the impulse arises in the ventricle and is propagated in a retrograde manner through the A-V junction and returns to the ventricle.

Terminology. The term "reciprocating rhythm" is applied to repeated cycles of tachycardia, and "reciprocal beat," to one cycle. The term "return extrasystole" has been used synony-

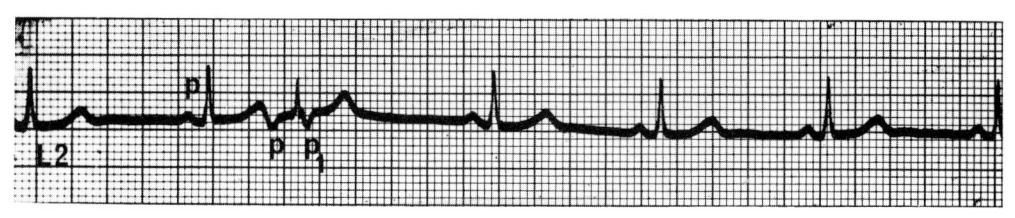

Figure 11–12. Atrial reciprocal beat. (Lead II.) Normal sinus rhythm. The complexes initiated by the inverted P (P-R interval, 0.14 second) probably represent an atrial premature beat. The following inverted P wave represents an atrial reciprocal beat (R-P, 0.08 second).

mously with "reciprocal beat," but this has the disadvantage in that "extrasystole" is used by some writers to mean an accurately coupled ectopic systole or an interpolated systole. The term "echo" is descriptive when the impulse originates in the atrium or ventricle and returns to activate the same chamber a second time but seems less so when the site or origin is in the A-V junction.

Etiology. Reciprocal rhythm appears chiefly in the presence of digitalis toxicity, coronary artery disease, and rheumatic myocarditis.

Diagnosis. The electrocardiographic diagnosis may be made, particularly in the presence of an A-V junctional rhythm, by the presence of an abnormally prolonged R-P interval (over 0.2 second) in which the retrograde P wave is followed by a second ventricular beat (Figs. 11–13, 11–14). This reciprocal beat is separated from the preceding beat by an interval of 0.5 second or less. The R-P interval of successive beats becomes increasingly longer, with the longest R-P interval yielding premature reciprocal beats.

Treatment. The treatment depends on the underlying clinical state and the cause, namely, digitalis toxicity, coronary artery disease, or other factors. Recently, propranolol has been shown to be particularly effective in the presence of reciprocal rhythm.

WIDENING OF QRS COMPLEXES

The QRS complexes may be widened and distorted in the presence of many factors, including (a) ventricular premature beats, (b) supraventricular premature beats and tachycardia (aberration), (c) delayed conduction during bradycardia (e.g., A-V junctional escape), (d) ventricular abnormality or dysfunction producing transient and frequently permanent bundle branch block, (e) drugs (quinidine, procaine amide), and (f) artificial pacemakers (see Chapter 37).

Prolongation in the width of the QRS complex depends on a variety of factors, which may be divided into: (a) functional alterations in the physiologic properties of the A-V junction and His-Purkinje system, and (b) organic cardiac changes. The most frequent functional alteration is propagation of an impulse during the partial refractory period of the A-V transmission system. Organic factors include: (a) the presence of cardiac hypertrophy or dilatation, (b) disease of the main bundle branches or their smaller subdivisions, and (c) a combination of "a" and "b."

The evidence concerning the modi-

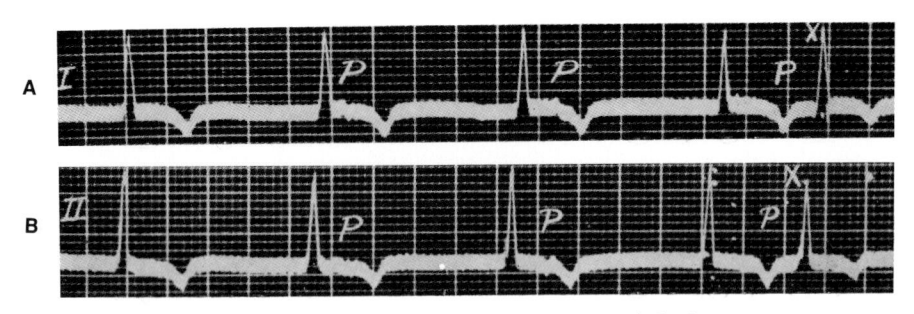

Figure 11–13. Reciprocal beats in a patient with A-V junctional rhythm.
(A) (Lead I) Shows low A-V junctional rhythm in which the QRS is followed by inverted P waves. Note the progressive lengthening of the R-P interval until a critical point is reached (X), when the re-entrant excitation wave finds the antegrade A-V pathway nonrefractory and gives rise to a contraction in the ventricle (reciprocal beat).
(B) (Lead II) Shows the same phenomenon at X.

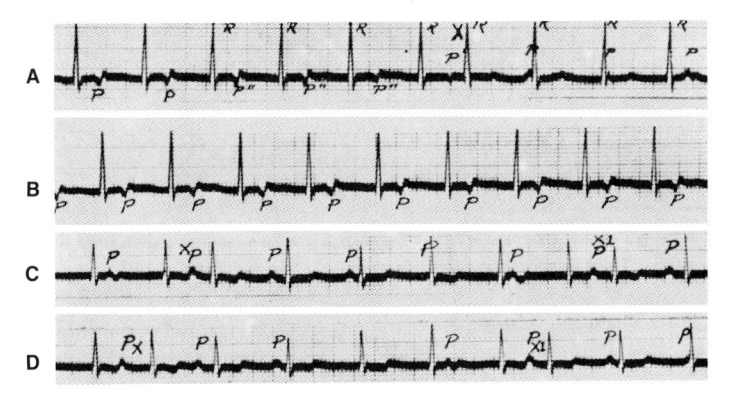

DISTURBANCES IN THE REGION OF THE A-V JUNCTION 157

Figure 11-14. A-V junctional rhythm, reciprocal beats, intermittent A-V dissociation and captured beats (lead II).

(A) Note the presence of "lower A-V nodal" rhythm in the initial six beats. There is a gradual increase in the R-P interval until in cycle X the R-P interval has increased to 0.32 second and is followed by a premature QRS complex, X (reciprocal beat). The remaining atrial beats in this strip are upright, indicating a sinus origin, the rate of which is slower than that of the ventricular cycles (the ventricular rate is 84 per minute; the atrial rate is 78 per minute). This represents a period of A-V dissociation.

(B) Shows resumption of a regular "lower A-V nodal" rhythm with an inverted P wave following the QRS complex at a fixed interval.

(C) A-V dissociation, at X: the P wave captures the ventricle (A-V dissociation with captured beats). Another captured beat is observed at X_1.

(D) A-V dissociation: ventricular capture occurs at X and X_1 and also in the cycle immediately following Px. Note that this cycle length is slightly shorter than that of the A-V nodal beats. Note the difference between reciprocal beats (which have also been considered to be captured beats) and the captured beats of A-V dissociation (so-called pseudoreciprocal beats). In the former, the P wave is inverted, indicating retrograde conduction with a return of the impulse to activate the ventricle; in the latter, the P wave is upright, indicating the usual type of antegrade conduction.

fications of the conducting fibers at rapid rates is complex; several points merit mention here. It has been shown experimentally that the refractory periods of the A-V junction, the bundle of His, and the bundle branches decrease at rapid rates (see Fig. 11-15); however, the cycle length decreases percentage-wise more rapidly than does the refractory period (especially in the right bundle branch), with the result that the refractory period of the conduction system may exceed the basic cycle length (see Fig. 11-15). Patients who manifest varying grades of myocardial abnormality may develop slowed conduction and QRS widening even at relatively slow rates. The factors precipating deviation from the normal conduction in the presence of arrhythmias may be classified into two groups, depending on whether the QRS widening is due to a derangement that resides primarily in the ventricular part of the conduction system or to a rapid or slow rhythm originating from a supraventricular pacemaker.

Supraventricular impulses may encounter refractoriness or block within the A-V conduction system and cause QRS widening in the presence of (a) atrial or junctional premature beats, in which the conduction may sometimes be aberrant, particularly if the premature beat occurs early in diastole during the relative refractory period of the bundle branches; (b) A-V junctional escape beats, in which QRS widening following a prolonged pause is due to aberrant transmission of the impulse through one of the branches of the bundle of His (usually the right bundle branch); (c) the W-P-W syndrome and other pre-excitation syn-

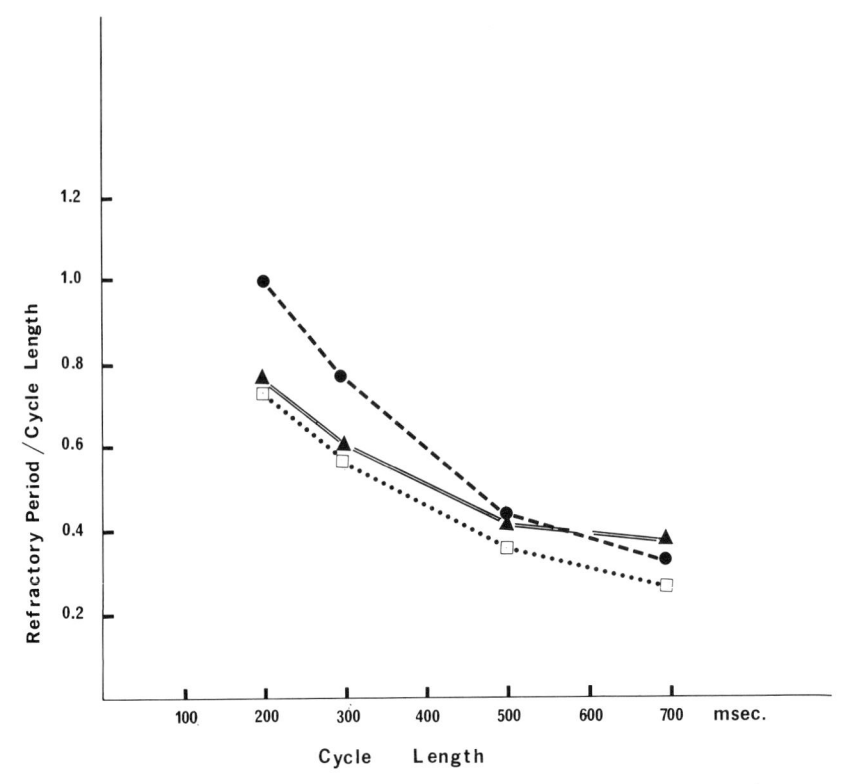

Figure 11–15. The relation of the length of the refractory period in various conduction tissues to cycle length. The circles are the A-V junctional values, the diamonds are the right bundle branch values, and the squares are the bundle of His values. The refractory period length is expressed as a fraction of the total cycle length on the ordinate. Note *that as the cycle length becomes progressively shorter (i.e., as the heart rate increases) the refractory period assumes a greater percentage of the cycle length.* (Compiled from data in Moe et al.: Circ. Res., 16:261, 1965.)

dromes in which fusion of the impulse transmitted through the aberrant pathway and the one propagated through the normal pathway occurs (see Chapter 13); (d) rapid heart rates (140 to 180 beats per minute), in which the QRS complexes may eventually widen to a level of 0.14 to 0.16 second, similar to that in bundle branch block (Figs. 11–16, 11–17, 11–18). This phenomenon exists because a critical heart rate has been observed above which recovery of the conduction system cannot be completed, thus resulting in aberrant conduction of the impulse; and (e) slow heart rates. In occasional subjects, when the heart rate drops below a critical level, QRS widening is observed that probably results from diastolic phase 4 depolarization and decremental conduction in the His-Purkinje system (Massumi, 1968).

Types of QRS Widening. QRS prolongation may be classified into three types, depending on their relationship to the heart rate: (a) those that occur with either slight or marked acceleration of the heart rate; (b) those that occur at slow heart rates; and (c) those cases in which the widening, which may be either constant or intermittent, occurs independently of the rate.

QRS Prolongation with Acceleration of the Heart Rate. A critical rate of recovery of conduction is observed in

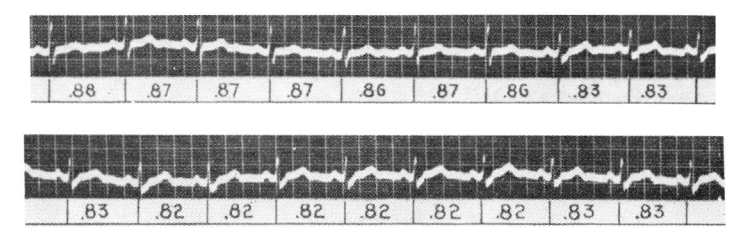

DISTURBANCES IN THE REGION OF THE A-V JUNCTION 159

Figure 11–16. Critical rate of intraventricular conduction.

Effect of ventricular rate on intraventricular conduction. Note that when the R-R interval is 0.86 second or more, the QRS complex measures 0.08 second. When the R-R interval is 0.83 second or less, the width of the QRS complex increases to 0.12 second.

The critical rate of intraventricular conduction is not a fixed figure for all hearts. It may vary considerably.

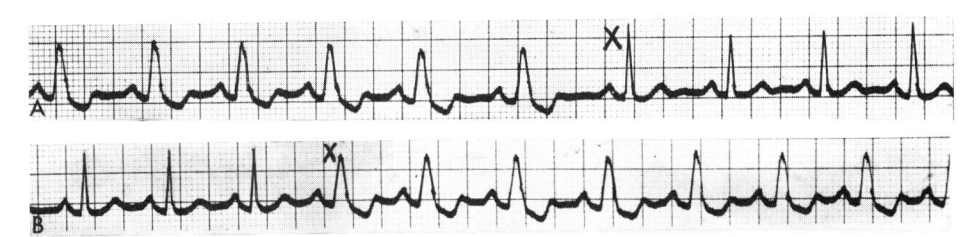

Figure 11–17. Spontaneous transition from bundle branch block to normal intraventricular conduction. (A and B represent a continuous lead II.) This tracing was taken from a patient with hypertensive heart disease of an advanced grade.

(A) Note conversion of bundle branch block to normal intraventricular conduction at X.

(B) Note return to bundle branch block at X again. A slight sinus arrhythmia is present. Several days later, the patient developed a permanent left bundle branch block.

Bundle branch block is not strictly rate-dependent, but it is rate-change-dependent, with two different levels of transition from normal conduction to bundle branch block and from bundle branch block to normal conduction. (See paper by Gardberg, M., and Rosen, I. L.: Amer. Heart J., 55:677, 1958.)

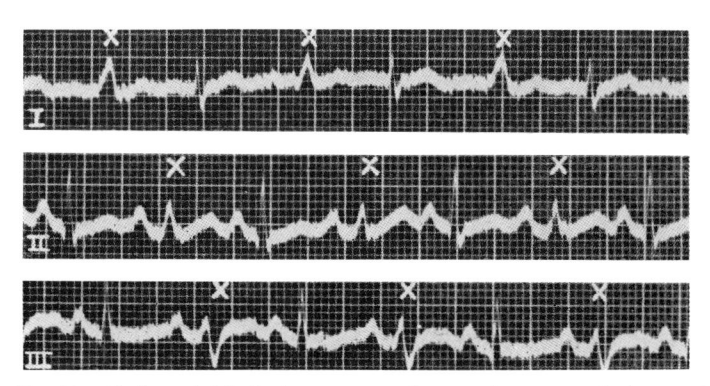

Figure 11–18. Bundle branch block alternating with normal intraventricular conduction. (Leads I, II, and III) Note normal QRS complexes alternating with those of bundle branch block. The interval between the normal and the widened QRS is slightly longer than that between the widened QRS and the following normal beat. P-R times are *constant;* R-R intervals are *constant* as well. This may be called 2:1 bundle branch block.

many hearts. Impulses falling during the effective refractory period of conduction will be completely blocked, and those occurring somewhat later, during the relative refractory period, will be conducted more slowly than normal (Fig. 11-19). The term "aberration" has been applied to those instances in which supraventricular impulses occurring at rapid rates or with a short cycle length following a long cycle length produce QRS widening (see p. 164): (1) the QRS widening occurs with only slight increments in rate (e.g., from 70 to 80 or 90 beats per minute); (2) the QRS widening does not depend on the occurrence of a short cycle length following a long one; (3) in general, derangements residing in the ventricular conduction system produce slowed conduction of supraventricular impulses when the heart rate increases; and (4) this pattern frequently progresses to complete bundle branch block. In some instances, especially with intermediate elevations of the heart rate, it is difficult to differentiate "bundle branch block associated with accelerated heart rate" from "aberration."

MECHANISMS. The mechanism of QRS widening with acceleration of the heart rate is complicated by several factors: (1) Since the right bundle branch ordinarily has the longest refractory period in the conduction system, block is most likely to occur there (Fig. 11-20), although it may also occasionally occur in the left bundle branch or in the subdivisions of either bundle branch. (2) The refractory period of each bundle branch is directly proportional to the cycle length of the preceding beat. (3) The refractory period changes relatively slowly after an alteration in the basic cycle length, a phenomenon which has been termed "warming up," and which possibly lasts over a period of several hundred beats. (4) The effects of premature beats (and hence, of tachycardia, since both diminish the cycle length) also depend upon their focus of origin, their position in the cardiac cycle, and the presence or absence of organic disease of the conduction system. If the greatest prolongation of refractoriness occurs in the bundle branches or their peripheral ramifications, QRS widening will result. Such individuals often have normal intraventricular conduction at slow heart rates (i.e., 60 per minute); but they show QRS widening at more elevated rates (see Figs. 11-16, 7-5).

In this light, rate-dependent bundle branch block, manifested by QRS widening and occurring with a slight increase in the heart rate (to 100 beats per minute or less) also implies the presence of cardiac abnormality, due to organic disease, functional alterations, or drug effects. When right bundle branch block develops with only moderate elevation in rate or incomplete RBBB is present at normal rates, complete non-rate-dependent RBBB is likely to develop. Dodge and Grant (1956) observed the latter sequence in 20 per cent of a series of 80 patients.

In occasional cases, 2:1 or 3:1 left

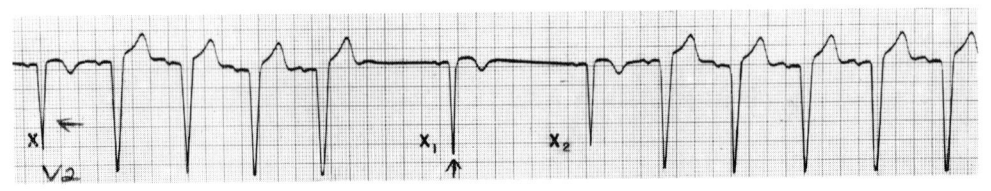

Figure 11-19. Widened QRS complexes, narrowing after long pause. Note the presence of widened QRS complexes, which measure 0.16 second. Note narrowing of the QRS complexes to 0.10 second at X_1 and X_2 following a long pause. This is due to S-A block which was observed in two cycles. X_2 is followed by a resumption of the pre-existent rhythm with widened QRS complexes.

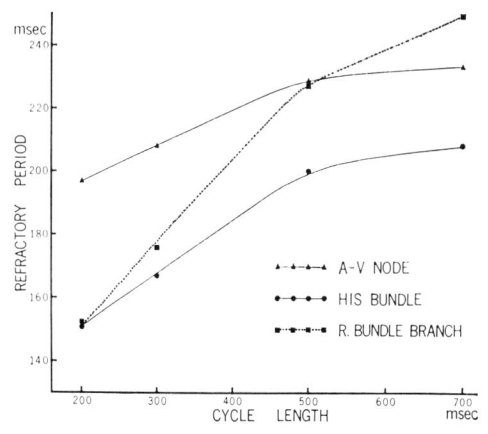

Figure 11-20. Apparent refractory periods of A-V node, His bundle, and right bundle branch as a function of basic cycle length. Open heart preparation. (Moe, G. K., Mendez, C., and Han, J. Circ. Res., 16:261, 1965.)

bundle branch block may occur with elevation of the heart rate; further acceleration causes complete LBBB.

On occasion, the critical heart rate for normal intraventricular conduction has been observed both clinically and experimentally to be lower for the return of normal conduction than it was for the initiation of abnormal conduction. If, for example, bundle branch block appears whenever the cycle length drops below 0.8 second, the conduction disturbance may persist until the cycle length exceeds 0.90 second. This difference has usually been attributed to the fact that the refractory period adjusts to rate changes only slowly ("warming up").

QRS Prolongation at Slow Rates. The subject of bradycardia-dependent bundle branch block has recently been reviewed (Massumi, 1968). The etiology is not clearly understood, although most instances reported to date have been in subjects with severe organic heart disease. At present, the most tenable explanation is that, during a long diastolic interval, phase 4 depolarization of automatic tissues in the bundle branches occurs, altering the excitability in that tissue. Both bundle branches possess automaticity (Hoffman and Cranefield, 1964), and conduction in them may be blocked if diastolic depolarization is sufficiently great.

QRS Prolongation Independent of Rate. Rate-independent QRS widening has considerable clinical significance for several reasons: (a) it frequently precedes the occurrence of complete bundle branch block; (b) sudden death may occur if a ventricular pacemaker does not emerge following the abrupt appearance of complete block; (c) the heart sounds may be altered; and (d) the same hemodynamic changes that accompany any alteration in intraventricular conduction occur (Fig. 11-21). Block of the bundle branches may occur intermittently owing to a number of factors other than rapid rates: (a) alteration in autonomic tone, (b) hemodynamic changes, and (c) effect of drugs.

In patients receiving antiarrhythmic drugs, the QRS widening in the electrocardiogram may manifest two patterns: (1) In the initial stages, widening may be present in only occasional ventricular beats, occurring during short intervals with a slight increase in rate, or may appear independent of it (Fig. 14-12). (2) Widened beats may then gradually increase in frequency until all are widened. These complexes usually appear with a rapid rate, and it may be difficult to differentiate them from ventricular premature beats and ventricular tachycardia.

Etiology and Clinical Significance. The etiology of rate-independent bundle branch block is a matter of some question. Seventy-five per cent of these patients have hypertension or coronary artery disease and, occasionally, normal intraventricular conduction is followed by widened QRS complexes as a result of exercise in subjects with the anginal syndrome. The presence or absence of cardiomegaly, however, appears to be the crucial factor in the clinical severity of the condition.

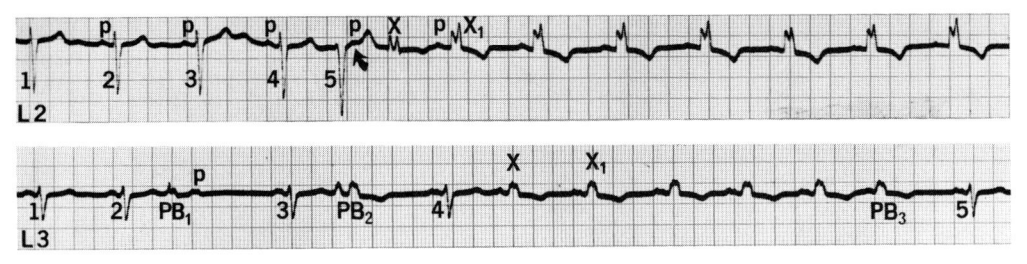

Figure 11-21. Intermittent bundle branch block (not rate-dependent).

(Lead 2) Four sinus beats (1 to 4) are followed by a premature beat, probably A-V junctional in origin with aberration (X). The next P wave (at arrow) occurs exactly on time and can be seen slightly changing the S-T segment of the premature beat. This P wave is conducted with a P-R time of 0.40 second and the QRS following is that of right bundle branch block (X) — this premature beat is therefore probably interpolated. Following this, sinus rhythm continues with all QRS complexes exhibiting right bundle branch block. The first QRS after the premature beat represents ventricular aberration (X₁). The morphology of the following QRS — slightly different from the first QRS — may be considered as rate-dependent right bundle branch block after a short cycle. In the remaining QRS complexes, the rate dependency cannot be evoked.

(Lead 3) The first premature beat (PB₁) with QRS aberration does not disturb the sinus rhythm, but the following P is blocked, resulting in a fully compensatory pause. The third sinus QRS is followed by a premature ectopic P wave (PB₂) with aberrant ventricular response. After a nonfully compensatory pause, a normal QRS-T complex appears. The following P wave (X) is premature and probably ectopic. The following four beats represents sinus arrhythmia terminated by an ectopic P wave (PB₃). All of these six beats resemble the right bundle branch block pattern. This observation illustrates how a block in the right bundle, once induced, may be self-perpetuating in following beats without being rate-dependent.

Other Types of Alteration in QRS Width

PARADOXICAL NARROWING OF QRS WITH SHORT CYCLE. Rarely, a paradoxical effect is observed when the widened QRS complex returns to a normal width following an interval that is shorter than that between the widened complexes (Fig. 11-22). This may be explained in the following ways: (a) the widened complexes at slower rates may have been due to a

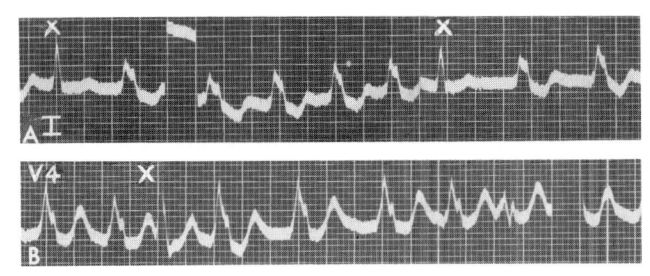

Figure 11-22. Following a run of aberrant, widened QRS complexes, note the occurrence of a QRS of normal width following a short pause.

A and B are taken from a patient with atrial fibrillation manifesting a relatively rapid ventricular rate. In cycles marked X, the QRS complexes following the short pause are narrower than the remaining complexes. This may be explained by the concept of supernormal recovery, as applied to the bundle branch fibers; thus, at this critical time, conduction is normal through the bundle branches. This has been described for other conduction tissues, but rarely for the bundle branches. An alternate explanation for the narrowed QRS would be that this is a premature beat arising from the upper midportion of the interventricular septum. Such an origin permits the impulse to travel simultaneously down both branches, thus producing a QRS complex of normal width. Other explanations of paradoxically non-aberrant QRS after a short cycle are longitudinal dissociation within one bundle branch, or the presence in one branch of two consecutive zones with different properties. (See Wellens, H.: Amer. Heart J., 77:158, 1969.)

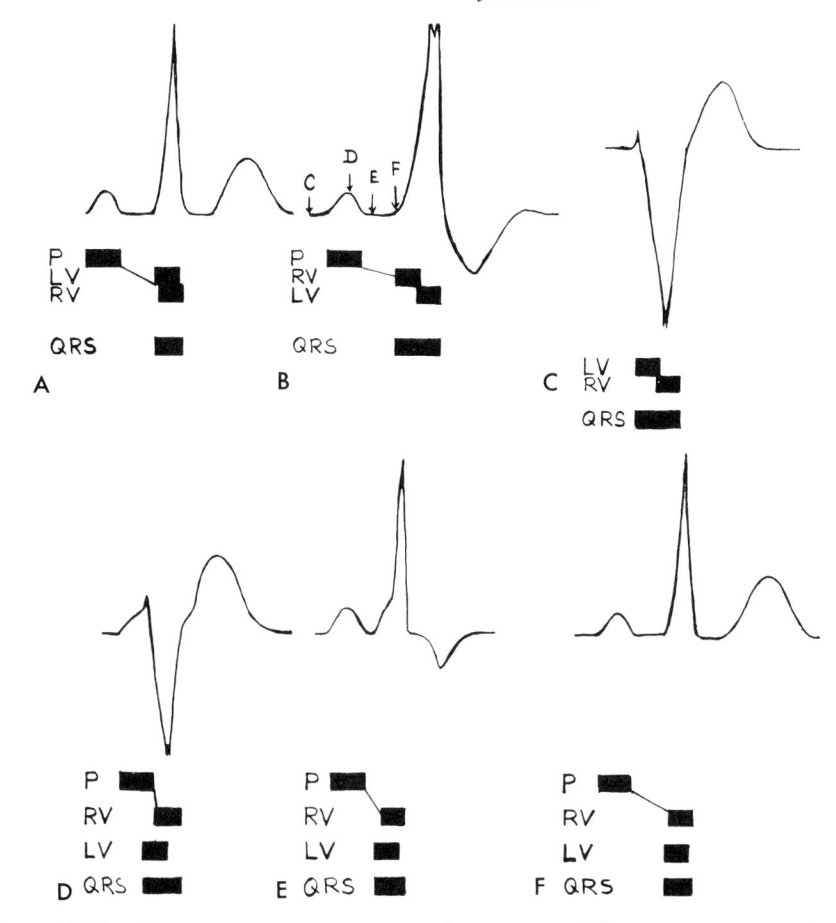

DISTURBANCES IN THE REGION OF THE A-V JUNCTION 163

Figure 11-23. Diagrammatic representation of various possibilities in intraventricular conduction with premature beats occurring in various portions of the cardiac cycle. Below each complex is shown in blocks the relative position of the P waves and their relation to left and right ventricular premature beats and the QRS complex.

(A) (Lead II) Normal QRS complex.

(B) Left bundle branch block pattern. (Lead II) The succession of events in the various chambers is noted in block form below. The activation wave travels from the atria to the right ventricle; delay occurs in the barrier zone of the septum before the left ventricle is activated. The various portions of the presystolic phase (phase 1) are labelled to show the effect of the timing of the premature beat (between the P and Q at points C, D, E and F) on the configuration of the QRS complex.

(C) Left ventricular premature beat occurring in phase 3 between T and P is activated first; after occurrence of the conduction delay in the septal zone, activation of the right ventricle takes place. The QRS is widened and aberrant, as in right bundle branch block.

From D to F are fusion beats between QRS of left bundle branch block and left ventricular premature beats.

(D) R wave of ventricular complex starting on the peak of the P wave (at D). The left ventricular events start immediately after the activation of the atria has begun. The main QRS deflection, therefore, is like that of a left ventricular premature beat.

(E) Left ventricular activation occurs immediately after the P wave (at E). W-P-W-like complexes occur (short P-R interval, widened QRS, and delta wave).

(F) Left ventricular premature beats occurring simultaneously with the beginning activation of the right ventricle at the beginning of the QRS complexes. P is conducted to the right ventricle. At the same time, the left ventricular events take place, so that the over-all activation of the heart closely resembles normal activation without bundle branch block. The P and QRS complex are inscribed in a normal fashion or only slightly aberrant. If the extrasystolic focus falls between D and E, narrowed complexes with changing morphology appear. (Muller, O. F., Cardenas, M., and Bellet, S.: Amer. J. Cardiol., 7:697, 1961.)

bradycardia-dependent bundle branch block; (b) supernormal recovery of the bundle branch fibers could account for it; (c) the narrowed QRS complexes could be the result of a premature beat arising from the upper midportion or the interventricular septum; (d) in the presence of bundle branch block, a premature beat arising in the contralateral ventricle, occurring between the P and Q, may bring about a fusion beat resulting in a QRS at normal or almost normal width (see Fig. 11–23).

In occasional instances, sympathomimetic agents, such as isoproterenol, and alkalinizing agents, such as sodium bicarbonate and molar sodium lactate, that speed conduction exert their effects by decreasing the refractory period of the conduction fibers, thus decreasing the QRS width (Fig. 11–24).

EFFECT OF CAROTID SINUS PRESSURE ON QRS WIDENING. The following are the most commonly observed effects of carotid sinus pressure on QRS widening changes: (1) there may be no effect; (2) with slowing of the heart rate, normal intraventricular conduction may be transiently restored; (3) occasionally, complete A-V block may result from a transient block of the unaffected bundle; and (4) ventricular fibrillation may occur as a rare complication. (See also p. 344.)

ABERRATION

GENERAL CONSIDERATIONS

Aberrant ventricular conduction is characterized by abnormal spread of the supraventricular impulse in the ventricle brought about by delayed activation of one of the branches of the bundle of His, with resultant widening of the ventricular complex. The right bundle branch is the branch most frequently involved (Fig. 11–25). Such impulses are to be differentiated from those originating in ectopic foci (premature beats or ectopic paroxysmal tachycardias) which they very frequently resemble. In the human subject, the effect of atrial pacing in producing aberration depends to some degree upon the control electrocardiogram, the atrial pacing rate, and the cardiac status prior to atrial pacing. For example, Cohen et al. (1968) studied this procedure in normal subjects with a normal electrocardiogram, and in those with left-axis deviation, left ventricular hypertrophy, and delay in the right bundle branch. In 20 of 52 subjects, they observed multiple patterns of aberrant conduction, the most frequent being straightforward RBBB in 31 cases, RBBB with left-axis deviation in 27, left-axis deviation in 14, inferior (rightward) axis deviation in 6, RBBB with inferior axis deviation in 7, and LBBB in 6 (Cohen et al., 1968).

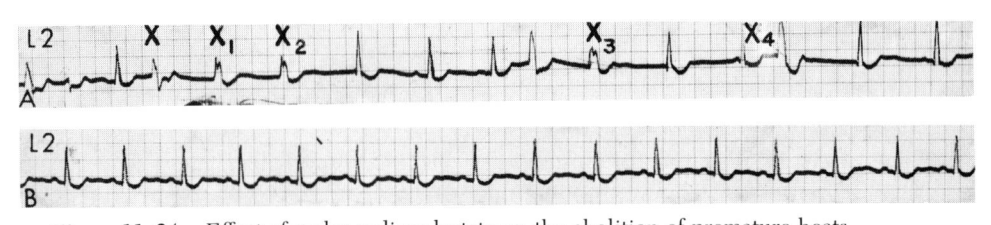

Figure 11–24. Effect of molar sodium lactate on the abolition of premature beats.
(A) The arrhythmia probably represents a parasystolic rhythm with periods of exit block and occasional fusion beats, for example, at X and X_4.
(B) After molar sodium lactate, note abolition of premature beats.

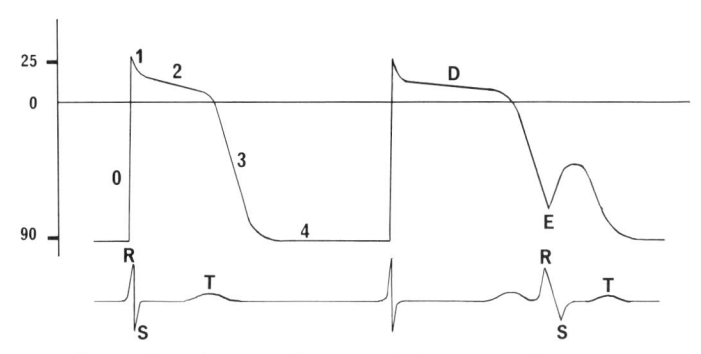

DISTURBANCES IN THE REGION OF THE A-V JUNCTION 165

Figure 11–25. Electrophysiologic mechanisms of aberration. The numbers refer to the phase of the transmembrane action potential. The situation in which a premature impulse discharging the ventricular fiber during the repolarization phase and in which phase 4 depolarization causes aberration has been illustrated in Figure 2–8 (p. 23). The long preceding cycle has produced an action potential with a prolonged phase 2 (D). Because of this widening of the action potential, the impulse arriving at (E) discharges the ventricular fiber during the repolarization phase. The resultant aberrant conduction is shown in the simultaneous electrocardiogram.

ELECTROCARDIOGRAPHIC CHARACTERISTICS

Gouaux and Ashman (1947) observed the presence of aberration when a beat with a short R-R interval followed a beat of a longer cycle (Ashman phenomenon). In this case, the long cycle predetermines a long refractory period so that the impulse arriving with the succeeding short cycle meets relatively refractory conduction which usually manifests itself in the right branch, thereby exhibiting a picture of RBBB. In fact, 85 per cent of aberrant complexes show an RBBB pattern. Furthermore, 70 per cent of aberrant beats showing the RBBB pattern in V_1 have a triphasic (rsR', rSR', or RsR') pattern, whereas the remaining 30 per cent show a mono- or diphasic pattern. (Sandler and Marriott, 1965). In 44 per cent of aberrant beats manifesting the RBBB pattern, the initial vector of the QRS complex was identical to the sinus beats.

DIFFERENTIAL DIAGNOSIS

The distinction between aberrant complexes and premature beats is often difficult. Certain electrocardiographic characteristics of these two groups may aid in the differentiation. The following favor the diagnosis of an ectopic rhythm: mono- or diphasic complexes in lead V_1; deep S waves in lead V_6; compensatory pauses after a complex; fixed coupling; and the presence of fusion beats, escape beats or parasystole. The following favor the diagnosis of aberration: a triphasic QRS pattern in lead V_1; an initial q wave in lead V_6; variable coupling; and a short cycle preceded by a long cycle.

SIGNIFICANCE

The diagnosis of aberration is important for several reasons. Although it usually signifies an abnormality in the intraventricular conduction, it has been held by some that aberration may in fact be a normal phenomenon (Berliner and Lewithin, 1945). However, there are certain factors which militate against considering aberration to be a strictly normal phenomenon: (1) it is rarely observed during exercise-induced tachycardias of up to 150 beats per minute or more in subjects with clinically normal hearts, particularly in the younger age groups; (2) the spontaneously occurring form seen at extremely elevated rates occurs in patients with atrial flutter or fibrillation and other types of myocardial abnormality; and (3) most experimental studies on human subjects have been performed by the use of rapid atrial pacing or the production of premature atrial beats. These procedures involve a type of stress on the A-V conduction system that does not necessarily occur under normal circumstances. Furthermore, aberration may obscure the site of origin of a supraventricular beat and may appear to be ventricular in origin. This is an important distinction to recognize.

THERAPY OF ABERRATION

Most important is to remove the cause, if it can be ascertained, particularly if it is the effect of drugs, e.g., procaine amide or quinidine, and to treat the underlying myocardial abnormality. Aberrant beats may respond somewhat differently to antiarrhythmic drugs as compared with premature beats, although occasionally their response to a therapeutic agent is similar. When quinidine or procaine amide is administered, the aberrant beats may disappear or tend to become widened still further due to the increase in the degree of intraventricular block. Diphenylhydantoin (Dilantin) would appear to be the preferred drug in such cases since it does not have the tendency to prolong the QRS interval.

When digitalis is given to such patients with atrial fibrillation, the aberrant beats may disappear or become less frequent, but in some instances, digitalis may be associated with short periods of grouping of these beats, resembling a paroxysmal tachycardia although the QRS complexes have the same configuration as that of the aberrant beats.

References

Barold, S. S., Linhart, J. W., Hildner, F. J., Narula, O. S., and Samet, P.: Incomplete left bundle branch block. A definite electrocardiographic entity. Circulation, 38:702, 1968.

Berliner, K., and Lewithin, P.: Auricular premature systole. I. Aberration of the ventricular complex in the electrocardiogram. Amer. Heart J., 29:449, 1945.

Bisteni, A., Sodi-Pollares, D., Medrano, G. A., and Pileggi, F.: Nerves Conceptos para el Diagnostico de las Extrasistoles Ventriculores. Arch. Inst. Cardiol. (Mexico), 27:46, 1957.

Bisteni, A., Sodi-Pollares, D., Medrano, G. A., and Pileggi, F.: A new approach for the recognition of ventricular premature beats. Amer. J. Cardiol., 5:358, 1960.

Cohen, S. I., Lau, S. H., Haft, J. I., and Damato, A. N.: Experimental production of aberrant ventricular conduction in man. Circulation, 36:673, 1967.

Cohen, S. I., Lau, S. H., Stein, E., Young, M. W., and Damato, A. N.: Variations of aberrant ventricular conduction in man: Evidence of isolated and combined block within the specialized conduction system. An electrocardiographic and vectorcardiographic study. Circulation, 38:899, 1968.

Damato, A. N., and Lau, S. H.: His bundle rhythm. Circulation, 40:527, 1969.

Damato, A. N., Lau, S. H., Berkowitz, W. D., Rosen, K. M., and Lisi, K. R.: Recording of specialized conducting fibers (A-V nodal, His bundle, and right bundle branch) in man using an electrode catheter technique. Circulation, 39:435, 1969.

DeFelice, L. J., and Challice, C. E.: Anatomical and ultrastructural study of the electrophysiological A-V node of the rabbit. Circ. Res., 24:457, 1969.

Dodge, H. B., and Grant, R.: Mechanism of QRS complex prolongation in man: Right ventricular conduction defects. Amer. J. Med., 21:535, 1956.

Fisch, C., and Knoebel, S. B.: Junctional rhythms. Prog. Cardiov. Dis., 13:141, 1970.

Gardberg, M., and Rosen, I. L.: Observations on conduction in a case of intermittent left bundle branch block. Amer. Heart J., 55:677, 1958.

Gouaux, J. L., and Ashman, R.: Auricular fibrillation with aberration simulating ventricular paroxysmal tachycardia. Amer. Heart J., 34:366, 1947.

Han, J., and Moe, G. K.: Cumulative effects of cycle length on refractory periods of cardiac tissue. Amer. J. Physiol., 217:106, 1969.

Hoffman, B. F., and Cranefield, P. F.: Physiological basis of cardiac arrhythmia. Amer. J. Med., 37:670, 1964.

Katz, L. N., and Pick, A.: Clinical Electrocardiography. Part I. The Arrhythmias. Philadelphia, Lea & Febiger, 1956.

Kistin, A. D.: Multiple pathways of conduction and reciprocal rhythm with interpolated ventricular premature systoles. Amer. Heart J., 65:162, 1963.

Lisi, K. R., Rosen, K. M., Lau, S. H., and Damato, A. N.: The electrophysiology of coronary sinus rhythm. Circulation, 39–40:III–34, 1969.

Massumi, R.: Bradycardia-dependent bundle-branch block. A critique and proposed criteria. Circulation, 38:1066, 1968.

Mirowski, M.: Left atrial rhythm: diagnostic criteria and differentiation from nodal arrhythmias. Amer. J. Cardiol., 17:203, 1966.

Moe, G. K.: The physiological basis of reciprocal rhythm. Prog. Cardiov. Dis., 8:461, 1966.

Pick, A., and Langendorf, R.: Recent advances in the differential diagnosis of A-V junctional arrhythmias. Amer. Heart J., 76:553, 1968.

Rosenbaum, M. B., Elizari, M. V., and Lazzari, J. O.: The mechanism of bidirectional tachycardia. Amer. Heart J., 78:4, 1969.

Sandler, I. A., and Marriott, H. J. L.: The differential morphology of anomalous ventricular complexes of RBBB-type in lead V$_1$. Circulation, 31:551, 1965.

Schamroth, L., and Dubb, A.: Escape capture bigeminy. Mechanisms in S-A block, A-V block, and reversed reciprocal rhythm. Brit. Heart J., 27:667, 1965.

Schamroth, L., and Yoshonis, K. F.: Mechanisms in reciprocal rhythm. Amer. J. Cardiol., 24:224, 1969.

Scherf, D., and Cohen, J.: Atrioventricular rhythms. Prog. Cardiov. Dis., 9:499, 1966.

Scherf, D., and Harris, R.: Coronary sinus rhythm. Amer. Heart J., 32:443, 1946.

Tawara, S.: Das Reizleitungsystem des Saugetierherzens. Jena, Gustav Fischer, 1906.

Truex, R. C., and Smythe, M. Q.: Recent observations on the human cardiac conduction system, with special considerations of the atrio-ventricular node and bundle. In Taccardi, B., and Marchetti, G. (eds.): Electrophysiology of the Heart. Oxford, Pergamon Press, 1964, pp. 177–198.

Urbach, J. R., Graurnan, J. J., and Strans, S. H.: Quantitative methods for the recognition of atrioventricular junctional rhythms in atrial fibrillation. Circulation, 39:803, 1969.

Waldo, A. L., Vitikainen, K. J., Harris, P. D., Malm, J. R., and Hoffman, B. F.: The mechanism of synchronization in isorhythmic A-V dissociation. Some observations on the morphology and polarity of the P wave during retrograde capture of the atria. Circulation, 38:880, 1968.

Wellens, H.: Unusual occurrence of non-aberrant conduction in patients with atrial fibrillation and aberrant conduction. Amer. Heart J., 77:158, 1969.

Chapter 12 *A-V Dissociation*

GENERAL CONSIDERATIONS
DEFINITION OF TERMS
  Dissociation
  Interference
  Ventricular Capture
  Atrial Capture
  Zone of Potential Dissociation
MECHANISMS PRODUCING A-V
  DISSOCIATION
INCIDENCE AND ETIOLOGY
TYPES OF A-V DISSOCIATION AND
  MODES OF ONSET

A-V Dissociation Presenting Deviations
  from Above Types
Other Types of Dissociation
AUSCULTATORY PHENOMENA
ECG IN A-V DISSOCIATION
DIFFERENTIAL DIAGNOSIS
DURATION AND FATE OF A-V
  DISSOCIATION
TREATMENT
PROGNOSIS

GENERAL CONSIDERATIONS

A-V dissociation consists in the completely independent beating of the atria and ventricles, each responding to its own pacemaker. Usually, the pacemaker controlling the atria is located in the S-A node, while that controlling the ventricles is located in the A-V junction or in the upper portion of the interventricular septum.

An important aspect of A-V dissociation is that it does not occur as a primary disturbance of rhythm, but arises secondary to some more fundamental disorder.

DEFINITION OF TERMS

Dissociation. The term "dissociation" refers in a general way to the presence in the same heart of two pacemakers with independent rhythmicity. This may refer to any combination of pacemakers, i.e., atrial, A-V junctional, and ventricular, although the most common type is A-V junctional. The term "A-V dissociation" most often implies that the atria, under the control of the S-A node, and the ventricles, under A-V junctional control, beat independently and that the ventricles usually beat faster than the atria. However, the atria may not necessarily be controlled by the S-A node and the ventricles may be controlled by a pacemaker other than the A-V junction. Deviations from the common type are discussed later (see p. 174).

The perpetuation of two rhythms depends upon the propagation of the two electrical impulses in such a fashion that each one produces a state of refractoriness to the electrical transmission of the other. It is about this process that most of the disputed terminology has arisen.

Interference. The term "interference" has been used in a different sense by different authors. (1) The most common use of this term is that in the presence of A-V dissociation the ventricles beat faster than the atria. When the P wave falls far enough beyond the QRS so that the junctional tissues are no longer refractory, the atrial impulse is conducted to the ventricles and the atrial rhythm thus "interferes" with the regular ventricular rhythm by producing an early

A-V DISSOCIATION

ventricular beat (captured beat). (2) The term is also used to mean the mutual extinction of two excitation fronts that meet in any portion of the heart. This form is seen in a "fusion" or summation beat. (3) When the A-V junction discharges its impulse just before the sinus impulse arrives, the latter impulse finds the A-V node refractory. The refractory junctional tissue, therefore, "interferes" with the propagation of the sinus impulse, so that the atrial and ventricular rhythms are dissociated.

All three types of "interference" can be observed. Whenever possible, it is preferable to use a more specific term, for example: (1) when one rhythm gains control of the other pacemaker, the terms "ventricular capture" or "atrial capture" are preferable; (2) when two wave fronts meet and extinction results, the term "fusion beat" best describes the result; and (3) when the A-V junction is refractory to the transmission of a sinus impulse, we shall simply use the term "A-V junctional refractory period."

Ventricular Capture. This occurs when, without a significant change in rate of either the atria or the ventricles, the R-P interval approaches a critical level so that the P wave finds the A-V junction nonrefractory and is conducted to the ventricle, producing a ventricular beat after an interval that is shorter than usual (Figs. 12–1, 12–2). With "ventricular capture," restoration to normal atrioventricular and intraventricular conduction may result; however, A-V conduction is frequently prolonged (Fig. 12–1).

Atrial Capture. Occasionally, during periods when the atria are under the control of a junctional or ventricular pacemaker, the sinus impulse may reach the atrial muscle during a nonrefractory phase and result in an atrial beat. This constitutes atrial capture by the S-A node. Conversely, when the atria are under the control of the sinus pacemaker during A-V dissociation, a retrograde impulse arising in the A-V junction or ventricles may reach the atria prior to the sinus impulse. The S-A node may be discharged or depressed by this impulse. This latter situation may result in atrial capture by a junctional or ventricular pacemaker. If the atrial capture is only partial and the two impulses meet in the atrial musculature, a fusion beat results.

Zone of Potential Dissociation. The period during which the sinus impulse can control the atria without interruption from an ascending A-V junctional impulse has been termed "the zone of potential dissociation" (Miller and

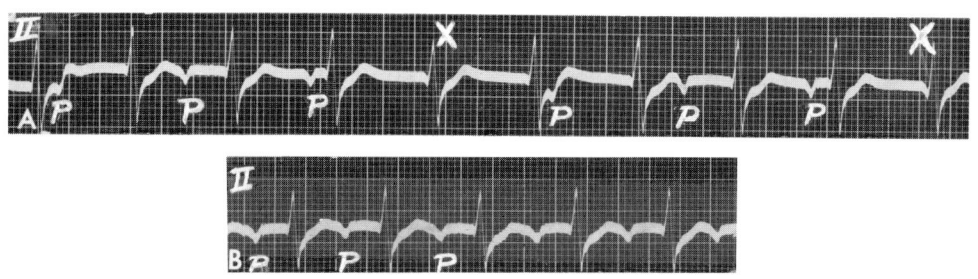

Figure 12–1. Incomplete A-V dissociation with captured beats. A and B represent a continuous lead I. The atrial rhythm is regular at a rate of 46 per minute and the ventricles beat at a rate of 50 per minute. At X, a captured normal sinus beat is seen. Note slight decrease in cycle length in this cycle. At X_1 a captured beat occurs; note the shortened R-R interval in this cycle and the slightly prolonged P-R interval. This is followed by lower nodal rhythm seen on strip B, clearly shown in the last three beats.

Figure 12-2. Incomplete A-V dissociation with captured beats.

(A) (Lead I) Note the relatively slow regular atrial rate at 48 per minute and the relatively more rapid ventricular rate at 56 per minute. These rhythms are entirely independent of each other; the P waves are upright, indicating a sinus origin. In the cycles marked X, the atrial beat occurs in that phase of the cardiac cycle which finds the A-V conduction system in a nonrefractory state, resulting in a ventricular response (captured beat). Note aberration of the QRS at X and X_2, but none at X_1.

(B) (Lead II) Note that in X and X_1 the QRS of the captured beats is somewhat different in contour from that of the other beats, indicating some alteration in the spread of the impulse through the A-V conduction system (aberration).

Sharrett, 1957). This zone is equal to the algebraic sum of the time for conduction from the sinus node to the A-V junction plus the time of retrograde conduction back to the atria.

MECHANISMS PRODUCING A-V DISSOCIATION

Dissociation may result from three different mechanisms: (1) slowing of the generation of impulse in the primary pacemaker of the heart; (2) acceleration, either paroxysmal or sustained, of impulse formation in the automatic tissue of the A-V junction or ventricles; and (3) permanent or intermittent failure of several successive primary pacemaker impulses, discharging at a normal rate, to reach or to cross the narrow atrioventricular bridge (Pick, 1963). If the failure of conduction is permanent, it is classified as a form of A-V block with concomitant A-V dissociation (Fig. 12-3).

INCIDENCE AND ETIOLOGY

The percentage varies from 0.48 per cent in 10,000 consecutive cases (Marriott et al., 1958) to 1.4 per cent in 50,000 cases (Katz and Pick, 1956). A-V dissociation always occurs secondary to some other disturbance in the function of the heart. Sinus slowing may be caused by "sinus arrhythmia," a compensatory pause following a premature atrial impulse, or any factor that decreases automaticity (i.e., decreased catecholamines, increased

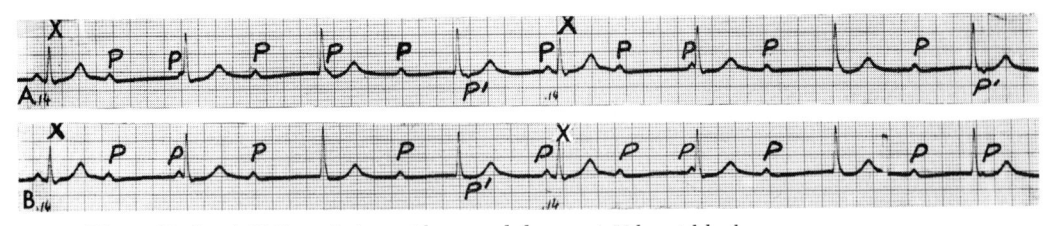

Figure 12-3. A-V dissociation with second degree A-V heart block.

(A and B) (Continuous strip, Lead II) The atrial rate averages 70 per minute; the ventricular rate is 37 per minute and is faster than half of the atrial rate. The QRS complexes following conducted P waves (at X) are of smaller amplitude. These P waves are preceded by an inverted P wave because of retrograde conduction; this represents an atrial capture (P'), which follows in a nonrefractory period of the atrium. A similar inverted P wave is observed (P') in B. No P wave occurs within 0.68 second after a nodal QRS is conducted; all P waves following a nodal QRS beyond 1.00 second are conducted.

A-V DISSOCIATION

vagal tone, electrolyte changes, toxic states, or the action of certain drugs, e.g., digitalis). A-V junctional acceleration may be caused by any factor that increases automaticity—acute rheumatic fever, acute infections, particularly diphtheria, scarlet fever, pneumonia, and typhus. Quinidine, procaine amide, protoveratradine, and influences exerted through the autonomic nervous system, such as forced inspiration, ocular pressure, carotid sinus sensitivity, and increased intracranial pressure, are causal factors. Failure of the impulse to cross the A-V junction may be caused by this tissue being in a refractory state following a previous junctional impulse, depression of conduction by digitalis and other drugs, or various forms of organic heart block. Digitalis toxicity notoriously acts by multiple mechanisms to produce A-V dissociation, including decreased automaticity of the A-V junction (Fig. 12-4).

TYPES OF A-V DISSOCIATION AND MODES OF ONSET

The varieties of A-V dissociation may be classified as: (1) complete or incomplete, and (2) persistent or transient. When A-V dissociation without capture of either pacemaker is observed in a long electrocardiographic tracing, "complete dissociation" is said to exist. On the other hand, incomplete dissociation is marked by several types of ventricular capture. An example might be the temporary incomplete A-V dissociation with ventricular captures in a patient with an A-V conduction block due to digitalis intoxication. The common types of A-V dissociation may be classified as follows:

(1) Depression of automaticity of the S-A node allows the impulses from the A-V junction to control the ventricles. Once the "escape beat" of the lower center occurs, it may result in the rhythmic activity of two independent foci, thereby maintaining the dissociation (Fig. 12-5). The dissociation is terminated when a sinus impulse occurs at such a point in the cardiac cycle that it can be propagated through the A-V junction (i.e., when the A-V junction is nonrefractory to impulses from the atrium) and results in a ventricular capture. This may occur, for example, after the disappearance of temporary sinoatrial block. The re-

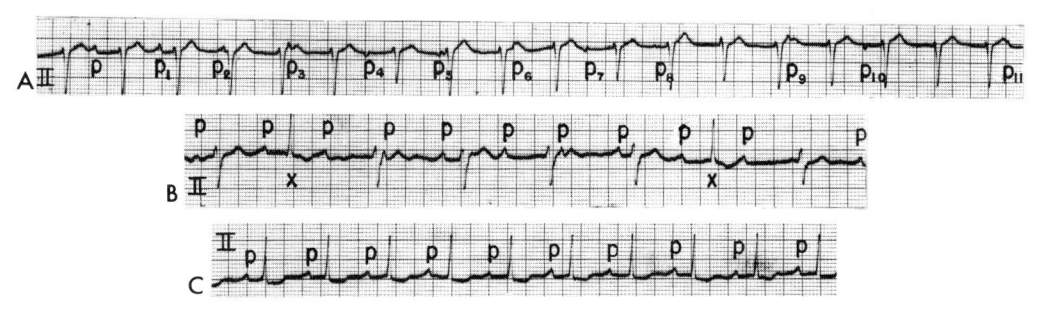

Figure 12-4. Incomplete A-V dissociation with wandering pacemaker caused by digitalis toxicity.

(A) Atrial rate is 79 per minute, ventricular rate, 100 per minute. Note alteration in the configuration of the P waves caused by a wandering pacemaker. The first three cycles (P to P_3) and P_9 and P_{11} show upright P waves and occur at a faster rate than the remaining cycles. P_4 to P_7 and P_{10} are inverted, and P_8 is diphasic. The QRS following P_4 and P_7 probably represent reciprocal beats.

(B) Digitalis is stopped. Atrial rate is 100 per minute; ventricular rate, 56 per minute. Incomplete A-V dissociation with occasional capture beats occur at X. Note the prolonged P-R interval, the lightly narrower QRS width, and the upwardly directed QRS with the conducted beats.

(C) Normal sinus rhythm with slightly prolonged P-R interval (0.24 second). Note the upwardly directed R waves, similar in configuration to the conducted beats in B.

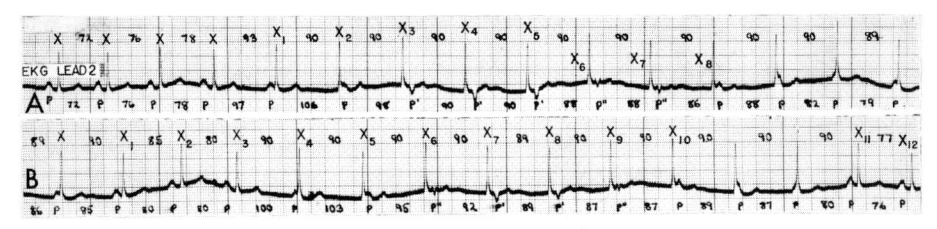

Figure 12–5. Continuous strip of lead II from patient with mitral stenosis. Shows sinus arrhythmia, A-V nodal escape, isorhythmic type of A-V dissociation and lower nodal rhythm. The numbers above the electrocardiogram denote R-R intervals; those below it denote P-R intervals in msec. P represents the sinus P wave; P′, retrograde nodal P wave; P″, fusion P wave.

(A) Note the first three cycles marked X show the normal sinus rhythm. (P waves are normal.) The QRS of X_1 and X_2 represent A-V nodal escape. Note the retrograde P wave in cycles X_3, X_4, and X_5. These are cycles of "lower" A-V nodal rhythm. Note the fusion P wave at X_6, X_7, and X_8. Note the variation in the P-P intervals in the initial part of the tracing, indicating the presence of sinus arrhythmia.

(B) Note the occurrence of the isorhythmic type of A-V dissociation in cycles X and X_1, the normal A-V conduction in X_2 and X_3, and an isorhythmic type of A-V dissociation in X_4 and X_5. A fusion P wave occurs at X_6, and retrograde P waves at X_7 and X_8. There is a fusion P wave at X_9, a return to upright P waves at X_{10}, and the restoration of normal sinus rhythm at X_{11} and X_{12}. (From Sackner, Somerson, and Bellet: Amer. J. Cardiol., 4:821, 1959.)

sumption of S-A nodal activity permits the S-A impulse to reach a position in the cardiac cycle so that it may be conducted (captured beat), with a resultant return to normal sinus rhythm (Fig. 12–6).

(2) Increased automaticity of the A-V junction to a level greater than that of the sinus pacemaker results in "usurpation"; this center then controls the ventricles (Fig. 12–7). This may occur when the junctional rate accelerates, with or without slowing of the sinus rate, or when both pacemakers are slowed or accelerated to an unequal degree (Miller and Sharrett, 1957). In this type, for example, a low junctional premature beat may occur at such a time that it extinguishes the sinus impulse by retrograde conduction or else leaves the A-V node refractory to the passage of a sinus impulse. If the second premature beat occurs early enough to produce the same effect, the resultant refractoriness is perpetuated, resulting in A-V dissociation.

(3) The term isorhythmic has been applied to A-V dissociation characterized by independent beating of the atria and ventricles at an almost identical rate. The P-R intervals are short, and the P waves often override the QRS complex. Captured beats are observed only rarely (Figs. 12–8, 12–9). This type of dissociation has had various explanations. Segers (1946), on the basis of work with amphibian hearts,

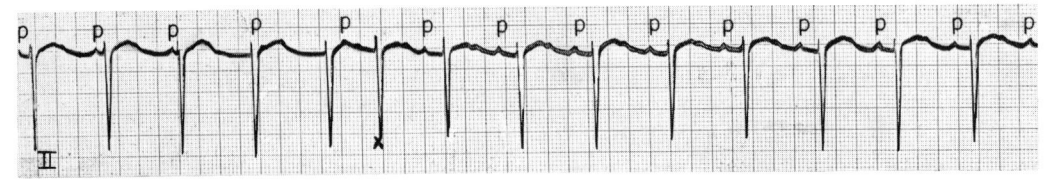

Figure 12–6. Incomplete A-V dissociation showing transition to normal sinus rhythm.
Note incomplete A-V dissociation in the initial four cycles; the atrial rate is 79 per minute and the ventricular rate is 81 per minute. A captured beat occurs at X, following which normal sinus rhythm is restored with a ventricular rate of 79 per minute and a P-R interval of 0.22 second.

A-V DISSOCIATION

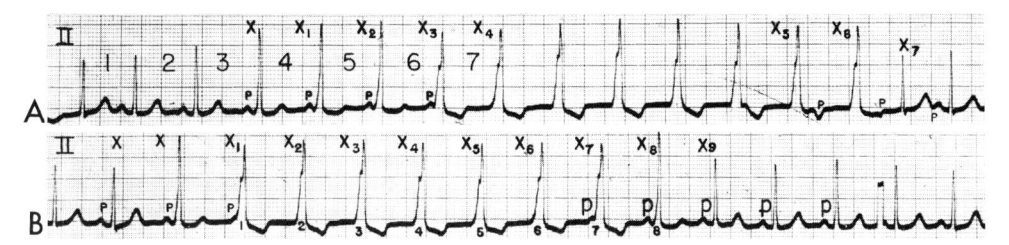

Figure 12-7. Intermittent A-V dissociation showing ventricular tachycardia and fusion beats.

(A) The atrial rate is slightly slower than the ventricular rate (atrial rate, 94 per minute, and ventricular rate, 100 per minute during period of A-V dissociation). The first three beats are normally conducted. From X to X_3, fusion beats with slight aberration of QRS are observed. Thereafter, 6 to the X_6 represent idioventricular beats. X_7 represents a fusion beat. The P wave following X_5 is an inverted P wave due to retrograde conduction. A normal upright P wave followed by a normally conducted beat is observed in the last QRS of the strip. It is preceded, following X_6, by an inverted P wave intermediate in form from the preceding one and the one following it. This represents a fusion beat.

(B) The above sequence is repeated in the first part of the strip (X to X_8). Normal sinus rhythm is restored at X_9.

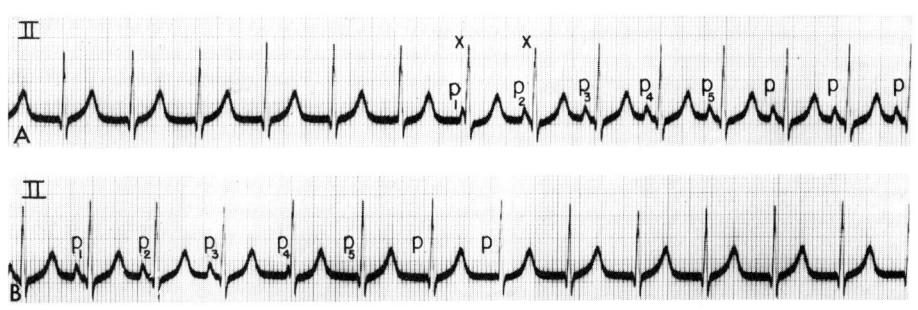

Figure 12-8. A-V junctional rhythm and A-V dissociation (isorhythmic type) observed during right cardiac catheterization.

(A) (Lead II) Note the appearance of A-V junctional beats occurring at a rate of 100 per minute from the beginning of the strip to the cycle marked X. The P waves are apparently buried in the QRS complex; however, at the first cycle marked X, P waves begin to emerge preceding the QRS complexes. The P-R interval gradually increases at P_1, P_2, and P_3. At P_4 and P_5 and in the following cycles, normal rhythm is restored with a P-R interval measuring 0.12 second.

(B) Shows the same process in reverse, namely, a normal P-R interval at P_1, P_2, and P_3, and sudden marked shortening of the P-R interval at P_4 and P_5 as the P wave becomes buried in the QRS complex with the occurrence of an A-V junctional rhythm towards the end of the strip.

Note that in A and B where no P waves are visible, A-V nodal rhythm without dissociation is probably present. The P waves are buried in the QRS (midnodal rhythm). The possibility of atrial standstill is unlikely.

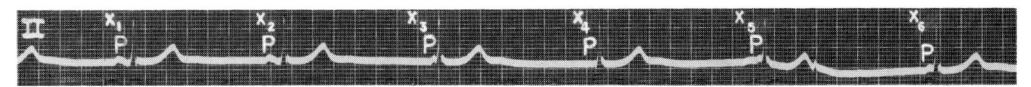

Figure 12-9. A-V dissociation of the isorhythmic type. At the beginning, a sinus bradycardia is present (both atrial and ventricular rates are the same, 38 per minute); at X_3 the atrial rate is slower; at X_5 and X_6, it is faster than the rate of the A-V rhythm. Note the normal P-R interval at X_1 (0.14 second) and X_2. At X_3, the P wave merges into the QRS complex, and at X_4 no P wave can be observed since it is probably buried in the QRS. At X_5, a small P wave is seen to emerge; this becomes larger at X_6.

proposed that synchronization occurred as a result of contact between two tissues with different rhythms, a process he called "accrochage." He observed that when two separate rhythmic cellular elements are placed in contact without true anatomic continuity, they tend to discharge their impulses at the same rate even though their initial rhythms differ.

A-V Dissociation Presenting Deviations from the Above Types. The following deviations from the above varieties may be frequently observed. Some of these might be easily anticipated. (a) The atria may be controlled, not by the S-A node, but by a lower pacemaker located in the coronary sinus region or in the A-V junction (Fig. 12–10). (b) The ventricles may be controlled not by the A-V junction, but by a ventricular pacemaker. (c) The type of A-V dissociation may change for a series of beats from one in which the rates deviate considerably from each other to one in which they are almost identical. (d) Instances may be observed in which the atria beat slightly faster than the ventricles. This situation may not be due to simple A-V dissociation but to A-V heart block combined with short periods of A-V dissociation. (e) A-V dissociation may be superimposed on a background of 2:1 A-V block. In these tracings the ventricular rate is slower than the atrial rate, but greater than the rate of conducted atrial impulses (Fig. 12–3). The differentiation of this type of dissociation from complete A-V heart block is discussed on page 138. (f) Forward conduction is often impaired in the presence of A-V dissociation. This is indicated by the following: the close relationship of the prolonged P-R interval and dissociation in rheumatic fever; and the fact that the P-R interval of the captured beat is often prolonged even when this beat does not occur particularly early in the cardiac cycle as shown by examples of concealed conduction observed in these cases. (g) Retrograde block is not absolute and retrograde conduction to the atria may occasionally occur. (h) Fusion beats may occur in A-V dissociation, in conjunction with any of the types mentioned. These beats represent partial dissociation or, from another point of view, partial capture and occur frequently during the transition between control of the heart by a single pacemaker (e.g, sinus or junctional) and A-V dissociation with two independent pacemakers.

Other Types of Dissociation. Other types of "dissociation" in which two or more pacemakers initiate impulses independent of each other include: (a) atrial dissociation; (b) junctional tachycardia without retrograde conduction, with the maintenance of normal sinus

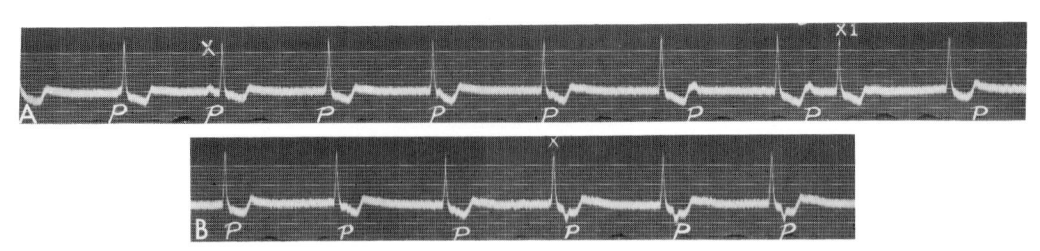

Figure 12–10. (A) Complete A-V dissociation. Both atrial and ventricular rhythms are slightly irregular. The atrial rhythm originates in the atria or in the A-V junction; the ventricular rhythm originates in the lower A-V junction. A-V junctional rhythm with 1:1 conduction to the ventricles and with 5:4 retrograde conduction to the atria (Wenckebach phenomenon, so-called "reversed Wenckebach") can be observed.

(B) First degree V-A block (the R-P interval measures 0.40 second) with an A-V nodal pacemaker. An alternate possibility is atrial flutter (200 per minute) with 2:1 A-V conduction.

pacemaker activity; (c) two junctional pacemakers beating independently (Fig. 12–10); (d) a rhythm arising from a ventricular focus; (e) complete A-V heart block; (f) two independent ventricular foci; and (g) A-V dissociation with ventricular parasystole.

AUSCULTATORY PHENOMENA

The auscultatory phenomena vary with the type and degree of dissociation. In the presence of A-V dissociation, there is a *variation* in the intensity of the first heart sound due to the difference in the time interval between the P wave and the QRS complex. When the P wave occurs much before the QRS complex, the first heart sound is faint, and when it is close to it, the sound is relatively more intense. This situation is similar to that which occurs in the presence of the A-V dissociation associated with complete A-V heart block. Alterations are also observed in the second heart sound. Alterations in intensity of cardiac murmurs are also observed, depending upon the proximity of the atrial to the ventricular beats.

ELECTROCARDIOGRAM IN A-V DISSOCIATION

There is an inconstant relationship between P waves and the adjacent QRS complexes; however, the atrial rate is usually slower than the ventricular rate. In each successive cycle, the P wave moves closer to the ventricular complex to its right and may ultimately coincide with or follow the QRS. When the P wave passes a QRS complex, the following events may occur in subsequent beats: (a) ventricular capture; (b) atrial capture; or (c) synchronization or "accrochage."

Inspection indicates that both atrial and ventricular cycle lengths are constant while bearing no relation to each other, unless a sinus arrhythmia is present. Usually, with a sufficiently long record, there appear to be repetitive "premature" QRS complexes of a supraventricular contour which represent "ventricular capture" beats. With these criteria fulfilled, the diagnosis of A-V dissociation is established. Occasionally, A-V dissociation may transiently develop into an A-V junctional rhythm for a varying number of cycles. This may be apparent from the fusion of the atrial and ventricular beats or by the transient appearance of inverted P waves; when they occur at almost identical rates, they may be superimposed, giving the appearance of a "mid" A-V junctional rhythm.

DIFFERENTIAL DIAGNOSIS

The following should be considered in the differential diagnosis of A-V dissociation: (a) First degree A-V heart block with a long P-R interval, with the P wave lying close to the preceding QRS. Tracings of this type closely resemble A-V dissociation with synchronization. However, the response to exercise, emotion, or atropine will alter the relationship of the P wave to the QRS and thus clarify the diagnosis. (b) Almost complete A-V heart block with V-A or A-V response. Differentiation of this condition from the type of A-V dissociation previously described has been briefly discussed by Miller and Sharrett (1957). The presence of complete or almost complete antegrade block with the occurrence of retrograde conduction may lead to A-V dissociation in reverse. (c) 2:1 A-V heart block with dissociation from complete A-V heart block with occasional ventricular captures. These two unusual conditions resemble each other, but careful study of the electrocardiograms will disclose differentiating features (see Fig. 12–3). In complete A-V heart block with occasional transmission of a sinus beat, the ventricular rate usually ranges from 30 to 36 beats per minute with only slight variation of the R-R interval. The QRS complex is often of the idioventricular type and is considerably widened. The atrial rate is frequently 3 to 5 times the ventricular rate and therefore two P-P cycles are shorter than one R-R cycle. When infrequent ventricular capture occurs (this may appear during a supernormal phase) the P-R interval is not fixed because of a varying refractory period of the A-V junction in the transmitted sinus beats. (d) A-V dissociation between S-A and A-V junctional rhythm with aberrant ventricular conduction. This may sometimes be confused with A-V dissociation between S-A and idioventricular rhythms. (e) Ventricular parasystole may rarely simulate A-V dissociation. The most important distinction is that in parasystole the rhythm of the lower center is slower than that of the upper one. The ventricular center is protected from the higher center by an entrance block; that is, there is unidirectional forward block into the parasystolic center, thereby preventing its capture. The impulses of the parasystolic focus, however, have free exit or egress when the ventricles are not in a refractory phase.

DURATION AND FATE OF A-V DISSOCIATION

Once initiated, A-V dissociation is usually brief or intermittent; it may be observed for a few cycles, a few minutes, hours, or days. It tends to be a transient condition and rarely persists without interruption for any appreciable time.

A-V dissociation may be terminated, transiently or permanently, by one of the following mechanisms: (a) When dissociation is due to an escape mechanism, it will of necessity be short-lived since the S-A pacemaker regains control of the heart after a few beats (Fig. 12-6). (b) Absolute or relative increase in atrial rate or decrease in A-V junctional rate, or a combination of both, may occur spontaneously or may be induced by conditions capable of suppressing or stimulating vagal or sympathetic mechanisms (e.g., therapeutic or toxic digitalis effects which disturb pacemaker activity). (c) Absolute or relative increase in the A-V junctional rate to overcome retrograde A-V block, thereby producing A-V junctional rhythm. This rhythm is usually transient and sinus rhythm usually supervenes. (d) Appearance of an atrial premature contraction, which effects an early discharge of the lower (junctional) pacemaker, thereby creating an opportunity for the sinus node to regain control of the heart (Figs. 12-6, 12-7). (e) Ventricular capture may discharge and depress the A-V junctional pacemaker, thus abolishing the A-V dissociation. Usually a ventricular capture has no effect on the S-A rhythm. (f) A delay in the appearance of the ventricular contraction until the time that it would be expected to appear following a ventricular "captured" beat. This results in a considerably prolonged ventricular cycle (increased R-R interval) and is attributed to the phenomenon of concealed conduction whereby the sinus impulse presumably penetrates the A-V junction, but because of distal refractoriness, cannot activate the ventricles. (g) A-V dissociation may be abolished by various maneuvers or drugs which affect the ectopic focus to a greater degree than the S-A node. Thus, normal sinus rhythm may be restored by forced breathing, carotid sinus pressure, exercise, change of posture, or the administration of atropine.

TREATMENT

A-V dissociation itself requires no therapy since it is always a secondary manifestation of an underlying cardiac disorder. Therapy should be directed to the underlying clinical state, drug effects, electrolyte imbalance, or acute rheumatic activity. Cessation of digitalis medication and potassium administration if the serum potassium is low may facilitate reversion to normal sinus rhythm. Often, mere omission of digitalis suffices. If digitalis is then re-administered, the use of a rapidly excreted form (Lanoxin) is preferable. Emergency therapy is rarely indicated except with rare types associated with a rapid ventricular rate.

PROGNOSIS

The prognosis in A-V dissociation per se with or without ventricular captured beats is generally good; much depends on the underlying clinical state and the precipitating cause (e.g., digitalis, infection). Because the heart rate usually does not vary unduly from the normal range, there is no serious concomitant disturbance in the cardiovascular hemodynamics. However, in that type which is accompanied by a rapid ventricular rate, particularly when digitalis-induced paroxysmal atrial tachycardia is associated with incomplete A-V heart block, the mortality is frequently high. A mortality of 58 per cent was reported in a series of 64 patients in whom this occurred (Jacobs et al., 1961). Of the patients with digitalis-induced A-V dissociation, 47 per cent expired as a result of their basic illness shortly after the onset of the arrhythmia (Jacobs et al., 1961). It is interesting that complications are seldom observed as a direct result of this condition. The presence of the A-V dissociation is a warning that there may be a serious derangement in myocardial function due to endogenous or exogenous factors, and if these are not corrected the outcome might be serious or at times fatal.

References

Jacobs, D. R., Donoso, E., and Friedberg, C. K.: A-V dissociation—a relatively frequent arrhythmia. Medicine, *40*:101, 1961.

Katz, L. N., and Pick, A.: Clinical Electrocardiography. Part I. The Arrhythmias. Philadelphia, Lea & Febiger, 1956.

Levy, M. N., and Edelstein, J.: Mechanism of synchronization in isorhythmic A-V dissociation. Circulation, *41–42:* III–99, 1970.

Marriott, H. J. L., and Menendez, M. M.: A-V dissociation revisited. Prog. Cardiov. Dis., 8:522, 1966.

Marriott, H. J. L., Schubart, A. F., and Bradley, S. M.: A-V dissociation: A reappraisal. Amer. J. Cardiol., *2*:586, 1958.

Miller, R., and Sharrett, R. H.: Interference dissociation. Circulation, *16*:803, 1957.

Pick, A.: A-V dissociation. A proposal for a comprehensive classification and consistent terminology. Amer. Heart J., 66:147, 1963.

Segers, M.: Les phénomènes de synchronisation an nivean du coeur. Arch. Int. Physiol., *54*:87, 1946.

Waldo, A. L., Vitikainen, K. J., Harris, P. D., Malm, J. R., and Hoffman, B. F.: The mechanism of synchronization in isorhythmic A-V dissociation. Some observations in the morphology and polarity of the P wave during retrograde capture of the atria. Circulation, 38:880, 1968.

Chapter 13 Pre-excitation Syndromes

GENERAL CONSIDERATIONS
ANATOMIC AND PATHOLOGIC
   CONSIDERATIONS
   Accessory Pathways
     Bundle of Kent
     Junctional Bypass Fibers
     Mahaim Fibers
   Relation of Pre-excitation Complexes to
     Types of Anomalous Pathways
     Classic W-P-W Syndrome
     Variants of Classic W-P-W Syndrome
LOWN-GANONG-LEVINE SYNDROME
WOLFF-PARKINSON-WHITE SYNDROME
   General Considerations
   Incidence and Etiology
   Electrocardiogram

   Diagnosis and Differential Diagnosis
   Types of W-P-W Complexes
   His Bundle Electrograms
Vectorcardiogram
Hemodynamics
   Correlation with Mechanical Events
Incidence and Mechanisms of Ectopic
     Rhythms in W-P-W
Treatment
   Drug Therapy
   Therapy in Drug-Resistant Subjects
     Cardioversion
     Use of pacemakers
     Surgical treatment
Prognosis

GENERAL CONSIDERATIONS

Pre-excitation occurs when the sinus impulse bypasses, partially or completely, the normal conduction pathway and activates the ventricular muscle earlier than would be possible if the impulse had traveled through the normal A-V junctional conduction system. This rapid transmission of the sinus impulse is accomplished over one or a combination of anomalous pathways: the bundle of Kent, the James fibers, and the Mahaim fibers (Fig. 13–1), which bypass various portions of the A-V junction.

Several different patterns of ventricular pre-excitation have been recognized from the electrocardiogram. These consist of: the classic W-P-W syndrome (including types A and B) which is characterized by a P-R interval of no more than 0.12 second, the presence of a delta wave, and QRS complexes of 0.12 second or more; various patterns of W-P-W syndrome, characterized by: (a) a P-R interval less than or equal to 0.12 second and a small delta wave with a QRS duration of 0.10 second, and (b) a P-R interval greater than 0.12 second, a delta wave, and a QRS duration greater than 0.12 second. The Lown-Ganong-Levine syndrome is characterized by a short P-R interval with a normal width QRS complex.

ANATOMIC AND PATHOLOGIC CONSIDERATIONS

The anatomic and pathologic considerations have revolved chiefly around the presence of accessory pathways. Kent first described an accessory bundle of conduction fibers between the atria and the ventricles in 1893. Since then, from time to time many

PRE-EXCITATION SYNDROMES

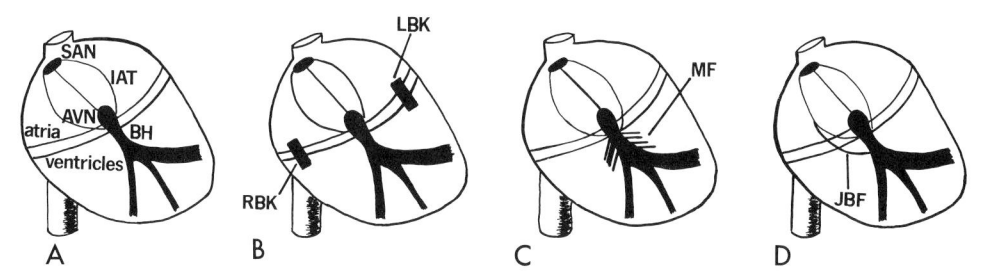

Figure 13-1. Diagrammatic representation of the anatomic pathways of the pre-excitation syndromes. SAN: sinoatrial node. AVN: atrioventricular node. BH: bundle of His. RBK: right bundle of Kent. LBK: left bundle of Kent. MF: Mahaim fiber. JBF: James "bypass" fiber.

(A) Schematic representation of the normal anatomy of the A-V conduction system. The atrial and ventricular muscle is separated by the fibrous skeleton of the heart; the internodal conduction pathways terminate at the A-V node, from which arises the bundle of His and from it the right bundle branch and the two main divisions of the left bundle branch.

(B) An accessory pathway (bundle of Kent) bypasses the A-V conduction system, causes early activation of a peripheral portion of the ventricle, and then produces the delta wave and pre-excitation.

(C) Mahaim fibers producing pre-excitation of a part of ventricular myocardium. The normal A-V delay may be preserved. This explains: (1) W-P-W with normal P-R interval, and (2) W-P-W with first degree A-V block.

(D) James fibers bypassing the A-V node and establishing connections with some portion of the A-V node or His bundle. This explains the Lown-Ganong-Levine syndrome: short P-R and normal QRS.

different mechanisms have been suggested as the underlying cause of these syndromes. The present theories may be divided into the following groups: those postulating (a) accessory pathways (bundle of Kent, Mahaim paraseptal fibers, and James' A-V junctional bypass fibers); and (b) abnormal conduction through normal pathways (Fig. 13-1).

Accessory Pathways. Considerable evidence has accumulated in recent years to make abnormal conduction through accessory pathways the favored theory (Lev, 1966; Cobb et al., 1968).

Bundle of Kent. It has been postulated that the bundle of Kent is in some way related to the W-P-W syndrome, but this does not rule out the possibility that pre-excitation results from other accessory pathways. Moreover, the exact role of the bundle of Kent in pre-excitation remains to be elucidated. Histologic examination of the bundle of Kent reveals that the fibers contain ordinary myocardial cells and not Purkinje cells. The tissue contained in the bundles, therefore, is a type ordinarily associated with relatively slow conduction (James, 1969).

Junctional Bypass Fibers. These comprise a direct anatomic connection between the S-A node and the A-V junction. While the majority of the fibers enter the crest of the A-V junction, several bypass the upper and central A-V junction and enter the lower third or may even connect directly with the bundle of His. Sherf and James (1969) suggest that, in acquired cases of pre-excitation syndromes due to rheumatic fever and myocardial infarction, the anatomic mechanism underlying the production of a pre-excitation syndrome may be a blocking of the anterior and middle atrial tracts, thus forcing the sinus impulse to be propagated over the posterior tract and thereby bypassing much of the A-V junction.

Mahaim Fibers. Mahaim and Clerc (1932) and others (Lev et al., 1966) have reported fibers connecting various portions of the conducting bundles to the interventricular septum. Conduction through A-V junctional bypass fibers and Mahaim fibers can result in pre-excitation that involves a septal or paraseptal focus. Lev and his associates have reported two cases of the W-P-W electrocardiogram pattern in which unusually profuse Mahaim fibers were found at autopsy (Lev et al., 1966). These fibers passed from the A-V junction and the length of the A-V bundle to the posterosuperior part of the muscular interventricular septum.

Relation of Pre-excitation Complexes to Types of Anomalous Pathways. Anomalous pathways, both congenital and acquired, may act to produce the characteristic pre-excitation syndromes. Although the mechanisms of all the various pre-excitation syndromes have not been proven beyond a doubt, extensive physiologic and pathologic investigations and observation during surgery on the human subject and in the dog offer plausible explanations for the electrocardiographic manifestations.

Classic W-P-W Syndrome. The classic form of the W-P-W syndrome, with short P-R interval, prolonged QRS complex, and delta wave, may occur as a result of the following accessory bundles, either individually or in combination: (1) the bundle of Kent alone, leading directly to the ventricular muscle; and (2) the Mahaim fibers, which could produce the delta wave of early ventricular depolarization and the prolonged QRS complex.

If the bundle of Kent were the sole mechanism, the atrial impulse would pass through the accessory fibers and reach the one ventricle, left or right, which is activated before the normally propagated impulse has been transmitted through the A-V junction. This mechanism results in a short P-R interval; from the original point of ectopic ventricular activation, the impulse spreads to both ventricles in an abnormal manner. While the impulse arising from the pre-excitation area is spreading, the impulse propagated through the A-V junction in the normal manner activates the remaining nonrefractory ventricular muscle. The summation of these two asynchronous impulses in the ventricles leads to the fusion beat; the prolongation of the QRS will be proportional to the asynchrony of the two impulses. When drugs such as quinidine and procaine amide block the accessory pathway, conduction can occur only through the normal conduction system.

These accessory pathways may be located in the left or right ventricle, thus producing different patterns. The W-P-W type A complexes apparently arise from pre-excitation of the left ventricle. In W-P-W type B syndrome, an area of the right ventricle near the A-V groove is activated 40 to 150 msec. earlier than if the activation had taken place over the normal A-V conduction system (Burchell et al., 1967; Durrer et al., 1970).

Variants of Classic W-P-W Syndrome. Those instances of pre-excitation which only partially fulfill the criteria of the W-P-W syndrome may be due to the same anomalous pathways; however, due to deviation from classic anatomic types or due to factors as yet poorly understood, conduction within them may be altered.

LOWN-GANONG-LEVINE SYNDROME

The mechanism underlying the production of short P-R intervals and normal QRS complexes may be either: (1) the James bypass fibers or the Mahaim fibers; and (2) accelerated conduction through normal pathways.

The QRS complex in the Lown-Ganong-Levine syndrome, unlike that of the W-P-W syndrome, is devoid of slurring and does not exceed 0.08 second in duration; there are short P-J and P-R intervals (0.08 to 0.12 second) which are strikingly constant over the course of years (Fig. 13–2). Ten per

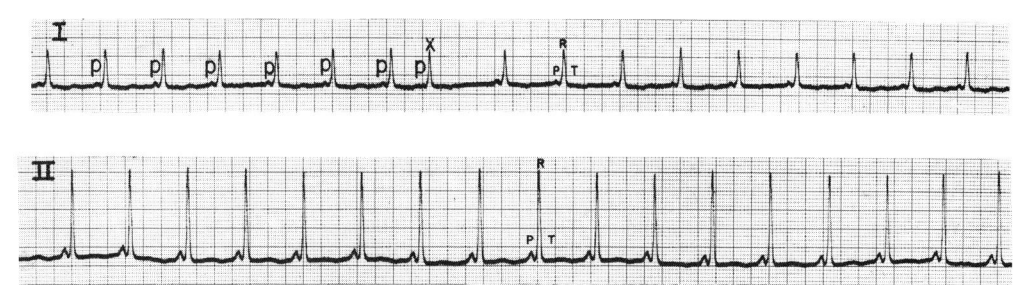

Figure 13–2. Short P-R and normal-width QRS (Lown-Ganong-Levine syndrome). Leads I and II show short P-R intervals (0.10 second) with upright P waves; the QRS complexes are of normal width. This has been explained in the past as being the result of accelerated conduction. However, recent data suggest that this is part of the Lown-Ganong-Levine syndrome (see p. 180) and may be explained by the short-circuiting of the portion of the A-V junction through the James fibers. Note the premature atrial beat at X in lead I.

cent of patients have paroxysmal tachycardia, compared with 0.5 per cent in a similarly selected control group of 200 with normal P-R duration (Lown et al., 1952). Among the 200 patients with short P-R intervals, 184 had normal QRS complexes and 16 had a W-P-W configuration. Massumi et al. (1970) have shown that cases of Lown-Ganong-Levine syndrome, when stressed by rapid atrial pacing, may develop the typical features of the W-P-W syndrome. The His bundle electrogram in these patients shows a shortened H-Q interval and a normal P-H interval.

WOLFF-PARKINSON-WHITE SYNDROME

General Considerations. This syndrome has assumed considerable importance because these subjects are susceptible to the development of paroxysmal acceleration of the heart beat, and the electrocardiogram frequently simulates that of severe heart disease, thus rendering its recognition of paramount importance.

The prognosis is particularly affected by the occurrence of arrhythmias, which, in addition to altering cardiovascular hemodynamics, are often refractory to treatment. The therapy of these ectopic tachycardias has been improved by the recent use of newer drugs, countershock, artificial pacemakers preset to interrupt episodes of tachyarrhythmia, and surgical interruption of the anomalous pathways (see p. 328).

Incidence and Etiology. Studies of large groups consisting of both healthy and hospitalized military personnel have yielded an incidence ranging from 0.1 to 3.1 per thousand (Averill et al., 1960; Chung et al., 1965; and Sears and Manning, 1964). The etiologic factors associated with W-P-W syndrome include: (a) the congenital type, seen most often in infants and children; and (b) the acquired type, observed frequently in the older age groups. This distinction has by no means been clearly established. It is felt that the appearance of W-P-W complexes at only certain times is the result of factors that tend to depress the normal pathways, thus permitting the accessory bundle to function. The fact that there is a high incidence of a congenital cardiac anomaly as an associated factor when it occurs in infancy and childhood has only recently been emphasized. Among 28 infants and children with the W-P-W syndrome, 13 had associated congenital cardiac anomalies; one had rheumatic heart disease. Of 83 subjects who had this syndrome with associated congenital heart disease, 24 had Ebstein's malformation. Occasional instances of familial occurrence of W-P-W have been reported. The mode of inheritance in reported cases has not been clearly established (Massumi, 1967).

Cardiac Status. Sixty to 70 per cent of adults manifesting the W-P-W syndrome have normal hearts; the corresponding range in children, however, is lower (32 to 58 per cent). Except for the limitations imposed by the occurrence of ectopic rhythms, the patients with normal hearts may live normal lives. The syndrome has been observed in healthy, vigorous athletes and others accustomed to strenuous activity. There is no evidence that the syndrome by itself leads to myocardial impairment. The chief complicating factor is the development of myocardial fatigue and exhaustion following frequent, prolonged seizures of tachyarrhythmias that are often refractory to treatment.

Roughly, one-third of adults with the W-P-W syndrome have associated organic heart disease. Paroxysmal tachycardia occurs in 70 per cent of patients with the W-P-W syndrome. A higher proportion of children than adults with the W-P-W syndrome suffer from organic heart disease; in one series of 48 children with W-P-W complexes, 20 (40 per cent) had accompanying organic heart disease (Swiderski, 1962).

Electrocardiogram

Diagnosis and Differential Diagnosis. The W-P-W syndrome presents the following characteristic electrocardiographic findings: (a) There is shortening of the P-R interval to 0.10 second or less; (b) There is widening of the QRS complexes to 0.11 second or longer; (c) In the typical case, widening of the QRS actually compensates for the shortened P-R, giving a normal P-J interval (this does not exceed 0.26 second); (d) The P wave is usually upright, although occasionally it may be inverted; (e) Notching or slurring is observed in the first portion of the QRS complex if the main deflection is upward; if the main deflection is downward slurring occurs on the descending limb; (f) S-T segment and T wave changes are observed, ranging from an S-T depression to a diphasic or inverted T wave; the degree of abnormality varies with the degree of widening of the ventricular complex; (g) There frequently occurs paroxysmal atrial tachycardia and occasional atrial fibrillation, flutter, and rarely, a pattern simulating ventricular tachycardia.

However, the following deviations from characteristic patterns are occasionally observed: (a) In the concealed W-P-W syndrome, the P-R interval is short, but the QRS is of normal duration; there is a prominent slur on the initial stroke of the QRS and the T wave may be normal. (b) There may be a progressive shortening of the P-R interval with a corresponding widening of QRS complexes ("concertina effect"); the reverse may also occur, viz., a typical W-P-W complex which in successive beats shows an increase in the P-R interval and decrease in QRS width, until both return to normal values. (c) During the paroxysm of tachycardia, the previously widened QRS may return to a normal width (not always) because the accessory pathway often cannot conduct impulses above a critical rate.

The following are aids in diagnosis: The P-R interval should be measured in all leads, since the characteristic findings of W-P-W may be typical in some but not in other leads. In doubtful cases, it is helpful if the electrocardiogram can be studied in relation to various procedures—exercise, drugs, and carotid sinus pressure.

Recently, atrial pacing has been found to be of value in confirming or excluding the diagnosis of W-P-W syndrome in patients who complain of

PRE-EXCITATION SYNDROMES

paroxysmal heart action or syncopal disorders but who have normal or equivocal electrocardiograms suggestive of the W-P-W syndrome in occasional records. By increasing the atrial rate or by inducing atrial beats of varying degrees of prematurity by artificial stimulation of the right atrium, it has been possible to induce QRS complexes that closely simulate those of the W-P-W type, and paroxysms of supraventricular tachycardia have developed. This method, recently employed, may be of considerable help in establishing an etiologic diagnosis in selected cases (Cheng, 1971).

From the electrocardiographic standpoint, the most common error in interpretation during normal sinus rhythm is that of bundle branch block, and during a rapid ectopic rhythm, the most common error is that of ventricular tachycardia. Because of the abnormal and often bizarre ventricular complexes, a mistaken diagnosis of coronary occlusion or other forms of heart disease may frequently be made.

Types of W-P-W Complexes. The precordial leads in association with W-P-W complexes can be divided into two groups (Rosenbaum et al., 1945): Group A shows large R waves, often double-peaked, over the right side of the precordium (Fig. 13–3). In Group B, leads over the right precordium are dominated by a large negative deflection. These findings suggest that the accessory pathway involves the left bundle of Kent in the first group and the right bundle of Kent in the second group.

His Bundle Electrograms. During sinus rhythm the onset of ventricular activation markedly precedes excitation of the His bundle spike, confirming that ventricular pre-excitation results from bypass of the normal A-V conduction system at least in certain patients (Castellanos et al., 1970; Weiss et al., 1969; Wallace et al., 1971). Castellanos and co-workers (1970) have shown that increasing the atrial rate by atrial pacing results in the onset of the delta wave substantially in advance of recorded activity from the bundle of His. This would indicate that pre-excitation of the ventricle occurs before electrical activity of the

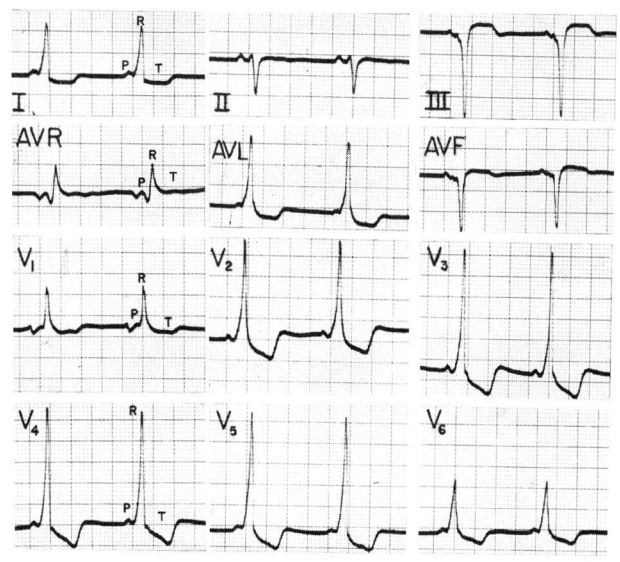

Figure 13–3. W-P-W syndrome—type A. Note the tall R waves on the right precordial leads, short P-R interval, widened QRS (V_1, V_2, V_3) with a positive delta wave in V_2 to V_6.

bundle of His and presumably is a consequence of early activation of the ventricle over some pathway at a distance from the bundle of His.

Vectorcardiogram. In certain doubtful instances of W-P-W syndrome, the vectorcardiogram may sometimes be helpful in confirming or excluding this syndrome. In W-P-W beats, this delay always appears at the very beginning of the loop; in true bundle branch block, right or left, the delay is seen somewhere in the mid-portion of the loop, while in the Wilson type of right bundle branch block, it is observed in the terminal portion. Although the delay is always manifest in the early part of the loop in the W-P-W syndrome, it may sometimes be observed in this portion of the loop in instances of intraventricular conduction disturbances independent of the W-P-W beats.

Hemodynamics
Correlation with Mechanical Events. Approximately one-half of patients with the W-P-W syndrome studied by means of phonocardiogram, carotid stethograms, and cardiac catheterization show deviations from normal mechanical events (March et al., 1960). These consist of early onset and completion of ejection of both ventricles, early completion of ejection in the left ventricle, and delayed onset of contraction on the contralateral side and possibly on the ipselateral side as well (three cases). The variable mechanical events result from differences of transmission time to the A-V node and to the site of entrance of the excitatory impulse from the anomalous pathway.

The occurrence of transient W-P-W complexes accompanied by marked widening is associated with transient but marked hemodynamic changes. The following alterations in the mechanisms of cardiac contraction were observed during the left bundle branch block pattern: the presence of delayed intraventricular conduction manifested by prolonged and deformed QRS complexes in the electrocardiogram tracing was accompanied by a significant fall in systolic blood pressures, which dropped from 110/4–24 to 92/4–22 in the left ventricle, from 108/60 to 90/54 in the ascending aorta, and from 130/52 to 110/48 mm. Hg in the brachial artery. The stroke volume was also decreased and the heart rate increased. The authors concluded that the force and intensity of left ventricle contraction and systolic ejection are significantly lowered with the onset of delayed conduction. A prolonged phase of isometric contraction was also observed, causing delay in onset and termination of systolic ejection. The ejection time, however, remained constant. These events probably cause delayed closure of the aortic valve, resulting in paradoxical splitting of the second heart sound, which is so often heard in such patients.

Incidence and Mechanisms of Ectopic Rhythms in W-P-W. From 40 to 80 per cent of subjects with the W-P-W syndrome suffer from an associated arrhythmia—usually premature and ectopic supraventricular beats, and/or paroxysmal tachyarrhythmias (Fig. 13-4). Paroxysmal atrial tachycardia is the most common and comprises 50 to 87 per cent of the associated arrhythmias. In addition, the following have been observed: varying degrees of P-R interval prolongation, partial A-V heart block with 2:1 response, incomplete A-V dissociation, wandering pacemaker, and ventricular fibrillation. The underlying mechanism for paroxysmal atrial tachycardia and atrial flutter in W-P-W was retrograde activation of the atrium through the accessory pathway. Burchell and his associates (1967) have provided direct evidence by electrode mapping of the sequence of activation at surgery for retrograde conduction through the accessory pathways. Castellanos and Castillo (1970), employing His bundle electrography, have shown that the

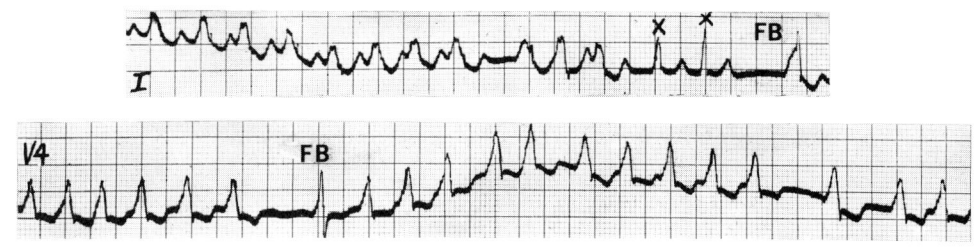

Figure 13-4. W-P-W beats associated with atrial fibrillation showing aberrant ventricular complexes and normally conducted beats. The QRS complexes are slurred, notched, and widened. Normally conducted beats are observed at X in lead I. At V_F following a long pause (V_F in lead I) beats transitional between the normal and widened QRS complexes are observed. Note the slurred initial portion of the QRS followed by a normal rapid upstroke with a termination as in a normal beat. Note the transitional beat (V_F) in lead I and in V_4 (fusion beat).

tachycardias associated with W-P-W result from a reciprocating mechanism involving both the normal A-V conduction system and the abnormal pathways. There is a critical period up to 280 msec. after the preceding QRS during which a premature beat can terminate the tachycardia, presumably by causing the accessory pathways to be refractory to the ensuing accelerated beat (Ryan et al., 1968).

One may readily anticipate on theoretical grounds that certain patients with the W-P-W syndrome would be susceptible to the development of ventricular fibrillation because of the combinations of rapid arrhythmias and the abnormal sequence of ventricular activation. This has been documented as the fatal mechanism in a number of human subjects with W-P-W (Kaplan and Cohen, 1969), as well as in a dog with this abnormality (Boineau et al., 1969). Several patients have been shown to suffer brief periods of ventricular flutter.

Treatment. In my experience, the episodes of tachycardia once having occurred are usually more difficult to treat than to prevent. The treatment is more satisfactory in those cases in which the QRS complexes approach the normal width than in those where the QRS complexes are markedly widened.

Drug Therapy. The effects of the various drugs employed are not always predictable by their pharmacologic action. In the presence of the W-P-W syndrome with sinus rhythm, no treatment is usually required; however, quinidine or procaine amide may occasionally be given to convert the W-P-W complexes to normal intraventricular conduction and, hopefully, as a prophylactic measure to prevent the ectopic tachycardias. During the rapid ectopic rhythm, digitalis is the drug of choice, but often even large doses fail to abolish the tachycardia. Atropine occasionally has the effect of reversion of the electrocardiographic pattern to normal as a result of its vagolytic action.

Quinidine and procaine amide tend to abolish the W-P-W syndrome by increasing the refractory period of the accessory pathway, thus permitting conduction over the normal pathway via the A-V junction. Other agents are ordinarily used when tachyarrhythmias have become established. Propranolol is an extremely valuable agent for terminating the tachycardia and for decreasing the incidence of episodes in patients with the W-P-W syndrome. Antithyroid drugs, particularly methimazole, are helpful in occasional refractory cases. The action of these drugs requires further study, particularly with reference to their effect on the conducting properties of the anomalous pathway.

Therapy in Drug-Resistant Subjects

CARDIOVERSION. Direct current cardioversion has been successful in terminating supraventricular tachycardia in the W-P-W syndrome. This method, although effective, has the drawback of not preventing recurrence of paroxysms.

USE OF PACEMAKERS. Attacks of supraventricular tachycardia in the W-P-W syndrome can be both initiated and terminated by appropriately timed pacemaker-induced atrial or ventricular premature beats (Durrer et al., 1967; Massumi et al., 1967). It appears that the pacemaker-induced premature beat causes the heart to be refractory to a subsequent ectopic beat. There is a critical period in which a premature impulse is able to interrupt the tachycardia—280 msec. after the QRS. Introduction of a ventricular premature beat causes early retrograde activation of the atria and stops the tachycardia (Ryan et al., 1968). Recently, patients with W-P-W and paroxysmal tachycardia have been treated by permanent artificial pacemakers with the electrodes attached to the left atrium. The pacemaker was turned off at all times except when the patient activated it during an episode by holding a magnet over the implanted power unit.

SURGICAL TREATMENT. The surgical treatment of W-P-W syndrome involves: (1) identifying and locating the anomalous pathways and (2) interrupting them surgically. At present, both procedures present certain problems.

Several techniques have been developed to identify and locate the anomalous pathways associated with the W-P-W syndrome. These procedures which map the spread of excitation across the heart include: (1) endocardial and epicardial mapping; and (2) precordial mapping. Mapping the spread of excitation over the precordium is a noninvasive technique which has usually been verified at surgery by epicardial mapping. Endocardial and epicardial mapping almost always identifies an area of pre-excitation; however, incision of the ventricular wall in this region does not uniformly abolish the W-P-W complexes (Castellanos and Castillo, 1970; Cole et al., 1970). To date, the techniques of endocardial and epicardial mapping have not proven conclusively to be valuable in locating the anomalous pathway of pre-excitation, but in the future these techniques may be modified and constitute a more reliable guide for detecting the site at which the anomalous pathway can be surgically interrupted.

Surgical treatment has been employed to control the paroxysmal tachycardia and abolish the W-P-W complexes by (1) production of complete heart block, which is subsequently treated with artificial cardiac pacing; and (2) interruption of the abnormal pathways, with a return to normal sinus rhythm or cessation of the ectopic tachycardia (ideal method). The former technique had been an early form of therapy but is not an ideal method, especially in a young patient, since it is not always successful in interrupting the anomalous pathways or even terminating the paroxysmal tachycardias. The second technique mentioned is still under investigation and shows promise for the future. Life-threatening supraventricular tachycardia associated with W-P-W was first treated by interruption of the atrioventricular conduction system in 1966 by Giannelli et al. (1967).

Permanent successful interruption of the accessory conduction apparently has been performed by Sealy and his colleagues (Cobb et al., 1968; Sealy et al., 1969). The pattern of cardiac excitation subsequently remained normal with abolition of both the W-P-W electrocardiographic findings and the tachycardia.

Selection of patients for surgical correction: The criteria for the selection of patients for surgical correction have recently been discussed by

Wallace et al. (1971). At present, this procedure should be offered only to patients who have symptoms that warrant such intervention and in whom pre-operative studies indicate a high likelihood that the anomalous pathway is a location that makes surgical division feasible. Because of the seriousness of the procedure, pre-operative study should be fairly extensive. The following findings should be evaluated: (a) The electrocardiogram shows a W-P-W syndrome, particularly type B, and the occurrence of frequent episodes of tachycardia that respond poorly to medical therapy. (b) The physiologic studies should include His bundle recordings which demonstrate that pre-excitation precedes electrical activity recorded from the bundle of His, and there should be evidence that during pacing the refractory period of anomalous pathways is sufficiently short so that rates in excess of 100 to 200 beats per minute can be induced by atrial pacing. (c) There should be available the necessary equipment and trained personnel who have experience in evaluating and using this technique, particularly multichannel hi-fidelity recording equipment and the technique of cardiac mapping.

PRESENT STATUS OF PRE-EXCITATION PATHWAYS. Although considerable advances have been made concerning the accelerated conduction which occurs during pre-excitation, the exact mechanisms, types, and combinations of pre-excitation are apparently more complicated than initially anticipated. In addition, not all of the ramifications have been definitely established. Further electrophysiologic and pathologic investigation will be necessary to clarify the pre-excitation pathways in their totality.

Prognosis. The prognosis of the W-P-W syndrome depends upon the following factors: (a) the condition of the heart, diseased or normal; and (b) the frequency of attacks of tachycardia, their duration, and the response to treatment. The present literature does not permit assessment of the added mortality rate of subjects with W-P-W; however, a prospective study in progress by the Aetna Insurance Company has found no increased mortality in 49 patients followed for 314 patient years, and young patients without episodes of tachycardia are considered normal insurance risks (Okel, 1968). An occasional paroxysm of tachycardia in a normal heart has no effect on the cardiovascular system and, as a rule, this group may lead normal, active lives.

However, in individual cases, prolonged episodes of tachycardia place considerable strain on the heart, particularly in infants or in patients suffering from underlying organic disease. In a recent review, 22 cases of sudden death due to the W-P-W syndrome were collected (Okel, 1968). Recent advances in the use of pacemakers and in surgical approaches may improve the prognosis in patients who suffer from repeated paroxysms of tachycardia or have organic heart disease.

References

Averill, K. H., Fosmoe, R. J., and Lamb, L. E.: Electrocardiographic findings in 67,375 asymptomatic subjects. IV. Wolff-Parkinson-White syndrome. Amer. J. Cardiol., 6:108, 1960.

Berkman, N. C., and Lamb, L. E.: The Wolff-Parkinson-White syndrome: Demonstrations in man. Circulation, 17:225, 1958.

Bleifer, S., Kahn, M., Grishman, A., and Donoso, E.: Wolff-Parkinson-White syndrome: a vectorcardiographic, electrocardiographic and clinical study. Amer. J. Cardiol., 4:321, 1959.

Boineau, J. P., et al.: An anatomic-electrophysiologic basis for the Wolff-Parkinson-White syndrome. Circulation, 39–40:III-48, 1969.

Burchell, H. B., Frye, R. L., Anderson, M. W., and McGoon, D. C.: Atrioventricular and ventriculoatrial excitation in Wolff-Parkinson-White syndrome (type B). Temporary ablation at surgery. Circulation, 36:663, 1967.

Castellanos, A., and Castillo, C.: The mechanism of Wolff-Parkinson-White syndrome as studied by His bundle recordings. Amer. J. Cardiol., 25:87, 1970.

Castellanos, A., Chapunoff, E., Castillo, C., et al.: His bundle electrograms in two cases of Wolff-Parkinson-White (pre-excitation) syndrome. Circulation, 41:399, 1970.

Castillo, C. A., and Castellanos, A.: His bundle recordings in patients with reciprocating tachycardias and Wolff-Parkinson-White syndrome. Circulation, 42:271, 1970.

Cheng, T. O.: Atrial pacing: Its diagnostic and therapeutic applications. Prog. Cardiov. Dis., 14:230, 1971.

Chung, K. Y., Walsh, T. J., and Massie, E.: Wolff-Parkinson-White syndrome. Amer. Heart J., 69:116, 1965.

Cobb, F. G., et al.: Successful surgical interruption of the bundle of Kent in a patient with W-P-W syndrome. Circulation, 38:1018, 1968.

Cole, J. S., et al.: The Wolff-Parkinson-White syndrome. Problems in evaluation and surgical therapy. Circulation, 42:111, 1970.

Dreifus, L. S., et al.: Control of recurrent tachycardia of W-P-W syndrome by surgical ligature of the A-V bundle. Circulation, 38:1030, 1968.

Durrer, D., and Roos, J. P.: Epicardial excitation of the ventricles in a patient with Wolff-Parkinson-White syndrome (type B). Circulation, 35:15, 1967.

Durrer, D., Schnilenburg, R. M., and Wellens, H. J. J.: Pre-excitation revisited. Amer. J. Cardiol., 25:691, 1970.

Durrer, D., Schoo, L., Schnilenburg, R. M., and Wellens, H. J.: Role of premature beats in the initiation and termination of supraventricular tachycardia in the W-P-W syndrome. Circulation, 36:644, 1967.

Giannelli, S., et al.: Therapeutic surgical division of the human conduction system. JAMA, 199:155, 1967.

James, T. N.: The Wolff-Parkinson-White syndrome. Ann. Intern. Med., 71:399, 1969.

Kaplan, M. A., and Cohen, K. L.: Ventricular fibrillation in the Wolff-Parkinson-White syndrome. Amer. J. Cardiol., 24:259, 1969.

Kent, A. F. S.: Researches on the structure and function of the mammalian heart. J. Physiol., 14:233, 1893.

Lev, M.: Anatomic considerations of anomalous AV pathways. In Dreifus, L. S., and Likoff, W. (eds.): Mechanisms and Therapy of Cardiac Arrhythmias. New York, Grune & Stratton, 1966.

Lev, M., Leffler, W. B., Langendorf, R., and Pick, A.: Anatomic findings in a case of ventricular pre-excitation (W-P-W) terminating in complete AV block. Circulation, 34:718, 1966.

Lown, B., Ganong, W. F., and Levine, S. A.: Syndrome of short P-R interval, normal QRS complex and paroxysmal rapid heart action. Circulation, 5:693, 1952.

Mahaim, I., and Clerc, A.: Nouvelle forme anatomique de bloc du coeur, a substituer an bloc dit d'arborisations (bloc bilateral manque). C. R. Soc. Biol. (Paris), 109:183, 1932.

March, H. W., Selzer, A., and Hultgren, H. N.: Mechanical events during anomalous atrioventricular excitation (W-P-W syndrome). Circulation, 22:784, 1960.

Massumi, R. A.: Familial Wolff-Parkinson-White syndrome with cardiomyopathy. Amer. J. Med., 43:951, 1967.

Massumi, R. A., Kostin, A. D., and Tawakkol, A. A.: Termination of reciprocating tachycardia by atrial stimulation. Circulation, 36:637, 1967.

Massumi, R., Timani, N., and Ali, N.: Patterns of atrioventricular (A-V) conduction studied by His electrography (HEG) in Wolff-Parkinson-White (WPW) syndrome and other types of short P-R intervals. Circulation, 41-42:III-66, 1970.

Okel, B. B.: The Wolff-Parkinson-White syndrome. Amer. Heart J., 75:673, 1968.

Rosenbaum, F. F., Hecht, H. H., Wilson, F. N., and Johnston, F. D.: The potential variation of the thorax and the esophagus in anomalous atrioventricular excitation (W-P-W syndrome). Amer. Heart J., 29:281, 1945.

Ryan, G. F., Easley, R. M., Zaroff, L. K., and Goldstein, S.: Paradoxical use of a demand pacemaker in treatment of supraventricular tachycardia due to the Wolff-Parkinson-White syndrome. Circulation, 38:1037, 1968.

Schamroth, L., and Coskey, R. L.: Reciprocal rhythm. The Wolff-Parkinson-White syndrome, and unidirectional block. Brit. Heart J., 31:616, 1969.

Sealy, W. C., Hattler, B. G., Blumenschein, S. D., and Cobb, F. R.: Surgical treatment of Wolff-Parkinson-White syndrome. Ann. Thorac. Surg., 8:1, 1969.

Sears, G. A., and Manning, G. W.: The Wolff-Parkinson-White pattern in routine electrocardiography. Can. Med. Assoc. J., 87:1213, 1964.

Sherf, L., and James, T. N.: A new electrocardiographic concept: synchronized sinoventricular conduction. Dis. Chest, 55:127, 1969.

Swiderski, J., Lees, M. H., and Nadas, A. S.: The Wolff-Parkinson-White syndrome in infancy and childhood. Brit. Heart J., 24:561, 1962.

Wallace, A. G., Boineau, J. P., Davidson, R. M., and Sealy, W. C.: Wolff-Parkinson-White syndrome. A new look. Amer. J. Cardiol., 28:509, 1971.

Weiss, M. B., Lau, S. H., Berkowitz, W. D., and Damato, A. N.: His bundle recordings and atrioventricular conduction in anomalous atrioventricular excitation. Circulation, 39-40:III-214, 1969.

Chapter 14 *Paroxysmal Ventricular Tachycardia*

GENERAL FEATURES
INCIDENCE AND ETIOLOGY
  Occurrence in "Normal Hearts"
MECHANISM
HEMODYNAMICS
PATHOLOGY
DIAGNOSTIC FEATURES
  Symptoms and Signs
  Electrocardiogram
  Types of Ventricular Tachycardia
    Common Type
    Repetitive Type
    Idioventricular Tachycardia
IDIOVENTRICULAR RHYTHM
T WAVE CHANGES FOLLOWING
  PAROXYSMAL TACHYCARDIA (ATRIAL,
  VENTRICULAR, OR JUNCTIONAL)

DIFFERENTIAL DIAGNOSIS OF
  VENTRICULAR TACHYCARDIA
  Supraventricular Arrhythmias Simulating
    Ventricular Tachycardia
  Ventricular Tachycardia Simulating
    Supraventricular Tachycardia
TREATMENT
  Drugs
  Overdrive Suppression
  Electric Countershock
COMPLICATIONS
PROGNOSIS

GENERAL FEATURES

Paroxysmal ventricular tachycardia is a relatively uncommon but serious arrhythmia. When six or more ventricular premature beats occur in succession, they may be said to constitute a paroxysm of ventricular tachycardia. The evolution of this type of tachycardia may sometimes be observed in serial tracings. Occasional ventricular premature beats present during periods of normal sinus rhythm or atrial fibrillation become more numerous and may be followed by coupled rhythm or premature beats occurring in sequences of two, three, or more. These episodes become more prolonged until a paroxysm results; this may last a few seconds, minutes, hours, days, or weeks. The danger lies not only in the frequent association of paroxysmal ventricular tachycardia with a severely damaged heart and the tendency for exhaustion of the heart muscle with resulting heart failure, but also in the tendency of the tachycardia to develop into ventricular fibrillation, a condition which usually results in fatality.

INCIDENCE AND ETIOLOGY

Ventricular tachycardia is observed in approximately 0.1 per cent of all arrhythmias encountered in a hospital population. This arrhythmia is more common in men (69 per cent) than women (31 per cent). Most cases appear between the ages of 40 and 80 years, with a peak incidence in the sixth decade (MacKenzie and Pascual, 1964).

Paroxysmal ventricular tachycardia almost always occurs in the presence of severe myocardial damage. The most important conditions associated with this arrhythmia are severe grades of hypertensive, rheumatic, or arteriosclerotic heart disease with or without myocardial infarction, severe infections, and toxic digitalis effects. Roughly, 35 per cent of patients with ventricular tachycardia had suffered a recent myocardial infarction. As many as 60 per cent of patients with acute myocardial infarction may have ventricular tachycardia at some time during their course (Cohn et al., 1966). Toxic digitalis effects are considered a causative factor in 25 per cent of the cases of ventricular tachycardia as reported in several series.

In addition, various stress situations and hypoxic states may precipitate paroxysmal ventricular tachycardia. These include the following: (a) the forced expiratory phase of the Valsalva maneuver; (b) electroshock therapy; (c) during cardiac catheterization; (d) immediately preceding and during Stokes-Adams attacks; (e) during the transition from a supraventricular tachycardia to normal sinus rhythm; and (f) following the infusion of certain drugs (epinephrine, quinidine, and procaine amide). That sympathetic activity may produce arrhythmias has been known for many years. However, a more specific relationship to paroxysmal ventricular tachycardia has only recently been appreciated (Wallace et al., 1967). In addition, it has been demonstrated that the heart is resistant to the development of ventricular tachycardia when deprived of its autonomic innervation.

Occurrence in "Normal Hearts." Occasionally, paroxysmal ventricular tachycardia may be observed in the absence of organic heart disease. Some authors have observed 5 to 17 per cent of patients to be in this category. A psychosomatic etiology has also been reported as a precipitating factor. The precipitation of bouts of paroxysmal ventricular tachycardia associated with emotional stress is occasionally encountered.

MECHANISM

Ventricular tachycardia may be said to consist of a series of successive ventricular premature beats. Such beats, occurring alone or in various combinations, are usually observed prior to an attack and often follow the paroxysm; they arise usually from the same focus as the beats of the paroxysm. The underlying mechanisms are similar to those of ventricular premature beats and include: (1) an ectopic focus firing at a rapid rate; (2) gross or microreentry, which is particularly likely to occur around infarcted tissue. The mechanism of re-entry, discussed under premature beats (see page 84), could also explain the occurrence of ventricular tachycardia; (3) a parasystolic focus may initiate the paroxysms if it is theorized that the parasystolic pacemaker initiates impulses at a rapid rate. This would presuppose the presence of an exit block which is normally operative and which tends to prevent the escape of impulses from the parasystolic pacemaker; when the block diminishes or disappears, it allows all of the ectopic impulses to give rise to premature beats, resulting in a paroxysmal tachycardia. The paroxysms may be initiated in the following ways: (a) If the ectopic activity occurs during the "vulnerable" phase of the cardiac cycle; this occurs at the end of the absolute refractory period, close to the peak of the T wave; (b) During a short hyperexcitable period or the vulnerable phase in early diastole, the ventricle becomes responsive to subthreshold stimuli; (c) Following a premature beat the threshold for successive premature beats may be lowered, leading to a paroxysm.

HEMODYNAMICS

In a study of the hemodynamic alterations caused by atrial and ventricular tachycardia of identical rates, it was found that the cardiac output, coronary blood flow, and mean arterial pressure undergo essentially the same changes in both forms of tachycardia; however, the effects of ventricular tachycardia are more marked (Wegria et al., 1958). Similarly, it has been demonstrated that artificial pacing from a site in one ventricular chamber, which results in an abnormal QRS complex, is accompanied by a decrease in cardiac output, whereas pacing at the bundle of His results in a normal QRS and normal output (Wallace, 1966).

During cardiac catheterization, the occurrence of a ventricular tachycardia is usually accompanied by a marked hypotension. When the paroxysms persist for a long period, certain circulatory adjustments are made. However, in the presence of coronary disease, this sudden decrease in coronary blood flow adds markedly to the degree of coronary insufficiency and may be fatal. There is usually a marked fall in cardiac output and consequently in cerebral as well as renal blood flow (Figs. 14-1, 14-2). This is probably due to the fact that ventricular tachycardia usually occurs in older patients, is accompanied by myocardial disease, often of a severe grade, and is often associated with profoundly deleterious hemodynamic effects.

PATHOLOGY

No distinct pathology is observed; it is that of the underlying conditions already mentioned (acute myocardial infarction, hypertension, rheumatic fever, or the result of toxic factors). The hearts are usually enlarged, dilated and flabby, and show marked degenerative changes.

DIAGNOSTIC FEATURES

The diagnosis of ventricular tachycardia may be made in the presence of one of the etiologic factors mentioned previously, by certain clinical features to be discussed, and by the electrocardiogram. The heart rate usually ranged from 140 to 180 beats per minute. The patients are usually in the older age group, present a history of severe myocardial damage (e.g., coronary artery disease, recent myocardial infarction, congestive heart failure, or

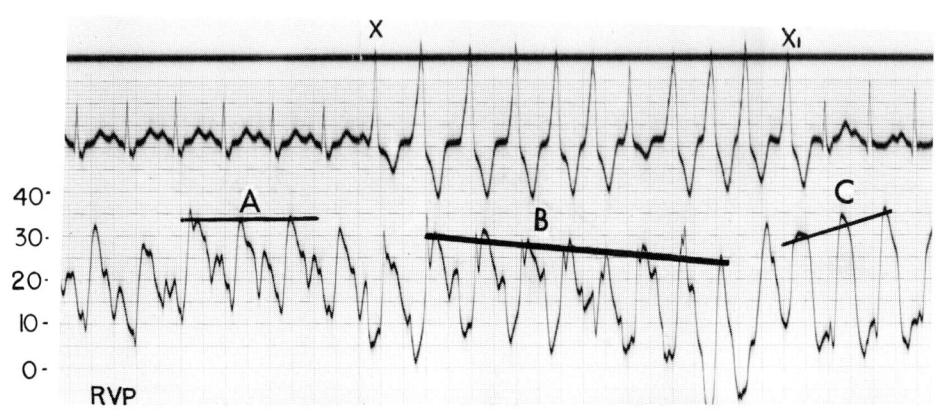

Figure 14-1. Effect of ventricular tachycardia on the right ventricular pressure. This record was taken during right heart catheterization. At A the ventricular rate is 136 per minute and the systolic pressure is 33 mm. Hg. During the onset of the ventricular tachycardia, starting at X, note the drop of the systolic blood pressure to about 25 mm. Hg. (at B). Following the cessation of the ventricular tachycardia at X_1, note the gradual restoration of the blood pressure to the control level (at C).

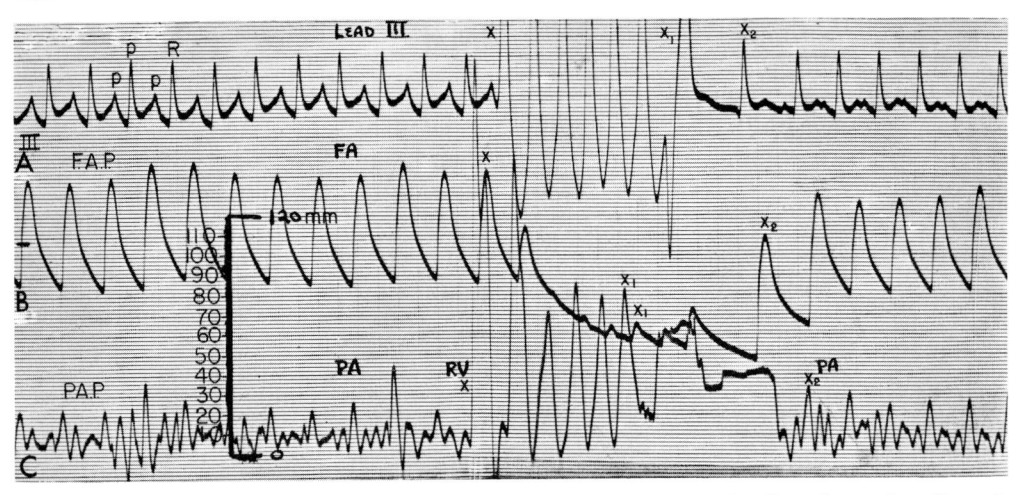

Figure 14-2. Cardiac catheterization in a patient with tetralogy of Fallot; shows the effect of ventricular tachycardia upon the systemic and the right ventricular blood pressure. This patient was 26 years of age; the diagnosis was ventricular septal defect, infundibular pulmonary stenosis, and cyanotic type of tetralogy of Fallot. A, B, and C show the simultaneous recording of the electrocardiogram (A), the femoral artery pressure (FAP) (B), and the pulmonary artery pressure (PAP) and right ventricular pressure (C).

(A) *The electrocardiogram* shows a simple tachycardia, rate 150 per minute. Note the occurrence of the ventricular tachycardia at X, showing markedly increased amplitude and bizarre and widened QRS complexes. Note the recurrence of a normal sinus rhythm at X_2 and the return of the blood pressure to control levels.

(B) *Femoral artery blood pressure.* The control blood pressure is 140/84. Note that with the occurrence of the ventricular tachycardia, there is a sudden fall in the femoral artery blood pressure, the maximum drop being 64/50. Note that with the re-establishment of normal sinus rhythm at X_2, the femoral artery blood pressure increases to 110/64 in the first beat and then increases to the control of 130/80.

(C) *Pulmonary artery blood pressure.* The control ranges from about 20 to 30 mm. systolic. Prior to the onset of the tachycardia, the catheter was pulled back into the right ventricle. Control *right ventricular pressure* shown at X was 200, and with the occurrence of ventricular tachycardia, there was a drop in the right ventricular pressure to a level of 70/0. This returned rapidly to control level pressures with the resumption of normal sinus rhythm.

Summary: The occurrence of a ventricular tachycardia in this patient with a tetralogy of Fallot resulted in a marked fall in femoral artery and the right ventricular pressure.

digitalis toxicity), and usually appear quite ill.

Symptoms and Signs. The symptoms observed during ventricular tachycardia resemble those of any ectopic rhythm, but are usually more marked because of the more severe hemodynamic alterations as compared to supraventricular arrhythmias and its more frequent appearance in severely damaged hearts. Commonly observed are substernal pain, dyspnea, syncopal attacks, especially in the upright position, and occasionally, sudden collapse or shock. In patients with either intermittent or persistent paroxysmal ventricular tachycardia uncomplicated by acute myocardial infarction, weakness and chest pain are equally apparent; dyspnea appeared most often in subjects with the persistent type of ventricular tachycardia. In the absence of adequate therapy, these tachycardias may last for days or weeks. Such subjects manifest a poor prognosis, complications are frequent, and death may be sudden. However, with the advent of recent therapeutic measures, the paroxysms may usually be controlled. The minor episodes, lasting only seconds or minutes, may present relatively mild symptoms even if repetitive. Roughly, one-half of patients with this arrhythmia manifest congestive heart failure.

The manifestations of the onset of ventricular tachycardia may not be remarkable in some patients who in the initial stage tolerate the tachycardia quite well. Palpitation, shortness of breath, weakness, and precordial pain may be the chief symptoms. When superimposed upon an acute myocardial infarction or congestive failure, the manifestations become more serious and if they persist may induce a shock-like state.

Prolonged periods of ventricular tachycardia have been noted to occur in patients with diseased hearts and rarely in patients with apparently normal hearts. Attacks which last longer than 24 hours are unlikely to remit spontaneously. With the recent development of improved methods of therapy, prolonged attacks are fortunately now rare.

The ventricular rate usually ranges from 140 to 180 beats per minute. Certain clinical features may lead one to suspect a ventricular origin of the tachycardia: (a) a changing intensity of the first heart sound as a result of the changing relationship between the atrial and ventricular contractions; (b) slight irregularity in cycle length which may range up to 0.03 second; and (c) at times, only one heart sound may be audible with each heart cycle, leading to an erroneous estimation (halving) of the ventricular rate.

After ten seconds of paroxysmal tachycardia, evidence of slow activity is observed in the electroencephalogram; after longer periods of tachycardia, the electroencephalogram assumes a flat appearance. These changes can very well be due to hypoxia, incident to a diminution of the cerebral blood flow during a paroxysm.

Electrocardiogram. The electrocardiographic criteria first described by Robinson and Herrmann (1921) still holds for most cases, that is: (a) the beats of the paroxysms must be ectopic in origin and must conform to those observed as isolated ventricular premature beats before the onset of the paroxysm; (b) the QRS complexes should be widened (0.12 second or more) and notched; (c) the first beat of the paroxysm should bear the same relationship to the preceding normal beat as a ventricular premature beat bears to the previous beat; and (d) the ventricles beat regularly, or only slightly irregularly, at a rate of 130 to 180 beats per minute, while the atria beat regularly, more slowly, and entirely independently of the ventricles. The diagnosis may be more definitely made when (e) occasional ventricular captures are observed, i.e., beats with a narrow QRS complex are conducted from the atria, and (f) ventricular fusion beats (from combined ectopic and sinus impulses) are present (this is practically diagnostic). In atrial fibrillation, aberrant beats with the configuration of right bundle branch block and, less commonly, of left bundle branch block are observed; these may simulate ventricular premature beats and paroxysms of ventricular tachycardia.

In doubtful cases, careful study of the initial beat of the paroxysm in all possible leads should be undertaken to determine whether a P wave precedes or is superimposed upon the QRS complex, indicating an atrial or A-V junctional origin (Kistin, 1966). The diagnosis of paroxysmal ventricular tachycardia may be suspected but should not be made unless it meets the aforementioned criteria (Figs. 14-3, 14-4, 14-5). In some cases, the diagnosis cannot be made with absolute certainty unless an esophageal lead is used or a His bundle electrogram is recorded by means of a catheter electrode during a paroxysm. This may help to determine the origin of the ectopic focus; in the supraventricular type the ventricular deflections arise proximal,

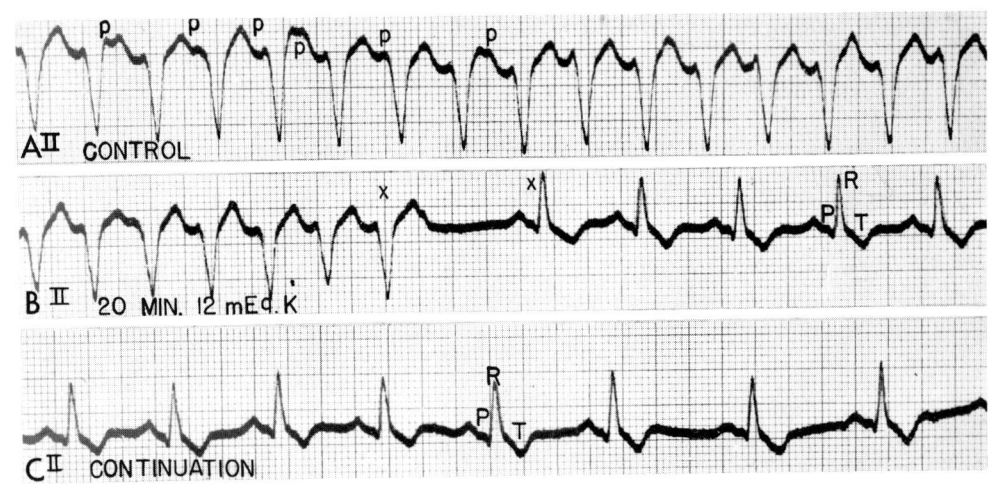

Figure 14-3. Probable ventricular tachycardia showing conversion to normal sinus rhythm.

(A) Note the rate of the tachycardia (167 per minute) with widening of the QRS complexes. The QRS width measures 0.12 second. Note the irregular type of notching of the T wave, indicating superimposed atrial complexes (P rate, 107 per minute). The differential diagnosis of A-V junctional tachycardia with ventricular aberration must be considered. In both cases there is a complete A-V dissociation during the paroxysm.

(B) Note the paroxysmal pause at X, followed by the resumption of normal sinus rhythm with a P-R interval of 0.18 second (after KCl).

(C) Note the arrhythmia and alterations in the P waves, indicating wandering of the sinus pacemaker.

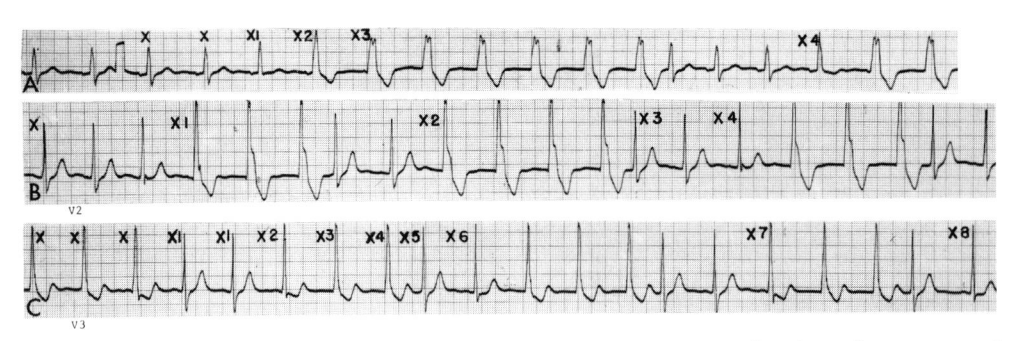

Figure 14-4. Periods of normal sinus rhythm showing beginning and ending of paroxysms of idioventricular tachycardia and fusion beats.

(A) (Lead III) Note normal sinus beats at X. The P waves are diphasic. Note the occurrence of widened QRS complexes with the rate of 75 per minute due to a ventricular tachycardia starting at X_3. X_2 is a beat of intermediate width. Another fusion beat is observed at X_4.

(B) (V_2) Shows two normal sinus beats and one fusion beat at X followed by widened QRS complexes, apparently ventricular in origin, starting at X_1. This is repeated at X_2 for a series of four beats with the resumption of normal sinus beats. A fusion beat is again at X_4.

(C) (V_3) Note the widened QRS complexes starting at X, followed by sinus beats at X_1, a fusion beat at X_2, widened QRS beats at X_3, a normal sinus beat at X_5, and a fusion beat at X_6. Two other fusion beats are observed at X_7 and X_8.

PAROXYSMAL VENTRICULAR TACHYCARDIA

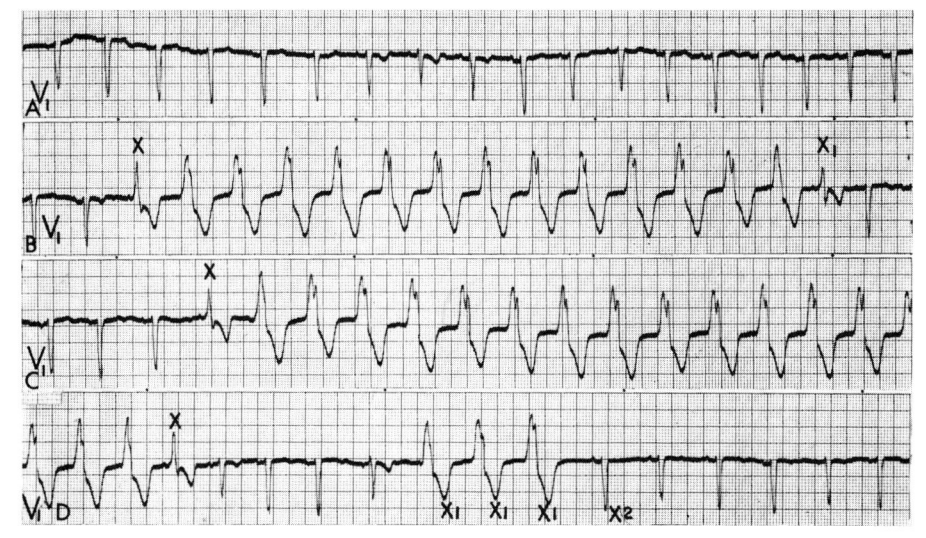

Figure 14–5. (All leads are V$_1$) Paroxysmal ventricular tachycardia, showing fusion beats, and beginning and ending of paroxysm.

(A) Heart rate is 91 per minute in the presence of sinus rhythm. Note inversion of T waves in three complexes in the middle of the strip.

(B) Note the occurrence of paroxysmal tachycardia with widened, aberrant QRS complexes with a ventricular rate of 100 per minute. Note the fusion beat (X) at the beginning of the paroxysm and (X$_1$) at the end of the paroxysm.

(C) Note the recurrence of a paroxysmal ventricular tachycardia following the fusion beat at X.

(D) Note the end of the paroxysm of tachycardia with a fusion beat at X and the restoration of normal sinus rhythm for four beats ending at X$_1$, followed by three ventricular ectopic beats (X$_1$); normal sinus beats starting at X$_2$ are observed at the end of the strip.

and in the ventricular type they occur distal to the bundle of His.

Types of Ventricular Tachycardia. These include varieties that range in rate from 60 to 100 beats per minute to 160 to 250 beats per minute.

Common Type. The common type is that in which all of the ventricular complexes present the same configuration with a rate over 110 and usually 130 to 180 beats per minute (Fig. 14–6). There is some variation in this group regarding the evolutionary stages preceding it, however. Parasystolic ventricular tachycardia consists of two separate pacemakers that remain independent of each other because the ectopic centers are protected by some form of block (see p. 116); both compete for control of the atria or ventricles. The cycle length may vary from a very short cycle length to a slower type in which the cycle length is a multiple of the normal. This phenomenon has been explained by the presence of an exit block. In the prefibrillatory type, the ventricular complexes vary between those of the common type and those of ventricular flutter (Figs. 15–1, 15–2). The ventricular rate ranges from 160 to 250 beats per minute. Such complexes are observed in severe hypoxic states and in other conditions associated with serious myocardial derangement, e.g., immediately preceding or during emergence from Stokes-Adams seizures. It is often premonitory to ventricular flutter or fibrillation, being a transition between normal sinus rhythm and these arrhythmias.

Repetitive Type. The repetitive type is characterized by short runs of ventricular premature beats occurring in groups of three to six complexes. They may be present for minutes, days,

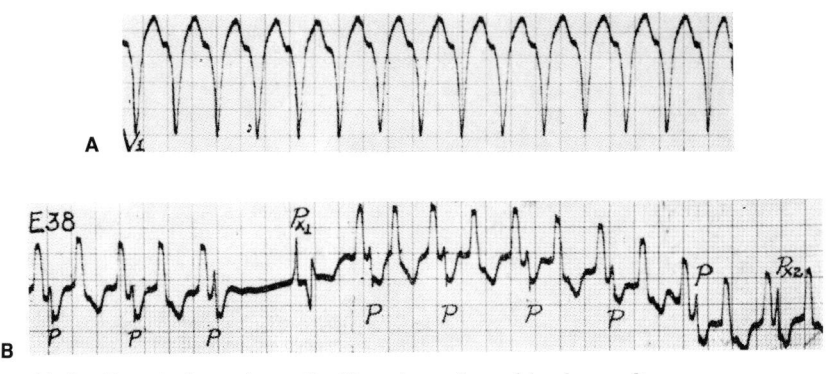

Figure 14-6. Ventricular tachycardia. V_1 and esophageal lead recording.

(A) (V_1) Note the presence of a regular paroxysmal tachycardia with a ventricular rate of 176 per minute. The QRS complexes are widened and notched, and no distinct P waves are observed.

(B) In the esophageal leads, the ventricular rate is 176 per minute, *the P waves are easily seen and occur at the rate of 88 per minute,* i.e., exactly a half of the ventricular rate. That means that every P wave is related to the preceding QRS—2:1 retrograde conduction. At P_{x1} following a long pause, there is a sinus escape (note different shape of QRS and P), followed by another run of ventricular tachycardia. P_{x2} resembles P_{x1} but apparently is not conducted. *Nodal tachycardia with aberration and 2:1 retrograde conduction cannot be ruled out.*

months, or even years. Sometimes this type may simulate the common type with periods of exit block (Fig. 14–7). This type is uncommon and the results of treatment are often unsatisfactory.

Idioventricular Tachycardia. Transient idioventricular tachycardia resembles idioventricular rhythm in many respects. Those cases in which the rate is quite slow (50 to 60 beats per minute) suggest an A-V junctional rhythm; however, the frequent ventricular fusion beats and the normal contour of the captured beats confirm a ventricular origin. This type of ventricular tachycardia has been studied by several workers and has been variously referred to as accelerated idioventricular rhythm, idioventricular rhythm in acute myocardial infarction, and slow ventricular tachycardia. Idioventricular tachycardia results from an enhancement of latent pacemaker fibers in the Purkinje network or from depression of the S-A node during bradycardia or the slow phase of sinus arrhythmia; thus, it differs from the common type of PVT. The ventricular rate ranges from 55 to 110 beats per minute; however, the paroxysm is observed only for short periods (up to 30 cycles) because of intermittent exit block or capture (see Fig. 14–8). Rothfeld et al. (1968) have recently studied this type in 100 consecutive patients followed by ECG monitoring during the postinfarction period. Thirty-six patients manifested one or more episodes of idioventricular rhythm (similar to "idioventricular tachycardia") with no apparent deleterious effect on survival. However, this condition should be watched carefully since its presence is associated with a significant abnormality.

This arrhythmia also occurs in patients with severe myocardial disease, especially acute myocardial infarction and digitalis intoxication (45 per cent of cases presented by Schamroth, 1968). This type of ventricular tachycardia rarely leads to ventricular fibrillation and thus does not usually pose a significant threat of sudden death. Since spontaneous termination is common, this arrhythmia usually requires no therapy; in fact, cardiosuppressive therapy may actually be contraindicated. It has been suggested that this rhythm is a protective mechanism against sustained bradycardia (Schamroth, 1968).

PAROXYSMAL VENTRICULAR TACHYCARDIA

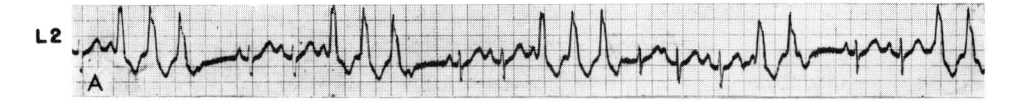

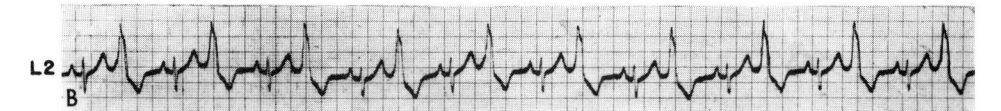

Figure 14-7. Ventricular parasystole appearing as ventricular premature contractions occurring in groups.

(A) Ventricular premature beats occurring in groups of two or three. These constitute a potential ventricular tachycardia. However, these complexes manifest an inconstant coupling and timing of premature beats, suggesting a parasystolic focus with exit block. Interectopic interval is 0.40 second between two successive beats and 2.00 seconds between groups of them.

(B) One hour after administration of 1 gm. procaine amide intramuscularly. Note that the ventricular ectopic beats no longer occur in groups, but are replaced by coupled rhythm (one ventricular premature beat occurring with each normal ventricular beat). The premature beats are followed by a fully compensatory pause. Here, the re-entry mechanism might be operative. However, the measurement shows the interectopic interval to be 1.20 seconds, *i.e.*, three times the short interectopic interval in A. It can be assumed, therefore, that the same parasystole persists as in A. This is an unusual example of parasystole with fixed coupling. The fixed relation of sinus and parasystolic rates (2:1) may be fortuitous or due to the effect of synchronization of both pacemakers. The effect of procaine amide may have resulted in a higher degree of exit block of the parasystolic impulses.

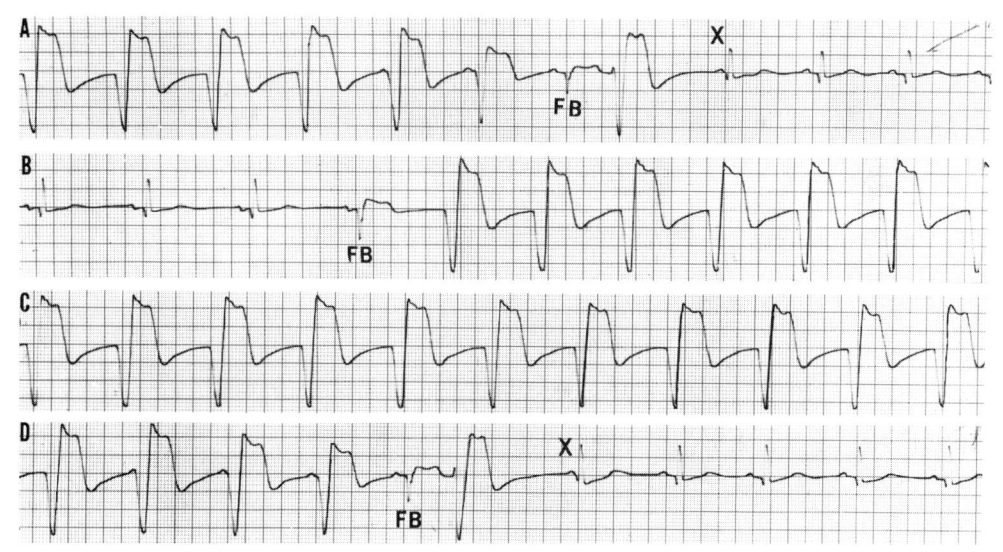

Figure 14-8. Idioventricular tachycardia. Note the presence of widened aberrant complexes with a ventricular rate of 60 per minute. A and B are continuous. C and D are continuous.

(A) FB is fusion beat. Note the occurrence of a normal sinus rhythm at the end of the strip. X shows a short P-R interval. In the remainder, the P-R interval is of normal length.

(B) Shows a fusion beat at FB followed by an idioventricular tachycardia with a rate of 60 per minute.

(D) Continuous record. FB represents a fusion beat and at X the P-R interval is short. The remaining QRS complexes are normal.

Although an idioventricular rhythm involves a less serious type of arrhythmia than the common type of ventricular tachycardia, it is not necessarily considered benign because it occurs on the basis of a serious pathophysiologic disturbance and may be associated with and lead to more serious types of ectopic tachycardias, i.e., a more serious type of ventricular tachycardia (Julian et al., 1970), and other serious disturbances in rhythm.

IDIOVENTRICULAR RHYTHM

Idioventricular rhythm is a form of autonomous ventricular beating with the pacemaker located in the Purkinje fibers of the ventricle. In this disturbance the ventricular pacemaker assumes control of the heart rhythm at a relatively slow rate, usually as a result of failure of the S-A nodal and A-V junctional pacemakers to function. This rhythm may occur transiently or for prolonged periods of time, and in some cases it may be permanent. It may be observed under the following conditions: (a) occasionally, in normal individuals following hyperventilation and breath-holding; (b) as a transient phenomenon following periods of hypoxia, particularly under anesthesia; (c) with certain types of bradycardia or the slow phase of bradyarrhythmia occurring in the immediate postinfarction period; (d) premonitory to or upon emergence from cardiac arrest; (e) in certain types of complete A-V heart block, especially the acquired type, which gives rise to a pacemaker below the bundle of His situated in the ventricular septum; (f) in the advanced stage of potassium intoxication; and (g) when an artificial pacemaker controls the ventricular rhythm by a directly placed electrode; this constitutes an artificial, not a spontaneous, form of idioventricular rhythm.

The electrocardiogram reveals widened and bizarre QRS complexes as in premature ventricular contractions (Fig. 14-9). When a complete A-V

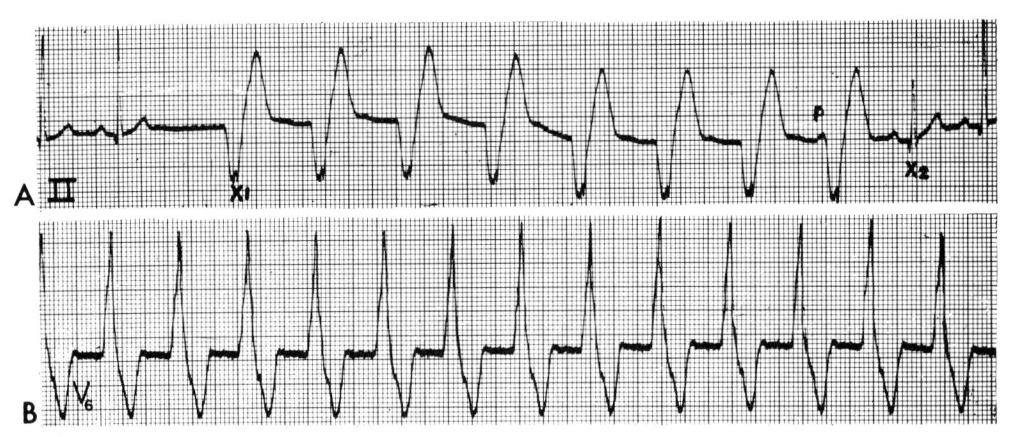

Figure 14-9. Idioventricular rhythm accelerating to ventricular tachycardia following hyperventilation.
(A) Shows an idioventricular rhythm following hyperventilation. Note the first normal cycle followed by widened QRS complexes of idioventricular beats without visible P waves. This continues until X_2, where a fusion beat is observed, indicating a ventricular origin of the ectopic rhythm.
(B) Shows widened QRS complexes (during period of hyperventilation) having a ventricular origin (ventricular tachycardia). (From Hiss, R. G., Averill, K. H., and Lamb, L. E.: Electrocardiographic Findings in 67,375 Asymptomatic Individuals. Part III: Ventricular Rhythms. In Lamb, L. E. (ed.): The First International Symposium on Cardiology in Aviation. Conducted at the School of Aviation Medicine, November 12-13, 1959. USAF Aerospace Med. Center (ATC), Brooks Air Force Base, Texas.)

PAROXYSMAL VENTRICULAR TACHYCARDIA 199

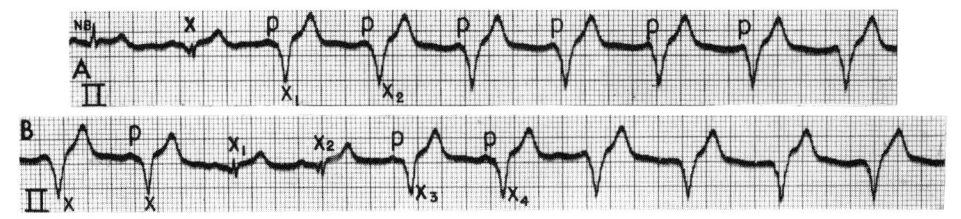

Figure 14–10. Ventricular rhythm (parasystolic idioventricular tachycardia).
(A) Note normal beat (NB) (rate 68 per minute) ventricular beats starting at X_1 (rate 79 per minute) and fusion beat at X.
(B) X and X are ventricular beats; X_1 and X_2 are fusion beats, and idioventricular tachycardia continues at X_3. (The actual rate may be twice the given value due to 2:1 exit block.)

heart block is not the cause of the idioventricular rhythm, occasional sinus beats will traverse the A-V junction and activate the ventricles. The resulting QRS complex serves to identify such a beat. However, at times, a sinus impulse occurring with an idioventricular beat will produce a fusion beat (Fig. 14–10). The resulting QRS complex will show features of both a supraventricular and a ventricular complex. In the absence of such fusion beats, it is often difficult to rule out an A-V junctional pacemaker with aberration or the pre-existence of a bundle branch block as the cause of the widened QRS.

Most instances of idioventricular rhythm represent a very serious type of cardiac abnormality and usually occur in subjects with severe underlying cardiac disease. In these cases, the treatment is that of the underlying disorder.

T WAVE CHANGES FOLLOWING PAROXYSMAL TACHYCARDIA (ATRIAL, VENTRICULAR, OR JUNCTIONAL)

Following attacks of rapid ectopic rhythms, particularly those of long duration, especially in older indi-

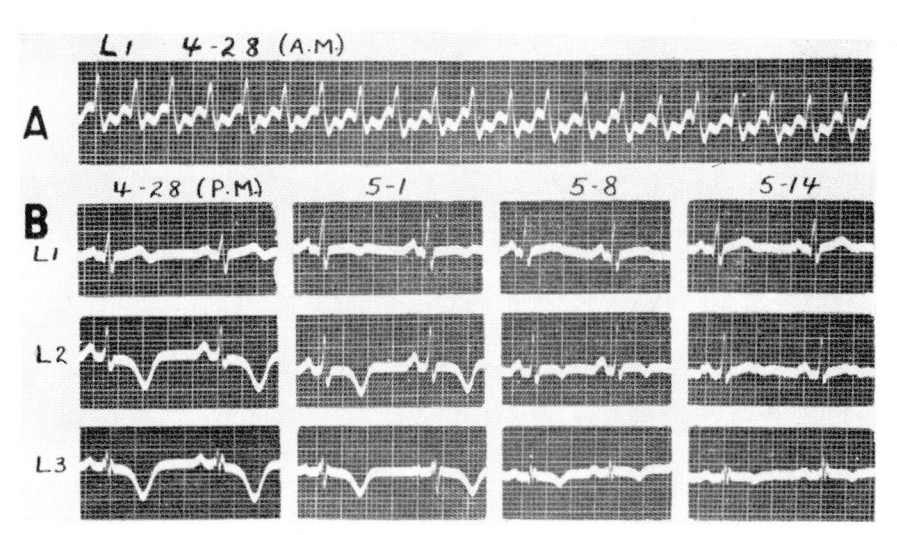

Figure 14–11. Post-tachycardia syndrome.
(A) Supraventricular tachycardia was present for ten days. (B) Following return to a normal sinus rhythm, note the marked T wave inversion in leads 2 and 3, which resembles that observed in the subacute stage of myocardial infarction. This persisted for five days and gradually returned to a normal configuration within two weeks.

viduals and in those with pre-existing heart disease, the electrocardiogram often shows inverted T waves in the limb and precordial leads which may resemble those seen in the subacute stage of myocardial infarction (Fig. 14–11). Indeed, in fatal cases of long-lasting tachycardia, diffuse areas of subendocardial fibrosis have been found at necropsy. This probably resulted from subacute coronary insufficiency. This state may well explain the symptoms usually associated with a prolonged tachycardia, viz., substernal pain, a temperature rise, leukocytosis, and a fall in blood pressure. Since the shock-like state incident to the tachycardia may eventuate in a myocardial infarction, the post-tachycardia T wave changes, because of their similarity to those of the subacute state of infarction, add to the difficulty in the differential diagnosis. The return of the electrocardiographic changes to normal often takes days or weeks. The cardiac effects of digitalis, quinidine, and procaine amide should be ruled out as productive of the electrocardiographic changes.

DIFFERENTIAL DIAGNOSIS OF VENTRICULAR TACHYCARDIA

All of the electrocardiographic manifestations of ventricular arrhythmias, except ventricular fibrillation, may be simulated by supraventricular arrhythmias (Kistin, 1966). The differential diagnosis between a supraventricular and a ventricular origin is often difficult to establish. If the appropriate data are available, it is often possible to prove that an arrhythmia with abnormal QRS complexes is supraventricular in origin; it is not possible to prove beyond a doubt that an arrhythmia is ventricular, except in ventricular fibrillation or when the arrhythmia is produced by artificial ventricular stimulation. Important information establishing the diagnosis can be derived from the history, the physical examination, the associated clinical state (especially acute myocardial infarction), and occasionally from the auscultatory phenomena. The reaction to parasympathetic stimulation and the results of other types of therapy, especially digitalis, are also important. The electrocardiographic patterns, especially those obtained during normal sinus rhythm and during the beginning or ending of a paroxysm, are of prime importance. Also, the use of esophageal leads is helpful in the differential diagnosis by demonstrating the atrial mechanism. The advent of His bundle recordings (see pp. 17 and 230) may allow more exact diagnosis of the origin of the tachycardia; however, data derived from this technique are rarely required for therapy.

Supraventricular Arrhythmias Simulating Ventricular Tachycardia. Many types of paroxysmal tachycardia considered to be ventricular in origin actually arise in the atria or A-V junction. Atrial arrhythmias may be and A-V junctional arrhythmias often are associated with abnormal QRS complexes as a result of incomplete recovery of the ventricular conduction fibers prior to the arrival of the next supraventricular impulse. This sequence may lead to an abnormal QRS pattern (e.g., RBBB pattern seen with PAT) (see Fig. 14–12).

In the presence of widened or abnormal QRS complexes, the following criteria suggest a supraventricular origin (Kistin, 1966): (a) the arrhythmia starts with an ectopic premature P wave which may be confirmed by esophageal or intra-atrial leads; (b) the QRS-to-P interval is too short to be explained by retrograde conduction from a ventricular focus; (c) the configuration of the QRS is the same as that which results from conduction from a known supraventricular site, before, during, or after the arrhythmia; (d) the P wave and QRS complex are so related as to suggest that the QRS complexes depend on supraventricular

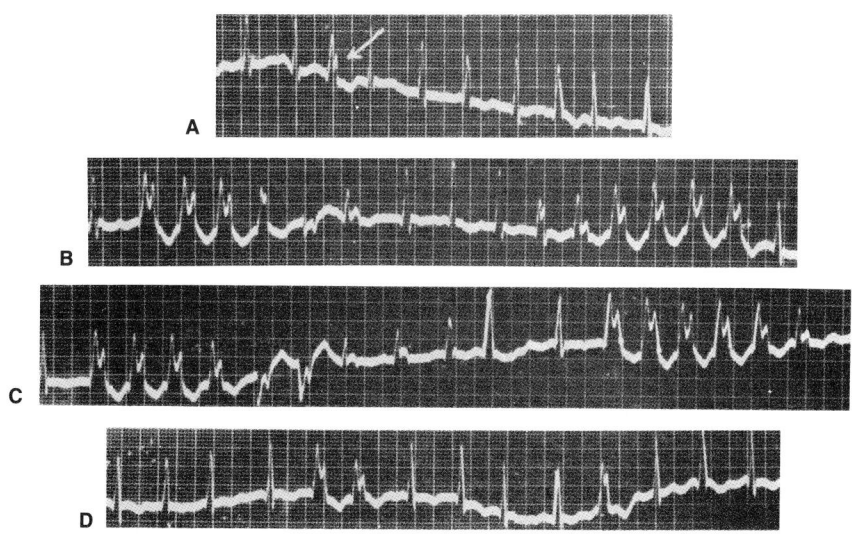

Figure 14-12. Atrial fibrillation with aberration simulating ventricular tachycardia; all tracings are Lead II.

(A) Before the administration of procaine amide (Pronestyl), the atria are fibrillating and some aberration of the ventricular complexes is seen. The arrow points to an aberrant beat.

(B) Fifteen minutes after the intramuscular injection of 1 gm. of procaine amide, the aberrant beats are more frequent and occur in runs constituting short paroxysms of tachycardia. Note that these aberrant beats are similar to the complex shown in A but are marked by increased widening of the QRS, which is a characteristic effect of procaine amide.

(C) Thirty minutes after the injection of procaine amide, the tracing is similar to B.

(D) Six hours after the injection of procaine amide, the ectopic beats are markedly reduced in frequency and the QRS is not as wide; however, they are still more frequent and the QRS is wider than those observed in the control tracing. (From Bellet, S., Zeeman, S. E., and Hirsch, S. A.: Amer. J. Med., 13:145, 1952.)

activity (i.e., intermittent block of conduction to the ventricles or Wenckebach phenomenon); (e) termination of the arrhythmia by carotid sinus pressure or administration of edrophonium; and (f) clearly establishing the type of atrial mechanism by esophageal leads may definitely rule out atrial tachycardia, junctional tachycardia, or atrial flutter. An atrial rate slower than the ventricular rate and A-V dissociation does not necessarily establish the diagnosis of ventricular tachycardia. It is sometimes impossible to differentiate a junctional tachycardia with widened QRS complexes from ventricular tachycardia. In our experience, a slower atrial than ventricular rate has, in most instances, occurred in a tachycardia of ventricular origin.

Ventricular Tachycardia Simulating Supraventricular Tachycardia. The occurrence of atrial beats with the atrial rate as rapid as the ventricular and bearing a constant relationship to the ventricular beat does not rule out a ventricular tachycardia, since these atrial beats may result from retrograde conduction; indeed, retrograde conduction is common (Kistin, 1966) (Fig. 14–13). However, this sequence is rare, and a ventricular origin is difficult to establish in such cases unless produced through direct ventricular stimulation by a pacemaker or during cardiac catheterization.

TREATMENT

The treatment of ventricular tachycardia depends on: (a) the type and duration; (b) the underlying cause (myocardial infarction, digitalis); (c) the as-

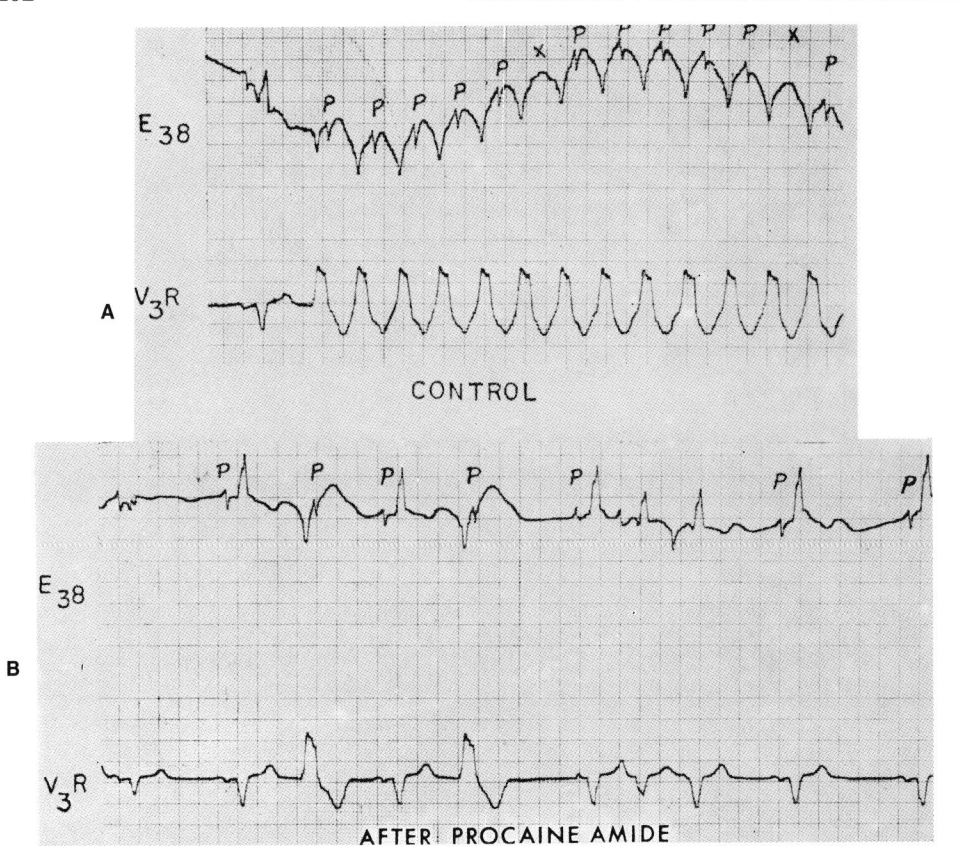

Figure 14-13. Ventricular tachycardia showing retrograde conduction.

(A) The esophageal lead taken at the atrial level is paired with a V$_3$R lead. Following a normal complex there is a run of ventricular premature beats constituting a paroxysm of ventricular tachycardia. It will be observed in the esophageal lead (E$_{38}$) that the QRS complex gives rise to a retrograde P wave and that the R-P interval becomes progressively longer until one drops out at X. This sequence is repeated at regular intervals. This represents a reverse Wenckebach phenomenon.

(B) After the administration of procaine amide (Pronestyl), there is a return of normal sinus rhythm which is interrupted by frequent ventricular premature beats. Note that the premature beats have the same configuration as the aberrant complexes of the paroxysm and are followed by retrograde P waves in lead E$_{38}$. Complex at X represents an atrial premature beat with ventricular aberration.

sociated clinical condition (dyspnea, cyanosis, congestive failure, precordial pain); and (d) the presence of hypotension or a shock-like state. These factors will help determine the seriousness, urgency, and intensity of the therapy. In the treatment of paroxysmal ventricular tachycardia, the methods of choice are the use of certain drugs, overdrive suppression by artificial pacemaker, and electric countershock.

Drugs. Of the drugs, lidocaine may be tried first and is often efficacious in controlling the arrhythmia. (The dose and administration of lidocaine are discussed on p. 362.) Other drugs include quinidine, procaine amide, propranolol, potassium salts, diphenylhydantoin (Dilantin), and bretylium. (Indications, dosages and routes of administration, and complications are discussed in Chapter 33.) However, if the patient is quite ill, e.g., with an acute infarction, and the response to therapy is not rapid, electric countershock should immediately be instituted (see p. 427).

Recently, the antiarrhythmic effects of lidocaine have become of great importance in the treatment of paroxysmal ventricular tachycardia. It is considered to be the drug of choice and is often used prior to electric countershock. It has particular efficacy in ventricular arrhythmias. Moreover, in therapeutic doses there is no evidence of myocardial depression of the type commonly observed with other antiarrhythmic drugs. Lidocaine should be administered via the intravenous route in a bolus of at first 50 and then 100 mg. It may be effective in as little as two minutes and suppresses the arrhythmia for periods up to 20 minutes. If tachycardia recurs, an I.V. drip at a rate of 1 to 8 mg. per minute of lidocaine may be administered for a period of up to 24 hours without ill effects. Recurrences may be treated with 1 mg./Kg. of lidocaine administered in an I.V. bolus. (This is further discussed on p. 362.)

Quinidine has long been used in the treatment of this arrhythmia. The intravenous route is attended by serious untoward effects and should be used only in cases of dire emergency; it must be given slowly and under electrocardiographic control. Intramuscular administration is less hazardous. The indications, plasma levels, mechanism of action, and toxic effects of quinidine are discussed on page 349.

Procaine amide (Pronestyl) is quite effective in the control of ventricular tachycardia. We have noted a favorable response in about 70 per cent of patients treated. For a rapid effect it may be given intramuscularly or intravenously. The former route is safer, since it is accompanied by a low incidence of hypotension and other side effects. Following conversion, the patient may be placed on an oral maintenance dose (250 to 500 mg., four times a day).

This drug is discussed fully in Chapter 33.

The use of diphenylhydantoin (Dilantin) in therapy of paroxysmal ventricular tachycardia is limited, since other agents are more effective. Bretylium has been shown to be effective in the conversion of ventricular tachycardia to normal sinus rhythm. Experience so far has not warranted its inclusion as a preferred drug in therapy. It is useful in subjects in whom the more traditional agents prove unsatisfactory. See Chapter 33 for a more complete discussion of bretylium. Most subjects with ventricular tachycardia do not respond to propranolol, but it is occasionally of use in cases resistant to other therapeutic agents. See Chapter 33 for a more complete discussion of propranolol.

With hypotension, vasopressor drugs are administered to maintain a minimal degree of blood flow to the vital organs, e.g., brain, heart, muscle, and kidney (see p. 327). The rapidity of administration depends on the condition of the patient and upon the blood pressure level prior to its infusion. Digitalis was apparently effective in converting the ectopic rhythm to normal when other drugs had failed. In these cases, a supraventricular origin could not always be excluded.

Overdrive Suppression by Artificial Pacemaker. Ventricular tachyarrhythmias may be terminated with overdrive suppression of the ectopic focus through atrial or ventricular pacing (DeSanctis and Kastor, 1968; Furman and Escher, 1970; Zipes et al., 1968). This technique is utilized as a temporary or as a permanent measure in cases of recurrent ventricular tachycardia resistant to other forms of therapy (see p. 407, Chapter 37).

Electric Countershock. Electric countershock has become the method of choice in the treatment of drug-resistant episodes of paroxysmal ventricular tachycardia and is considered of special use in ventricular tachycardia accompanying coronary occlusion (Fig. 14–14). In ventricular tachycardia due to toxic digitalis effects, electric countershock should not be used since it may have no effect and may result in ventricular fibrillation.

In the absence of more efficacious modes of therapy, a blow to the precordium may terminate episodes of paroxysmal ventricular tachycardia. However, since this maneuver may precipitate ventricular fibrillation, it should be undertaken only if the patient manifests evidence of marked hemodynamic dysfunction; a defibrillator should be available. Pennington et al. (1970) have reported termination of 12 episodes of paroxysmal ventricular tachycardia occurring in five patients by using the thump method. The sharp thump to the chest through electromechanical transduction provides a low energy depolarizing current to the heart, thereby probably disrupting the re-entry pathway.

Occasionally, one encounters patients with short paroxysms or continuous paroxysms of ventricular tachycardia who are refractory to the usual types of therapy. Although they may respond to electric countershock, the restoration to normal sinus rhythm is only temporary and within a few hours the tachycardia recurs. In such cases one must therefore depend on drugs or other therapy to maintain normal rhythm. The results obtained are often unsatisfactory. Many of these cases occur in patients with an advanced grade of myocardial abnormality and extensive coronary artery disease with healed infarction. These subjects are often nonreactive or react unsatisfactorily to the usual medication previously mentioned—quinidine, procaine amide, lidocaine, diphenylhydantoin, bretylium, and propranolol. In such cases the following steps should be considered: (1) re-evaluate the myocardial state; (2) rule out the presence of electrolyte imbalance; (3) correct hypoxia or hyperventilation; (4) occasionally the arrhythmia may be controlled by a pacemaker inserted either in the atrium or ventricle starting with an initial overdrive (see p. 407); and (5) consider that occasionally these episodes are the result of excessive sympathetic tone. Tapazole has been successful in decreasing episodes because of its antithyroid effect; however, this effect takes three weeks to become apparent. Propranolol or alprenolol, which has very little negative inotropic effect, may be tried. Stellate ganglionic block or sympathectomy has been of help in the experimental animal and in some human cases. Recently, instances have been reported where excision of the infarcted area has abolished the ventricular tachycardia after all other measures have failed.

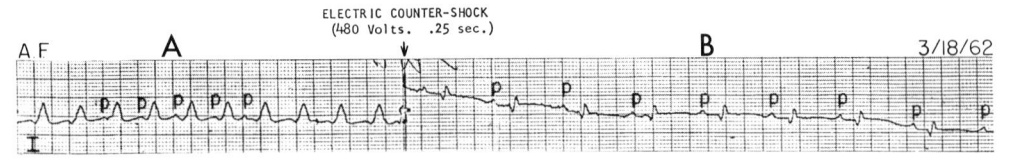

Figure 14–14. Effect of electric countershock in a patient with ventricular tachycardia refractory to drug therapy. (Lead I)

(A) Taken from a patient, age 75, with a ventricular tachycardia refractory to the usual methods of therapy. Note the ventricular rate of 145 per minute with markedly widened QRS complexes and P waves occurring at a slower rate independent of the ventricular complexes (complete A-V dissociation).

(B) After the electric countershock (480 volts, 0.25 second). Note the restoration of a normal sinus rhythm with a P-R interval of 0.24 second. (From Medow, A., and Dreifus, L. S.: Amer. J. Cardiol., 11:87, 1963.)

COMPLICATIONS

The most serious complications are the precipitation of ventricular fibrillation and death. The following additional complications of ventricular tachycardia may be noted: (a) alternation of the heart (electrical or mechanical) has been observed; (b) hypoxia and necrosis in the subendocardial zone of the heart muscle may occur; (c) a previous area of infarction may increase in size because of the increased cardiac work and the resultant hypoxic state; (d) mural thrombi may form in the ventricle resulting in secondary pulmonary and systemic embolism; and (e) renal tubular necrosis may result from a prolonged shock-like state.

PROGNOSIS

In general, the prognosis depends on the type of ventricular tachycardia, the rate during the paroxysm, its duration, the underlying pathologic state, and the response to therapy. The outlook is quite serious in the prefibrillatory type. The presence of heart failure or a shock-like state adds to the gravity of the situation, so that even if the patient recovers from the paroxysm the amount of damage incurred is so great that death will be hastened following its termination. Fortunately, the prognosis has been improved by the use of cardioversion, certain new developments in drug therapy, and the advent of electrocardiographic monitoring in coronary care units so that attacks are treated more promptly.

From the standpoint of prognosis, the patients may be divided into three main groups: (1) Patients with apparently normal hearts or with little evidence of disease. Such cases are relatively uncommon. The prognosis in these subjects is good, particularly if the attacks are controlled; however, the risk of ventricular fibrillation cannot be minimized. (2) Patients in whom the paroxysms are the result of a severe toxic factor, i.e., severe infections or drug toxicity (digitalis, quinidine, or procaine amide). The paroxysms disappear as the cause is removed. (3) Patients who have severe heart disease; these constitute the preponderant group. Many of these subjects have sustained a recent myocardial infarction or manifest evidence of severe coronary artery disease. The prognosis is quite poor in this group. Eighty per cent in Strauss' series (1930) died within a period of only 24 hours. Cooke and White (1943) observed that half of their group died within three weeks of the paroxysm and those who recovered died a few months later, the longest survival being 18 months. The prognosis has improved in recent years with the advent of improved methods of therapy and the use of monitoring devices, especially in the CCU. Lown and associates (1967) reported 17 deaths among 84 patients (20.2 per cent) who manifested ventricular tachycardia in the immediate postinfarction period, an excess of two deaths over that expected from the average mortality (17.7 per cent) in their entire series.

References

Campbell, M.: Inversion of T waves after long paroxysms of tachycardia. Brit. Heart J., 4:49, 1942.

Cass, R. M.: Repetitive tachycardia. A review of 40 cases with no demonstrable heart disease. Amer. J. Cardiol., 19:597, 1967.

Cohn, L. J., Donoso, E., and Friedberg, C. K.: Ventricular tachycardia. Prog. Cardiov. Dis., 9:29, 1966.

Cooke, W. T., and White, P. D.: Paroxysmal ventricular tachycardia. Brit. Heart J., 5:33, 1943.

Corday, E., et al.: Alternating failure of mechanical response to electrical depolarization (the aformed phenomenon) — a new phenomenon in cardiac arrhythmias. Abstr. 18th Annual Scientific Session, Amer. Col., Cardiol., Amer. J. Cardiol., 23:108, 1969.

DeSanctis, R. W., and Kastor, J. A.: Rapid intracardiac pacing for treatment of recurrent ventricular tachyarrhythmias in the absence of heart block. Amer. Heart J., 76:168, 1968.

Easley, R. M., Jr., and Goldstein, S.: Differentiation of ventricular tachycardia from junctional tachycardia with aberrant conduction. Circulation, 37:1015, 1968.

Furman, S., and Escher, D. J. W.: Temporary transvenous pacing. *In* Principles and Techniques of Cardiac Pacing, New York, Harper & Row, 1970.

Julian, D. G., Vellani, C. W., Godman, M. J., and Terry, G.: Prolongation of QRS duration in acute myocardial infarction. Prog. Cardiov. Dis., 13:56, 1970.

Katz, M. J., and Zitnik, R. S.: Direct current shock and lidocaine in treatment of digitalis-induced ventricular tachycardia. Amer. J. Cardiol., 18:552, 1966.

Kistin, A. D.: Problems in the differentiation of ventricular arrhythmias from supraventricular arrhythmias with abnormal QRS. Prog. Cardiov. Dis., 9:1, 1966.

Lown, B., et al.: Unresolved problems in coronary care. Amer. J. Cardiol., 20:494, 1967.

MacKenzie, G. J., and Pascual, S.: Paroxysmal ventricular tachycardia. Brit. Heart J., 26:441, 1964.

Muller, O. F., Cardenas, M., and Bellet, S.: QRS alterations produced by auricular and ventricular paroxysmal tachycardia in the presence of bundle branch block pattern: An experimental study in dogs. Amer. J. Cardiol., 7:697, 1961.

Pennington, J. E., Taylor, J., and Lown, B.: Chest thump for reverting ventricular tachycardia. New Eng. J. Med., 283:1192, 1970.

Robinson, G. C., and Herrmann, G. R.: Paroxysmal tachycardia of ventricular origin and its relation to coronary occlusion. Heart, 8:59, 1921.

Rothfeld, E. L., Zucker, I. R., Parsonnet, V., and Alinsonorin, C. A.: Idioventricular rhythm in acute myocardial infarction. Circulation, 37:203, 1968.

Schamroth, L.: Idioventricular tachycardia. J. Electrocardiol., 1:205, 1968.

Strauss, M. B.: Paroxysmal ventricular tachycardia. Amer. J. Med. Sci., 79:337, 1930.

Wallace, A. G.: Personal communication cited in McIntosh, H. D., and Morris, J. J., Jr.: The hemodynamic consequences of arrhythmias. Prog. Cardiov. Dis., 8:330, 1966.

Wallace, A. G., et al.: The electrophysiologic effects of beta-adrenergic blockade and cardiac denervation. Bull. N.Y. Acad. Med., 43:1119, 1967.

Wegria, R., Frank, C. W., Wang, H. H., and Lammerent, J.: Effect of atrial and ventricular tachycardia on cardiac output, coronary blood flow and blood pressure. Circ. Res., 6:624, 1958.

Zipes, D. P., et al.: Treatment of ventricular arrhythmia by permanent atrial pacemaker and cardiac sympathectomy. Ann. Intern. Med., 68:591, 1968.

Chapter 15 *Ventricular Flutter and Fibrillation*

ETIOLOGY
FACTORS AFFECTING THE
  VENTRICULAR FIBRILLATION
  THRESHOLD
HEMODYNAMICS
CARDIAC MECHANISMS PRECEDING
  ONSET OF VENTRICULAR
  FIBRILLATION
MECHANISMS UNDERLYING
  VENTRICULAR FIBRILLATION

CLINICAL DIAGNOSIS
ELECTROCARDIOGRAM
TREATMENT
SEQUELAE FOLLOWING
  RESUSCITATION FROM VENTRICULAR
  FIBRILLATION
PROGNOSIS

Ventricular flutter and fibrillation, together with asystole, are the most dangerous of the cardiac arrhythmias. Indeed, it has been estimated that fibrillation is the terminal cardiac event in 40 to 50 per cent of all patients; the remainder manifest asystole. Ventricular fibrillation is closely allied with cardiac arrest—one mechanism often develops into the other. In fact, which of the two is considered to be present after cardiovascular collapse often depends on the timing of the electrocardiogram. The exact occurrence of ventricular flutter and fibrillation and its relation to cardiac arrest as well as to the clinical picture can best be studied by continuous electrocardiographic monitoring. In one series (Adgey et al., 1969), when an electrocardiogram was obtained within four minutes of the onset of symptoms, the majority of patients (91 per cent) manifested ventricular fibrillation; after four minutes, 82 per cent manifested cardiac standstill. Therefore, many facets of these two mechanisms may be considered together since the clinical manifestations and immediate treatment, except for defibrillation, are quite similar.

Attitudes toward ventricular fibrillation have undergone a striking change in recent years. Formerly considered to be a terminal mechanism in an irreversibly damaged heart, it is now known that ventricular fibrillation may occur unexpectedly in hearts with relatively little, slight, or moderate degrees of organic damage, resulting from various acute changes caused by hypoxia and enhanced sympathetic tone (with or without myocardial infarction) or other factors that tend to cause instability of the ventricular fibers or inhomogeneous conduction through the ventricular musculature.

The abolition of ventricular fibrillation with restoration of normal sinus rhythm results in a resumption of normal function without necessarily decreasing the longevity of the patient. Resuscitation may prove successful in the majority of patients: as many as 80 per cent of patients who develop this arrhythmia while recovering in a coronary care unit from an otherwise uncomplicated myocardial infarction may be resuscitated with restoration of normal sinus rhythm and may survive. In these cases, the long-term prognosis is not necessarily affected by the occurrence of ventricular fibrillation during the acute postinfarction period.

ETIOLOGY

The causes of ventricular fibrillation in humans are not always clear cut, and, except under ideal circumstances, there are few opportunities to study the causative factors in the individual patient. Most patients who develop ventricular fibrillation suffer from either an acute myocardial infarction or chronic organic heart disease (especially hypertensive, rheumatic, or atherosclerotic types). Ventricular fibrillation is observed in roughly 8 to 10 per cent of patients with acute myocardial infarction, most often within the first four hours following the occlusion. Hypoxia and heightened autonomic activity in the postinfarction period play an important role. In addition, severe emotional upsets in a predisposed subject may be the immediate cause of increased autonomic tone which may precipitate ventricular fibrillation. Sympathetic activity tends to enhance the automaticity of ventricular pacemaker tissue and to increase the excitability and conductivity of the myocardium; thus, it predisposes to the development of ventricular premature beats and runs of ventricular tachycardia. Increased vagal stimulation results in increased temporal dispersion of repolarization which is conducive for microre-entry circuits.

Ventricular fibrillation may occasionally be initiated by an electrical impulse delivered during repolarization (downsweep of the T wave), either by an artificial pacemaker, electric countershock, or a premature beat (QRS or T phenomenon).

Ventricular fibrillation often occurs during various types of surgery (see Chapter 25), especially during cardiac procedures. The primary factor may be the anesthesia, surgical trauma, or inadequate coronary perfusion. Hypothermia, occasionally employed during surgery, is an occasional cause of ventricular fibrillation. This arrhythmia develops commonly when the body temperature falls below 28°C.

A wide variety of drugs have been implicated in the production of ventricular fibrillation: (a) anesthetics (cyclopropane and chloroform); (b) sympathomimetic agents; (c) quinidine, procaine amide, and other antiarrhythmic agents; (d) digitalis; and (e) radiopaque substances used in angiography.

Poor design and improper grounding of common electrical hospital devices may lead to ventricular fibrillation. Various instruments including electrocardiograms, dye injection through an intracoronary catheter, densitometer, and a soldering iron have been implicated in producing ventricular fibrillation (Briller, 1966).

Ventricular fibrillation may also occur in persons struck by lightning. It has been postulated that the lightning discharge simultaneously causes violent ventricular contraction, arrest of the respiratory center, and a shock-like state.

Trauma from severe blows to the chest, knife and bullet wounds without cardiac tamponade, and direct mechanical irritation during cardiac catheterization may also result in ventricular fibrillation (see Chapter 26).

Relatively rare instances of spontaneous ventricular fibrillation have been documented in human subjects with no indication of myocardial abnormality, drug effects, or trauma (Stern, 1957).

FACTORS AFFECTING THE VENTRICULAR FIBRILLATION THRESHOLD

The ventricular fibrillation threshold (VFT) is the minimum amount of current which will cause ventricular fibrillation when applied to the ventricles. Factors which will decrease the VFT, therefore, will predispose toward the development of ventricular fibrillation. Some of the clinically significant factors which depress the VFT are discussed later.

It is well known that the ischemic process associated with coronary occlusion and resulting myocardial infarction lowers the fibrillation threshold. The VFT is also decreased by metabolic acidosis (Gerst et al., 1966) and the following drugs: sympathomimetics, anesthetic agents (cyclopropane, halothane), digitalis, nicotine and caffeine (Bellet et al., 1971, 1972). The VFT is increased with metabolic alkalosis (Gerst et al., 1966) and following the administration of lidocaine.

HEMODYNAMICS

The arterial blood pressure may be partially maintained with ventricular flutter. However, the circulation effectively ceases with the onset of ventricular fibrillation, and unless blood flow to vital organs is restored, this arrhythmia terminates rapidly in death.

CARDIAC MECHANISMS PRECEDING ONSET OF VENTRICULAR FIBRILLATION

Although ventricular fibrillation may occur without an initiating arrhythmia, it is usually preceded by a variety of mechanisms, including: (a) lability of the ventricular rate; (b) development of ventricular premature beats, either singly or in groups; (c) the appearance of bizarre and deformed ventricular complexes with prolonged QRS segments and progressive T wave inversion; and (d) runs of ventricular tachycardia.

These observations are in keeping with the hypothesis that an ectopic focus is created which is responsible for occasional premature beats which increase in frequency and that ventricular fibrillation results if these premature beats occur at a sufficiently rapid rate in a setting encouraging microre-entry.

MECHANISMS UNDERLYING VENTRICULAR FIBRILLATION

Ventricular fibrillation is caused by factors which cause fibers to be out of phase at a time when the refractory period is shortened (Burn, 1961). Under these conditions impulses arising from one or several foci cannot be conducted normally and the presence of areas of refractory tissue results in disorganized conduction and in the creation of multiple microre-entry circuits. This electrophysiologic inhomogeneity then tends to perpetuate itself. These conditions have also been found to occur following one or more premature ventricular beats or an accelerating ventricular tachycardia. Several of the etiologic factors discussed previously similarly cause inhomogeneities in the refractory periods and conduction in the ventricles. Thus, following myocardial infarction, the effects of ischemia are not necessarily uniform over the entire heart, and varying degrees of circulatory impairment lead to nonuniform depolarization and repolarization.

CLINICAL DIAGNOSIS

The diagnosis of ventricular fibrillation should be suspected when there is sudden disappearance of a palpable pulse and audible heart sounds and the blood pressure becomes unobtainable, especially during surgery and the administration of certain types of anesthesia (particularly in patients with coronary artery disease, or following myocardial infarction). These manifestations are compatible with ventricular fibrillation or cardiac standstill. Since the initial therapeutic approach to these two conditions is essentially the same, closed chest compression should be instituted without delay (see p. 328).

A clinical diagnosis of terminal ventricular fibrillation cannot be made with certainty. It may be suspected when some of the etiologic factors mentioned previously are present: coronary occlusion, digitalis toxicity, or electric shock. A clinical diagnosis of transient ventricular fibrillation may be suspected in any patient with complete heart block who is subject to syncopal attacks and whose heart rate at the time of emergence from the attack ranges from 80 to 110 per minute. A definitive diagnosis can be established by an electrocardiogram but can be immediately made by the use of a hand-held oscilloscope placed over the upper chest (Semler).

ELECTROCARDIOGRAM

The transition from ventricular tachycardia to ventricular flutter and fibrillation may be followed in the experimental animal and occasionally in man, particularly during Stokes-Adams seizures. The QRS complexes of ventricular tachycardia become widened and more aberrant until they appear as regular, continuous waves of large amplitude at a rate of 180 to 250 per minute. This stage is called ventricular flutter (Fig. 15–1). Except for the increased amplitude, they bear a striking resemblance to the waves of atrial flutter. The T waves and S-T segments cannot be differentiated from the QRS complexes. As these complexes become more aberrant and irregular in rhythm and form, ventricular fibrillation is said to be present. The stage between ventricular flutter and fibrillation may be called "impure ventricular flutter" (Fig. 15–2).

Ventricular fibrillation is character-

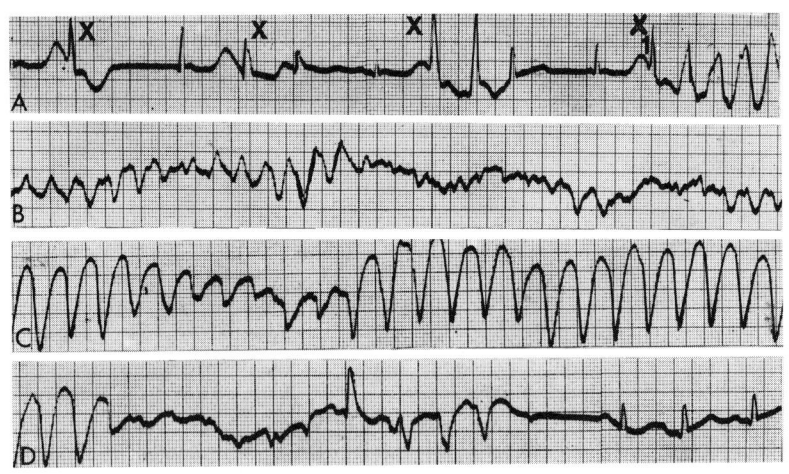

Figure 15–1. Shows onset and offset of ventricular flutter and ventricular fibrillation.

(A) Note presence of aberrant QRS complex at downstroke of T wave at X and presence of numerous idioventricular beats following the cycle with a long Q-T segment at X_1. Note that the premature beats follow close upon the peak of the T waves and that at X they initiate a paroxysm of ventricular flutter.

(B and C) Note changes from ventricular flutter to ventricular fibrillation.

(D) Note the resumption of normal sinus rhythm with normal Q-T length and absent U wave at the end of the strip.

VENTRICULAR FLUTTER AND FIBRILLATION

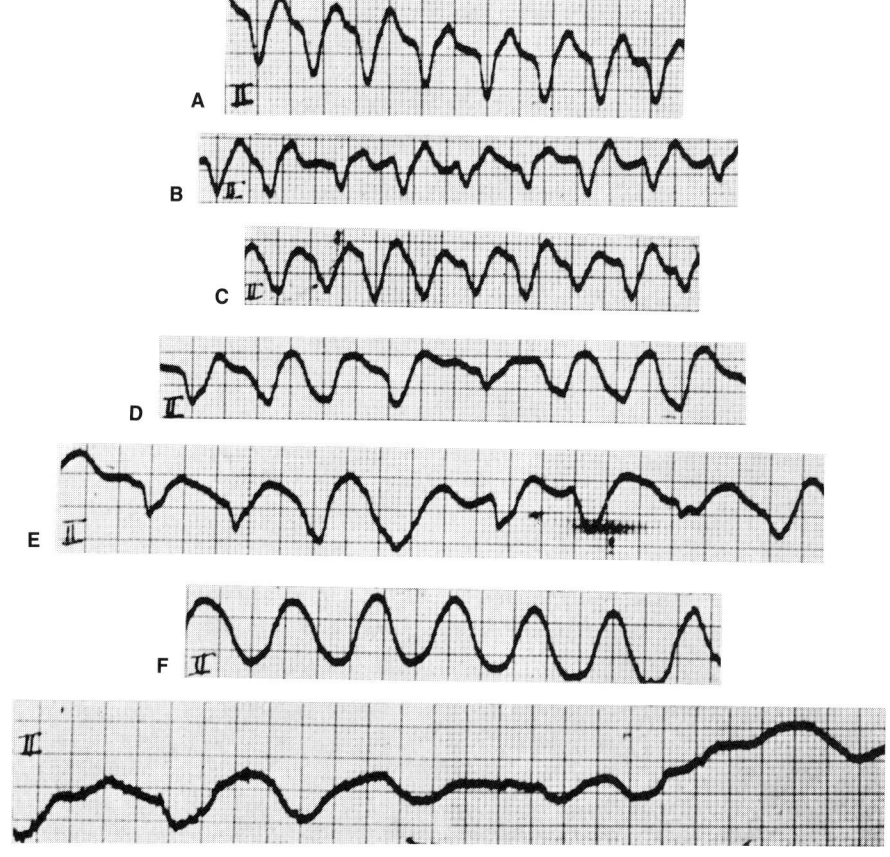

Figure 15–2. Transition of ventricular tachycardia to ventricular flutter and fibrillation following the administration of procaine amide (dying heart). (A to G represent a continuous strip of Lead II.) Patient, age 70, with arteriosclerotic heart disease was observed to be almost in extremis with a tachycardia (strip A) that was considered to be probably ventricular in origin. He was given 400 mg. of procaine amide intravenously in a period of about three to four minutes. This patient was one of the first in which this drug was used in our laboratory.

(B) Note the increase in aberration of the ventricular complexes.
(C) Increased widening of the ventricular complexes.
(D) Increase in abnormality, suggesting beginning of ventricular fibrillation.
(E) The irregularity is well marked and the ventricular complexes are more bizarre.
(F) This may be considered to be representative of ventricular flutter at a rate of 120 per minute.
(G) A slow and irregular ventricular rate of the dying heart.

ized by bizarre ventricular oscillations without a suggestion of a QRS or T wave; the waves are very coarse and irregular and range from 150 to 300 per minute. They are characterized by varying amplitude, contour, and spacing and, except for increased amplitude, resemble those of atrial fibrillation. The waves may be divided into several stages: (a) coarse fibrillation; (b) fine fibrillation in which the rate is higher; (c) a terminal stage, characterized by slow, extremely aberrant complexes.

TREATMENT

With the increased knowledge of the premonitory and initiating mechanisms and the increasing use of monitoring devices, the prevention of ventricular fibrillation assumes crucial importance. The active treatment of ventricular fibrillation depends on the setting in which ventricular fibrillation occurs, whether inside or outside of the hospital, and the immediacy of diagnosis and institution of therapy. It consists of cardiopulmonary resuscitation, direct-current countershock, and the use of certain drugs (see Chapter 38).

The result of treatment depends upon several factors: (a) the underlying disease state, (b) the incidence of complications, and (c) the rapidity with which treatment is begun (treatment must be started within four minutes of the onset of fibrillation). The training of paramedical personnel to promptly defibrillate subjects in special areas (e.g., factories, sports stadiums, and the like) and in mobile coronary care units will probably increase survival from unexpected ventricular fibrillation.

Prophylaxis entails prompt and vigorous efforts whenever any of the precipitating factors or premonitory arrhythmias discussed previously appear. Hypoxia, toxic drug effects, electrolyte disturbances, and the potentially dangerous premonitory arrhythmias — ventricular premature beats and ventricular tachycardia — should particularly be avoided or corrected. Thus, prophylactic measures for the prevention of ventricular fibrillation include a cautious approach to certain etiologic situations, particularly surgery, and the use of those drugs which raise the fibrillation threshold or abolish arrhythmias that may evolve into ventricular fibrillation.

During surgery, anesthetics that predispose to the development of ventricular fibrillation should be avoided, as well as all the other possible etiologic factors discussed earlier. An increased index of suspicion that serious ectopic rhythms might develop must be considered in the following subjects: (a) patients in the older age group, especially those undergoing prolonged operations; (b) those undergoing chest surgery, especially cardiac surgery; (c) those with advanced heart disease; (d) individuals with a past history of ectopic rhythms; (e) those with coronary artery disease; and (f) patients with any of the following electrocardiographic findings: W-P-W syndrome, A-V heart block, or bundle branch block.

Lidocaine increases the ventricular fibrillation threshold (VFT) to a substantial degree and is thus the drug of choice in treating the premonitory ventricular arrhythmias. It has been established that bretylium has an antifibrillatory action and reduces the incidence of ventricular fibrillation following electrical stimulation or coronary artery ligation (Bacaner, 1966). The dosage, routes of administration and side effects are discussed on p. 371. Propranolol is a beta-adrenergic blocking agent that has an antifibrillatory effect. It is uncertain whether this effect is due to its adrenergic blocking properties or to the direct actions of the drug, i.e., quinidine-like effect. The introduction of Practolol, a pure, beta-blocker without quinidine-like effects, may prove to be a better drug. Quinidine and procaine amide manifest only moderate efficacy in the prevention of ventricular fibrillation.

The active therapy once the arrhythmia is present is defibrillation. Successful external defibrillation requires application of the countershock within four minutes; this limitation can be met by the use of cardiac monitoring, which allows immediate recognition of cardiac arrest and identification of the arrhythmia.

PROGNOSIS

The prognosis depends on the underlying disease state of the heart, on the immediacy and efficacy of treatment of the fibrillatory episode, and on the severity of the patient's acute condition as manifested by heart failure or shock. Analysis of mortality rates suggests that the prognosis is poor for patients who had signs of cardiac decompensation prior to the occurrence of ventricular fibrillation. However, among patients without such signs, the expected long-term survival is about 85 per cent. This agrees with the 83 per cent long-term survival in the group studied by Lawrie et al. (1968). Of 23 patients from the working population, 14 have returned to work, including three to manual trades. These results emphasize that the occurrence of ventricular fibrillation during the acute stage of myocardial infarction does not necessarily influence the long-term prognosis, provided cardiac failure is not present.

References

Adgey, A. A. J., et al.: Management of ventricular fibrillation outside hospital. Lancet, *1*:1169, 1969.
Alexander, S., and Ping, W. C.: Fatal ventricular fibrillation during carotid stimulation. Amer. J. Cardiol., *18*:289, 1966.
Bacaner, M.: Bretylium tosylate for suppression of induced ventricular fibrillation. Amer. J. Cardiol., *17*:528, 1966.
Bellet, S., DeGuzman, N. T., Kostis, J. B., Roman, L., and Fleischmann, D.: The effect of cigarette smoke inhalation on VFT in normal dogs and dogs with acute myocardial infarction. Amer. Heart J., *83*:67, 1972.
Bellet, S., Roman, L., DeGuzman, N. T., Horstmann, E., and Kostis, J. B.: Effect of caffeine on the VFT in normal dogs and dogs with acute myocardial infarction (in press), 1971.
Briller, S. A.: Electrocution hazards. *In* Dreifus, L., and Likoff, W. (eds.): Mechanisms and Therapy of Cardiac Arrhythmias. New York, Grune & Stratton, 1966, p. 542.
Burgess, M. J., Abildskov, A., and Millar, K.: Early time course of fibrillation threshold in experimental coronary occlusion. Circulation, *41–42*:III–141, 1970.
Burn, J. H.: The cause of fibrillation. Can. Med. Assoc. J., *84*:625, 1961.
Chardack, W. M.: Fibrillation in empty and loaded ventricles. Arch. Surg., *93*:795, 1966.
Danese, C.: Pathogenesis of ventricular fibrillation in coronary occlusion: perfusion of coronary arteries with serum. JAMA, *179*:52, 1962.
Gerst, P. H., Fleming, W. H., and Malm, J. R.: Increased susceptibility of the heart to ventricular fibrillation during metabolic acidosis. Circ. Res., *19*:63, 1966.
Han, J.: Ventricular vulnerability during acute coronary occlusion. Amer. J. Cardiol., *24*:857, 1969.
Han, J., Garcia de Jalon, P. D., and Moe, G. K.: Adrenergic effects on ventricular vulnerability. Circ. Res., *14*:516, 1964.
Han, J., Malozzi, A. M., and Lyons, C.: Ventricular vulnerability to paired-pulse stimulation during acute coronary occlusion. Amer. Heart J., *73*:79, 1967.
Harris, A. S., Estandia, A., and Tillotson, R. F.: Ventricular ectopic rhythm and ventricular fibrillation following cardiac sympathectomy and coronary occlusion. Amer. J. Physiol., *165*:505, 1951.
Lawrie, D. M., et al.: Ventricular fibrillation complicating acute myocardial infarction. Lancet, *2*:523, 1968.
Lown, B., Kleiger, R., and Williams, J.: Cardioversion and digitalis drugs. Changed threshold to electric shock in digitalized animals. Circ. Res., *17*:519, 1965.
Maling, H. M., and Moran, N. C.: Ventricular arrhythmias induced by sympathomimetic amines in unanesthetized dogs following coronary artery occlusion. Circ. Res., *5*:409, 1957.
Palmer, D. G.: Interruption of T waves by premature QRS complexes and the relationship of this phenomenon to ventricular fibrillation. Amer. Heart J., *63*:367, 1962.
Pantridge, J. F., and Adgey, A. A. J.: Pre-hospital coronary care. The mobile coronary care unit. Amer. J. Cardiol., *24*:666, 1969.
Schaal, S. F., Wallace, A. G., and Sealy, W..C.: Protective influence of cardiac denervation against arrhythmias of myocardial infarction. Cardiov. Res., *3*:241, 1969.
Scherf, D.: The mechanism of flutter and fibrillation. Heart Bull., *16*:88, 1967.
Stern, T. N.: Paroxysmal ventricular fibrillation in the absence of other disease. Ann. Intern. Med., *47*:552, 1957.
Wolff, G. A., Veith, F., and Lown, B.: A vulnerable period for ventricular tachycardia following myocardial infarction. Cardiov. Res., *2*:111, 1968.

Chapter 16 *Cardiac Arrest*

GENERAL CONSIDERATIONS
TYPES OF CARDIAC ARREST
INCIDENCE AND ETIOLOGY
PATHOPHYSIOLOGY
DIAGNOSIS
   In the Operating Room
   Outside the Operating Room
TREATMENT OF CARDIAC ARREST
CARDIAC COMPLICATIONS
   Closed-Chest
   Open-Chest

CEREBRAL COMPLICATIONS OF
   CARDIAC ARREST
CRITERIA OF DEATH
PROGNOSIS FOLLOWING CARDIAC
   ARREST
   Cardiac Arrest in the Operating Room
   Resuscitation in the Coronary Care Unit
   Resuscitation Elsewhere in Hospital
   Results Outside Hospital
THE TERMINAL ELECTROCARDIOGRAM

GENERAL CONSIDERATIONS

The term "cardiac arrest" is usually used to mean clinical cessation of cardiac activity, causing sudden and often unexpected failure of effective circulation. Since respiratory failure is an important causative factor of cardiac arrest, and since it follows circulatory arrest within a matter of 20 to 30 seconds in any case, the more inclusive term "cardiopulmonary arrest" is preferable and is often employed (Jude, 1969).

The term "cardiac arrest" may be used in the literal sense meaning cessation of electrical activity of the heart as determined by the electrocardiogram. Clinically, the term is applied to the syndrome characterized by the cessation of purposeful cardiac activity with no peripheral blood pressure. This may be the result of ventricular fibrillation or cardiac arrest in various combinations and sequences. In this section the term is used in one or the other connotation, but cardiac arrest (absence of electrical activity) occupies a prominent role.

Cardiac arrest has become a topic of prime importance because of the recent development of effective resuscitation methods and the experience that the prompt institution of therapy may avert a fatal outcome. Cardiac arrest is frequently the terminal mechanism in desperately ill patients. However, in this discussion we are primarily concerned with its sudden appearance in less severely ill patients during the course of anesthesia or surgery, following certain clinical conditions, and under unexpected circumstances in apparently healthy subjects or in the presence of minimal cardiac abnormality.

TYPES OF CARDIAC ARREST

Cardiac arrest in the human may be divided into the following categories: (a) primary cardiac arrest, (b) cardiac arrest as part of general circulatory failure, (c) cardiac arrest secondary to or coincident with respiratory failure, and (d) induced cardiac arrest during cardiac surgery.

INCIDENCE AND ETIOLOGY

Cardiac arrest is most commonly encountered during surgery and as a result of serious heart disease, either acute or chronic. It may also occur under totally unpredictable circumstances.

The factors that predispose to cardiac arrest include: (a) pathologic states of the heart or cardiac dilatation; (b) acute conditions (e.g., severe chest trauma, overwhelming systemic infections, pulmonary embolism); (c) advanced age; (d) long-lasting nonphysiologic position of the patient; (e) hypoxia; (f) acute myocardial infarction; (g) electrolyte disturbances, particularly hyperpotassemia and hypocalcemia; (h) hypercapnea; (i) vagal reflexes; (j) drugs and anesthetic agents; (k) electric shock; (l) direct myocardial irritation; and (m) combinations of factors. Some cases of cardiac arrest occur without an apparent etiology.

In one study, the following etiologic factors were observed in 100 consecutive patients who developed cardiac arrest following admission to a medical intensive care unit: (a) myocardial infarction, 63 cases; (b) atherosclerotic, hypertensive, and valvular heart disease, 19 cases; (c) cerebrovascular disease, 4; (d) pulmonary embolism, 4; and (e) miscellaneous group, 10 (Linko et al., 1967).

Some of the important precipitating factors of unexpected cardiac arrest include: (a) Valsalva maneuver during defecation; (b) excitement or anxiety and severe mental stress in susceptible patients; (c) early ambulation after prolonged periods of bed rest accompanied by a vasodepressor or postural type of hypotension; (d) the development of ectopic rhythms (e.g., ventricular tachycardia, ventricular fibrillation, sinus arrest); (e) parasympathetic activity, from whatever cause (e.g., carotid sinus pressure), especially in the presence of hypoxia, hypercapnea, or hyperpotassemia, resulting in sudden depression of pacemaker activity with cardiac standstill or ventricular fibrillation; (f) the effect of drugs (e.g., digitalis, quinidine, procaine amide, potassium, and respiratory depressants); (g) hypoglycemia, leading to ectopic rhythms; and (h) convulsive seizures accompanying tetanus or epileptic forms of attack.

In addition, cardiac arrest may be precipitated unexpectedly during many therapeutic procedures. Cardiac arrest has been observed under the following circumstances: (a) during angiography; (b) during delivery and other gynecologic procedures; (c) following rectal examination in elderly patients; (d) during the rapid infusion of certain antiarrhythmic drugs; and (e) during urologic examination (i.e., urethral catheterization) (Stephenson, 1969). Cardiac arrest also occurs in victims of drowning and other catastrophic accidents.

PATHOPHYSIOLOGY

The greatest danger of cardiac arrest lies in the extremely limited time within which the circulation may be safely restored, owing to the poor tolerance of certain cells to hypoxia. Cardiac arrest and its resultant hypoxia must be corrected in three to four minutes if residual neurologic changes are to be avoided. Profound hypothermia may prolong this period considerably; however, this is rarely immediately available and is associated with hazards of its own (e.g., hypotension and ventricular fibrillation).

DIAGNOSIS

In the Operating Room. The diagnosis of cardiac arrest during cardiac or thoracic operations is easy because the heart is either exposed or available to palpation. It should be diagnosed during any operative procedure when there is sudden cessation of the pulse, inaudible heart sounds, an absent blood pressure, and the development of apnea. It may occur completely without warning, but in most instances there may be some premonitory signs, e.g., bradycardia, tachycardia, or premature beats (Fig. 16–1). Early detection of changes in cardiac rhythm is possible by use of a cathode ray oscilloscope or by continuous monitoring on tape.

Outside the Operating Room. The diagnosis of cardiac arrest outside the operating room is somewhat more difficult. It should be suspected if heart sounds are absent and the blood pressure is unobtainable or if respirations have ceased. These episodes of unexpected cardiac arrest are often preceded by a convulsive seizure.

When a patient has no audible heart beat and an absent pulse, the diagnosis of cardiac arrest is usually made. However, studies with continuous electrocardiography show that the cardiac mechanisms may be those of cardiac arrest, ventricular fibrillation, or a slow idioventricular rhythm. Recently, such studies in 132 critically ill patients who were continually monitored before and at the time of mechanical cardiac arrest showed ventricular fibrillation in 56 instances (43 per cent) and ventricular standstill in 76 instances (57 per cent) (Camarata et al., 1970). In such instances, it is often suggested that the patient be defibrillated if no electrocardiographic records are available because time is of the essence.

Recently, Semler et al. (1970) have developed an instant cardiac sensor to record the electrocardiogram in less than three seconds. This consists of a portable, battery-operated oscilloscopic type instrument which is placed over the sternum without need of electrodes, paste, or patient preparation. This instrument by itself records the rhythm on an oscillating needle, and if time permits, it may be connected with an oscilloscope or an elec-

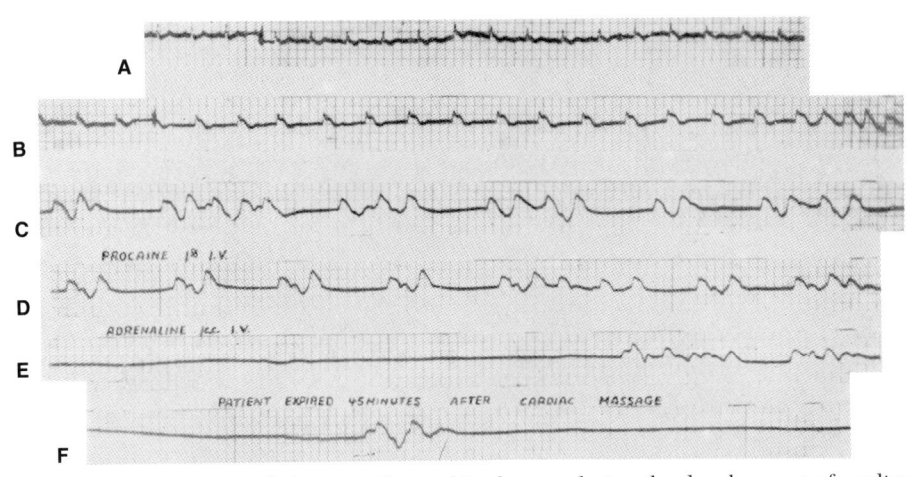

Figure 16–1. Evolution of electrocardiographic changes during the development of cardiac arrest at operation (continuous Lead II).
(A) Taken prior to the beginning of cardiac arrest. Soon after the beginning of this strip, note the inversion of T waves followed by slight elevation of the S-T segment at the end of the strip.
(B) Shows increasing elevation of the S-T segment associated with atrial standstill. The ventricular rate increases toward the end of the strip.
(C) Note the increasing aberration of the ventricular complexes and irregularity of the ventricular rate.
(D) Further aberration of ventricular beats following administration of procaine amide.
(E) Long periods of standstill with beginning ventricular fibrillation (after epinephrine).
(F) Long pause, two ventricular beats, and cardiac standstill.

trocardiograph. Differentiation of ventricular fibrillation from asystole can be made instantly. This would obviate the application of the defibrillator to patients with asystole or slow idioventricular rhythm.

Since one has relatively little time in which to resuscitate the heart, therapy should be started immediately.

The outline of therapy for closed-chest cardiopulmonary resuscitation is discussed in Table 16-1. (See also Fig. 16-2.)

TREATMENT OF CARDIAC ARREST

Cardiac arrest is a medical emergency for which effective treatment needs to be instituted within three to four minutes of onset in order to prevent permanent cerebral damage. Several developments, particularly the effective techniques for closed chest cardiac compression, the capacitor discharge defibrillator, and efficient pacing devices, have advanced treatment so that many patients may recover completely.

Because cardiac arrest may occur at any time, it is imperative that nurses, physicians, and other hospital personnel be taught the technique of treating cardiac arrest early in their training. This is the area in which the greatest advances can and must be made. A planned regimen is necessary, and instruments should be placed strategically. Although it may not fit every case, an orderly regimen should be prepared that will be suitable for most cases.

CARDIAC COMPLICATIONS

Closed-Chest. As many as half of the patients in whom closed-chest resuscitation is performed suffer some form of injury associated with this procedure. Rib fractures are most com-

Table 16–1. **PROCEDURE OF CLOSED CHEST CARDIOPULMONARY RESUSCITATION**

1. *Diagnosis*
   a. Made on physical findings
   b. DO NOT DELAY INITIATION OF RESUSCITATION TO OBTAIN ECG
2. *Call for Assistance:* note exact time
3. *Deliver a Direct and Vigorous Thump to Precordium*
4. *Ventilation*
   a. Check for and maintain an open airway
   b. Give artificial ventilation. DO NOT USE ENDOTRACHEAL TUBE AT THIS POINT DUE TO VAGAL REFLEXES AND THE TIME CONSUMED IN THE PROCEDURE
   c. If alone, ventilate five or six times and then begin cardiac compression; after each 15 compressions, ventilate twice
   d. When the anesthesiologist arrives, he continues artificial ventilation or assisted respiration by whichever technique is indicated
5. *External Cardiac Compression*
   a. Place patient on a *firm surface*
   b. Maintain a rate of 60 compressions per minute
   c. Carotid pulse should be used to monitor the efficacy of the compression
6. *Drug Therapy:* (Once effective cardiorespiratory assistance has been established, drugs may be used to treat circulatory collapse)
   a. Open and maintain route(s) for rapid administration of drugs
   b. Agents to increase myocardial contractility
      1. Epinephrine
      2. Isoproterenol
      3. Norepinephrine
      4. Metaraminol
   c. Agents to reverse acidosis and increase ventricular beating
      1. Sodium bicarbonate
      2. Calcium gluconate
7. *Definitive Treatment*
   a. Administer a cardioactive drug (See 6b)
   b. Establish electrocardiographic diagnosis (by ecg or Semler technique, p. 216)
      1. Beware of artefacts of precordial compression
      2. Asystole requires pacing (external or transvenous) (see Chapter 37)
      3. Fibrillation requires defibrillation (see Chapter 38)
8. *Maintain Postresuscitative Care*
   a. Prevention of recurrence of cardiac arrest
   b. Maintenance of circulation
   c. Prevention of CNS damage

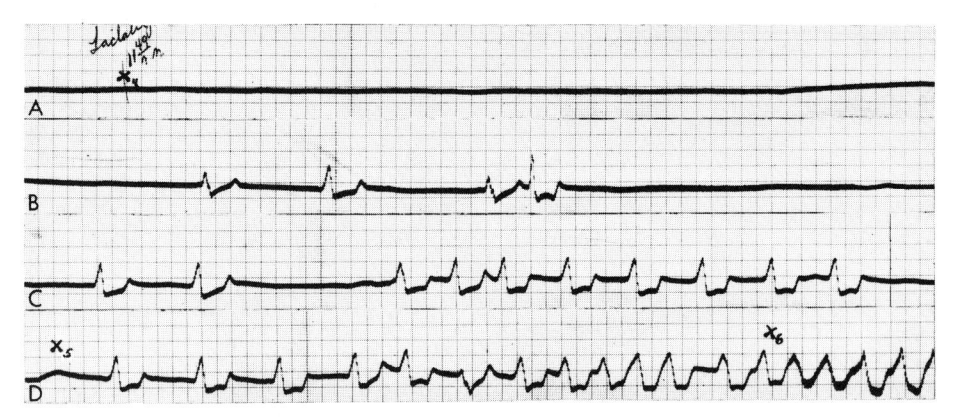

Figure 16-2. Patient, 73 years, manifesting terminal episodes of cardiac arrest. Following the infusion of molar sodium lactate, note resumption of idioventricular beats in B, which become more frequent in C and D. The rate increases in D although the complexes are bizarre. Although the electrocardiogram shows evidence of ventricular oscillations, the heart was in standstill at this time and showed only minute fibrillary twitchings. It should be emphasized that the presence of electrocardiogram deflections even of a relatively normal contour does not necessarily coincide with an effective ventricular contraction; they may be observed in the presence of cardiac standstill.

mon. Sternal fractures occur with a roughly equal frequency. Fat emboli from bone marrow have been observed to occur in about 10 per cent of patients resuscitated (Baringer et al., 1961). More serious complications include trauma to the liver (which occurs in roughly 2 per cent of patients and, less commonly, trauma to the spleen, inferior vena cava, and aorta (Nelson and Ashley, 1965; Paaske et al., 1968). Although complications are common, they generally do not have great significance. It has been estimated that 1 per cent of patients resuscitated in this manner showed serious complications that could have in themselves resulted in death (Paaske et al., 1968). While these should be kept in mind, this consideration should in no way restrict therapy.

Open-Chest. The complications of open-chest cardiac resuscitation are (a) direct trauma to the heart; and (b) the operative risk involved in thoracotomy. Rupture or lacerations of the myocardium, pericardial tamponade, herniation of the heart, and epicardial hemorrhage have been reported (Stephenson, 1969).

CEREBRAL COMPLICATIONS OF CARDIAC ARREST

Brain damage due to thrombosis of cerebral vessels and brain damage due to hypoxia and subsequent disturbances in cerebral metabolism may occur after either method of resuscitation. The residual deficit may consist of loss of recent memory, inability to relearn, emotional lability, and intellectual impairment with loss of integrative ability. In one series of 552 patients resuscitated by the closed-chest method, 11 subjects demonstrated irreversible cerebral damage. In most of these subjects, the damage could be explained as caused by either delayed treatment or advanced age (Johnson et al., 1967).

Cardiac arrest is followed by various alterations in the mental and emotional state. Many patients demonstrate a mild to severe organic brain syndrome following resuscitation, which usually clears with the passage of time (Druss and Kornfeld, 1967). Serious cerebral complications have been estimated to occur in roughly 2 per cent of patients who are resuscitated successfully.

CRITERIA OF DEATH

Recent advances, particularly in the field of cardiac transplantation, have raised the question of what signs constitute definitive evidence of death. Several criteria have been proposed, particularly the combination of certain signs referable to the absence of central nervous system function—complete unresponsiveness to external stimuli, total absence of spontaneous movements, and total absence of reflexes for 24 hours. An isoelectric electroencephalogram cannot be interpreted with certainty and therefore is not a good criterion of death if the patient has ingested drugs such as barbiturates or is being treated by hypothermia. The aforementioned criteria are obviously far more rigorous than those commonly employed in the presence of cardiac arrest, since the signs of hypoxic cerebral damage discussed previously indicate a grave prognosis even in the presence of activity in the EEG. However, when cerebral activity has been specifically depressed, as by an overdose of barbiturates, a flat EEG should not be considered evidence of cerebral death, since full mental recovery may occur.

PROGNOSIS FOLLOWING CARDIAC ARREST

The clinical diagnosis of cardiac arrest includes patients in whom the electrocardiogram demonstrates ventricular fibrillation as well as true arrest or asystole. In fact, most instances of acute arrest probably begin as ventricular fibrillation and progress to asystole with the passage of time. When asystole has supervened before resuscitation begins, the chance of successful resuscitation is much diminished (Adgey et al., 1969). If, however, asystole is the initial mechanism, resuscitation may be successful in an appreciable proportion of patients—the reports ranging from 2 to 15 per cent (Hollingsworth, 1969; Stephenson, 1969). Long-term prognosis has been investigated when arrest occurs in the following situations:

Cardiac Arrest in the Operating Room. Recent experience indicates that resuscitation may be successful in as many as 75 per cent of patients who experience cardiac arrest during surgery (Jude, 1969). If, however, the cardiac arrest occurs as a result of myocardial infarction during surgery, the prognosis is poor. The patient may be operated upon again with no apparent increase in risk. If possible, however, the etiologic factors in the initial cardiac arrest should be avoided at the second operation.

Resuscitation in the Coronary Care Unit. The prognosis following resuscitation in the coronary care unit is discussed in more detail on page 306. Reports of 20 to 40 per cent survival have been reported for patients in whom arrest did not occur in the operating room (Flynn and Fox, 1967). The principal function of the coronary care unit now should be in prevention of cardiac arrest as well as the prompt resuscitation of the patient who has already suffered arrest.

Resuscitation Elsewhere in Hospital. When resuscitation is begun efficiently within the first four minutes following the onset of cardiac arrest, the success rate in obtaining immediate recovery and the long-term prognosis for these patients may be good but are not comparable to those obtained in the coronary care units. Delay in the institution of therapy often occurs, with disastrous results.

Results Outside Hospital. These are considered in some detail under Mobile Coronary Care Units, page 307.

THE TERMINAL ELECTROCARDIOGRAM

The common pathophysiologic feature of terminal arrhythmias is the reduction of hemodynamic performance below that which is essential to provide adequate blood flow to the essential organs, especially the brain and the heart itself. In addition to ventricular fibrillation and asystole, disturbances of rhythm that cause inadequate blood flow consist of: (1) severe tachyarrhythmias, especially ventricular tachycardia; and (2) severe bradyarrhythmias, especially those with transient brief periods of ventricular asystole. Although death or at least neurologic dysfunction becomes inevitable after, at most, four minutes of total circulatory collapse, the period of circulatory arrest that can be tolerated is markedly reduced in individuals with severe pre-existing cardiac derangement.

The terminal mechanism is not easily determined unless one fortuitously has an electrocardiographic recorder connected to the patient at that time. Its elucidation has been facilitated by the use of continuous electrocardiographic monitoring.

The terminal cardiac mechanism depends principally upon whether: (1) the arrhythmia occurs suddenly in an individual whose cardiac function has been at least minimally adequate or occurs at the termination of a progressively worsening cardiac derangement; (2) the subject had pre-existing conduction defects predisposing to ventricular asystole; (3) cardiovascular collapse is to some degree secondary to respiratory or peripheral vascular failure; and (4) the electrocardiogram is obtained promptly or is recorded after a period of delay.

Ventricular fibrillation or ventricular asystole are the usual terminal mechanisms in most instances of sudden circulatory arrest. However, when death occurs slowly over a period of minutes or hours, the following sequence of events is frequently observed: (1) sinus slowing, leading to atrial standstill; (2) slow A-V junctional rhythm; (3) idioventricular rhythm with ventricular premature beats and occasionally ventricular tachycardia terminating in ventricular fibrillation, and finally ventricular standstill; or (4) with a slow idioventricular rhythm the ventricular complex becomes more aberrant and widened, and the terminal mechanism is that of ventricular standstill (see Fig. 37–15).

References

Adelson, L.: A clinicopathologic study of the anatomic changes in the heart resulting from cardiac massage. Surg., Gynec., Obstet., 104:513, 1957.

Adgey, A. A. J., et al.: Management of ventricular fibrillation outside hospital. Lancet, 1:1169, 1969.

Ad Hoc Committee on Cardiopulmonary Resuscitation of the Division of Medical Sciences, National Academy of Sciences, National Research Council: Cardiopulmonary resuscitation. JAMA, 198:372, 1966.

American College of Cardiology, Conference Report: Training techniques for the coronary care unit. Amer. J. Cardiol., 17:736, 1966.

American College of Cardiology, Sixth Bethesda Conference: Early care for the acute coronary suspect. Amer. J. Cardiol., 23:603, 1969.

Baringer, J. R., Salzman, E. W., Jones, W. A., and Friedlich, A. L.: External cardiac massage. New Eng. J. Med., 265:62, 1961.

Bellet, S., and Wasserman, F.: Indications and contraindications for the use of molar sodium lactate. Circulation, 15:591, 1957.

Birch, L.: The need for training, retraining, and testing trainees in cardiopulmonary resuscitation. In Gordon, A. S. (ed.): Cardiopulmonary Resuscitation: Conference Proceedings. Washington, D.C., National Research Council, 1967.

Camarata, S., Weil, M. H., Shubin, H., and Hanashiro, P. K.: Hemodynamic documentation of cardiac arrest in 132 patients. Amer. J. Cardiol., 26:627, 1970 (Abst.).

Druss, R. G., and Kornfeld, D. S.: Survivors of cardiac arrest. JAMA, 201:291, 1967.

Editorial: Complications of cardiac massage. Brit. Med. J., 1:68, 1969.

Editorial: EEG signs of death. Brit. Med. J., 2:318, 1968.

Elain, J. O.: Principles and practice of cardiopulmonary resuscitation. In Gordon, A. S. (ed.): Cardiopulmonary Resuscitation: Conference Proceedings. Washington, D.C., National Research Council, 1967.

Flynn, R. L., and Fox, S. M.: Coronary care unit programs in the United States. Israel J. and Sci., 3:279, 1967.

Guzman, S. V., DeLeon, A. C., Jr., West, J. W., and Bellet, S.: Cardiac effects of isoproterenol, norepinephrine, and epinephrine in complete A-V heart block during experimental acidosis and hyperkalemia. Circ. Res., 7:666, 1959.

Hollingsworth, J. H.: The results of cardiopulmonary resuscitation: A 3-year university hospital experience. Ann. Intern. Med., 71:459, 1969.

Johnson, A. L., Tanser, P. H., Ulan, R. A., and Wood, T. E.: Results of cardiac resuscitation in 552 patients. Amer. J. Cardiol., 20:831, 1967.

Jude, J. R.: Cardiopulmonary arrest and resuscitation. In Gibbon, J. H., Jr., Sabiston, D. C., Jr., and Spencer, F. C. (eds.): Surgery of the Chest. Philadelphia, W. B. Saunders, 1969.

Killip, T., III, and Kimball, J. T.: Treatment of myocardial infarction in a coronary care unit. A two year experience with 250 patients. Amer. J. Cardiol., 20:457, 1967.

Linko, E., Koskinen, P. J., Siitonen, L., and Ruosteenoja, R.: Resuscitation in cardiac arrest. An analysis of 100 successive medical cases. Acta Med. Scand., 182:611, 1967.

Medical Tribune: Electrocerebral silence 24 hours is held proof. May 12, 1969.

Nelson, D. A., and Ashley, P. F.: Rupture of the aorta during closed-chest cardiac massage. JAMA, 193:681, 1965.

Paaske, F., Hansen, J. P. H., Koudahl, G., and Olsen, J.: Complications of closed-chest cardiac massage in a forensic autopsy material. Dan. Med. Bull., 15:225, 1968.

Ruth, H., Bukley, M. L., and Keown, K.: Cardiac asystole. JAMA, 164:831, 1957.

Semler, H. J., Lauer, K. E., and Smith, L. D.: Stat—electrocardiography in cardiac arrest. Amer. J. Cardiol., 26:668, 1970 (Abst.).

Seppala, K., and Yli-Uotila, R.: Cardiac arrest. Resuscitation results. Acta Med. Scand., 181:385, 1967.

Stephenson, H. E.: Cardiac Arrest and Resuscitation. Ed. 3. St. Louis, C. V. Mosby, 1969.

Chapter 17 *Alternation of the Heart*

GENERAL CONSIDERATIONS
ETIOLOGY AND CLINICAL
  SIGNIFICANCE
TYPES OF ALTERNATION
  Electrical Alternation
  Alternation in the Various Phases of the Electrocardiogram
MECHANISMS INVOLVED IN
  ALTERNATION
  Partial Asystole

Hyposystole
Supernormal Strong Beat
Anatomic Rotation Hypothesis
Alternation in Single Fibers
CLINICAL FEATURES
DIAGNOSIS
  Differential Diagnosis
THERAPY
PROGNOSIS

GENERAL CONSIDERATIONS

The term alternation, as originally used, indicated an alternation in the force or strength of the pulse in the presence of a regular cardiac rhythm, arising usually in a normal pacemaker. At present, this term has a broader connotation, suggesting alternation of the heart as a whole or of any of its chambers.

ETIOLOGY AND CLINICAL SIGNIFICANCE

The diagnosis of "alternation of the heart" is of considerable clinical and prognostic importance. Its presence usually indicates the existence of myocardial damage, often of a severe grade, and usually suggests a poor prognosis. This state, as far as the author knows, has not been encountered in a normal heart except under conditions of stress, i.e., a rapid heart rate. The portion of the heart that is the seat of disease or under strain is mirrored by the type of alternation observed.

The following conditions will produce the common type of alternation (pulsus alternans) involving the left ventricle: coronary artery disease, coronary occlusion, aortic insufficiency, aortic stenosis, hypertension, myocarditis, congestive failure, digitalis toxicity, and pericardial disease. The following conditions tend to produce alternation involving particularly the right ventricle: pulmonary hypertension incident to pulmonary disease, congenital heart disease, and any other condition causing right ventricular strain.

TYPES OF ALTERNATION

The following types of alternation may be observed: (1) Mechanical alternation, which may involve the left or right ventricle, or left or right atrium. This is manifested by alternation in the strength of contraction of the chambers and may be associated with alternation in the intensity of heart sounds. (2) Electrical alternation, which may involve any portion of the electrocardiogram: the P wave, P-R interval, QRS complexes, Q-T interval, or the T wave. Electrical alternation may occur independently of, or in association with, mechanical alternation. (3) Combination of mechanical and electrical alternation.

Electrical Alternation. Electrical alternation of the amplitude or contour of the various phases of the electrocardiogram includes alternation not only of the QRS complexes, but of the P waves, P-R interval, or U waves. Alternation of the T wave with or without QRS changes is the most frequent type (Fig. 17–1).

Electrical alternation has, in general, the same significance as mechanical alternation. The differential diagnosis of electrical alternation includes the following: bigeminal pulse, which can be differentiated by the type of irregularity (premature beats); the effects of respiration, which produce variation in voltage that do not occur in regular alternating cycles; bidirectional complexes as observed in junctional tachycardia; and alternating bundle branch block.

Alternation in the Various Phases of the Electrocardiogram. Clinically, alternation may also be manifested in any of the components of the electrocardiogram. Alternation of the P wave has been observed in electrocardiographic tracings taken directly from the atria during cardiac catheterization in both the experimental animal and in the human subject. An analogous phenomenon, alternation of the intraventricular conduction, has also been observed previously in cases of intermittent bundle branch block (Langendorf, 1958). Alternation in the amplitude of the R wave is not present equally in all leads; it may be observed in precordial leads when it is not present in limb leads; marked alternation may also be observed in intracardiac leads, although only slight alternation may appear in standard electrocardiographic leads. In two infants with pulsus alternans, Bertrand et al. (1959) found that, although only very slight electrical alternation could be seen in the standard electrocardiographic leads, marked alternation was present in the R waves of intracardiac leads.

Alternation of the T wave with or without the QRS is the most frequent type observed. A case of postextrasystolic U wave alternans that most likely was due to depletion of potassium has been reported (Mullican and Fisch, 1964).

MECHANISMS INVOLVED IN ALTERNATION

Various differing theories have been proposed to explain the mechanisms involved in alternation. Some of these follow:

Partial Asystole. The theory most accepted at the present time is that of Gaskell (1882) and Hering (1913). These authors concluded, as the result of animal experiments, that in alternation, portions of the heart muscle possess a lowered excitability and can respond only to every second impulse, while the remaining tissue responds to every impulse. Thus the alternation is the result of fewer fibers participating in the ventricular contraction

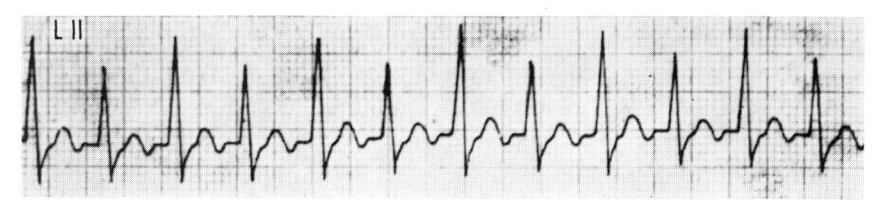

Figure 17–1. Electrical alternans (Lead II). Note the alternation in amplitude of the QRS complexes in a patient with atrial tachycardia. The rate is 160 per minute.

during the weak beat, followed by a full contraction of all fibers with the strong beat. Recently, as a result of His bundle electrogram recordings, it has been suggested that alternation may be associated with changes in A-V and intraventricular conduction. Alternation may result from rhythmic conduction disturbances which cause effective contractions to alternate with ineffective contractions; this may be produced by partial bundle branch block. Since the recovery period is shorter following functional blockade, it is reasonable to postulate that blockade may cause a weakened pulse, and the subsequent impulse finds the conduction system fully recovered and thus causes a normal contraction.

Hyposystole. The theory of hyposystole was first suggested by Wenckebach (1901). After premature beats, the first sinus beat following the compensatory pause puts out a greater volume of blood than the normal beat, leaving a decreased residual volume for the next beat. The decreased initial volume is then increased and a large beat follows. Repetition of this sequence results in alternation of the ventricular contraction. Whether this is due to alternation in the amount of residual blood present in the heart, to an alternation in the strength of the ventricular contraction, or to a combination of both factors, has been a matter of controversy (Fig. 17-2).

Supernormal Strong Beat. Pulsus alternans may better be regarded as a coupling of weak and supernormal beats instead of a coupling of weak and normal contractions. The mechanism for the production of this supernormal beat is still open to question.

Anatomic Rotation Hypothesis. Certain mechanical phenomena, such as alternating intensity of the pericardial friction rub, pulsus alternans, and the alternation of heart murmurs, are occasionally observed and may coincide with the mechanical rotation of the heart, thereby altering the relation of the heart to the chest wall.

Alternation in Single Fibers. The following types of electrical alternation have been produced in single ventricular fibers by means of triiodothyronine, thyroxine, and acute anoxia: alternation in (a) the rate of depolarization, (b) the rate of repolarization, (c) the magnitude of the action potential, and (d) hyperpolarization.

CLINICAL FEATURES

Alternation may be observed at normal, slow, or fast heart rates. The type seen with a slow heart rate is usually associated with a serious myocardial abnormality. When observed with a rapid heart rate, e.g., paroxysmal atrial tachycardia, the prognosis may not be serious, since the alternation usually disappears as the heart rate slows. It may appear after exercise, indicating an inability of the heart to respond normally to effort, or it may occur with congestive failure. The phenomenon is diminished or even abolished by recumbency, exercise, digitalis, norepinephrine, transfusion of blood, and the application of external vascular support (McIntosh, 1960).

Although the cycle length in alternation varies little, slight differences occasionally may be noted in alternate beats. Strong beats are followed by shorter cycles, and the weak beats, by longer cycles, the differences being usually about 0.01 to 0.03 second in duration. At very rapid heart rates, slight alternation in cycle length may contribute to the development or increased severity of the mechanical alternation (Friedman, 1956).

DIAGNOSIS

The presence of alternation should be suspected in those patients with a condition predisposing to or manifest-

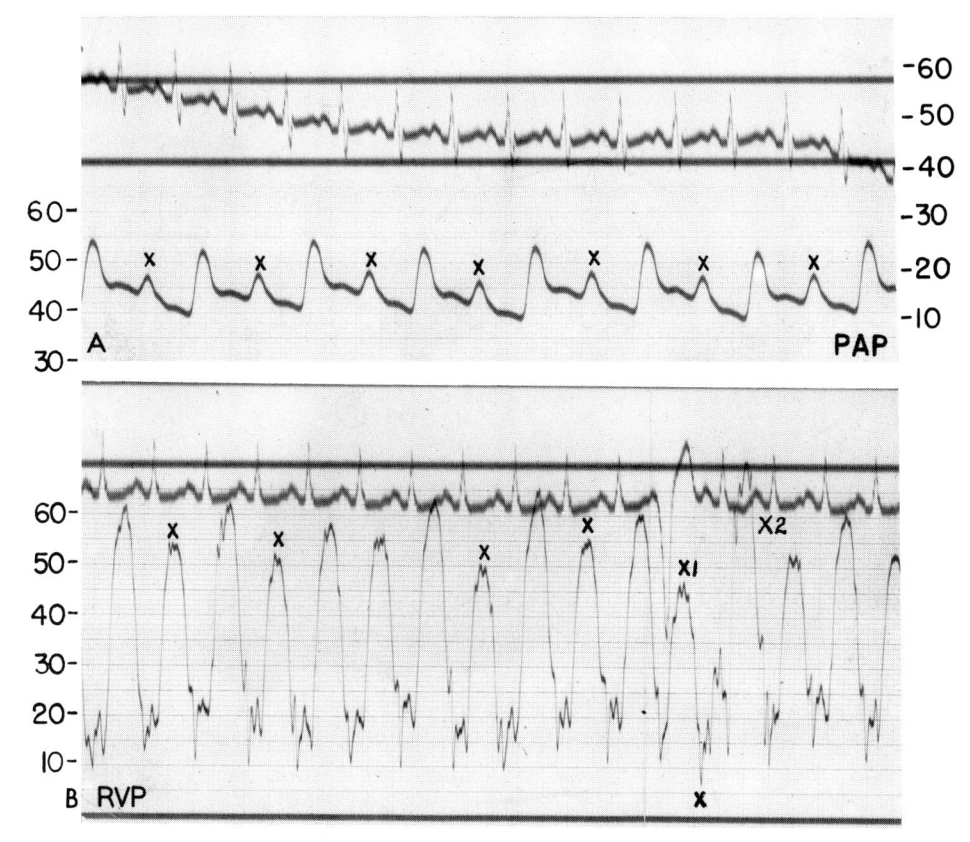

Figure 17-2. Alternation of right ventricular pressure curve. Taken from a patient 48 years of age with muscular dystrophy.

(A) Pulmonary artery pressure. (The ventricular rate is 136 per minute.) Note the alternation in the amplitude of the pulmonary artery pressure curve. The pressure in the high amplitude waves measures 55 mm. and the lower amplitude waves measure 48 mm.

(B) Right ventricular pressure. Note the alternation in the amplitude of the ventricular beats. The pressure in the high amplitude beats is 62 mm. and in the low amplitude beats 57 mm. at X.

Note the fall in pressure with the premature beat at X_1 and the increase in amplitude of the pressure curve in the following beat (X_2).

ing evidence of left ventricular strain (e.g., coronary occlusion, coronary artery disease, hypertension, aortic insufficiency or stenosis, the presence of a rapid ectopic rhythm). Pulsus alternans may be induced in susceptible individuals by the use of certain stress mechanisms. In subjects with myocardial abnormality (exertional dyspnea, nocturnal dyspnea, coronary artery disease), pulsus alternans has been induced by atrial pacing (rate 110/minute) (Cheng, 1971).

The following procedures may be used in establishing the diagnosis of alternation of the heart: (1) Palpation of the pulse may reveal alternate strong and weak beats in a patient with a regular rhythm; (2) Alternation in the intensity of heart sounds may be detected by auscultation or by graphic recording (Fig. 17-3); (3) Alternation may also be detected by intracardiac phonocardiography and blood pressure tracings (Fig. 17-2); (4) Electrical alternation may be observed in the electrocardiogram. It is important that the precordial as well as the limb leads be taken since alterna-

226   ALTERNATION OF THE HEART

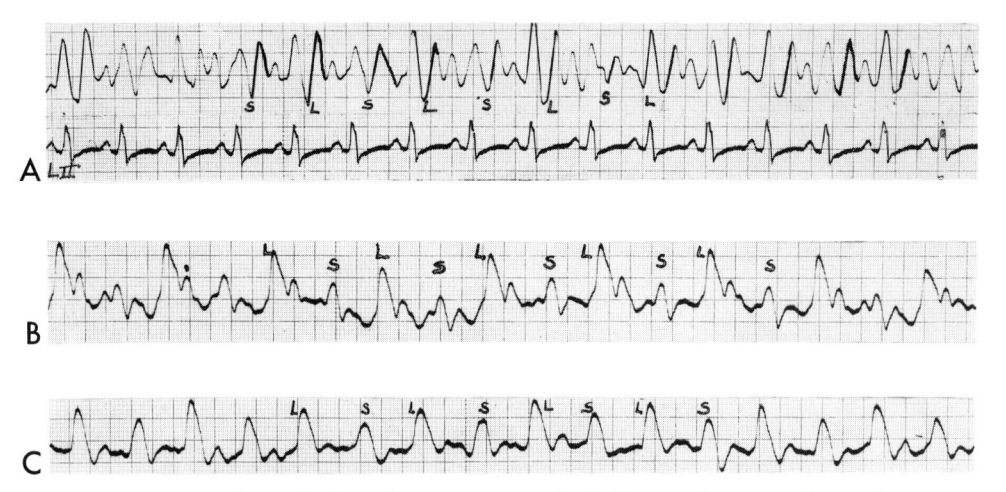

Figure 17-3. Mechanical pulsus alternans seen on the ballistocardiogram and on pulse tracings. The patient is a 45-year-old man with previous hypertension and a myocardial infarction.

(A) Simultaneous ballistocardiogram and electrocardiogram. Note the definite tendency for the amplitude of I-J (dark lines) to alternate. (Small I-J waves are marked S, and larger, L.) This cannot be attributed to respiratory variation, but is a manifestation of pulsus alternans.

(B) Pulsus alternans seen in the carotid artery record.

(C) Pulsus alternans seen in the femoral pulse record. Note the alternation of small cycles (S) and large cycles (L).

tion may be missed in some leads (Figs. 17-1, 17-4).

Differential Diagnosis. Pseudoalternation may involve the following conditions: (a) coupled rhythm, which results in alternating strong and weak beats and may be differentiated from true alternation by the irregularity of rhythm in the former; (b) pseudoalternation, alternation of 3:1 and 2:1 or other combinations of A-V heart block that may appear in alternate cycles, may be easily differentiated with the electrocardiogram; (c) the changes produced in systolic pressure by respiration, especially when the respiratory rate is about one-half the

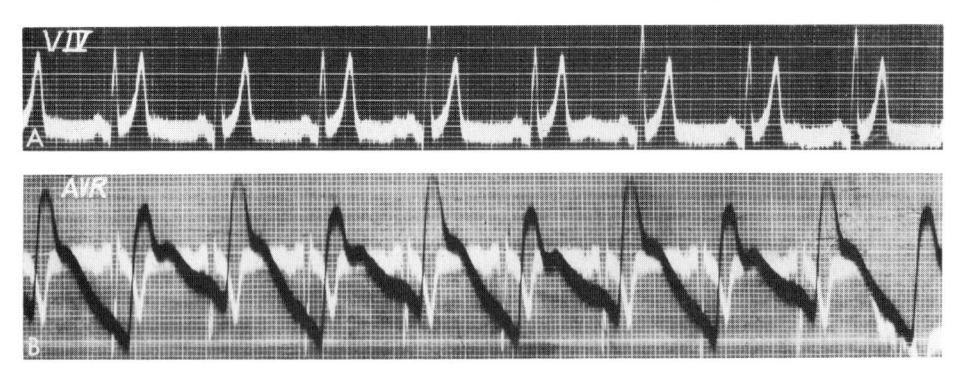

Figure 17-4. Electrical and mechanical alternation in the same patient.

(A) (V$_4$) From a patient during the early stages of acute myocardial infarction. Note the extremely tall T waves often observed in the acute stage. There is an alternation of the amplitude of the R waves. This alternation was not observed in the limb leads.

(B) Brachial pulse taken simultaneously with aVR. Note the alternation in the amplitude of the pulse waves. The evidence of electrical alternation is less evident in this lead.

heart rate, may be revealed by temporarily controlling the respiratory rate; (d) a dicrotic pulse palpated at the wrist is often confusing; pulsus alternans may be ruled out by the fact that the pulse rate would be twice the apical heart rate; (e) alternation of the "a" wave of the jugular pulse may be due to factors other than alternation of the atrium, e.g, right ventricular alternation, especially in the presence of tricuspid insufficiency, or 2:1 A-V heart block with every other atrial contraction occurring against a closed tricuspid valve; and (f) alternation of normal sinus beats and premature beats.

THERAPY

There is no specific therapy for alternation itself; the therapy is that of the underlying disease or abnormality.

Certain drugs, however, are effective in the abolition of alternation. The reversion of pulsus alternans to a normal series of mechanical contractions has been observed by the action of mephentermine (Oppenheimer et al., 1957). Mephentermine acts by increasing conduction velocity; it shortens the refractory period and A-V conduction time and thus tends to abolish the conditions producing the alternation. Other more commonly used drugs may also abolish alternation by improving cardiac function.

PROGNOSIS

From the prognostic standpoint, patients with alternation may be divided into two groups, namely, those with a rapid ventricular rate, i.e., paroxysmal tachycardia, and those with a slow heart rate. In the first group, the alternation usually results from cardiac strain incident to the rapid rate and disappears when the rate returns to normal. These hearts are not necessarily severely diseased, and the prognosis may not be serious. In the second group, where the alternation occurs with a slow heart rate, the hearts are usually seriously damaged and the prognosis is usually poor. In such instances, life expectancy is usually about one to two years, even if at the time of onset of the pulsus alternans there is no other evidence of sufficiently severe disease to warrant such a grave prognosis.

References

Badeer, H. S., et al.: Factors affecting pulsus alternans in the rapidly driven heart and papillary muscle. Amer. J. Physiol., 213:1095, 1967.

Bertrand, C. A., Zohman, L. R., and Williams, M. H.: Intracardiac electrocardiography in man. Amer. J. Med., 26:534, 1959.

Cheng, T. O.: Atrial pacing: Its diagnostic and therapeutic applications. Prog. Cardiov. Dis., 14:230, 1971.

Chung, K. Y., Walsh, T. J., and Massie, E.: Electrical alternans: A report of 12 cases. Amer. J. Med. Sci., 248:220, 1964.

Cohen, S. I., Lau, S. H., Berkowitz, W. D., and Damato, A. N.: Alternating patterns of ventricular excitation during alternate induced atrial premature beats ("alternation"). Circulation, 39–40:III–60, 1969.

Cohn, K. E., Sandler, H., and Hancock, E. W.: Mechanisms of pulsus alternans. Circulation, 36:372, 1967.

Cossio, P., Lascalea, M., and Fongi, E. G.: Alternation of the heart sounds. Arch. Intern. Med., 58:812, 1936.

DeRabago, P., Kohout, F. W., and Katz, L. N.: An unusual case of pulsus alternans recorded during cardiac catheterization from the pulmonary and systemic blood vessels. Amer. Heart J., 49:472, 1955.

Feldman, L.: Electrical alternans with pericardial effusion. Amer. Heart J., 15:100, 1938.

Friedman, B.: Alternation of cycle length in pulsus alternans. Amer. Heart J., 51:701, 1956.

Gaskell, W. H.: Rhythm of heart of frog and nature of action of vagus nerve. Phil. Trans. Roy. Soc., 173:993, 1882.

Hering, H. E.: Zur-Erklarung des Herzalternans. Z. exp. Path. Therap., 12:325, 1913.

Kleinfeld, M., and Stein, E.: Electrical alternans of components of action potential. Amer. Heart J., 75:528, 1968.

Langendorf, R.: Alternation of A-V conduction time. Amer. Heart J., 55:181, 1958.

McIntosh, H. D.: Discordant pulsus alternans. Circulation, 21:214, 1960.

Morris, R. S.: Clinical notes of pulsus alternans. JAMA, 87:463, 1926.

Mullican, W. S., and Fisch, C.: Postextrasystolic alternans of the U wave due to hypokalemia. Amer. Heart J., 68:383, 1964.

Oppenheimer, M. J., Lynch, P. R., and Ascanio, G.: Action of mephentermine on arrhythmias due to pulsus alternans rapidly discharging single atrial foci and prolonged P-R intervals. Amer. J. Physiol., 191:481, 1957.

Segers, M.: The alternans of A-V conduction time. Arch. Mal. Coeur, 44:525, 1951.

Spodick, D. H., and St. Pierre, J. R.: Pulsus alternans: physiologic study by non-invasive techniques. Amer. Heart J., 80:766, 1970.

Wenckebach, K. F.: Zur Analyse des unregelmassigen Pulsus. IV. Ueber den Pulsus Alternans. Z. klin. Med., 44:218, 1901.

Chapter 18 — Methods Employed in ECG Diagnosis of an Arrhythmia

METHODS OF DIAGNOSIS
  P Waves
  P-R Interval
  QRS Complex
  T-Wave
CONDITIONS SIMULATING
  ARRHYTHMIAS

Electrocardiogram
LONG-TERM MONITORING
  Contourography
COMPUTERS
  Uses in Arrhythmia Detection

An arrhythmia may be suspected when there is a rate above 120 or below 40 beats per minute even with a regular rhythm or when there is any irregularity of the rhythm, an alteration in the shape of P waves or QRS complexes, or a variation in the relation between the P wave and the QRS complex.

If an arrhythmia is present, a general survey of records should be made to determine the following: the presence of the dominant rhythm (e.g., normal sinus rhythm, atrial tachycardia, atrial flutter). Subsidiary rhythms (e.g., premature beats, A-V block) should also be ascertained. Long strips should be taken from several leads, especially one in which QRS and P waves are best shown (the latter are usually best recorded with V_3R). In some cases, certain maneuvers and techniques may be employed to help elucidate the underlying cardiac mechanism. These include exercise, atrial pacing, carotid sinus pressure, breath-holding, administration of atropine, and other methods discussed in this chapter. In the electrocardiographic diagnosis, the use of calipers and a magnifying glass may be of help.

METHODS OF DIAGNOSIS

The atrial and ventricular rate should be determined, and any irregularity should be noted.

P Waves. (1) If P waves are present, determine whether they are normal or abnormal (e.g., inverted or altered in form as compared to the normal or dominant rhythm). (2) Note if the atrial rate is normal or slow or rapid and if the rhythm is regular. (3) If the atrial rhythm is regular, is the rapid rate a simple multiple of the slow rate? (4) Other factors to be considered are: (a) Is the P wave always followed by a QRS complex? (b) Are P waves and QRS complexes unrelated? (c) If related, is the P-R interval constant? (d) Is the irregularity phasic; is it related to the phases of respiration? (e) Do the P waves vary in contour?

P waves may be absent in mid A-V junctional rhythm or atrial standstill (see Fig. 11–1). Moreover, the P waves may be obscured by superimposition on the T wave or the terminal portion of the QRS complex (see Fig. 18–1). The constancy of the P-R or R-P intervals should be determined. P waves

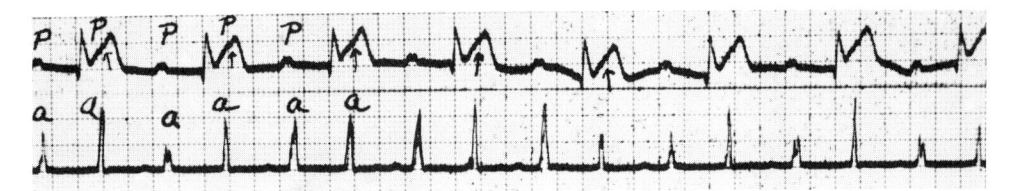

Figure 18-1. Second degree A-V heart block. Tracings from a 53-year-old man with acute inferior infarction. The original electrocardiographic diagnosis was first degree A-V heart block. The Doppler tracing shows large "a" waves with a rate double that of the QRS. Careful inspection shows slight notching in the T wave due to a superimposed P wave (at arrow). The ventricular components of the Doppler tracing have been eliminated by a change in the direction of the ultrasound beams.

may be replaced by flutter (F or P waves) or fibrillation (f waves) (see Chapters 6 and 7). It is important to note that P waves may at times be confused with U waves or artifacts (see Fig. 18-2).

The buried P wave presents a particular problem. The methods of determining the atrial mechanism at slow or fast rates when the P waves are not clearly shown are: (1) recording of leads V_3R, II, or III; (2) recording esophageal (Fig. 18-3) or right intra-atrial leads taken simultaneously with another lead, e.g., V_3R; (3) carotid sinus pressure; (4) exercise; (5) administration of atropine in the presence of slow rates; (6) recording from intra-atrial electrode (Fig. 18-4); and (7) recording a Doppler "amplitude tracing" simultaneously with the electrocardiogram (Figs. 18-1, 18-5, 18-6).

P-R Interval. In examining the P-R interval, which is measured from the beginning of the P wave to the beginning of the QRS complex, one must decide whether it is normal, prolonged, or shortened (accelerated conduction or pre-excitation syndrome). It should also be noted whether the P-R interval is constant or if there is a progressive lengthening from beat to beat. If the P wave progressively approaches closer to the QRS complex, in some cycles it may be hidden within the QRS, e.g., as in A-V dissociation.

As discussed previously, the P-R interval contains many electrical events that are not apparent on the scalar electrocardiogram (see Fig. 2-5). This electrical activity can be recorded with His bundle electrography, a new technique that has recently been introduced (Damato et al., 1969; Scherlag et al., 1970). The His bundle recording is of value in (1) differentiating complex junctional, retrograde, and reciprocal rhythms; (2) establishing the site of block in the A-V junction; and (3) the diagnosis of aberration (ventricular or supraventricular origin of a tachyarrhythmia) (see Chapter 11). Moreover, in cases of A-V heart block, His bundle electrography is occasionally useful in the evaluation of therapy and prognosis.

QRS Complex. When studying the QRS complex, the rate and the rhythm (regular or irregular) should be noted. Is the ventricular rate normal, slow, or rapid; is it identical to the atrial rate? Is it slower or more rapid than the atrial rate? If the rhythm of the QRS complexes is irregular, the cause should be sought; such irregularity may be due to sinus arrhythmia, sinoatrial block, atrial fibrillation, A-V dissociation, junctional escape, or atrial, junctional, or ventricular tachycardia. The diagnostic features of atrial, junctional, and ventricular tachycardia have been discussed under their respective chapters. The characteristic morphology of the QRS complex, whether normal, narrow, or widened, must be determined. Is the abnormal complex due

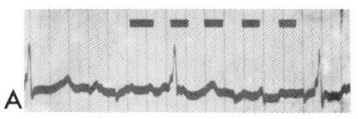

Figure 18-2. Artifacts.

(A) Loose electrode plus the effect of the lead marker produced movements in the baseline which simulate and may be mistaken for atrial activity.

(B) Loose electrode producing oscillations simulating multiple ventricular premature contractions.

(C) Wandering baseline due to patient coughing.

(D) Wandering baseline (due to patient moving his hands) which renders visualization of individual P and T waves difficult.

(E) Electrical interference (60 cycle) due to improper grounding and loose connection gives wandering baseline.

(F) (Patient's) tremor gives rise to a fuzzy baseline and obscures T and P waves.

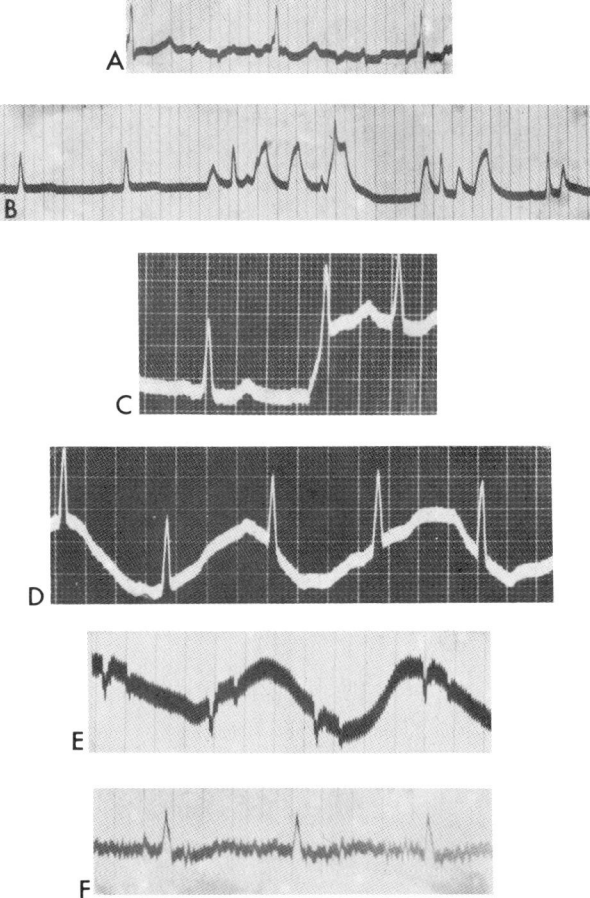

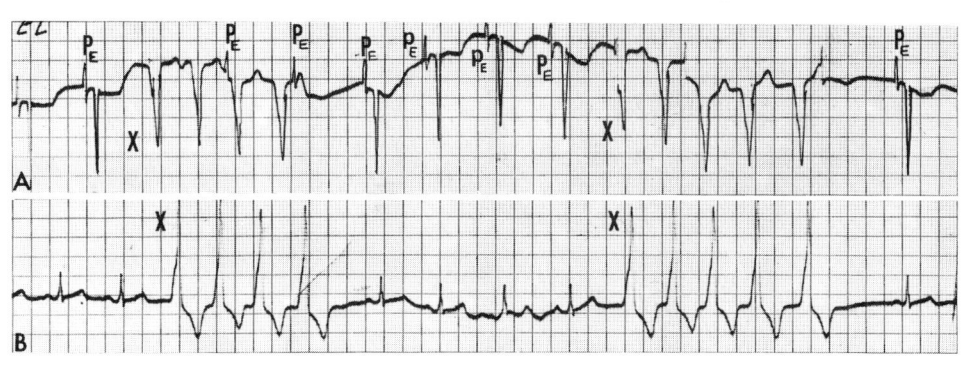

Figure 18-3. Shows ventricular tachycardia in lead II taken simultaneously with esophageal leads. Note that the atrial beats (P_E) occur regularly at a slower rate (84/minute) than that during the periods of ventricular tachycardia (140/minute).

(A) (Esophageal lead) note the P waves (P_E) with a normal P-R interval of 0.16 second in the normal beats. In the aberrant beats the ventricular rate is 140 per minute and the atrial rate is 84 per minute. Note the series of four complexes of the ventricular tachycardia occurring regularly at X at the initial and at the terminal part of the strip.

(B) (Lead II) Shows the typical normal complexes with a paroxysm of ventricular tachycardia at X in the initial part and at the terminal part of the strip. The rate is identical to that shown above with the esophageal leads. However, the P waves are not shown in lead II but are clearly delineated in the esophageal leads, thus helping to establish a diagnosis of ventricular tachycardia.

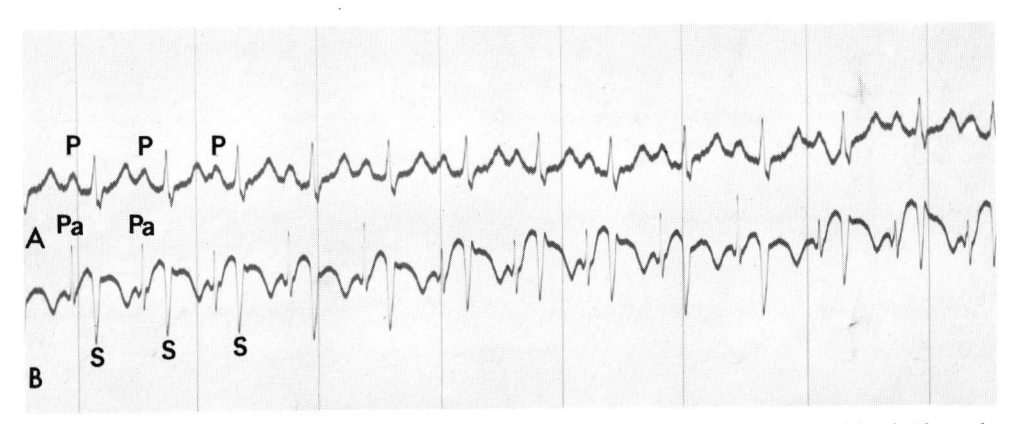

232   METHODS EMPLOYED IN ECG DIAGNOSIS OF AN ARRHYTHMIA

Figure 18-4. Electrocardiogram, lead II taken simultaneously with a right atrial lead. The right atrial lead is taken through a platinum tip electrode catheter positioned in the right atrium. Note the normal P wave and P-R intervals in the top tracing (A). In the intra-atrial electrocardiogram (B), note the atrial deflection consisting of a sharp, upward spike followed by a smaller downward deflection (Pa), whereas the QRS complex is defined by a QS type of deflection. This method helps to delineate the P waves more clearly than in the usual electrocardiogram.

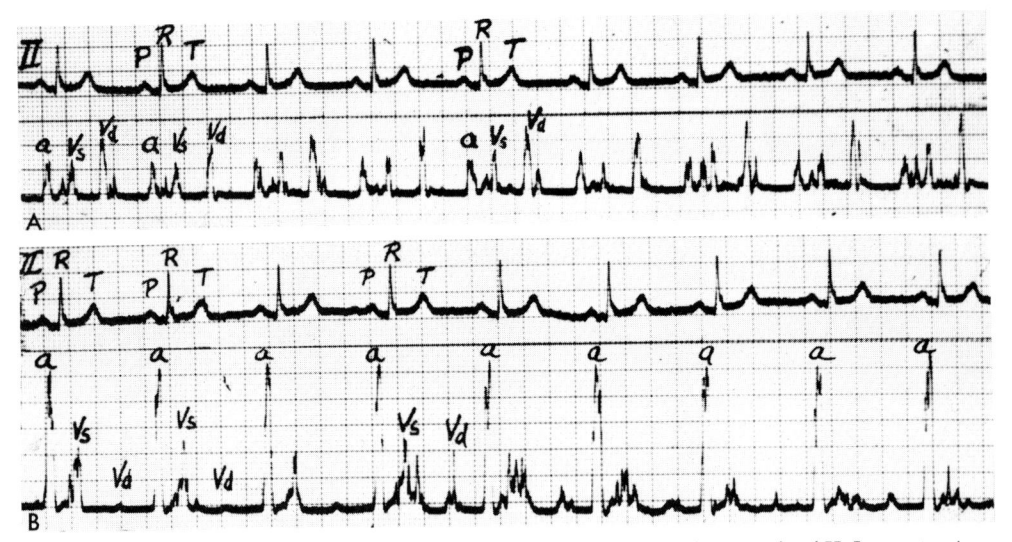

Figure 18-5. (A) *Normal sinus rhythm.* Upper tracing: electrocardiogram, lead II. Lower tracing: Doppler tracing taken at the fourth right intercostal space close to the sternum. Note the components of the Doppler tracing ("a," "v_s," and "v_d") and their relationship to the P, QRS, and T waves of the electrocardiogram.

(B) Tracings taken on the same patient as A. The patient has been placed in the right lateral decubitus position. Note the increased amplitude of the atrial component ("a") of the Doppler tracing.

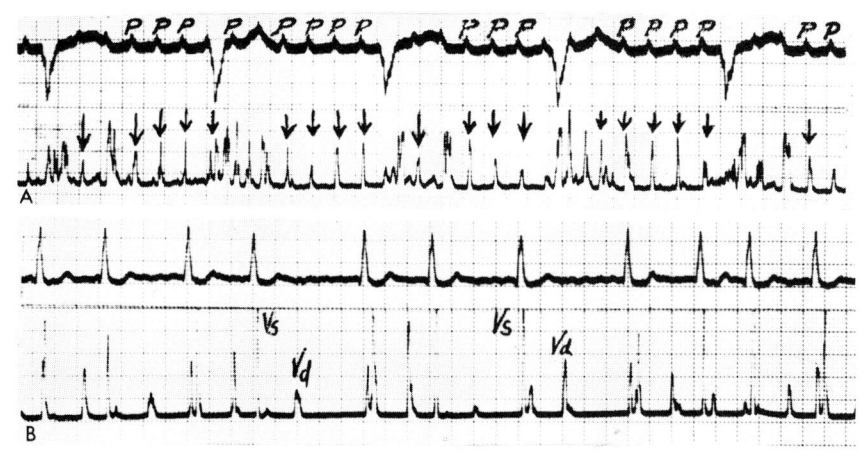

Figure 18-6. (A) Atrial flutter. Tracing from a man, 70 years of age, with arteriosclerotic heart disease and congestive failure. The distance between the thick lines represents 0.2 second. The "a" wave (at arrows) on the Doppler tracing corresponds to the P waves of the electrocardiogram. Components "v_s" and "V_D" are also recognized.

(B) Atrial fibrillation. Tracing from a patient with hypertensive and arteriosclerotic heart disease and congestive failure. The Doppler tracing consists of deflections "v_s" and "v_d" only. The atrial component ("a") is absent.

to a premature beat, an idioventricular beat with a slow rate, an aberrant complex with a fast rate, or the presence of fusion beats?

If premature beats are present, one must determine (a) the site (atrial, junctional, or ventricular); (b) whether they are unifocal or multifocal; (c) whether they are coupled (fixed or not); (d) the presence of a parasystolic rhythm; (e) fusion beats, and (f) if the ectopic beats occur in groups.

T Wave. When observing the T waves, one should look for a long QT and prominent U waves. P waves may occur between QRS and T, on the peak of T, or superimposed on the descending limb of T. The T wave may be inverted after a ventricular premature beat. The configuration of the S-T segment may suggest digitalis effect. Q-T prolongation may suggest hypoxia or electrolyte imbalance.

The foregoing data will aid in determining: (a) the nature of the arrhythmia; (b) a possible etiologic factor (certain types of myocardial disease, electrolyte imbalance, drug effects, especially digitalis); (c) the nature of the atrial or ventricular mechanisms; and (d) the urgency of and the best approach to therapy.

CONDITIONS SIMULATING ARRHYTHMIAS

When examining a patient or an electrocardiogram, one must be aware that certain conditions which do not involve the heart may simulate arrhythmias. The conditions simulating cardiac arrhythmias may be divided into two categories: (1) subjective and (2) electrocardiographic. Subjective manifestations include symptoms of palpitation, rapid beating of the heart, sensation of the "heart turning over," and a sense of palpitation in the region of the epigastrium and lower part of the chest.

Electrocardiogram. The electrocardiographic records may simulate an arrhythmia under the following conditions: (a) tremor of various types, particularly that of Parkinson's disease (which may disappear from the electrocardiogram during sleep); (b) hiccough; (c) artifact in the machine, which may result in an extra stimulus at various periods of time; however, these stimuli do not have the characteristic configuration of the QRS complex; (d) poor electrocardiographic connection or temporary interruption of connection presenting the appearance of cardiac arrest on the electrocardiogram; (e) interference with other electrical apparatus; (f) connection from an outside person, as for example, while taking a precordial lead; in these instances, the electrocardiogram of the technician may be superimposed upon that of the patient; and (g) diaphragmatic flutter.

The electrocardiograph machine may produce several types of artifacts, either as a result of malfunction or improper adjustment. Furthermore, a shifting baseline may make interpretation impossible especially when only a short tracing is available for analysis. Loose electrodes may simulate many types of arrhythmias (Fig. 18–2). Premature beats and extra atrial activity are particularly simulated by movement of a loose or improperly applied electrode.

Disturbances in diaphragmatic motility can be divided into two groups: (1) clonic contractions (hiccough, diaphragmatic flutter), and (2) tonic contractions (as seen in tetany, tetanus, rabies, strychnine poisoning). Diaphragmatic flutter (Figs. 18–2, 18–7) is usually distinguished from persistent hiccough by the higher frequency of the diaphragmatic contractions and by the absence of the inspiratory sound (due to insufficient or nonsynchronous opening of the glottis) which is observed in the former.

Clinically, the synchronous form of diaphragmatic flutter may present a problem in differential diagnosis, although auscultation will usually establish its extracardiac origin. The mechanism of synchronous diaphragmatic flutter is unknown, but the following theories have been postulated: (a) the current of ventricular depolarization actually stimulates the left phrenic nerve; (b) the baroreceptors in the carotid sinus, aortic arch, and cardiac chambers may abnormally connect with phrenic nuclei, explaining why alteration in heart rate would lead to identical alteration in the rate of diaphragmatic flutter; and (c) the patient demonstrating this entity has an abnormally increased number of preganglionic sympathetic fibers innervating the diaphragm.

Fluoroscopic examination of diaphragmatic movements is one of the most important methods for diagnosis. One may see rapid movement of one or both leaves of the diaphragm.

LONG-TERM MONITORING

Cardiac monitoring, the observation or recording of the electrocardiogram over long periods of time, has found widespread use in coronary care units, in general intensive care units, during surgery, and in the immediate postoperative period. This type of monitoring usually employs an oscillo-

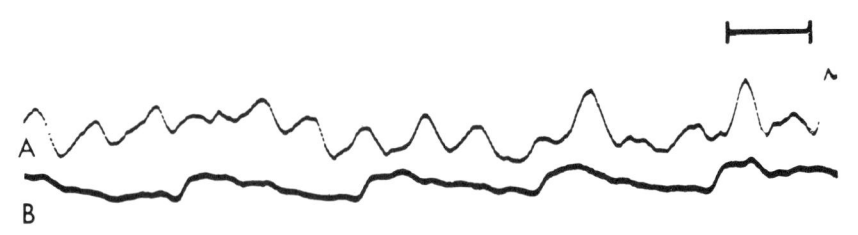

Figure 18–7. Tracings obtained during a paroxysm of diaphragmatic flutter. (A) Epigastric beats. (B) Apexcardiogram. (From Rigatto, M., and De Medeiros, N. P.: Amer. J. Med., 32:103, 1962.)

A   B

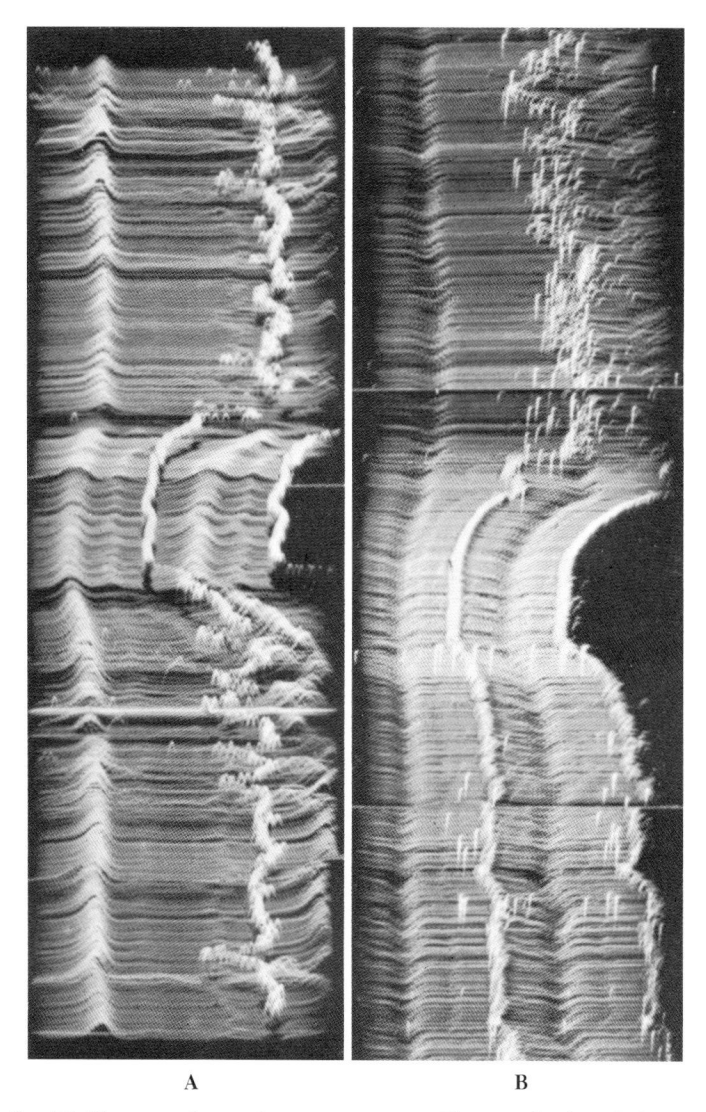

Figure 18-8. (A) Electrocardiographic contourogram. This is a display of electrocardiograms for a ten-minute period, from top to bottom, showing reaction to rest, exercise and again rest. The horizontal scale is linear with time in the cardiac cycle with each sweep starting at a specific epoch, an R wave, and continuing for two cardiac cycles. The vertical scale is linear with time during the study combined with the amplitude of the electrocardiogram. The intensity is a function of the electrocardiographic amplitude.

(B) Contourogram with derivative emphasis. In addition to showing again three periods of rest, exercise and rest, this illustration emphasizes premature ventricular contractions by adding to the intensity modulation signal used in A, the first time derivative of the electrocardiogram. The bright vertical lines are thus produced by the PVCs. (From Webb, G. N.: Bull. Johns Hopkins Hosp., *116*:211, 1965.)

scope by which visual observation is available; it often also entails the permanent brief recording (two minutes or less) during periods of alarm and during rapid or slow rates and irregular rhythms. This method of monitoring should be distinguished from the type that includes continuous recording on tape over long periods (6 to 24 hours).

The most important purpose of long-term monitoring is the detection of arrhythmias during various times of the day and night and their association with selective activities of the subject. Continuous electrocardiographic observation can be used to determine the cause of syncopal attacks, fainting episodes, dizziness, and precordial pain. It is used in monitoring astronauts, pilots, automobile drivers, and scuba divers; and it can be employed to record the electrocardiogram of patients performing various tasks under various types of stress, including exercise.

The radioelectrocardiograph is particularly useful in studying the cardiac effects *during* exercise, inasmuch as previously only postexercise effects could be observed (Bellet et al., 1961; 1962). The electrocardiographic tracing is not materially altered by this technique (see Fig. 20-3). The progressive electrocardiographic changes occurring during exercise or normal daily activity may be monitored and a more complete approach to a patient's cardiac status may be made.

The Holter technique has also provided considerable information relative to arrhythmias and other electrocardiographic changes occurring during various daily activities (e.g., certain stressful situations — physical and emotional).

Contourography. In evaluating a patient's progress over a long period of time (12 to 24 hours), contourography, a method of organizing and compressing physiologic data in order to simplify visual evaluation, may be helpful (see Fig. 18-8). The contourogram is produced by the organization and display of repetitive events (e.g., electrocardiographic cycles) by means of an oscilloscope.

COMPUTERS

The computer has been increasingly employed in electrocardiographic diagnosis; however, its use in the diagnosis and recording of arrhythmias represents a new phase of this development.

Uses in Arrhythmia Detection. Continuous monitoring of each patient by a nurse or physician using conventional electrocardiographic equipment is too costly in time and personnel to be feasible. Monitoring the heart rate by simple equipment which can sound an alarm for bradycardia or tachycardia is not specific enough to be truly a great aid in avoiding or recognizing promptly specific arrhythmias. Therefore, several types of monitoring and diagnosing equipment have been developed: (1) the simplest type of equipment is the small hybrid computer combining analog and digital circuitry. This monitor recognizes only the QRS complex and measures the QRS duration and R-R interval. The use of this type of monitor is predicated on the fact that beats originating from an abnormal ventricular focus produce widened QRS complexes, thus detecting the most important disturbances leading to ventricular tachycardia or fibrillation. (2) More sophisticated monitors have been developed which diagnose premature ventricular beats, premature atrial beats, bigeminy, trigeminy, multifocal premature ventricular contractions, and ventricular tachycardia as well as ventricular asystole. These monitors, however, do not recognize P waves. In one study, the premature atrial contractions, premature ventricular contractions, bradycardia, and tachycardia were recognized with a reliability of 95 per cent and bundle branch block and sinus arrhythmias with 80 per cent reliability. (3) More advanced monitoring systems, now under development, are able to analyze P waves as well as QRS complexes; however, for these systems a large-scale digital computer is necessary.

There are still many difficulties with the electronic interpretation of the electrocardiogram and more particularly in arrhythmia analysis. The P wave is difficult to analyze since it has an amplitude of 100 microvolts in most leads and the noise level is approximately half of that value; therefore the P wave may be evasive at times. It may be erroneously categorized as a QRS complex if it is peaked. In atrial fibrillation, atrial flutter, or junctional rhythms in which retrograde P waves may be superimposed on any portion of the cycle, the P waves may be even more difficult to distinguish. Furthermore, only 5 to 10 seconds of any one lead are sampled and thus complex arrhythmias usually detected with rhythm strips are missed.

The accuracy of a computer system is of extreme importance and the present systems are not as good as one might wish. Although in one series the computer was correct in 91 per cent of the tracings and only omitted in 7 per cent of the diagnosis in which it was present, it missed the diagnosis of bundle branch block in 12 per cent of cases and myocardial infarction in 7 per cent of the cases in which these were present. Moreover, the computer reported these two conditions twice as often as they were actually present (Pordy et al., 1967). At present, due to this high number of both false positives and false negatives, equivocal tracings should be re-evaluated by a cardiologist in order to prevent medicolegal complications.

Caceres and Hochberg (1970) have analyzed the correlation between physician and computer interpretations of electrocardiographic tracings and have presented recommendations for improving the latter. They emphasize that in many situations human interpreters disagree over criteria for certain diagnoses, and that although the computer makes errors, these are more easily defined and corrected.

The use of computers in clinical medicine has many implications and raises many problems. Equipment failure looms as an ever-present problem in the increasing use of automated systems in medicine. At present, there are no efficient data-reduction systems for economically and conveniently storing and retrieving all the data collected. With continuous monitoring of many parameters, undoubtedly a great deal of superfluous information will be generated. A major problem lies in the training of physicians in the use and acceptance of computer-aided monitoring in diagnosis.

Finally, the legal implications of who will be responsible for errors in processing activities and the possibility of wide dissemination of confidential material raise other problems. Since computers have not been widely used to date, many of the potential medicolegal problems have not yet been encountered. However, although the use of computers will subject physicians to greater legal exposure, it appears that computers may also reduce the risk of malpractice by aiding in patient care.

In spite of these problems, computer monitoring of arrhythmias appears to be an aid in the care of seriously ill patients, which may significantly decrease the death rate attributable to their presence. Although computer applications to arrhythmias are still in the formative stages, it is apparent that these systems will aid in monitoring and diagnosing the cardiac rhythm.

The present availability and economics of this technology make it primarily a tool of clinical investigation; however, developments in computer design and refinement of programming during the next decade may enable the widespread use of this technique.

Computers are now being used in the education of physicians and nurses. Programmed instruction controlled by computers enables students to progress at their own rate and allows branching and individualized programs of study in the recognition and therapy of arrhythmias.

References

Barnes, B. A.: Computer and clinical medicine. Postgrad. Med., 37:597, 1965.

Bellet, S., Deliyiannis, S., and Eliakim, M.: The electrocardiogram during exercise as recorded by radioelectrocardiography; comparison with the postexercise electrocardiogram (Master two-step test). Amer. J. Cardiol., 8:385, 1961.

Bellet, S., Eliakim, M., Deliyiannis, S., and LaVan, D.: Radioelectrocardiography during exercise in patients with angina pectoris. Circulation, 25:5, 1962.

Bellet, S., and Kostis, J.: Study of the cardiac arrhythmias by the ultrasonic Doppler method. Circulation, 38:721, 1968.

Bellet, S., Roman, L., Kostis, J., and Slater, A.: Continuous electrocardiographic monitoring during automobile driving. Studies in normal subjects and patients with coronary artery disease. Amer. J. Cardiol., 22:856, 1968.

Caceres, C. A., and Hochberg, H. M.: Performance of the computer and physician in the analysis of the electrocardiogram. Amer. Heart J., 79:439, 1970.

Damato, A. N., et al.: Study of atrioventricular conduction in man using electrode catheter recordings of His bundle activity. Circulation, 39:287, 1969.

El Sherif, N., El Ramly, Z., and Sorour, A. H.: Oesophageal electrocardiography in the study of cardiac arrhythmias. Brit. Heart J., 31:414, 1969.

Graber, A. L., and Sinclair-Smith, B. D.: Paroxysmal flutter of the diaphragm. Amer. J. Cardiol., 15:252, 1965.

Irons, G. W., Ginn, W. M., and Orgain, E. S.: Contribution of the platinum-tipped electrode catheter to the diagnosis of cardiac arrhythmias. Amer. J. Cardiol., 21:894, 1968.

Pordy, L., et al.: Computer analysis of the electrocardiogram: A joint project. J. Mt. Sinai Hosp., 24:69, 1967.

Rigatto, M., and DeMedeiros, N. P.: Diaphragmatic flutter: Report of a case and review of literature. Amer. J. Med., 32:103, 1962.

Riseman, J. E. F., and Sagall, E. L.: Diagnostic problems resulting from improper electrocardiographic technique. JAMA, 178:110, 1961.

Scherlag, B. J., Narula, O. S., Lister, J. W., and Samet, P.: Analysis of atrioventricular conduction by direct intracardiac recordings. Mt. Sinai J. Med., 37:266, 1970.

Slater, A., and Bellet, S.: An underwater temperature telemetry system. Med. Biol. Engineer., 7:633, 1969.

Switzer, J. L.: Unilateral paroxysmal diaphragmatic flutter: Response to quinidine. Gastroenterology, 31:79, 1956.

Yokoi, M., et al.: On-line computer diagnosis of arrhythmias on ECG using small scale digital computer system. Jap. Circ. J., 33:129, 1969.

Chapter 19 *Syncopal Attacks*

GENERAL CONSIDERATIONS
ETIOLOGIC FACTORS
CARDIAC CAUSES
   Primary Factors
   Reflex Factors
   Cardioauditory Syndrome
POSTURAL SYNCOPE
   Treatment

DIAGNOSIS OF ETIOLOGY OF
   SYNCOPAL ATTACKS
DIFFERENTIAL DIAGNOSIS
COMPLICATIONS OF FAINTING
PROGNOSIS

GENERAL CONSIDERATIONS

Dizziness and fainting, with or without convulsions, are common clinical manifestations of cardiovascular disease, but only recently have many of the causative factors been elucidated. Fainting, or syncope, refers to a transient phenomenon characterized by a brief loss of consciousness and is nearly always the result of cerebral hypoxia. Syncopal attacks or episodes of unconsciousness are not uncommon and may appear in normal subjects at one or more periods of their lives due to a variety of causes. In a group of 871 college students with an average age of 21.1 years, 47.1 per cent had experienced at least one episode of loss of consciousness (Williams and Allen, 1962). Of these, 74.3 per cent were caused by trauma to the head, intake of alcohol, pain, postural change, and infection, in that order. In older subjects the incidence is increased and other factors, especially cardiovascular, are frequently causative.

Syncopal attacks may be classified by their duration into three types: (a) slight grade, usually described by the patient as "dizzy spells," "giddiness," "faintness," "spots before the eyes," or "lightheadedness"; (b) mild grade, which is characterized by loss of consciousness for a few seconds; and (c) severe grade, characterized by syncopal episodes or convulsive seizures which usually occur when the cerebral hypoxia persists for 10 to 15 seconds.

ETIOLOGIC FACTORS

The unconscious episodes may be triggered by one or various combinations of the following: (a) cerebral vasoconstriction due to hypocapnea; (b) previous or concomitant exposure to increased gravitational force (G); (c) hypoglycemia; (d) hyperventilation; (e) ectopic rhythms; and (f) the use of certain drugs (digitalis, coronary and peripheral vasodilators, antihypertensive and tranquilizing agents). Anxiety, anger, and states associated with hypoxia may contribute to diminished cerebral activity. The removal of one or more of these factors might prevent the unconscious episode.

Certain arrhythmias result in a diminished cerebral blood flow. This tends to occur with slow heart rates, particularly when associated with hypotension; however, it may also occur in the presence of extremely rapid heart rates. It is a matter of general experience that ectopic rhythms may produce a reduction in the cerebral blood flow sufficient to cause cerebral ischemia. Hemiplegia has been observed immediately following tachyarrhythmias. This is even more apt to occur in the upright position and in the presence of pre-existing cerebral arteriosclerosis. I have observed instances in which rapid ectopic rhythms in subjects between 65 and 75 years of age resulted in the production of syncopal attacks, convulsive seizures, and psychotic episodes. These recurred during repeated episodes of tachycardia, followed by a remission with a return to a normal sinus rhythm. In experimental animals, frequent premature atrial beats have been found to cause a 7 per cent reduction of the internal carotid blood flow, while frequent premature ventricular beats cause an average reduction of 12 per cent (Corday and Irving, 1960). In addition, the average reduction in the cerebral blood flow during paroxysms of rapid supraventricular tachycardia is 14 per cent and atrial fibrillation caused an average reduction of 23 per cent in cerebral blood flow. As the ventricular rate rises to 180 per minute, the cerebral blood flow frequently increases; however, above this rate, the cardiac output decreases as does the cerebral blood flow. The greatest reduction in the internal carotid flow occurs when the ventricular rate exceeds 190 per minute; this reduction ranges between 40 and 75 per cent (Corday and Irving, 1960).

Recently, techniques have been devised to measure phasic coronary blood velocity in man by the use of a Doppler ultrasonic flowmeter catheter system (Benchimol et al., 1969, 1971). This data obtained relates closely to the blood flow. By this method, it has been shown that ventricular premature beats and ventricular tachycardia result in diminished forward blood flow and stroke output and that a reduced coronary blood flow contributes to the impaired ventricular performance during these arrhythmias (Benchimol and Desser, 1971). The altered central flow velocity events are closely paralleled by carotid blood flow as well as providing evidence for dysfunction of the organ supplied by these vessels during ventricular arrhythmias (Benchimol and Desser, 1971).

The various types of syncope may be classified under the following headings: (a) cerebral causes, (b) cardiac causes, (c) postural syncope, (d) fainting secondary to respiratory and pulmonary disorders, (e) psychogenic factors, and (f) general factors. The important etiologic factors are listed on page 239.

CARDIAC CAUSES

Disturbances in the heart per se are a most important cause of syncopal attacks. Approximately one-third of patients with syncope have evidence of either cardiac disease or a disorder of the heart beat. Unless surrounded by unmistakable evidence of its etiology, syncope should warrant a search for cardiac abnormalities, which may be either a causative or coexistent factor.

The cardiac causes of syncope will be discussed under the following headings: (1) *primary factors* — (a) disturbances in the S-A node (sinus pauses and cardiac standstill); (b) disturbances in the A-V node and bundle of His; (c) ectopic rhythm with rapid ventricular rate; (d) congenital heart disease; (e) coronary occlusion; (f) valvular lesions; (g) ball valve thrombosis in the left atrium; (h) cardiac tamponade; (i) dissecting aneurysm; and (2) *reflex factors*, leading to carotid sinus syncope.

Primary Factors. When the S-A node fails to function as the pacemaker, lower centers in the heart may then assume this role, usually the A-V junction or a lower ventricular center. If the sinus pauses are prolonged or if for some reason these centers fail to immediately assume the function of pacemaker, syncopal attacks may occur.

Cardioauditory Syndrome. Recently, the cardioauditory syndrome has been observed in a group of subjects who presented with marked QT prolongation and deafness with clinically normal hearts (Jervell and Lange-Nielsen, 1957). QT prolongation and deafness has also be observed in subjects with congenital heart disease. A third syndrome has been observed in children (Ward, 1964) and adults (Garza et al., 1969) who present the same phenomena but without deafness. These subjects show a marked susceptibility to the development of syncopal attacks due to the occurrence of episodes of ventricular tachycardia and ventricular fibrillation (Karhunen et al., 1970).

When disease exists in the A-V node and bundle of His, there are periods when the impulse from the atrium to ventricle is transmitted with difficulty and, at times, not at all. Sudden cessation of the heart beat may occur during the transition from partial to complete A-V heart block until the ventricular pacemaker assumes its role in initiating ventricular beating.

The sudden development of cardiac tamponade may alter cardiovascular dynamics by interfering with the inflow of blood into the right heart when the intrapericardial pressure exceeds the intra-atrial pressure. The decrease in the venous return results in a precipitous drop in the cardiac output and consequently in the cerebral blood flow. The most frequent causes of acute cardiac tamponade are rupture of the ventricle following myocardial infarction or a stab wound in the heart.

In addition, a dissecting aneurysm may produce syncopal attacks when it involves the arch of the aorta with encroachment upon the innominate and carotid arteries, thus leading to diminished cerebral blood flow and cerebral hypoxia.

Reflex Factors. Syncopal attacks may occur as a result of various reflex factors. The most thoroughly studied mechanism is that involving the parasympathetic effect, which travels by various afferent pathways and is mediated by the carotid sinus mechanism.

The carotid sinus syndrome is defined as the occurrence of cerebral ischemic symptoms precipitated by a hypersensitive carotid sinus reflex. It is characterized by episodes of dizziness or faintness, or periods of unconsciousness, which are usually brief but may be accompanied by convulsive seizures. These manifestations are not an uncommon cause of distressing and disabling symptoms in the middle-aged and elderly (Hutchinson and Stock, 1960). The diagnosis is established only if external stimulation of the affected sinus reproduces exactly, in whole or in part, the spontaneous symptoms of which the patient complains.

These cases may be divided into types according to the circulatory changes considered responsible for the attacks: (a) The cardioinhibitory type is due to cardiac inhibition resulting in abrupt slowing or standstill. These attacks may be prevented or abolished by sympathomimetic drugs or atropine; (b) the depressor type of carotid sinus syncope is attributed to peripheral vasodilatation accompanied by a slow heart rate and fall in blood pressure. Although the cardiodepressor type is much less common, recent studies have shown that it is not uncommon to see both varieties in the same patient.

The electrocardiogram during episodes of cardioinhibitory carotid sinus syncope may show the following mechanisms: (a) complete cardiac standstill; (b) marked ventricular slowing with a maintenance of atrial beats; (c) complete A-V heart block with slow ventricular rate of 10 to 20/min.; (d) sinus bradycardia with atrial standstill and episodes of ventricular escape; (e) associated ectopic

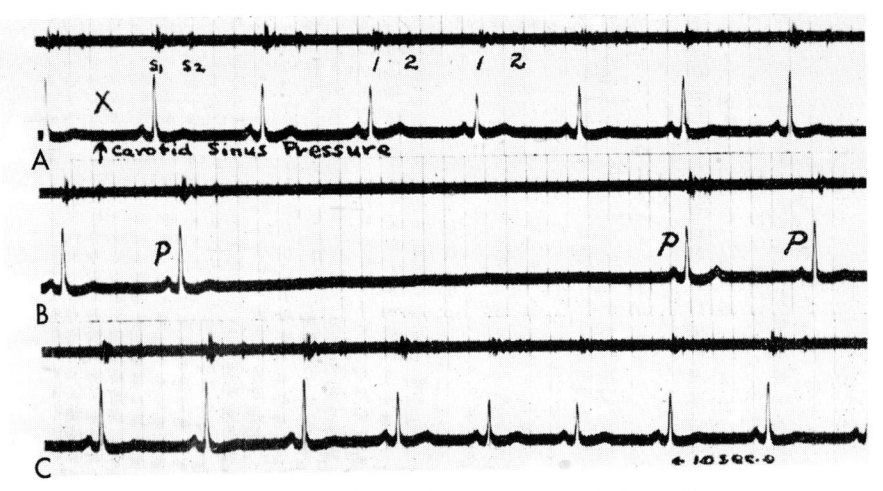

Figure 19-1. Cardioinhibitory type of carotid sinus syncope. A, B, and C represent a continuous tracing of lead I, taken simultaneously with the heart sounds at the apex. Carotid sinus pressure was applied at X of strip A. Note the cessation of the heart sounds and electrical activity for 5 seconds in strip B and the resumption of cardiac beating at the end of strip B and slight speeding of the rate in strip C. Note that there is no change in the character of the first heart sound following the long period of asystole in strip B.

rhythms such as multiple premature beats, ventricular tachycardia, and ventricular fibrillation. The period of slowing in (b) and (d) may range from six to ten seconds and is always followed by a period of simple sinus bradycardia. Associated with the cardiac slowing is a marked hypotensive effect which always outlasts the influence on the heart rate. Since most of these tests are performed in the recumbent position, it must be assumed that the hypotensive effect would be more marked were the patient sitting or standing (Figs. 19-1, 19-2).

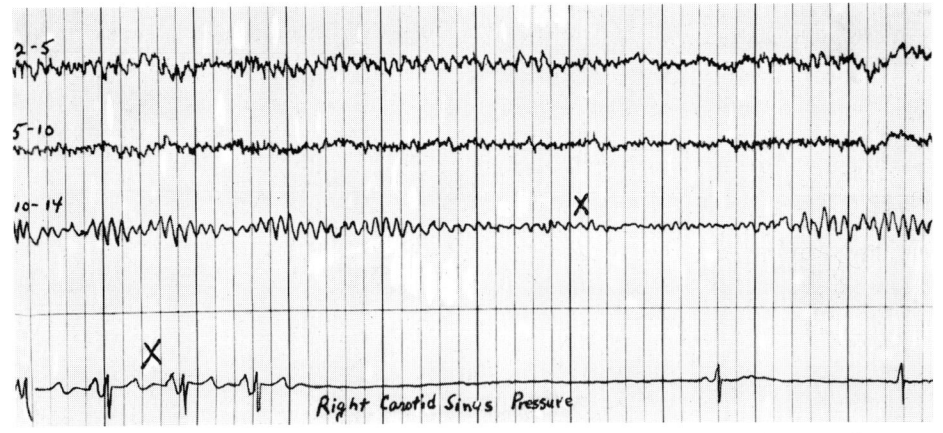

Figure 19-2. Cardioinhibitory type of carotid sinus syncope (electrocardiogram taken simultaneously with electroencephalogram).

The upper tracings represent the electroencephalogram taken at the positions noted simultaneously with the electrocardiogram. Note that following right carotid sinus pressure (X) there is a prolonged asystole in the electrocardiogram. Following a short but definite latent period, low voltage waves appear in the electroencephalogram at X (10-14). Slow, high voltage waves in the electroencephalogram characteristic of anoxia are often observed at the end of a period of cardiac standstill.

The following procedures are frequently efficacious in the treatment of the cardioinhibitory type of syncope: (a) *Use of drugs.* Atropine is only of temporary help, since its action is transient and it has unpleasant side effects. More effective are sympathomimetic drugs (Hutchinson and Stock, 1960) which tend to neutralize parasympathetic effects, e.g., ephedrine sulfate (25 mg., three to four times daily). (b) *Artificial pacemaker.* Unless the manifestations of the disease are transient or yield dramatically to medical therapy in four to seven days, artificial pacing is the therapy of choice. Syncopal episodes can be frequent, severe, and unpredictable, and death may occur in any attack. I have observed many such subjects in whom an artificial pacemaker has prevented further seizures. Ventricular pacing is the method usually recommended (see p. 413).

POSTURAL SYNCOPE

Normally, a change from the recumbent to the upright position is accompanied by a slight rise in blood pressure (10 to 15 mm. Hg) and a transient tachycardia, which lasts but a few minutes. The maintenance of the blood pressure in the upright position is mediated by the sympathetic system of the brain and spinal cord, which acts by effecting a certain degree of arterial and venous vasoconstriction, particularly in the blood vessels of the splanchnic area and the lower extremities. Furthermore, there is a reflex increase in the heart rate, occurring concurrently with the vasoconstriction, and reflex augmentation of respiration, which facilitates the return of blood to the right heart by the rhythmic changes in the intrathoracic and intraabdominal pressure. The presence of normal muscle tone is an additional important factor. Failure of these mechanisms would result in a pooling of blood in the lower part of the body, a decrease in venous return, a fall in cardiac output, and a fall in blood pressure leading to a decreased cerebral blood flow, thus precipitating a fainting attack. This sequence of events occurs in postural hypotension.

There are many types of syncope in which posture is an important or accessory factor in inducing the attack. While other conditions (e.g., coronary occlusion, cardioinhibitory type of carotid sinus syncope, rapid ventricular rate) are the principal causes in the cases discussed previously, posture may be an important predisposing factor. Despite the presence of the primary cause of the syncope, fainting would not often occur in the recumbent position. However, those states in which posture alone, uncomplicated by other factors, is the primary cause of the attack are discussed under postural hypotension. Postural hypotension will be described under two headings: (a) vasopressor type of postural hypotensive syncope, which is by far the most frequent of all types encountered; and (b) orthostatic hypotension.

The vasodepressor type of syncope is characterized by fainting in the erect position and is usually the result of hearing bad news, the sight of blood, severe pain, fear, hot environment, and the like. It is due to a dilatation of the vessels in the lower part of the body and requires no special therapy. Occasionally, the vasodepressor type occurs in association with the cardioinhibitory type of syncope.

The primary disturbance is related to a failure of the blood pressure regulating mechanism to function normally in the erect position, with pooling of blood in lower portions of the body due to loss of muscle, venous, and arteriolar tone. The actual loss of consciousness is due to diminished cerebral blood flow resulting from diminished cardiac output and systolic pressure insufficient to raise the blood from the heart to the brain. The unconsciousness is an expression of acute cerebral hypoxia. The attacks in most instances are transient, lasting but a few moments, and the blood pressure usually returns to its original level within minutes. However, I have observed instances in normal hearts where the hypotension persisted for several hours, accompanied by notable R-ST segment deviation in the electrocardiogram. In diseased hearts and in the older age groups, the electrocardiographic alterations may persist for several days; indeed, these as well as syncopal attacks of other etiologies may precipitate episodes of coronary insufficiency or even an acute myocardial infarction.

In orthostatic hypotension, the normal physiologic reactions to a change from the recumbent to the upright position do not occur. In these subjects, the blood pressure falls 20 to 40 mm. Hg or more when an upright position is assumed. This may lead to dizziness or fainting spells. The syncopal attacks are more easily produced when the patient stands quietly.

A significant rise in the venous concentration of epinephrine and norepinephrine occurs in normal subjects who manifest an adequate hemodynamic response to the assumption of the upright position. These changes in the plasma norepinephrine concentration correlate well with changes in arteriolar tone, as judged by maintenance of the diastolic pressure level. Hickler et al. (1959) presented data supporting the concept that norepinephrine release by the sympathetic nerves is the important factor in this homeostatic mechanism. A failure of this catecholamine response may be a cause of the postural type of syncope.

The clinical states in which orthostatic hypotension is observed include disease in the sympathetic nervous system or structural damage to the neural pathways concerned with maintenance of the peripheral vasomotor tone. Orthostatic hypotension is particularly likely to occur in tabes dorsalis and other diseases of the spinal cord (e.g., peripheral neuritis and poliomyelitis) and in Addison's disease, following sympathectomy for hypertension, in asthenic patients and in those patients who have been maintained in the recumbent position for prolonged periods. It may also appear during pregnancy; in the presence of venous defects in the legs (patients with varicose veins resulting in excessive pooling of blood in the lower extremities); during physical exhaustion in patients with fatigue, in starvation; and after the use of drugs such as the nitrites, tetraethylammonium chloride, guanethidine, and other antihypertensive agents.

Treatment. The treatment of the syndrome is usually unsatisfactory. However, the following methods of therapy should be tried: (a) treatment of the underlying cause if ascertainable; (b) avoidance of situations and drugs that tend to precipitate attacks; (c) bandaging of the lower extremities and use of an abdominal support; (d) use of an antigravity suit of the type worn by pilots flying at high altitudes — this has only recently been employed successfully; (e) use of the "head-up" bed at night; (f) administration of sympathomimetic drugs, e.g., ephedrine and hydroxyamphetamine or methylphenidate hydrochloride (Ritalin); (g) a regimen of increased intake of sodium chloride (12 gm. daily), which leads to an increase in total blood volume and in the volume of extracellular fluid, the latter mostly in the lower extremities; and (h) the administration of 9-alphafluorohydrocortisone, a salt-retaining hormone of the adrenal gland.

DIAGNOSIS OF ETIOLOGY OF SYNCOPAL ATTACKS

The most common types of syncopal attacks are vasodepressor and hysterical types and those due to hyperventilation. Less common are those due to vagal reflexes, cardiac causes (Stokes-Adams syndrome, paroxysmal tachycardia), and postural hypotension. The age and sex are of some importance; the vasodepressor and hysterical types usually occur early in life. Vasodepressor syncope is more common among men; hysterical syncope and hyperventilation are more common in women. When repeated fainting episodes occur later in life, one should suspect cerebrovascular disease or hyperactive vagal reflexes.

In evaluating syncopal episodes it is well to remember that during an asystole of less than 5 seconds' duration, it is usually possible to produce syncope only in the standing position. A longer period of asystole may not produce symptoms in the recumbent position. If a syncopal attack occurs, in order to rule out cerebrovascular disease, atropine should be administered to the patient (1.0 mg. intravenously). If the syncopal attacks are of the cardioinhibitory type, they will not be produced under these conditions. On the other hand, if the cause is an occlusion of one of the carotid arteries, atropine will not prevent these attacks. During these studies, recordings of the electrocardiogram, electroencephalogram, and blood pressure are desirable. The results of stimulation of the carotid sinus may be misleading due to the presence of coincidental carotid sinus sensitivity, which has no definite bearing on the spontaneous syncope developed by the patient (carotid sinus sensitivity is relatively common, while carotid sinus syncope is infrequent). Furthermore, the application of firm and sustained pressure may interfere with the cerebral circulation and thus simulate the reflex type.

To evaluate the postural effects in a case of syncope, the blood pressure and pulse are obtained after 10 to 15 minutes of recumbency and after tilting the patient 60 to 75 degrees on a tilt table. The blood pressure and pulse are recorded immediately after the position is changed and at frequent intervals for about 10 to 15 minutes thereafter. With true postural hypotension the fall in blood pressure may be slight (10 to 15 mm. Hg), moderate (15 to 25 mm. Hg), or marked (40 to 60 mm. Hg).

To further evaluate a syncopal episode, the patient while being monitored by an electroencephalogram and electrocardiogram should hyperventilate in the recumbent position and thereafter in the sitting position. One often encounters a fall in blood pressure with the development of a fainting episode. At this time, the electrocardiogram may show A-V junctional or an idioventricular rhythm. The electroencephalogram will also show low frequency, high amplitude waves typical of hypoxia; these are also seen with cardioinhibitory types of syncope. One should remember that these actions may occur in normal subjects and do not necessarily indicate the cause of the fainting episode. In hysterical individuals, unconsciousness usually occurs without alterations in the electroencephalogram. The response may of course be due to acapnia, which may cause marked slowing of the waves of the electroencephalogram. The electroencephalogram taken between attacks in patients who complain of fainting is generally normal. However, if the episodes relate to structural or toxic changes in the brain, abnormalities are noted.

The electrocardiogram taken during a syncopal attack yields extremely valuable information. If the heart is implicated, it may show the following: cardiac standstill, ventricular standstill, ventricular fibrillation, rapid ventricular rates with ectopic rhythms such as atrial flutter with 2:1 A-V heart block, paroxysmal tachycardia, or extremely slow heart rates (36 or less per minute) usually associated with hypotension. Recently, the use of monitoring devices which may be attached to the patient for periods of eight hours or more have been of considerable help in determining the exact cardiac mechanism during spontaneous episodes.

DIFFERENTIAL DIAGNOSIS

Syncope and convulsive seizures, which are often manifestations of cerebral hypoxia, represent a symptom complex that may result from many factors other than those caused primarily by cerebral ischemia. Among these are epilepsy, vertigo, narcolepsy, cataplexy, and familial periodic paralysis. A distinction between the various syndromes is difficult because all have some characteristics in common. For example, in certain types of syncope, convulsive seizures occur which are indistinguishable from those of epilepsy.

COMPLICATIONS OF FAINTING

The complications of fainting are numerous; some may be serious. These include bodily injury, which may involve bone fractures and even death if the attack occurs while the person is engaged in driving an automobile or in certain occupations. They may result in vascular thrombosis (cerebral, cardiac or other viscera). Even though the patient recovers completely, repeated episodes may create serious anxiety and fear.

PROGNOSIS

The prognosis depends on the underlying cause of the attacks, their frequency, the pre-existing cardiovascular status, and response to therapy. In many instances, the fainting episodes may not be particularly serious, e.g., in occasional vasodepressor, orthostatic, and hysterical episodes. Under these conditions, the patient should be told that these attacks are not of serious import. The chief risk lies in the environmental circumstance. In general, as soon as the victim is placed in the recumbent position, recovery takes place. However, in older patients and those with vascular disease the possibility of secondary thrombotic complications should be considered. In the forms of syncope associated with heart disease, the prognosis is more ominous. The severity of the underlying heart lesion and particularly the presence of complete A-V heart block has much to do with the ultimate prognosis. The course in patients with Stokes-Adams disease is discussed on page 141.

References

Benchimol, A., and Desser, K. B.: Ventricular function in the presence of ventricular arrhythmias. Presented at the 25th Hahnemann Symposium, Cardiac Arrhythmias: Pathophysiology, Pharmacology and Management, Phila., Sept. 21–25, 1971.

Benchimol, A., Stegall, H. F., and Gartlan, J. L.: New method to measure phasic coronary blood velocity in man. Amer. Heart J., 81:93, 1971.

Benchimol, A., Stegall, H. F., Maroko, P. R., Gartlan, J. L., and Brener, L.: Aortic flow velocity in man during cardiac arrhythmias measured with the Doppler catheter-flowmeter system. Amer. Heart J., 78:649, 1969.

Botticelli, J. T., Keelan, M. H., Rosenbaum, F. F., and Lange, R. L.: Circulatory control in idiopathic orthostatic hypotension (Shy-Drager syndrome). Circulation, 38:870, 1968.

Braunwald, E., et al.: Congenital aortic stenosis. I. Clinical and hemodynamic findings in 100 patients. Circulation, 27:426, 1963.

Corday, E., and Irving, D. W.: Effect of cardiac arrhythmias on the cerebral circulation. Amer. J. Cardiol., 6:803, 1960.

Dermksian, G., and Lamb, L. E.: Cardiac arrhythmias in experimental syncope. JAMA, 168:1623, 1958.

Engel, G. L.: Fainting, 2nd ed. Springfield, Ill., Charles C Thomas, 1962.

Frick, M. A.: 9-Alpha-fluorohydrocortisone in the treatment of postural hypotension. Acta Med. Scand., 179:293, 1966.

Gale, G. E., Bosman, C. K., Tucker, R. B. K., and

Barlow, J. B.: Hereditary prolongation of QT interval. Study of two families. Brit. Heart J., 32:505, 1970.

Garza, L. A., McNamara, D. G., Nora, J. J., Vick, R. L., and Sommerville, R. J.: Familial repolarization myocardiopathy. Amer. J. Cardiol., 23:112, 1969.

Glick, G., and Yu, P. N.: Hemodynamic changes during spontaneous vasovagal reactions. Amer. J. Med., 34:42, 1963.

Goodall, McC., Harlan, W. R., Jr., and Alton, H.: Noradrenaline release and metabolism in orthostatic (postural) hypotension. Circulation, 36:489, 1967.

Goodall, McC., Harlan, W. R., Jr., and Alton, H.: Decreased noradrenaline (norepinephrine) synthesis in neurogenic orthostatic hypotension. Circulation, 38:592, 1968.

Hickler, R. B., Wells, R. E., Tyler, H. R., and Hamlin, J. T.: Plasma catecholamine and electroencephalographic response to acute postural change. Amer. J. Med., 26:410, 1959.

Hutchinson, E. C., and Stock, J. P. P.: The carotid sinus syndrome. Lancet, 2:445, 1960.

Jervell, A., and Lange-Nielsen, F.: Congenital deaf-mutism, functional heart disease with prolongation of the Q-T interval, and sudden death. Amer. Heart J., 54:59, 1957.

Karhunen, P., Luomanmaki, K., Heikkila, J., and Eisalo, A.: Syncope and Q-T prolongation without deafness: The Romano-Ward syndrome. Amer. Heart J., 80:820, 1970.

Karp, H. R., Weissler, A. M., and Heyman, A.: Circulatory and electroencephalographic changes associated with loss of consciousness in vasodepressor syncope. J. Clin. Invest., 38:1016, 1959.

Ward, O. C.: A new familial cardiac syndrome in children. J. Irish Med. Assoc., 53:104, 1964.

Weiss, S., and Ferris, E. G.: Adams-Stokes syndrome with transient complete heart block of vagovagal reflex origin. Arch. Intern. Med., 54:931, 1934.

Williams, R., and Allen, P.: Loss of consciousness: incidence, causes, and electroencephalographic findings. Aerospace Med., 33:545, 1962.

Chapter 20: Stress Tests Producing Arrhythmias: Exercise, Emotion, Respiratory Maneuvers, and Atrial Pacing

INTRODUCTION
EXERCISE
  Hemodynamic Effects
  The ECG During the Period of Exercise
  Relation of Exercise to Arrhythmias
    Relation of Premature Beats to Exercise
    Relation of A-V Conduction Disturbances to Exercise
    Other Arrhythmias and Exercise
    Arrhythmias Induced by Isometric Exercise
EMOTIONAL STRESS
RESPIRATORY MANEUVERS
ATRIAL PACING

INTRODUCTION

Many patients with a history of palpitation or syncopal attacks often present a normal rhythm at the time of the initial examination. However, cardiac arrhythmias are often precipitated by certain stress factors. Stress may be the result of mental tension, drugs, or physical exercise. The following easily available stress procedures may be employed: (1) physical exercise; (2) emotional stress; (3) certain respiratory maneuvers, such as the Valsalva maneuver, breath-holding after deep inspiration, and hyperventilation (see p. 253); and (4) atrial pacing (see discussion on p. 254).

EXERCISE

The relationship between exercise and arrhythmias is a particularly important one and depends on many different factors: the state of the patient's heart (normal or diseased), his age, the physical condition, the type of exercise and the rapidity with which it is performed, and whether or not the patient is accustomed to performing exercise of the type employed. The effects of exercise on the heart involve the central nervous system, the endocrine system and certain alterations in biochemistry, and other body functions related to the heart and other portions of the circulatory system. These as well as other factors tend, in turn, to influence the hemodynamic events.

Exercise manifests the following effects: (1) decrease in vagal tone; (2) increase in circulating catecholamines and sympathetic tone; and (3) increase in plasma cortisol and growth hormone levels. These factors tend to increase the cardiac rate and output. The increase in HGH levels and the subsequent elevation of free fatty acid (FFA) levels is associated with a decrease in the respiratory quotient leading to an increase in the combustion of fat to provide the energy required for muscular effort. During the period of exercise, FFA levels decrease; they increase above the pre-exercise control level during the immediate postexercise period. The biochemical effects of exercise result from hypoxia, hypercapnea, and increase in serum lactic acid. These factors, acting directly and reflexly on the centers in the brain which control or modify cardiac function, are largely responsible for the effects of exercise on the heart.

Hemodynamic Effects. During exercise, the cardiac output increases often to six times the normal resting value. This is due mainly to an increase in heart rate; it is also associated with increased venous return caused by vigorous muscular contractions, increased depth and frequency of respirations, and rise of capillary and venous pressure. The systolic blood pressure rises, and the diastolic falls; however, the mean pressure does not change significantly. The oxygen uptake parallels the increased cardiac output and coronary blood flow. The increased cardiac output is the result chiefly of the tachycardia. In trained athletes, there is in addition an increase in stroke volume. The response to exercise of patients with myocardial abnormalities varies somewhat from the normal group.

Detailed studies of the effect of exercise on normal human subjects and in those with myocardial disease were performed by Donald et al. (1955). These authors found that in healthy human subjects performing exercises equal to walking 1.5 to 5 m.p.h., the cardiac output rises to a peak within one minute, remains stable during the period of exercise, and returns to a steady resting state within one minute of termination of the exercise. Cerettelli (1966) has shown that in the kinetics of the transition from rest to exercise, the plateau or "steady state" at the peak of cardiac output is reached at about the same time as oxygen uptake reaches its peak plateau, and that the final level of cardiac output is closely related to the intensity of exertion. Figure 20–1 shows the initial rise in cardiac output, the peak or "steady state" plateau, the return to resting state after termination of the exercise, and the concurrent increase in oxygen uptake. Coronary blood flow is increased in normal human subjects during exercise; however, cardiac work increases more than the myocardial oxygen consumption, indicating an increase in left ventricular efficiency.

The response to exercise of patients with myocardial abnormalities varies somewhat from that of the normal group. For example, the response of patients with mitral stenosis differs from that of normal subjects in that many of the patients are incapable of raising their cardiac output to any significant degree, and when this occurs, there is a delay in the achievement of the peak. There is also a delay in the return of the cardiac output to the control level following cessation of the exercise. A similar response is observed in hypertensive patients with exertional dyspnea and cardiac enlargement. In patients with myocardial disease, the work and the efficiency of the left ventricle fails to increase adequately in response to exercise.

The studies mentioned above indicate, as might be expected, that the heart is under maximal strain during the first minute of exercise when the metabolic demands are higher than normal but the compensatory mechanisms are still not entirely operative. It is of interest that the electrocardiographic changes frequently appear during the first minute of exercise and disappeared thereafter, in spite of continued exercise. In patients with severe myocardial disease, the changes do not regress, but usually increase as exercise continues and, sometimes, are even more pronounced in the postexercise period. The latter phenomenon may be due to the decrease in pulse rate and the fall of cardiac output

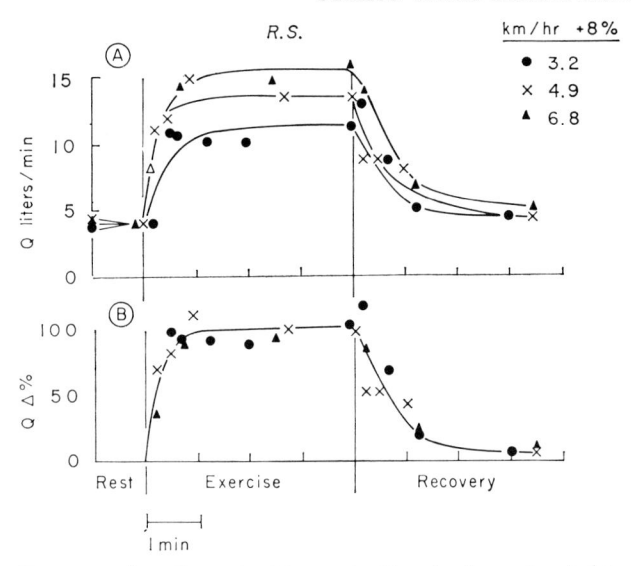

Figure 20–1. Response of cardiac output to constant levels of exercise. Subject exercised at three rates of work. (A) Increase in cardiac output (in liters) shows increasing flows with higher rates of work. (B) Increase of cardiac output in response to exercise occurs in two phases: a rapid initial increase over first 30 seconds, during which about 90 per cent of the total increase occurs, and a second phase of slow increase in cardiac output to peak levels, followed by a plateau at that level. The initial, rapid response is thought to be due to reflexes arising both from the cortex (anticipating exercise before it begins) and from chemoreceptors in the circulation (responding to altered metabolism of O_2 and CO_2). (From Cerretelli, P.: In Anderson, K. L. (ed.): Physical Activity in Health and Disease. Universitetsforlaget, Oslo, 1966, pp. 15–18.)

and coronary blood flow prior to recovery of the myocardium from the increased metabolic demands of exercise. In addition, the sustained local cardiac effects of the exercise, hypoxia, and accumulation of metabolites are present for some time after the exercise is over.

The Electrocardiogram During the Period of Exercise. The electrocardiographic recording during the period of exercise is best accomplished by the technique of radioelectrocardiography using a telemetering apparatus. The absence of a cable connected between the subject and the recording machine permits the recording of exercise performance at a distance up to 500 feet or more from the recording apparatus without electrical interference. The electrical impulses picked up by the electrodes are delivered by the connecting wires to the transmitter which is usually placed in the patient's pocket. The electrocardiogram is broadcast on a radio frequency beam and picked up by the receiver which may be situated close to or at a distance from the patient. The information is then fed into an oscilloscope or a conventional electrocardiogram for continuous monitoring or may be recorded on magnetic tape (Fig. 20–2).

Relation of Exercise to Arrhythmias. It has been known for a long time that exercise may produce ectopic rhythms or may abolish or modify such rhythms if they are already present. This is of considerable importance. Sudden deaths occasionally reported following more or less strenuous exercise are usually attributed to coronary insufficiency. However, some of them are probably due to the occurrence of tachyarrhythmias with the superimposition of coronary insufficiency.

Relation of Premature Beats to Exercise. The following patterns of response of premature beats to exercise may be noted: (a) premature beats present in the resting state unaffected

STRESS TESTS PRODUCING ARRHYTHMIAS

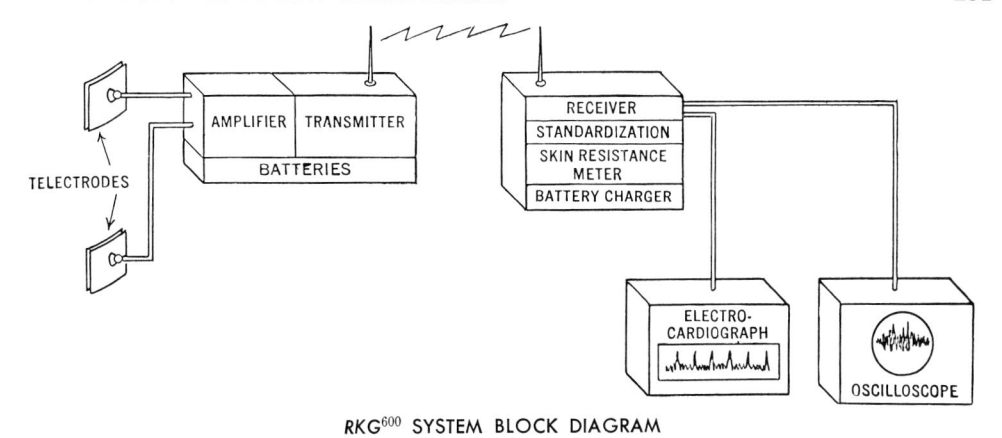

RKG⁶⁰⁰ SYSTEM BLOCK DIAGRAM

Figure 20-2. Diagrammatic scheme of apparatus used in radioelectrocardiography. Impulse is transmitted from electrodes to the transmitter, where it is amplified and broadcast on a certain wave length to be picked up by the receiver. It is then fed to a conventional electrocardiograph or oscilloscope and may also be tape recorded. (From Bellet, S., Deliyiannis, S., and Eliakim, M.: Amer. J. Cardiol., 8:385, 1961.)

by exercise (uncommon); (b) premature beats present in the resting state which are abolished by exercise (most common). Premature beats are usually abolished by exercise. These manifestations are observed not only in normal subjects but also in patients with various types of cardiac abnormalities (Bourne, 1927); (c) premature beats which are precipitated by or increased with exercise. In this discussion, the term "produced by exercise" refers to the actual period of exercise or to the immediate postexercise period. In most of the cases studied thus far, premature beats produced by exercise are most marked during the actual period of exercise and usually disappear or are less marked in the postexercise period (Bellet, unpublished observations) (see Fig. 20-3).

Figure 20-3. Production of premature beats during the period of exercise. Taken by radioelectrocardiography during Master two-step test. (A) Control shows sinus arrhythmia and bradycardia, rate 58/minute. (B) Note increase in rate to 84/minute. (C) Note the occurrence of premature beats after 138 seconds of exercise (X and X₁). (D) Note the paroxysm of tachycardia (supraventricular) at 156 seconds of exercise, starting at X and X₁. Note single supraventricular premature beat one minute after exercise. (E, F) Note the absence of premature beats in the postexercise period (two and five minutes).

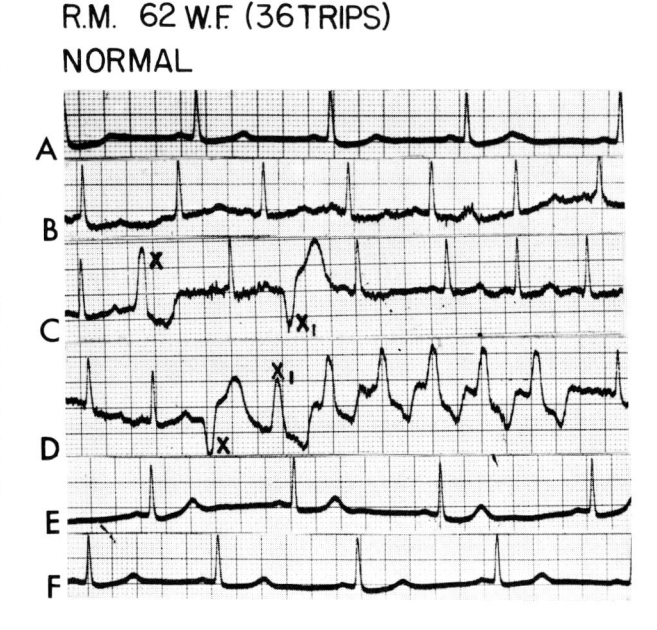

R.M. 62 W.F. (36 TRIPS)
NORMAL

The significance of premature beats initiated during exercise is a matter of some controversy. The question continually arises as to whether such occurrences are to be regarded as normal or abnormal findings. Premature beats may be precipitated following moderate to strenuous exertion in apparently normal subjects (Mattingly et al., 1954; Master et al., 1957; Lepeschkin and Surawicz, 1958; Lamb and Hiss, 1962); however, these may belong in a special category. They are usually observed in young subjects and may be the result of increased reactivity to catecholamines, recent infections, or excessive amounts of nicotine or caffeine.

Arrhythmias occurring after exercise are much more apt to appear in subjects with myocardial disease rather than in those without it. For example, 309 subjects with known heart disease and 164 without heart disease were submitted to treadmill exercise stress with the following results: 27 of the patients with heart disease (9 per cent) and two (1.5 per cent) of the normal subjects developed transient arrhythmias (Gooch and Evans, 1968). The following is a summary of our experience (Bellet, unpublished observations). In normal subjects, aged 17 to 25, moderately severe exercise results in the production of a tachycardia, with the heart rate increasing to as much as 160 to 180 per minute. However, arrhythmias are quite rare in this group. In an examination of 200 subjects by means of a double Master two-step test, we observed isolated beats in only two individuals. Unless associated with unusual circumstances (e.g., strenuous exercise, physical exhaustion, toxic states, drugs, excessive intake of caffeine), the precipitation of numerous premature beats or a paroxysmal tachycardia by exercise is, in our opinion, evidence of some degree of deviation from the normal. The basis for this belief is the fact that (a) we have been unable to produce premature beats or paroxysmal tachycardia (except in rare instances) in young normal subjects, but have produced them frequently in patients with myocardial abnormality; and (b) they occur at a time when there is an increased strain on the heart and they are frequently associated with other types of abnormalities, namely, alterations of the R-ST segment, T waves, and so forth.

Relation of A-V Conduction Disturbances to Exercise. Alteration of the P-R interval during exercise has been infrequently studied. It is often difficult to obtain exact values for the P-R time at high pulse rates and, occasionally, no distinct P-R interval can be seen. The available studies reveal the following: In all age groups and in both sexes, regardless of the initial value at rest, the P-R interval decreases to the value of 0.11 second during work performed up to a heart rate of 170 beats per minute. This is significant, since if a prolonged P-R interval at rest is due solely to pathology of the A-V node, the P-R interval should show either no change or a further increase after exercise. Less frequently, it decreases during exercise (release of vagal effect); but in these instances, normal values are seldom obtained, and a secondary increase for the P-R interval beyond the initial prolonged value at rest usually occurs several minutes after exercise.

Other observers have found that the P-R interval is decreased during the period of exercise to a greater extent than would be expected to occur as a result of the observed elevation of the heart rate. In addition, it may be independent of the latter in the period immediately following exercise (Bengtsson, 1956). This additional decrease is probably the result of an increase in sympathetic tone.

Increase of the P-R interval during exercise with an increase in heart rate has been observed in several cases. Following the exercise, the heart rate decreases and the P-R interval may become longer than at rest, particularly in untrained or vasolabile persons. The increase does not exceed 0.02 second or the absolute value of 0.22 second. That partial A-V heart block may be converted to a higher degree of block by exercise was reported by Scherf and Boyd (1946).

Other Arrhythmias and Exercise. Atrial fibrillation has been observed following strenuous exercise in apparently normal subjects. Atrial fibrillation has occurred after long distance walking and ski races in exhausted persons (Scherf and Schaffer, 1952; Hay and Jones, 1927).

The effects of exercise on pre-excitation vary considerably; however, usually this is unaffected by exercise. The experience in 28 cases follows: (a) with no pre-excitation at rest, pre-excitation appeared during exercise (two cases); (b) pre-excitation present at rest disappeared during exercise and returned after exercise (eight cases); (c) pre-excitation was not affected by the exercise (eighteen cases) (Sandberg, 1961).

Arrhythmias Induced by Isometric Exercise. Isometric exercise has been observed to have a significant effect on left ventricular function. The occurrence of arrhythmias during maximum handgrip contraction has recently been studied (Matthews et al., 1971). Fifty-eight patients with a variety of heart diseases, but who manifested no arrhythmias at rest, were studied during sustained 25 per cent and 50 per cent maximum, voluntary, handgrip contraction during cardiac catheterization and by noninvasive techniques. These results were compared with the results obtained during graded bicycle exercise. During handgrip, arrhythmias were observed in 37 per cent of patients during catheterization and 26 per cent with noninvasive study. These included atrial arrhythmias in 12 per cent; ventricular in 33 per cent; ventricular tachycardia in 16 per cent; and pulsus alternans in 13 per cent. With dynamic exercise, 13 per cent of 45 patients developed arrhythmias. The results of these studies indicate that a high incidence of cardiac arrhythmias occurred during sustained isometric exercise, and it is suggested that this may be a hazardous form of exercise for certain individuals.

EMOTIONAL STRESS

The effect of emotions and mental stress on the heart rate has been recognized for years, since the heart is one of the most sensitive targets for stimuli of psychic origin. It is known that emotional factors, especially fear, anxiety, and sudden anger, or marked excitement can precipitate various arrhythmias (Bellet and Roman, 1970; Bellet et al., 1968; Stevenson et al., 1949). This is probably due to increased sympathetic tone and catecholamine release which accompanies the emotional stress, resulting in, among other changes, increased work of the heart and increased myocardial oxygen consumption (see p. 27).

RESPIRATORY MANEUVERS

Respiration is known to affect the heart rate in healthy subjects and leads to the well-known respiratory arrhythmia. Changes are due to vagal reflexes initiated by stimulation of stretch receptors in the lung and visceral pleura, venous return secondary to variations in the intrathoracic pressure, and hypoxia and other alterations in the blood gases. Respiratory maneuvers, like breath holding after deep inspiration, Valsalva, or hyperventilation, frequently result in electrocardiographic changes, especially marked sinus bradycardia associated with junctional or ventricular escapes, A-V dissociation with nodal or idioventricular rhythm, transient A-V block, and even prolonged sinus arrest with syncope (Bellet and Roman, 1970).

Some subjects are particularly sensitive to vagal stimulation and the other aforementioned changes which occur during respiratory maneuvers. In such subjects, breath holding, the Valsalva maneuver, or hyperventilation may produce syncope or even sudden death. The detection of such arrhythmia-prone subjects by recording the electrocardiogram during various respiratory maneuvers is, therefore, of interest in the investigation of the mechanism of syncopal attacks of unclear etiology. Also, as stressed by Lamb et al. (1958), detection is of special importance in the medical evaluation in airplane pilots or deep-sea divers, in whom breath holding and deep inspiratory movements are common.

ATRIAL PACING

Atrial pacing as a modality for stressing the heart was only recently introduced (Benchimol and Ligget, 1966; Samet et al., 1966; and Sowton et al., 1967). The technique for atrial pacing consists of using a bipolar electrode catheter or a multiple electrode catheter which is introduced percutaneously through the femoral vein and advanced under fluoroscopic control into the right atrium (Cheng, 1971). The preferred position is one in which one or both electrodes are positioned against the lateral wall of the upper third of the right atrium. Electrode stimulation is carried out by an external battery-driven pulse generator. This method is quite simple and safe.

This method has the advantage in that it increases the heart rate without requiring physical effort on the part of the patient and it may be terminated as soon as untoward manifestations appear. It can be used in patients with poor exercise tolerance or in those who cannot achieve an adequate exercise level because of dyspnea, claudication, or other handicaps.

Some of the information that might be obtained through atrial pacing follows: (1) Induction of premature beats or paroxysms of atrial tachycardia with an increase in the heart rate.

(2) Induction of varying degrees of A-V heart block as the rate is increased. This may be physiologic above a certain rate (130/min.), but it is abnormal if it occurs at pacing at relatively slow rates (below 100/min.).

(3) Induction of pulsus alternans in patients with no clinical evidence of heart failure. For example, patients with symptoms of dyspnea or exertion, paroxysmal nocturnal dyspnea, or evidence of angina develop pulsus alternans after atrial pacing at 110/minute (the resting rate was 75/min.) (Cheng, 1971).

(4) Diagnosis of W-P-W syndrome: Atrial pacing is of value in helping to establish the diagnosis of the W-P-W syndrome in patients with suggestive but atypical ECG evidence who present a history of paroxysmal tachycardia. Atrial pacing may be performed (a) by increasing the heart rate, or (b) by producing atrial premature beats of varying degrees of prematurity by artificial stimulation of the right atrium. In this manner, both a delta wave and paroxysmal tachycardia have been produced (Cheng, 1971).

(5) Significance of certain types of bilateral bundle branch block: Although it is known that some patients with right bundle branch block and left-axis deviation may develop the Stokes-Adams syndrome and transient or permanent complete A-V heart block, it is difficult to determine the individual patients in whom this will occur. Atrial pacing up to 180/min. has been shown to be of help in this regard by producing intermittent complete A-V heart block in some of this group (10 per cent). This could help to pinpoint the patient who may require prophylactic pacemaker insertion.

(6) In the diagnosis of "sick sinus syndrome" and for indications relative to the type of therapy involved, atrial pacing is of help in the following way: In clinically normal hearts, the interval between the last pacing impulse and the onset of the first intrinsic P wave ranged from 0.8 to 1.1 seconds (mean 0.9 second), whereas in patients with clinical evidence of sinoatrial disease this interval was 1.6 to 7.0 seconds. Moreover, atrial pacing is a useful, provocative test for studying A-V nodal function. If delay in A-V conduction occurs with pacing below 130 per minute, it suggests the presence of potential A-V nodal disturbances, and such patients would require a ventricular rather than an atrial pacemaker.

References

Andersen, K. L.: The cardiovascular system in exercise. In Falls, H. B. (ed.): Exercise Physiology. New York, Academic Press, 1968.

Barger, A. C., Richards, V., Metcalfe, J., and Gunther, B.: Regulation of the circulation during exercise: cardiac output (direct Fick) and metabolic adjustments in the normal dog. Amer. J. Physiol., 184:613, 1956.

Bellet, S.: Clinical Disorders of the Heart, 3rd Ed., Philadelphia, Lea & Febiger, 1971.

Bellet, S., and Roman, L.: Stress electrocardiography in the diagnosis of arrhythmias. Geriatrics, 25:102, 1970.

Bellet, S., Roman, L., Kostis, J., and Slater, A.: Continuous electrocardiographic monitoring during automobile driving. Amer. J. Cardiol., 22:856, 1968.

Benchimol, A., and Ligget, M. S.: Cardiac hemodynamics during stimulation of the right atrium, right ventricle, and left ventricle in normal and abnormal hearts. Circulation, 33:933, 1966.

Bengtsson, E.: Exercise electrocardiogram in healthy children and in comparison with adults. Acta Med. Scand., 154:225, 1956.

Bourne, G.: Classification of premature ventricular beats. Quart. J. Med., 20:219, 1927.

Cerretelli, P.: In Andersen, K. L. (ed.): Physical Activity in Health and Disease. Oslo, Universitetsforlaget, 1966.

Cheng, T. O.: Atrial pacing: Its diagnostic and therapeutic applications. Prog. Cardiov. Dis., 14:230, 1971.

Cornil, A., DeCastes, A., Copinschi, G., and Frankson, J. R. M.: Effect of muscular exercise on the plasma level of cortisol in man. Acta Endocrinol., 48:163, 1965.

Donald, K. W., Bishop, J. M., Cumming, G., and Wade, O. L.: Effect of exercise on cardiac output and circulatory dynamics of normal subjects. Clin. Sci., 14:37, 1955.

Dunn, F. L., and Beenken, H. G.: Short distance radio telemetering of physiological information. JAMA, 169:1618, 1960.

Friedberg, S. J., Harlan, W. R., Trout, D. L., and Estes, E. H.: The effect of exercise on the concentration and turnover of plasma nonesterified fatty acids. J. Clin. Invest., 39:215, 1960.

Gooch, A. S., and Evans, J. M.: Treadmill ECG helps detection of arrhythmias. Med. Tribune, p. 27, Dec. 9, 1968.

Hay, J., and Jones, H. W.: Trauma as a cause of auricular fibrillation. Brit. Med. J., 1:559, 1927.

Hurst, V. W., III, and Nutter, D. O.: Quantitation of arrhythmias during a controlled exercise stress in normal young men. Circulation, 35–36:II–147, 1967.

Jones, W. B., and Reeves, T. J.: Total cardiac output response during four minutes of exercise. Amer. Heart J., 76:209, 1968.

Lamb, L. E., Dermksian, G., and Sarnoff, C. A.: Significant cardiac arrhythmias induced by common respiratory maneuvers. Amer. J. Cardiol., 2:563, 1958.

Lamb, L. E., and Hiss, R. G.: Influence of exercise on premature contractions. Amer. J. Cardiol., 10:209, 1962.

Lepeschkin, E., and Surawicz, B.: Characteristics of true-positive and false-positive results of electrocardiographic Master two-step exercise tests. New Eng. J. Med., 258:511, 1958.

Master, A. M., Field, L. E., and Donoso, E.: Coronary artery disease and "two-step" exercise test. New York State J. Med., 57:105, 1957.

Matthews, O. A., Atkins, J. M., Houston, J. D., Blomqvist, G., and Mullins, C. G.: Arrhythmias induced by isometric exercise (handgrip). Clin. Res., 19:23, 1971.

Mattingly, T. W., Fancher, P. S., Bauer, F. L., and Robb, G. P.: Army Medical Service Graduate School Research Report, Washington, D.C., Walter Reed Army Medical Center, Sept. 21–24, 1954.

Porter, W. B.: The probably grave significance of premature beats occurring in angina pectoris induced by effort. Amer. J. Med. Sci., 216:509, 1948.

Rumbal, C. A., and Acheson, E. D.: Electrocardiograms of healthy men after strenuous exercise. Brit. Heart J., 22:415, 1960.

Rushmer, R. F., Smith, O. A., Jr., and Franklin, D. L.: Mechanisms of cardiac control during exercise. Circ. Res., 7:603, 1959.

Samet, P., Castillo, C., and Bernstein, W. H.: Hemodynamic sequelae of atrial, ventricular, and sequential atrioventricular pacing in cardiac patients. Amer. Heart J., 72:725, 1966.

Sandberg, L.: Studies on electrocardiographic changes during exercise tests. Acta Med. Scand., 169 (Supp. 365):1–117, 1961.

Scherf, D., and Boyd, L. J.: Clinical Electrocardiography. Philadelphia, J. B. Lippincott, 1946.

Scherf, D., and Schaffer, A. I.: The electrocardiographic exercise test. Amer. Heart J., 43:927, 1952.

Sowton, G. E., Balcon, R., Cross, D., and Frick, M. H.: Measurements of the angina threshold using atrial pacing. A new technique for the study of angina pectoris. Cardiov. Res., 1:301, 1967.

Stevenson, I. P., Duncan, C. H., Wolff, S., et al.: Life situations, emotions, and extrasystoles. Psychosom. Med., 11:257, 1949.

Wyndham, C. H., and Ward, J. S.: An assessment of the exercise capacity of cardiac patients. Circulation, 16:384, 1957.

Chapter 21 *Pregnancy*

ETIOLOGY
TYPES OF ARRHYTHMIAS
　Premature Beats
　Supraventricular Tachycardia
　Ventricular Tachycardia
Atrial Flutter
Atrial Fibrillation
A-V Heart Block
Cardiac Arrest

Arrhythmias are not infrequently observed during pregnancy. They may be precipitated in a previously normal heart, but occur more frequently in the presence of pre-existing heart disease especially in association with heart failure.

ETIOLOGY

Many alterations in the heart and circulation, occurring during the various stages of pregnancy, are important in the production of arrhythmias, particularly in the presence of pre-existing disease. The heart rate increases gradually and returns toward the pre-pregnant control level at term. The maximal increase occurs in the seventh and eighth months and averages 10 beats per minute. The cardiac output is increased in pregnancy to levels approximately 30 to 50 per cent above the nonpregnant control level. The peak increase occurs during the twenty-fifth to thirty-second weeks of pregnancy; then the values gradually return toward normal prior to term. The mechanisms for this increment include an increase in maternal oxygen consumption, hypervolemia, and an arteriovenous (A-V) shunt in the placenta.

The cardiac work further increases during the second stage of labor, as manifested by the sudden rise in blood pressure, pulse, and cardiac output. Although this occurs in the normal pregnancy, its effect is greater in the patient with rheumatic, hypertensive, or thyroid heart disease, particularly in the presence of congestive heart failure. Reflexes arising from the abdomen, anemia, psychogenic factors, and idiopathic myocardial degeneration, which is observed in rare cases, are other important factors involved in the production of arrhythmias.

TYPES OF ARRHYTHMIAS

All of the various clinical disorders of the heart beat have been observed in pregnant patients with previously normal hearts as well as those with organic heart disease. Although observed during routine electrocardiographic examination, additional arrhythmias may be detected by continuous monitoring. Premature atrial and ventricular beats are the most common. Paroxysmal atrial tachycardia, atrial flutter, and atrial fibrillation are relatively rare, except in patients with rheumatic mitral disease. Their occurrence in such patients may precipitate congestive heart failure and result in death.

Premature Beats. Premature atrial or ventricular beats are not uncommon during pregnancy and the puerperium.

Premature beats may arise in the atria, A-V junction, or the ventricles. They may occur occasionally, every second beat (bigeminy), or every third beat (trigeminy) (Mendelson, 1956).

In patients with occasional or frequent premature beats existing before pregnancy, one may anticipate that this ectopic rhythm will become more marked or lead to paroxysmal tachycardia (atrial, ventricular, or junctional) during the course of pregnancy. In such instances, one should consider this possibility, anticipate its presence, and be prepared to institute therapeutic measures following its inception. Occasional premature beats require no specific therapy. Multiple premature beats constitute a potential hazard in the development of atrial or ventricular tachycardia and should be treated. The actual presence of one of the tachyarrhythmias demands vigorous treatment.

In general, occasional premature beats have no special obstetric significance. If the premature beats are frequent and disturbing to the patient, it is suggested that procaine amide be employed in a dose of 0.25 to 0.5 gm., three to four times daily, or antazoline (Antistine, 100 to 200 mg., three times a day). Quinidine is contraindicated because of its tendency to induce premature labor. Digitalis is of no benefit unless the patient is in heart failure. Propranolol should not be administered during pregnancy because its effects on the fetus are not known.

Supraventricular Tachycardia. Paroxysmal atrial or junctional tachycardia is rare during pregnancy. The clinical manifestations are similar to those described in Chapter 9; however, they are apt to be more marked in the latter stages of pregnancy. Collapse during labor or immediately thereafter, although most naturally attributed to some obstetric complication, may be precipitated by an ectopic rhythm. The diagnosis should be suspected in the presence of a regular cardiac rhythm with a heart rate of 140 to 220 per minute.

The therapy is generally similar to that noted in the section on paroxysmal tachycardia (see page 108). Prophylaxis includes the avoidance of undue physical and mental strain. Should episodes of this arrhythmia occur, it is advisable to digitalize the patient or use procaine amide. Quinidine should be avoided for the reasons previously mentioned. Patients with W-P-W syndrome should be given digitalis if subject to recurrent attacks. In cases that are refractory to drug therapy, countershock has been employed, without harm to the fetus.

The prognosis depends upon the underlying condition of the heart, the duration of the tachycardia, and the results of treatment. Since most of these cases respond to therapy, the prognosis is usually favorable.

Ventricular Tachycardia. Ventricular paroxysmal tachycardia is relatively rare during pregnancy and is usually associated with a serious type of heart damage, particularly coronary artery disease. The occurrence of ventricular paroxysmal tachycardia during labor is a serious complication, especially in diseased hearts.

Lidocaine given intravenously under continuous monitoring is probably the drug of choice. Procaine amide is the drug of second choice. Electric countershock may be safely employed if the aforementioned measures are unsuccessful (Vogel et al., 1965). The prognosis depends upon the underlying condition of the heart, the duration of the tachycardia, and the results of therapy. With the recent improvement in the therapeutic regimen, the possibility of conversion to normal sinus rhythm is usually quite good. In patients whose history indicates a serious circulatory response to these attacks, it may be well to consider Cesarean section as the method of delivery, unless the disturbance is readily controllable by drugs or electric countershock.

Atrial Flutter. Atrial flutter occurs rarely in pregnancy. It is usually associated with organic heart disease but may occasionally occur in otherwise normal hearts. Atrial flutter with 1:1 conduction represents a serious complication.

Therapy is aimed toward controlling the ventricular rate by digitalis and restoring normal sinus rhythm by other antiarrhythmic agents. The arrhythmia, when resistant to medical therapy, may be successfully terminated by electric countershock. Countershock has been employed in six cases of arrhythmias during pregnancy without harm to either the patient or to the fetus (Sussman et al., 1966; Vogel et al., 1965).

Atrial Fibrillation. Atrial fibrillation constitutes a serious complication to the pregnant woman. Such patients should be carefully observed and treated during the period of gestation. A complication that may occur is embolism, systemic or pulmonary. During pregnancy, two types of atrial fibrillation are observed: (1) chronic atrial fibrillation which has existed prior to pregnancy and which is usually associated with rheumatic heart disease; and (2) atrial fibrillation occurring initially during the period of pregnancy, usually following moderate or severe nervous strain, infection, or Graves' disease. The group in which atrial fibrillation first occurs during pregnancy is significantly more susceptible to heart failure than the group that has had a history of atrial fibrillation.

A pregnant patient with atrial fibrillation should be digitalized to lower the ventricular rate to about 70 to 80 beats per minute. Because of the attendant risk during the initial period of observation and occasional complications of reversion, attempts should not usually be made to restore normal sinus rhythm.

A-V Heart Block. First degree A-V heart block is occasionally observed in pregnancy, under the following conditions: (1) rheumatic heart disease (inactive), usually present prior to the pregnancy; (2) acute rheumatic fever or reactivation of an old carditis (rarely observed during pregnancy); (3) myocarditis due to nonspecific infections; and (4) digitalis effects. Prolongation of the P-R interval is of interest chiefly from a diagnostic standpoint and requires no specific therapy except that required for the underlying clinical state. Second degree A-V heart block is rare during pregnancy.

Complete A-V heart block observed during pregnancy is usually of the congenital variety and only rarely the result of rheumatic fever, diphtheria, or unknown factors. The symptoms may vary from a completely asymptomatic bradycardia to episodes of Stokes-Adams attacks due to ventricular standstill or paroxysmal ventricular tachycardia. Congenital A-V heart block may occur as an isolated finding but usually appears in conjunction with other congenital cardiac lesions (see section on congenital A-V heart block, p. 262). Uncomplicated cases do fairly well throughout pregnancy and usually give birth to live, healthy children. The relatively benign nature of this condition has been repeatedly emphasized (Kenmure and Cameron, 1967); however, those patients with acquired complete A-V heart block are more susceptible to the development of heart failure during pregnancy. In one study, 20 per cent of these patients had heart failure, while only 5 per cent of the patients with congenital complete A-V heart block manifested heart failure (Mendelson, 1956).

There is no specific indication for interruption of pregnancy on the basis of A-V heart block. The indications are those of the underlying cardiovascular state and the presence of heart failure. Cesarean section is advised only if obstetric indications are present, since vaginal delivery has not been associated with any unusual morbidity or mortality.

The treatment of heart block during pregnancy is similar to that in the nonpregnant patient and consists of the administration of isoproterenol for very slow rates, atropine, ephedrine, and so forth. In the presence of marked bradycardia and syncopal attacks, the insertion of cardiac pacemakers is indicated (Berestka and Spellacy, 1967). Two patients with complete A-V heart block in pregnancy whose prior pregnancies were complicated by Stokes-Adams episodes during the second stage of labor have been reported. By the use of a transvenous cardiac pacemaker, their subsequent labors were managed without incident and the patients manifested no postpartum complications (Schonbrun et al., 1966).

Cardiac Arrest. Cardiac arrest is relatively rare during pregnancy. The following possible etiologic factors have been suggested: (a) multiple drug therapy in premedication, (b) the hypotensive influence of tranquilizing agents, (c) prolonged labor, (d) severe anemia, and (e) unreplaced acute blood loss (Gold et al., 1961).

Patients with a serious arrhythmia or hemorrhage who are in a state of shock or who have sustained a myocardial infarction should be admitted into an intensive care facility where they can be carefully watched and where continuous monitoring and resuscitative equipment are readily available. If arrest does occur, treatment includes closed-chest cardiac resuscitation, electrical defibrillation, and drug therapy. Electric countershock has been employed successfully to terminate ventricular fibrillation without any disturbance in the fetal electrocardiogram (Curry and Quintana, 1970).

References

Berestka, S. A., and Spellacy, W. N.: Complete heart block associated with pregnancy and treated with an internal pacemaker. Lancet, 87:461, 1967.

Curry, J. J., and Quintana, F. J.: Myocardial infarction with ventricular fibrillation during pregnancy treated by direct current fibrillation with fetal survival. Chest, 58:82, 1970.

Gold, E. M., Jacobziner, H., Pakter, J., and Stone, M. L.: Cardiac arrest in obstetrics. JAMA, 175:1065, 1961.

Kenmure, A. C. F., and Cameron, A. J. V.: Congenital complete heart block in pregnancy. Brit. Heart J., 29:910, 1967.

McMillan, T. M., and Bellet, S.: Ventricular paroxysmal tachycardia: Report of a case in a pregnant girl of 16 years with apparently normal heart. Amer. Heart J., 7:70, 1931.

Mendelson, C. L.: Disorders of the heart beat during pregnancy. Amer. J. Obstet. Gynec., 72:1268, 1956.

Mendelson, C. L.: Cardiac Disease in Pregnancy. Philadelphia, F. A. Davis, 1960.

Schonbrun, M., Rowland, W., and Quiroz, A. C.: Complete heart block in pregnancy; successful use of an intravenous pacemaker in 2 patients during labor. Obstet. Gynec., 27:243, 1966.

Spritzer, R. C., et al.: Serious arrhythmias during labor and delivery in women with heart disease. JAMA, 211:1005, 1970.

Sussman, H. F., Duque, D., and Lesser, M. E.: Atrial flutter with 1:1 A-V conduction. Dis. Chest, 49:99, 1966.

Vogel, J. H. K., Pryor, R., and Blount, S. G., Jr.: Direct-current defibrillation during pregnancy. JAMA, 193:970, 1965.

Chapter 22 Congenital Cardiac Anomalies

GENERAL CONSIDERATIONS
FAMILIAL OCCURRENCE OF ARRHYTHMIAS
ARRHYTHMIAS IN CONGENITAL HEART DISEASE

Congenital Complete A-V Heart Block
Congenital Partial A-V Heart Block
Other Cardiac Arrhythmias

GENERAL CONSIDERATIONS

The arrhythmias observed in association with congenital cardiac anomalies depend largely on the type of anomaly present. They are due to one or a combination of factors: (a) congenital malformation with disturbance in the normal distribution of the automatic centers and conduction tissue; (b) strain on various chambers of the heart because of septal and valvular defects, with resulting hypertrophy or dilatation of the cardiac chambers (e.g., the right atrium, right ventricle or left ventricle); (c) inflammatory changes with fibrosis; and (d) hypoxia, especially after effort or excitement.

When arrhythmias occur in the presence of serious anomalies, they add to the strain of an already overburdened heart. Therefore, their appearance is serious and the indications for therapy are often urgent. A discussion of the familial occurrence and arrhythmias encountered in congenital cardiac anomalies follows.

FAMILIAL OCCURRENCE OF ARRHYTHMIAS

A familial occurrence of certain arrhythmias has been observed in successive generations. They may appear in conjunction with congenital anomalies or independently of clinical manifestations of their presence. This, however, does not rule out the possible presence of microscopic abnormalities in some of the conduction pathways.

The following arrhythmias occurring independently of demonstrable cardiac anomalies have been observed to have a familial occurrence: (1) sinus tachycardia, (2) atrial fibrillation, (3) paroxysmal atrial tachycardia, (4) junctional tachycardia, and (5) multifocal premature ventricular beats (Harris, 1970). In addition, the familial occurrence of several other arrhythmias has been linked to either a gross or microscopic lesion. These include: (1) bradycardia and Stokes-Adams seizures, (2) impaired atrioventricular conduction, (3) bundle branch block, (4) complete A-V heart block, and (5) sudden death (Harris, 1970). In the families in which A-V conduction disturbances have been reported, varying stages from first degree block to complete block have been observed. The pathologic lesions in these cases vary from well-recognized anomalies (i.e., atrial septal defect) to rare anomalies (e.g., complete absence of the A-V node or hypoplasia of the bundle branches). There does not appear to be a pattern of inheritance common to all familial occurrences of arrhythmias. Each case appears to be individual and the modes of inheritance vary from sex-linked recessive to autosomal dominant.

ARRHYTHMIAS IN CONGENITAL HEART DISEASE

Congenital Complete A-V Heart Block. Among all cases of complete A-V heart block, 8 to 36 per cent are of congenital origin. An underlying congenital origin is often difficult to definitely establish in infants and younger children because of the possibility that an infection (rheumatic, diphtheritic, or the like) is superimposed on a congenital anomaly. The congenital variety of complete A-V heart block may be associated with the following defects: ostium primum, atrial septal defect, congenitally corrected transposition of the great arteries with ventricular inversion, single ventricles, ventricular septal defect (especially if the membranous septum is involved), and single atrium.

In cases in which the conduction system has been studied histologically, congenital or fibrotic disruptions in continuity have been observed between the A-V junction and the bundle of His. In addition, absence of the A-V junction with complete separation of the atria from the bundle of His is stated to have been present in some cases. Complete A-V heart block has also been observed in association with congenital anomalies in which no conduction system studies have been made to date, e.g., congenital aneurysm of the pars membranacea, tricuspid atresia, mitral atresia, aortic stenosis or atresia, tetralogy of Fallot, Eisenmenger's syndrome, bicuspid aortic valve with sclerosis and calcification, fibroelastosis, and fetal coarctation. In rare instances, normally formed but enlarged hearts have been the seat of congenital heart block.

The clinical manifestations vary with the heart rate and associated cardiac lesions. There may be no symptoms associated with these lesions in isolated cases. Following exertion or crying spells, a transient right-to-left shunt may occur in those cases in which a septal defect exists. This may result in the precipitation of syncopal or convulsive episodes secondary to cerebral hypoxia. The ventricular rate in congenital complete A-V heart block varies with the age of the patient. In infancy, it may range from below 50 to 80 per minute; in early childhood, from 50 to 60 per minute. In young children, a slow rhythm under 70 per minute should suggest the possibility of congenital complete A-V heart block, particularly if the rhythm accompanying the slow rate is regular. The effect of exercise and atropine upon the heart rate of children differs from that usually seen in adults with complete A-V heart block in that a slight acceleration of 10 to 20 beats per minute is more apt to occur in children than in adults (see pp. 124 to 139 for complete discussion) (Fig. 22-1).

The following diagnostic criteria have been established for the diagnosis of complete A-V heart block of congenital origin: (a) bradycardia noted at an early age; (b) absence of history of infectious disease that might otherwise explain the heart block; (c) A-V heart block proved by graphic methods in a young person; and (d) the presence of congenital cardiac anomaly or syncopal attacks during childhood.

The differential diagnosis involves particularly the presence of persistent slow heart rates. A sinus bradycardia and partial A-V block (2:1, 3:1) may be ruled out by the electrocardiogram. The differentiation between acquired and congenital complete heart block may sometimes be quite difficult; however, the aforementioned criteria,

CONGENITAL CARDIAC ANOMALIES

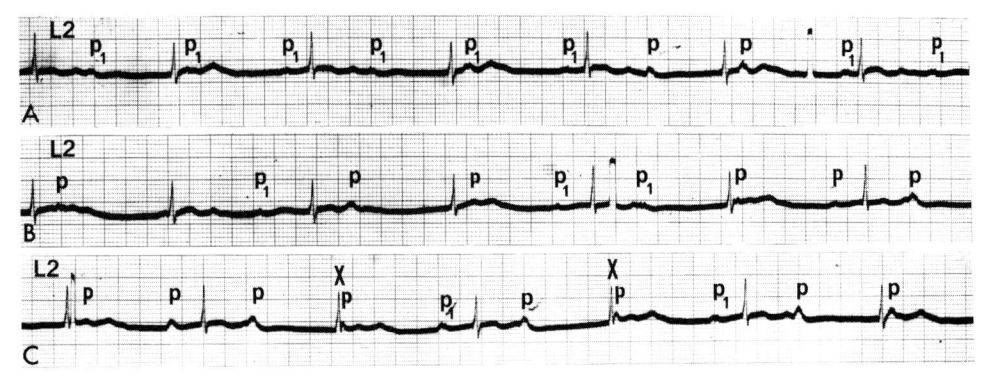

Figure 22-1. Complete A-V heart block from a 13-year-old male subject with congenital heart disease. Note the narrow QRS width, the regular ventricular rate of 47 per minute, and the atrial rate of 72 per minute. There is no relationship between the atrial and ventricular rhythms. The P-P intervals are slightly irregular; the cycle lengths of the P waves including the QRS are shorter than those between the QRS complexes (ventriculophasic sinus arrhythmia). Two types of P waves are observed: P and P_1, indicating an origin from the different foci.

In C, the QRS complexes marked at X, are probably the result of impulses due to slightly different activation of the A-V junction as compared to the control.

particularly the electrocardiogram, may be extremely helpful. The ventricular rate in congenital heart block is generally 40 to 80 beats per minute and the QRS complex is usually supraventricular in form. This would indicate that the dominant impulse center is located above the bifurcation of the bundle of His and that the excitatory process propagates through the ventricular myocardium in a relatively normal sequence.

The treatment of congenital complete A-V heart block is discussed on page 270. The prognosis depends on the type (nodal or an idioventricular origin), the heart rate, its reaction to exercise, associated congenital anomalies, and the incidence of Stokes-Adams seizures. The prognosis is good in the presence of narrow QRS complexes with a ventricular rate of 40 to 60 per minute which increases with exercise. It is poor in infants in whom the ventricular rate is very slow (<36 per minute). In a series of 192 patients with congenital complete A-V heart block, the greatest risk of death was observed to occur during the first six months of life. Furthermore, of the 30 deaths in the series, 22 were associated with congenital cardiac anomalies that contributed directly to death. The natural history of congenital complete A-V heart block has been improved by cardiac surgery (in the presence of an identifiable anomaly) and by pacemakers (in the presence of heart failure or Stokes-Adams attacks) (Engle et al., 1970).

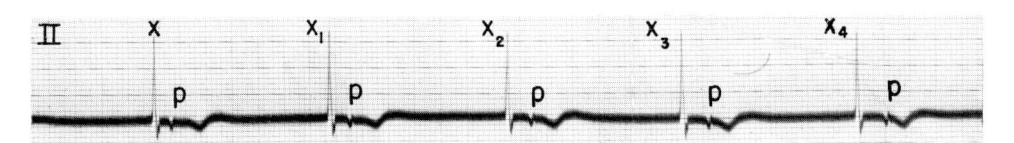

Figure 22-2. A-V junctional rhythm with retrograde conduction. From a seven-year-old child with congenital cardiac anomaly. Note the inverted P waves following the QRS complexes, with the gradually increasing R-P intervals (0.14 at X, 0.15 at X_1, 0.18 at X_2, 0.20 at X_3, 0.21 at X_4). The ventricular rate is 44 per minute.

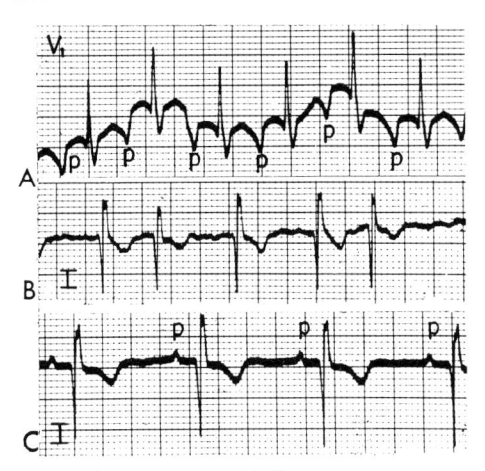

Figure 22-3. Atrial flutter occurring in a child, age 6, with tetralogy of Fallot. Conversion to normal sinus rhythm.

(A) (V₁). Note the presence of atrial flutter with a 2:1 A-V conduction. The ventricular rate is 130 per minute and the atrial rate is 260 per minute. (B) (Lead I). Shows conversion to atrial fibrillation by digitalis. (C) (Lead I). Shows restoration of normal sinus rhythm.

Congenital Partial A-V Heart Block. Prolongation of the A-V conduction time (P-R interval) is relatively common in association with certain congenital heart lesions. The association of prolonged P-R interval with ostium primum defects is common. An increased P-R interval is also found in association with an ostium secundum defect (about 10 per cent), patent ductus arteriosus (10 to 20 per cent), Ebstein's anomaly (25 per cent), severe pulmonary stenosis (30 per cent), complete transposition with ventricular inversion (75 per cent), double outlet right ventricle and high pulmonary blood flow (60 per cent), adult type coarctation (10 per cent), and ventricular septal defect (15 per cent) (Burch and DePasquale, 1967).

Other Cardiac Arrhythmias. Premature beats, atrial flutter, atrial fibrillation, and junctional rhythms have been reported at an early age due to anatomic lesions or indirect effects (hypoxia or atrial and ventricular strain). Precipitation of a rapid heart rate in a patient with a congenital anomaly imposes a serious additional burden on the heart (Figs. 22-2, 22-3).

The Wolff-Parkinson-White syndrome may be associated with a congenital cardiac anomaly, and it may lead to paroxysmal atrial tachycardia and occasionally atrial fibrillation. This syndrome is associated most commonly with Ebstein's anomaly. It has also been reported in conjunction with subaortic stenosis and corrected transposition of the great arteries with ventricular inversion (Burch and DePasquale, 1967) and rarely accompanying complete transposition with ventricular septal defect.

Atrial fibrillation is uncommon with congenital heart disease, except with atrial septal defect. It is observed in 20 per cent of patients with large atrial septal defects. In these cases, atrial fibrillation correlates well with elevation of the left atrial pressure, left atrial enlargement, and the patient's age.

References

Amarasingham, R., and Fleming, H. A.: Congenital heart disease with arrhythmia in a family. Brit. Heart J., 29:78, 1967.

Bacos, J. M., Eagan, J. T., and Orgain, E. S.: Congenital familial nodal rhythm. Circulation, 22:887, 1960.

Bizarro, R. O., et al.: Familial atrial septal defect with prolonged atrioventricular conduction. A syndrome showing the autosomal dominant pattern of inheritance. Circulation, 41: 677, 1970.

Burch, G. E., and DePasquale, N. P.: Electrocardiography in the Diagnosis of Congenital Heart Disease. Philadelphia, Lea & Febiger, 1967.

Engle, M. A., Ehlers, K. H., and Frand, M.: Natural history of a congenital complete heart block, a cooperative study. Circulation, 41–42:III–112, 1970.

Gazes, P. C., Culler, R. M., Taber, E., and Kelly, T. E.: Congenital familial cardiac conduction defects. Circulation, 32:32, 1965.

Harris, W.: The cardiovascular system. In Goodman, R. M. (ed.): Genetic Disorders of Man. Boston, Little, Brown & Co., 1970. pp. 219–222.

Kahler, R. L., Braunwald, E., Plauth, W. H., Jr.,

and Morrow, A. G.: Familial congenital heart disease. Amer. J. Med., *40*:384, 1966.

Khorsandian, R. S., Moghadam, A., and Muller, O. F.: Familial congenital A-V dissociation. Amer. J. Cardiol., *14*:118, 1964.

Morquio, L.: Sur une maladie infantile et familiale caracterisee par des modifications permanentes du pouls, des modifications syncopales et epileptiformes. Arch. Med. Enf., *4*:467, 1901.

Paul, M. H., Rudolph, A. M., and Nadas, A. S.: Congenital complete atrioventricular block: Problems of clinical assessment. Circulation, *18*:183, 1958.

Tikoff, G., Schmidt, A. M., and Hecht, H. H.: Atrial fibrillation in atrial septal defect. Arch. Intern. Med., *121*:402, 1968.

Tsagaris, T. V., Bustamante, R. A., and Friesendorff, R. A.: Familial heart disease. Dis. Chest., *52*:153, 1967.

Wallgren, G., and Agorio, E.: Congenital complete A-V block in three siblings. Acta paediat., *49*:49, 1960.

Chapter 23 Arrhythmias in Infants, Children, and in the Fetus

GENERAL CONSIDERATIONS
ETIOLOGY AND INCIDENCE
ARRHYTHMIAS ENCOUNTERED IN
  INFANCY AND CHILDHOOD
  Premature Beats
  Paroxysmal Tachycardia
  Atrial Flutter
  Atrial Fibrillation
  A-V Heart Block
  Cardiac Arrest

ELECTROCARDIOGRAMS OF THE FETUS
  General Considerations
  Arrhythmias Encountered in the Fetus
CARDIO-AUDITORY SYNDROME
  General Considerations
  Genetic Factors
  Clinical Findings
  Electrocardiogram
  Therapy
  Prognosis

GENERAL CONSIDERATIONS

Abnormalities of rhythm are not uncommon in infancy and childhood, but they differ in many respects from those observed in adults. The principal differences are related to etiology, the less stable autonomic system of childhood, and the greater facility of conduction through the A-V junction at high rates. In addition, the types of arrhythmias, their incidence, course, prognosis, and therapeutic regimen differ somewhat from those encountered in adults.

One may observe the following: sinus arrhythmia; S-A heart block; premature beats; shifting pacemaker from the S-A to the A-V node (this occurs rather commonly when the vagus is unusually active); atrial tachycardia and atrial flutter; arrhythmias arising in the A-V junction or the bundle of His; various grades of A-V heart block (partial and complete), although the higher degrees of block are less frequently encountered (Keith et al., 1967).

Although the therapeutic measures employed are similar, the response often differs. In our experience, infants and children demonstrate a less predictable and less satisfactory response to therapy than adults. The proper use of digitalis, quinidine, procaine amide, and more recently, lidocaine and propranolol form the basis of successful therapy (see Chapters 32 to 34). Recently, synchronized direct current countershock has been increasingly used to terminate tachyarrhythmias in infants and children and is now considered an accepted type of current therapy (White and Humphries, 1967).

ETIOLOGY AND INCIDENCE

The important etiologic factors are congenital and rheumatic heart disease, viral infections, malnutrition, and neurogenic disturbances. Head trauma and cardiac surgery or catheterization are occasional factors. A frequent association has been observed between neonatal arrhythmias and mothers who are elderly primiparas (Lundberg, 1963). Toxic digitalis effects play a minor role and the degenerative states, including hypertension and coronary artery disease, of such prime importance in the genesis of arrhythmias in adults, are virtually absent.

As in adults, the causative factor is not definitely ascertainable in a large number of instances. Evidence of abnormalities in function and structure may, however, become more apparent as the individual grows older. Furthermore, other etiologic factors may appear and assume prominence in later decades.

Since many cases pass unrecognized, the incidence of arrhythmias is probably greater than the data presently available would indicate. In fact, rapid ectopic rhythms are probably one of the important unrecognized causes of sudden death in infants and children. Long-term monitoring, commonly employed in adults in intensive care units, has only recently been used in infants and children, except under special circumstances in a hospital setting. Where the electrocardiograms of infants and children have been monitored over long periods, a significantly higher incidence of arrhythmias has been observed (Morgan and Guntheroth, 1965) (see below).

ARRHYTHMIAS ENCOUNTERED IN INFANCY AND CHILDHOOD

Premature Beats. The three main types of premature beats—atrial, junctional, and ventricular—are observed. They are not common in infancy and childhood and usually have little clinical significance. If premature ectopic beats occur in a child demonstrating no untoward symptoms, treatment usually is not necessary since the condition will probably rectify itself as the child grows older. When the ectopic beats occur frequently, therapy directed to the abolition of the arrhythmia is indicated in addition to treatment of the underlying clinical state. This may include the administration of quinidine or procaine amide. (Fig. 23–1)

Paroxysmal Tachycardia. Although paroxysmal tachycardia is relatively infrequent, it is probably the most common type of rapid heart action en-

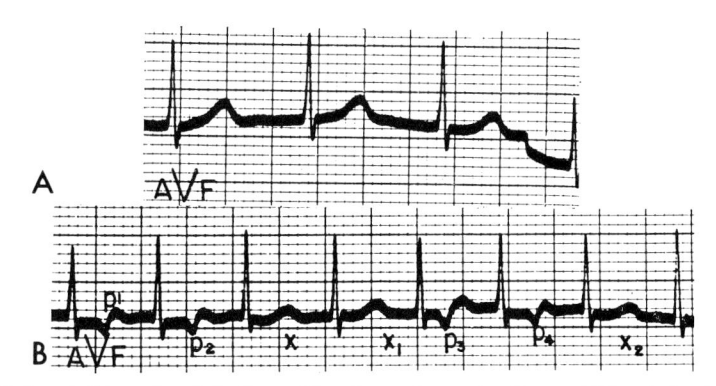

Figure 23–1. A-V junctional rhythm with retrograde conduction and Wenckebach phenomenon, taken from a child, 2½ years of age.

(A) The cardiac rate is 100 per minute. Note the absence of P waves, probably the result of an A-V junctional rhythm.

(B) Note the absence of P waves in cycles X, X_1, and X_2. Note the retrograde P waves (P_1, P_2, P_3, and P_4). These are due to retrograde conduction in the presence of a "lower" A-V junctional rhythm. The R-P interval is short in the cycle with P_3 and longer with P_4 (Wenckebach phenomenon, so-called reverse Wenckebach).

countered in the newborn or in young children. The most common types of paroxysmal tachycardia encountered are those of supraventricular origin, usually paroxysmal atrial tachycardia, atrial flutter and rarely those of a junctional origin. A ventricular origin is rare; as in adults, a positive diagnosis is difficult to establish unless encountered during cardiac catheterization or cardiac surgery (Fig. 23-2). As a result of physiologic differences in the A-V junction of children as compared to adults, supraventricular tachycardias of infants and children with atrial rates of as high as 300 will usually be conducted through an efficient A-V junction with resulting 1:1 ventricular response.

The etiology of these tachyarrhythmias is similar to that mentioned for arrhythmias in general. In this age group more specific factors include cardiac catheterization, surgery, certain drugs such as digitalis, anesthetic agents, and tumors in and around the heart (especially in the region of the S-A node and the A-V junction). The W-P-W syndrome is not rare in infants (Gleckler and Lay, 1952).

About 10 per cent of the cases manifest no symptoms, the tachycardia being discovered only during routine physical examination. However, the majority, especially the very young infants, appear quite ill; their color is often ashen gray, their skin is cold and damp, and cyanosis is frequently present. The infant is usually restless and irritable, and the respirations are rapid and labored. At times, a hacking cough may appear and the abdomen may be distended. Fever may be present, but this usually indicates the existence of an infection that may have actually initiated the arrhythmia, or it may result from congestive failure with complicating pneumonitis. The clinical picture may closely resemble a severe pneumonia or septicemia. The heart is usually enlarged, and transient functional murmurs may appear. Congestive failure, although infrequent in adults, is a relatively common complication of paroxysmal atrial tachycardia in children.

Often the paroxysms end spontaneously. An initial attempt to bring the rate to normal may be made by carotid sinus pressure. Digitalis is the drug of choice in infants and children; it is successful in terminating 80 per cent of episodes (Keith et al., 1967). The most commonly employed digitalis preparation in pediatric use is oral digoxin. The digitalizing dose in infants under one year of age is 0.04 mg./lb. of body weight. One-half the

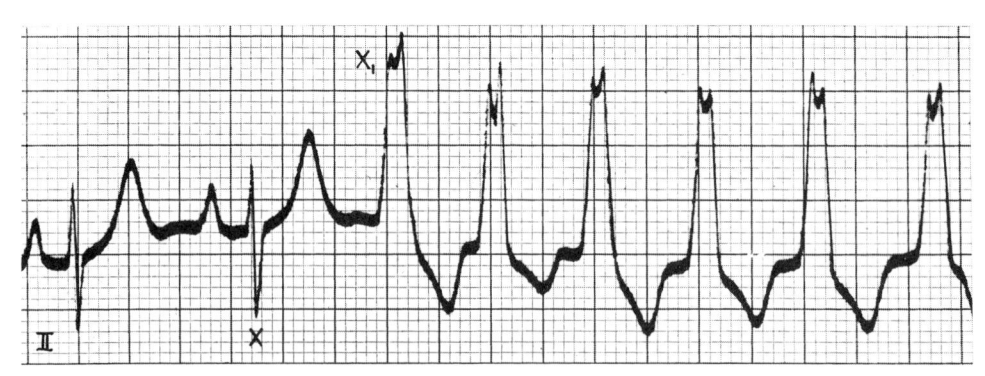

Figure 23-2. Ventricular tachycardia (Lead II). Taken from a child six years of age during right heart catheterization. Note the normal cycle at X and the paroxysm of ventricular tachycardia starting at X_1. During the paroxysm the QRS complexes are widened and notched and are followed by inverted T waves.

calculated dose is given initially, followed by one-quarter dose at two consecutive four- to six-hour intervals.

Quinidine and procaine amide seem to be particularly effective in the treatment of supraventricular as well as ventricular tachycardias. The dose of quinidine must be determined by clinical trial; the usual dosage in children is 3 mg./lb. of body weight every two hours for four to five doses or until the tachycardia stops. Maintenance of careful clinical and electrocardiographic observation is advisable in order to prevent serious toxic effects. Procaine amide hydrochloride may be administered intramuscularly, but rarely intravenously, with constant electrocardiographic monitoring. Propranolol is often efficacious in the therapy of paroxysmal tachycardias that have proven refractory to digitalis. It is particularly effective in the treatment of digitalis-induced arrhythmias. Successful conversion of various paroxysmal tachycardias to normal sinus rhythm have been observed in infants and children.

Atrial Flutter. Atrial flutter is rare in the pediatric age group. Etiologic factors include upper respiratory infections and other infections, diphtheria, pertussis, pneumonia, and bronchitis associated with otitis media. The manifestations of atrial flutter vary greatly; however, they are generally similar to those of the paroxysmal tachycardia. The occurrence of this arrhythmia in association with congenital heart disease presents a serious complication. The diagnosis is suspected clinically by the presence of a tachycardia (rate of 200 to 350 per minute) and is definitely established by finding characteristic F waves in the electrocardiogram.

Electrical countershock is the therapy of choice in children as in adults. Digitalis is successful in slowing the ventricular rate and abolishing the flutter only in approximately a third of cases (Keith et al., 1967).

Atrial Fibrillation. Atrial fibrillation, which is not uncommon in adults, is infrequent in infants and children. When it is present it is almost always associated with a severe grade of myocardial disease. The most important etiologic factors are rheumatic heart disease (atrial fibrillation occurs in 1 to 2 per cent of cases) (Paul, 1966); digitalis intoxication; hypopotassemia; congenital heart disease, especially with interatrial septal defects; thyrotoxicosis (Keith et al., 1967); and tumors of the atria.

Treatment usually entails full digitalization, followed by quinidine in an attempt toward conversion to normal sinus rhythm. In refractory cases or where conversion is considered urgent, direct current countershock should be employed (White and Humphries, 1967) and quinidine used to maintain normal sinus rhythm after conversion.

The onset of this arrhythmia in children frequently carries ominous prognostic implications. In one group, the average survival after onset of atrial fibrillation was eight months in children between 9 and 12 years of age and 30 months in the adolescents (Gibson, 1941).

A-V Heart Block. A-V conduction disturbances are apparently not uncommon in infants and children (Ayers et al., 1966; Nakamura and Nadas, 1964). The normal upper limit for the P-R interval varies from 0.14 second in infancy to 0.18 second in adolescence. Prolongation of the P-R interval beyond this range constitutes first degree A-V heart block (see page 121).

First degree heart block is commonly found in association with rheumatic heart disease, occasionally with diphtheria, and in association with some types of congenital heart disease, including patent ductus arteriosus, atrial septal defect, Ebstein's anomaly, and corrected transposition of the great vessels. Second degree A-V heart block may be seen in similar conditions and also after the intracardiac trauma of surgical repair of atrial or ventricular septal defects, with hypoxia, and with digitalis intoxication.

Complete or third degree A-V heart block most commonly has a congenital etiology, although it has also been noted in association with viral myocarditis (Nakamura and Nadas, 1964) and diphtheria and following cardiac surgery, especially with correction of an interventricular septal defect. Intrauterine infection has been suggested as a causative factor in some cases of congenital complete heart block.

The clinical manifestations depend on the underlying etiology, the severity of the block, and the associated cardiovascular state. The manifestations of first and second degree heart block are those of the underlying etiology. The course and prognosis depend on the etiology, the site of the block in the A-V junction, the cardiac adaptation to stress, and the occurrence of Stokes-Adams attacks which are usually rare (see Chapter 10) (Nakamura and Nadas, 1964).

The therapy depends on the underlying cause and clinical manifestations. Heart failure should be treated by administration of isoproterenol and diuretics. This by itself will improve the cardiac state and often abolish heart failure. An artificial pacemaker may be indicated (see Chapter 37). Although digitalis may be administered in small doses, it may be given with greater impunity after pacemaker insertion. Stokes-Adams attacks may be treated initially with isoproterenol or ephedrine to increase cardiac automaticity. During an attack, a vigorous thump on the precordium frequently restores cardiac beating.

Cardiac Arrest. Cardiac arrest arises nearly three times as frequently in infants as in all other age groups (Rackow et al., 1961). Because infants and children possess a high degree of vagal tone, they are apt to develop episodes of cardiac slowing accompanied by sinus pauses. Thus, surgery and anesthesia in infants are not uncommonly complicated by cardiac arrest. Emergency therapy in infants consists of closed-chest cardiac compression with both thumbs pressing on the midsternum. Flexing the lower extremities upon the chest has frequently been successful in cardiac resuscitation in infants and children. Older children may be treated with cardiac compression techniques similar to those used in adults (see page 217). Mouth-to-mouth ventilation should be applied simultaneously until positive pressure respiration is instituted. When these techniques are employed in the early stages before the occurrence of prolonged hypoxia, recovery with little or no neurologic impairment should result.

ELECTROCARDIOGRAMS OF THE FETUS

General Considerations. Fetal electrocardiography represents an objective method of studying the developing heart in the fetus. The key factors facilitating progress in this area are a combination of improved instrumentation and improved biophysical techniques. Although still largely in a developmental stage, fetal electrocardiography has already furnished the cardiologist and obstetrician with an invaluable tool in the diagnosis of cardiac arrhythmia in the fetus before and during labor. Furthermore, the fetal electrocardiogram can help to reveal the presence of congenital heart disease and to determine whether a fetal malformation has occurred during the course of a maternal illness or infection.

With present techniques, the earliest demonstration of the fetal electrocardiogram has been at 11 weeks. Many other successful recordings have been made at 12, 13, and 14 weeks, and increasing numbers at later peri-

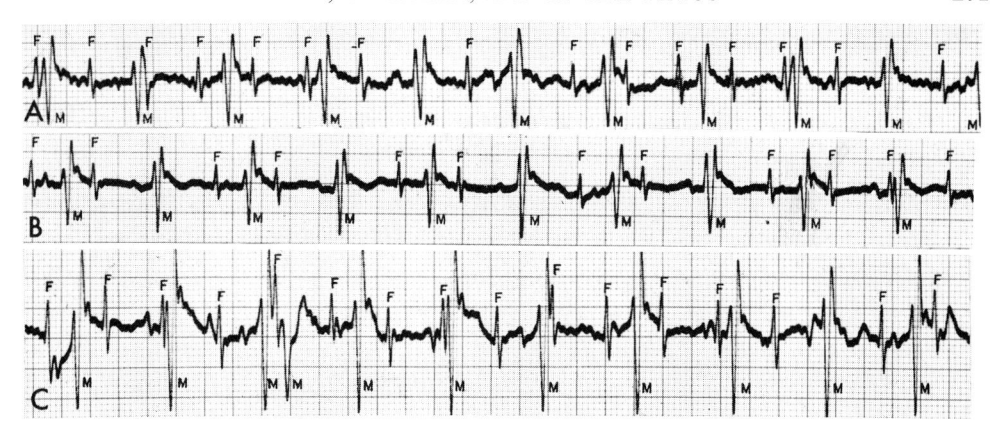

ARRHYTHMIAS IN INFANTS, CHILDREN, AND IN THE FETUS 271

Figure 23-3. Fetal electrocardiogram. The maternal heart rate (M) is 92 per minute and the fetal heart rate (F) is 140 to 160 per minute. Note that the fetal beats are easily distinguishable from the maternal beats. Note 3:2 "synchronization" of both rhythms in B (every third F buried in M). (This tracing was taken by the technique of radioelectrocardiography—see Chapter 20.)

ods of gestation. The fetal electrocardiogram in the human is recorded through the intact maternal abdomen. A telemetering technique has been used with which 99.1 per cent positive tests have been obtained (Kendall et al., 1962). The percentage of positives, i.e., the accuracy of the fetal electrocardiogram, increases rapidly after the seventeenth week until at about 22 weeks the peak is reached with very nearly 100 per cent positives (Fig. 23-3). At present, positive records cannot dependably be obtained with a living fetus of less than 22 weeks.

Arrhythmias Encountered in the Fetus. Transient bradycardias as low as 70 beats per minute or transient tachycardias up to 200 per minute are observed occasionally during the period of gestation and during labor (Figs. 23-4, 23-5). A-V junctional

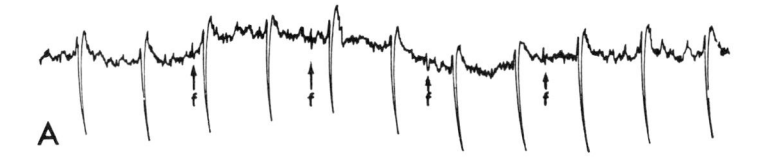

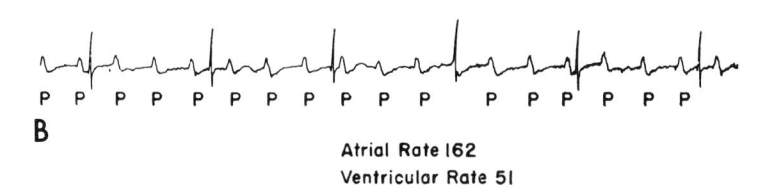

Atrial Rate 162
Ventricular Rate 51

Figure 23-4. Antenatal diagnosis of complete heart block with the fetal electrocardiogram. (A) Fetal electrocardiogram showing fetal complexes occurring at a slow fixed rate, slower than the maternal rate.
(B) The newborn electrocardiogram confirms the existence of heart block, showing complete A-V dissociation. (From Larks, S. D.: Fetal Electrocardiography: The Electrical Activity of the Fetal Heart, 1961. Courtesy of Charles C Thomas, Publisher, Springfield, Illinois.)

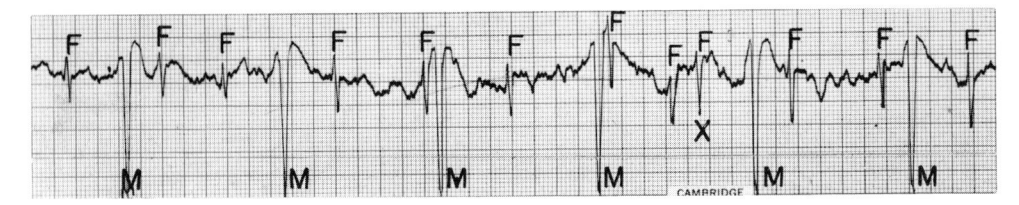

Figure 23-5. Fetal electrocardiogram showing premature beats. This tracing was taken during the eighth month of pregnancy (F, fetal; M, maternal). The patient gave birth to a normal child and there was no evidence of abnormality or ectopic rhythm thereafter. The maternal heart rate is 43 per minute with a regular rhythm. The fetal rhythm is slightly irregular and the rate is about 72 per minute. Note premature beats preceding X. (This tracing was taken by the technique of radioelectrocardiography—see Chapter 20.)

escape rhythm has been observed in the fetus during periods of sinus bradycardia. Paroxysmal tachycardia of supraventricular origin with heart rates ranging from 210 to 240 beats per minute has been observed (Urbach et al., 1966). Atrial fibrillation occurs only rarely in the fetus; however, it carries an extremely serious prognosis (Urbach et al., 1966). It is believed to be a primary factor in the death of the fetus.

Figure 23-4 demonstrates a case of complete A-V heart block as diagnosed prenatally with the fetal electrocardiogram. Various degrees of A-V block in the fetus occur most commonly during periods of vagal stimulation. There is evidence to suggest that A-V block occurs normally in the fetus during vagal stimulation but may be indicative of congenital heart disease when it is sustained.

Bradycardia alone or in association with other fetal cardiac arrhythmias and tachycardia, in addition to alterations in the S-T segments and T waves of the fetal electrocardiogram, have been considered ominous signs.

CARDIO-AUDITORY SYNDROME

General Considerations. The cardio-auditory syndrome, also called the surdo-cardiac syndrome, presents a characteristic set of signs and symptoms with onset in infancy and childhood. These subjects suffer from congenital deafness and attacks of syncope (Stokes-Adams attacks) or milder episodes resembling angina pectoris. Two types have been described: (1) marked Q-T prolongation and deafness occurring in subjects with clinically normal hearts (most common); and (2) Q-T prolongation and deafness occurring in subjects with congenital heart disease. In addition, a third very similar syndrome has been described in children and adults with no auditory impairment. These latter patients have a tendency to develop paroxysmal ventricular fibrillation.

Genetic Factors. The cardio-auditory syndrome appears to be an autosomal recessive trait which occurs more commonly in situations of parental consanguinity. The syndrome without deafness is thought to be transmitted as a dominant trait (Barlow et al., 1964).

Clinical Findings. Approximately 20 cases of cardio-auditory syndrome have been reported. Most have been in females ranging in age from infancy to 12 years of age at the time of onset. Its initial appearance in adult life has also been described (James, 1967). The most common types associated with deafness characteristically developed their initial syncopal attacks in infancy and childhood. They suffered from repeated brief episodes and in many instances experienced a lessening of symptoms with increasing age (Jervell et al., 1966).

Various degrees of syncopal attacks have been observed: (a) episodes without loss of consciousness; (b) those with loss of consciousness and recovery; and (c) those terminating fatally. Mild attacks without loss of consciousness may cause the child to sit quietly, in evident pain, and hold his chest, mimicking an anginal episode.

In the series by Garza et al. (1969), four factors appeared capable of precipitating attacks which ended in death: (1) an increase in systemic blood pressure with pressure-induced extrasystoles; (2) increase in serum potassium; (3) an early extrasystole (R on T syndrome); and (4) sinus tachycardia when the sinus impulse reaches the ventricles still in a depolarized state.

Electrocardiogram. The electrocardiogram shows characteristic findings. The Q-T interval is prolonged often to a considerable degree; however, the prolongation may be transient. The Q-T interval is further prolonged by exercise, epinephrine, and quinidine and tends to decrease following digitalization. Sinus pauses have been noted in some cases (James, 1967). The T wave may be abnormal; it may be negative in lead I and aVL; diphasic in the precordial leads; and bizarre, often of considerable amplitude in leads II, III, aVF, V_1, V_2, and V_3. The T waves vary in appearance from one examination to another and usually become more abnormal with exercise.

Therapy. To date, therapy has generally proven unsatisfactory. Digitalis has been given to shorten the Q-T interval, but it is doubtful whether it has any actual effect on the other manifestations, and it may prove dangerous because it produces ventricular premature beats (James, 1969). Propranolol has been suggested to suppress the syncopal episodes; however, it also may predispose to the development of premature beats by producing a sinus bradycardia. Sympathomimetic drugs aggravate the condition. A stress-free life is recommended because of the tendency for excitement or fright to precipitate the episodes. Because of this association, James has proposed the investigation of drugs known to suppress paroxysmal discharges from the central nervous system as well as to decrease cardiac automaticity, particularly phenobarbital and diphenylhydantoin (James, 1969). Children with repeated syncopal attacks have been treated by pacemaker implantation, but this procedure is relatively unsatisfactory because of the age of the patients and the danger (because of the long Q-T interval) of a pacemaker impulse falling in the vulnerable period.

Prognosis. The prognosis is poor; seven of 18 reported cases have died between the ages of three and 14. In the cases with unimpaired hearing, the prognosis appears to be similar; however, some patients have survived to the fourth and fifth decade.

References

Ayers, C. R., Boineau, J. P., and Spach, M. D.: Congenital complete heart block in children. Amer. Heart J., 72:381, 1966.

Barlow, J. B., Bosman, C. K., and Cochrane, J. W. C.: Congenital cardiac arrhythmias. Lancet, 2:531, 1964.

Cohen, L. S., Samet, P., and Yeh, B. K.: Analysis of A-V conduction in children using His bundle electrograms. Circulation, 41-42: III-80, 1970.

Garza, L. A., et al.: Familial repolarization myocardiopathy. Amer. J. Cardiol., 23:112, 1969.

Gibson, S.: Auricular fibrillation in childhood and adolescence. JAMA, 117:96, 1941.

Gleckler, W. J., and Lay, J. V. M.: Wolff-Parkinson-White syndrome and paroxysmal tachycardia in infancy. JAMA, 150:683, 1952.

James, T. N.: Congenital deafness and cardiac arrhythmias. Amer. J. Cardiol., 19:627, 1967.

James, T. N.: QT prolongation and sudden death. Mod. Conc. Cardiov. Dis., 38:35, 1969.

Jervell, A., and Lange-Nielsen, F.: Congenital deaf-mutism, functional heart disease with prolongation of the Q-T interval, and sudden death. Amer. Heart J., 54:59, 1957.

Jervell, A., Thingstad, R., and Endsjo, T.: The Surdo-cardiac syndrome. Three new cases of congenital deafness with syncopal attacks and Q-T prolongation in the electrocardiogram. Amer. Heart J., 72:582, 1966.

Keith, J. D., Rowe, R. D., and Vlad, P.: Heart Disease in Infancy and Childhood, 2nd ed. New York, Macmillan, 1967. pp. 1049–1075.

Kendall, B., Farrell, D. M., and Kane, H. A.: Fetal radioelectrocardiography: A new method of fetal electrocardiography. Amer. J. Obstet. Gynec., 83:1629, 1962.

Lundberg, A.: Neonatal asphyxia with atrial flutter. Acta Pediat., 52:531, 1963.

Morgan, B. D., and Guntheroth, W. G.: Cardiac arrhythmias in normal newborn infants. J. Pediat., 67:1199, 1965.

Nakamura, F. F., and Nadas, A. S.: Complete heart block in infants and children. New Eng. J. Med., 270:1261, 1964.

Paul, M. H.: Cardiac arrhythmias in infants and children. Prog. Cardiov. Dis., 9:136, 1966.

Rackow, H., Salanitre, E., and Green, L. T.: Frequency of cardiac arrest associated with anesthesia in infants and children. Pediatrics, 28:697, 1961.

Urbach, J. R., Zweizig, H. Z., Loveland, M. W., and Lambert, R. L.: Monitoring of fetal and neonatal arrhythmias. In Dreifus, L. S., Likoff, W., and Moyer, J. H.: Mechanisms and Therapy of Cardiac Arrhythmias. New York, Grune and Stratton, 1966.

White, R. I., Jr., and Humphries, J. O'N.: Direct current electroshock in the treatment of supraventricular arrhythmias. J. Pediat., 70:119, 1967.

Chapter 24 *Endocrine Disturbances*

THYROID DISEASE
  Hyperthyroidism
  Myxedema
HYPER- AND HYPOPARATHYROIDISM

HYPOGLYCEMIA
ADRENAL DYSFUNCTION
  Addison's Disease
HEMOCHROMATOSIS

Endocrine disorders produce their effect by hypo- and hyperactivity. Discussed in this chapter are those endocrine disorders most commonly observed to be associated clinically with arrhythmias. Of these disorders, the most important is thyroid heart disease. Others discussed briefly in this section include adrenal dysfunction, acromegaly, and parathyroid disorders. Some of these arrhythmias are the result of indirect effects on the autonomic nervous system and electrolyte imbalance.

THYROID DISEASE

Hyperthyroidism. The most frequently observed arrhythmia in hyperthyroidism is sinus tachycardia in which the rate ranges from 130 to 170 beats per minute. Atrial fibrillation, however, is the most important of the arrhythmias observed in hyperthyroidism. In one series of 402 cases (Dratchinskaja and Andrejeva, 1956), it appeared in 43 (10.7 per cent). Atrial fibrillation observed in this state possesses the following characteristics: (a) although it may be paroxysmal in the early stages of the disease, it is usually of the established form during the thyrotoxic state; (b) the ventricular rate is rapid and does not respond as well to the effects of digitalis as that of euthyroid patients; and (c) it usually disappears spontaneously as the thyroid state returns to normal.

The following are possible mechanisms for the atrial fibrillation of hyperthyroidism: (a) the thyroid hormone causes an increase in the rate by direct action; (b) increased atrial excitability has been related to increased oxygen consumption and the increased basal metabolism in the atria; and (c) augmented venous return to the heart may result in mechanical stimulation of the atrial muscle surrounding the entrance to the great veins.

Atrial flutter is seen much less commonly but has the same significance as atrial fibrillation. Other atrial arrhythmias, such as atrial premature beats or paroxysmal atrial tachycardia, are infrequently observed. Ventricular arrhythmias are uncommon in hyperthyroidism.

Some hyperthyroid patients manifest a prolonged P-R interval; however, most return to normal A-V conduction when they are euthyroid (Busnardo and Carenza, 1968; Rosenblum and Delman, 1963). This P-R prolongation may be related to a selective localization of thyroid hormone in the A-V conduction system (as has been demonstrated in thyrotoxic experimental animals), exerting a direct

275

toxic effect on this tissue (Busnardo and Carenza, 1968).

Upon reduction of the hyperthyroidism or restoration of the euthyroid state, atrial fibrillation often spontaneously reverts to normal rhythm. Thus, this should be the primary therapeutic goal. The ventricular rate in atrial fibrillation due to thyrotoxicosis responds poorly to digitalis. A dosage higher than that ordinarily required in the euthyroid state is necessary to slow the ventricular rate. Quinidine is usually ineffective in converting atrial fibrillation to normal rhythm in the hyperthyroid state. However, if the atrial fibrillation persists in the euthyroid state, the ventricular rate usually shows a good response to digitalis, and quinidine is again effective in restoring the rhythm to normal.

Myxedema. Arrhythmias are only occasionally observed in myxedema. The heart rate is usually slow. The P-R interval is at the upper normal limits and is occasionally prolonged to about 0.30 second or longer; this prolongation may persist or disappear following thyroid therapy. Complete A-V heart block has also been reported. Other arrhythmias, i.e., paroxysmal atrial fibrillation, flutter, and tachycardia, as well as junctional tachycardia have been observed in myxedema. Usually, all of these arrhythmias revert to normal sinus rhythm after treatment of the thyroid disease.

HYPER- AND HYPOPARATHYROIDISM

The parathyroids function as the primary hormonal regulators of body calcium. Therefore, the electrocardiographic changes that accompany hyperparathyroidism are essentially those that arise with hypercalcemia. Conversely, the changes accompanying hypoparathyroidism are those arising from hypocalcemia (see Chapter 29).

HYPOGLYCEMIA

Hypoglycemia is a relatively uncommon but important cause of ectopic rhythms. Some of the important causes of hypoglycemia include: (a) excessive doses of insulin in diabetics; (b) spontaneous hypoglycemia due to lack of food intake or endocrine disturbances; and (c) the rare type due to a tumor of the islets of Langerhans.

In the younger age groups with normal hearts, the occurrence of ectopic rhythms is relatively infrequent and appears only after large doses of insulin, as for example, during insulin shock therapy (Bellet et al., 1939). However, in elderly diabetic patients with clinical evidence of coronary arteriosclerosis or angina pectoris, rather alarming symptoms may be observed with hypoglycemia (Soskin et al., 1933). The following changes in rhythm are noted: (a) striking sinus arrhythmia; (b) premature beats (atrial, ventricular, and junctional in origin); and (c) atrial fibrillation. These changes tend to return to normal after glucose administration.

Recently, Read and Doherty (1969) administered 0.3 units/Kg. of regular insulin as part of a Hollander test following vagotomy. They observed the following electrocardiographic changes: 60 patients exhibited varying degrees of ST-T changes, "U" waves, premature atrial and ventricular contractions, A-V dissociation, nodal rhythm, atrial tachycardia, and sinus tachycardia. The greatest fall in blood glucose occurred at 30 to 60 minutes (mean 45 minutes) to a level of 8 to 50 mg. per cent (mean 29.9 mg. per cent) (Read and Doherty, 1969). These alterations are ascribed to the following factors: (a) The hypoglycemia per se tends to increase cardiac work at a time when there is a decrease in available energy in the form of combustible glucose in the heart. (b) Increased secretion of catecholamines is compensatory to the hypoglycemia.

ADRENAL DYSFUNCTION

The adrenal medulla is in effect a ganglion of the sympathetic nervous system which releases epinephrine and small amounts of norepinephrine in response to nervous impulses. This results in an elevation of the circulating catecholamine levels which may, if sufficiently great, exert a positive inotropic and chronotropic effect on the heart. The effects on automaticity, excitability, conductivity, and contractility have already been discussed (Chapter 2).

The adrenal cortex plays an important role in the maintenance of normal cardiovascular function. Mineralocorticoids such as aldosterone maintain intravascular fluid volume by their actions on the kidney. The most important function of adrenocortical hormones is the role of cortisol in maintaining the reactivity of vascular smooth muscle to norepinephrine and epinephrine (Williams, 1968).

Addison's Disease. In Addison's disease, the heart is small in size paralleling the course of the disease. Hypotension, characteristic of the chronic form of the disease as well as the acute crisis, is also the most constant cardiovascular manifestation. The accompanying weakness of adrenal insufficiency frequently overshadows cardiac symptoms in the untreated patient, but dyspnea and palpitation are common complaints.

Postmortem examination reveals an atrophic heart with no specific histologic alterations (Gould, 1953). Electrocardiographic tracings in Addison's disease have shown in order of frequency: (a) flat or inverted T waves; (b) a prolonged Q-T interval; (c) low voltage QRS complexes; (d) prolonged P-R and QRS intervals; (e) a depressed RS-T segment; and (f) prominent U waves (Friedberg, 1966). Many of these changes are undoubtedly related to the alterations of potassium and sodium metabolism associated with this disease.

HEMOCHROMATOSIS

Cardiac involvement in hemochromatosis has been emphasized in recent years. Morphologic examination reveals the presence of hemosiderin in the muscle cells of the heart as well as in histiocytes infiltrating the interstitial spaces. Varying degrees of fibrosis also exist.

Hemochromatosis of the heart is manifested during life by paroxysmal atrial fibrillation, flutter, and tachycardia. Various degrees of A-V block are found as well (Petit, 1945). Ventricular premature beats are occasionally observed (Levin and Golum, 1953), but ventricular tachycardia seems very rare (Lewis, 1954). The most common electrocardiographic abnormality seen is low voltage throughout all leads (Horns, 1949).

References

Arnsdorf, M. F., and Childers, R. W.: Atrial electrophysiology in experimental hyperthyroidism in rabbits. Circ. Res., 26:575, 1970.

Bellet, S., Freed, H., and Dyer, W. W.: Electrocardiogram during insulin shock treatment of schizophrenia and other psychoses. Amer. J. Med. Sci., 198:533, 1939.

Busnardo, B., and Carenza, P.: Hyperthyroidism, possible cause of A-V conduction prolongation. Cuore e Circol., 52:146, 1968.

Dratchinskaja, E. S., and Andrejeva, M. P.: The fibrillation arrhythmias in thyrotoxicosis. Its origin and treatment. (Russian Text.) Probl. Endokrinol. Gormontherapii., 2:50, 1956.

Egeli, E. S., and Berkmen, R.: Action of hypoglycemia on coronary insufficiency and mechanism of ECG alterations. Amer. Heart J., 59:527, 1960.

Friedberg, C. K.: Diseases of the Heart. 3rd Ed. Philadelphia, W. B. Saunders, 1966.

Gould, S. E. (ed.): Pathology of the Heart. Springfield, Ill., Charles C Thomas, 1953.

Hansen, J. E.: Paroxysmal ventricular tachycardia associated with myxedema: A case report. Amer. Heart J., 61:692, 1961.

Horns, H. L.: Hemochromatosis. Amer. J. Med., 6:272, 1949.

Leak, D., and Starr, P.: The mechanism of arrhythmias during insulin-induced hypoglycemia. Amer. Heart J., 63:688, 1962.

Leonard, J. J., and deGroot, W. J.: The thyroid state and the cardiovascular system. Mod. Conc. Cardiov. Dis., 38:23, 1969.

Levin, E. B., and Golum, A.: The heart in hemochromatosis. Amer. Heart J., 45:277, 1953.

Lewis, H. P.: Cardiac involvement in hemochromatosis. Amer. J. Med. Sci., 277:544, 1954.

Petit, D. W.: Hemochromatosis with complete heart block with a discussion of cardiac complications. Amer. Heart J., 29:253, 1945.

Read, R. C., and Doherty, J. E.: Cardiovascular effects of induced insulin hypoglycemia in man. Circulation, 39–40:III–167, 1969.

Rosenblum, R., and Delman, A. J.: First-degree heart block associated with thyrotoxicosis. Arch. Intern. Med., 112:488, 1963.

Soskin, S., Katz, L. N., Strouse, S., and Rubinfeld, S. H.: Treatment of the elderly diabetic patients with cardiovascular disease; Available carbohydrate and blood sugar level. Arch. Intern. Med., 51:122, 1933.

Williams, R. H. (ed.): Textbook of Endocrinology. Philadelphia, W. B. Saunders, 1968.

Chapter 25 Anesthesia and Surgery

GENERAL CONSIDERATIONS
PATHOPHYSIOLOGY
ARRHYTHMIAS OBSERVED DURING SURGERY
  General (Nonthoracic) Surgery
  Noncardiac Thoracic Surgery
  Cardiac Surgery
  The Postoperative Period
TREATMENT

GENERAL CONSIDERATIONS

The many alterations in body function that occur during anesthesia and surgery make this an ideal situation for the occurrence of arrhythmias. These changes in function include the development of hypoxia, alterations in vagal and sympathetic tone, electrolyte alterations, and other factors mentioned in the following pages.

The subject of cardiac arrhythmias during anesthesia and surgery has recently assumed increased importance because: (a) they are encountered with increased frequency, partly because of the greater number of surgical procedures, particularly in older and poor-risk patients, and the increase in thoracic surgery, especially cardiac surgery; (b) many of these arrhythmias are serious and may lead to complications, such as shock-like states, ventricular fibrillation, and cardiac arrest; (c) continuous monitoring devices which are commonly employed allow immediate diagnosis; and (d) new methods of therapy are available that may be life-saving (Fig. 25–1).

General anesthesia produces various physiologic alterations which provide a "fertile ground" for the development of arrhythmias. All general anesthetics cause some degree of central nervous system depression. The effect is proportionate to the arterial concentration of the agent.

Surgical anesthesia is usually achieved with the blood pressure unaltered or only slightly decreased. Occasionally, an increase of blood pressure may be observed which is often caused by carbon dioxide retention or stimulation in a patient who has not been sufficiently anesthetized. Deep anesthesia may depress the heart and the vasomotor center to a degree that the blood pressure may be markedly lowered. The effect on cardiac output during anesthesia depends on the interrelation of many physiologic mechanisms and on the particular agent used. An increase in the level of circulating catecholamines during induction and the early stages of anesthesia may cause the cardiac output to rise.

General anesthesia unaccompanied by a catecholamine response produces a dilatation of peripheral vessels which at first is accompanied by an increased blood flow. This initial increase may last throughout the duration of a minor procedure but results in a diminished blood flow during longer procedures. The initial vasodilatation probably originates from a central depression of vasomotor tone. The splanchnic vessels constrict and compensate for vasodilatation in the skin and skeletal musculature so that the total peripheral resistance may remain unchanged. However, blood flow to the viscera, including the kidneys, decreases.

Furthermore, many anesthetic agents have been said to "sensitize"

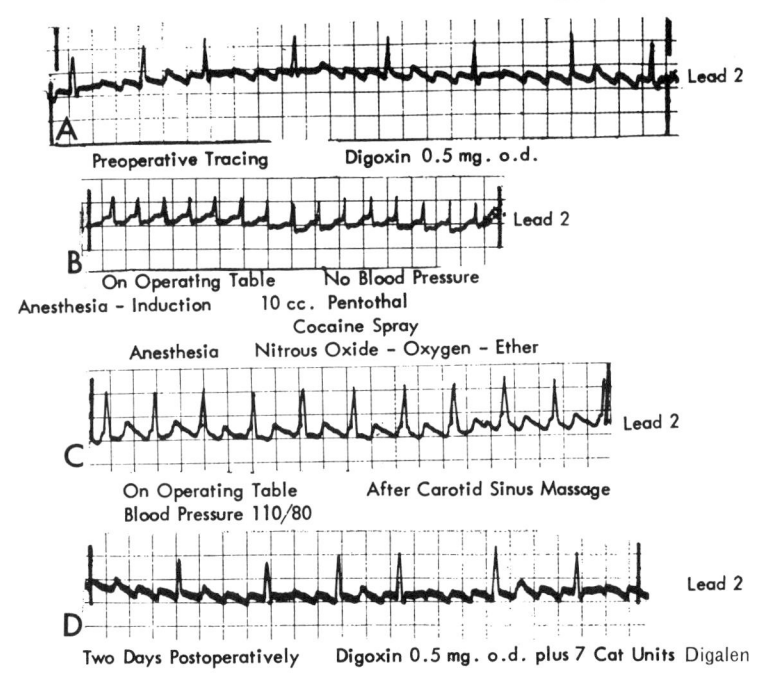

Figure 25-1. Electrocardiograms during the development of shock due to atrial flutter with 1:1 ventricular response during induction of anesthesia. Note the value of monitoring in immediate diagnosis and therapy.

The patient, 58 years of age with arteriosclerotic heart disease, was known to have atrial flutter; the ventricular rate had been controlled (at a rate of 80 per minute), by digoxin 0.5 mg. per day. Conversion to normal sinus rhythm had been attempted with quinidine on several occasions without success.

(A) Note the presence of an atrial flutter with varying degrees of block, 4:1 to 2:1 (with a ventricular rate ranging between 75 and 100 per minute).

(B) On the operating table, after induction of anesthesia, note that the ventricular rate had increased to 290 per minute. The patient developed a state of shock due to the 1:1 conduction and the high ventricular rate.

(C) Following carotid sinus massage and after the intravenous administration of Cedilanid (0.8 mg.), the ventricular rate decreased to 150 per minute due to a decrease of A-V conduction from 1:1 to 2:1.

(D) Two days later, note the presence of atrial flutter with varying degrees of A-V heart block similar to the control.

This series of tracings illustrates the value of monitoring the patient during anesthesia and surgery by (a) diagnosis of the presence of, and exact type of, ectopic rhythm and (b) the administration of appropriate therapy and noting its effect. This regimen was life-saving in this patient. The operation was performed two weeks subsequently without mishap.

the myocardium to the arrhythmogenic actions of catecholamines. On the other hand, some anesthetics such as ether may prevent the occurrence of arrhythmias and thus can be said to exert a protective effect (Katz and Epstein, 1968). By pooling various studies, Katz and Epstein (1968) were able to devise a classification of anesthetic agents in descending order with respect to "sensitization": trichloroethylene, ethyl chloride, cyclopropane, halothane, chloroform, methoxyflurane, and fluoroxine. However, these agents have never been compared in a single study, and these results indicate no more than a general trend.

PATHOPHYSIOLOGY

During anesthesia and surgery, the factors which might contribute to alterations in cardiac function include: the previous condition of the heart, the type and length of the operation, the type and duration of anesthesia, electrolyte disturbance, and perhaps most important, the degree of hypoxia.

Hypoxia during anesthesia is an important contributory factor toward both arrhythmogenesis and mortality. Vulnerability to hypoxia is increased because anesthetic agents modify the body's response to hypoxia by counteracting the normal circulatory compensatory mechanisms. The body has recourse to two systems in trying to compensate for hypoxia—the pulmonary and circulatory systems. The pulmonary response is unspectacular with mild hypoxia. The body can improve oxygen uptake only minimally by hyperventilating, by increasing the tidal volume, or by increasing the pulmonary blood flow proportionate to an increase in ventilation (Bendixen and Laver, 1965). However, such measures will only result in an increase in arterial oxygen concentration if the patient is severely hypoxemic.

The circulatory response to hypoxia consists of local and general changes (Bendixen and Laver, 1965). The local response of every tissue except the pulmonary circulation to hypoxia is vasodilatation. Local hypoxia is still considered the most powerful vasodilatation stimulus in every vascular bed except the cerebral, where carbon dioxide retention is equally strong. The effect is to augment blood flow, thereby increasing the pressure gradient between blood and tissue which improves oxygen transfer. The systemic response to hypoxia is first to mobilize blood from various vascular beds and increase cardiac output, and then, through sympathetic control of the vasculature, to redistribute blood according to highest priority needs (i.e., heart, brain, and pulmonary beds) (Bendixen and Laver, 1965).

The etiology of hypoxia in anesthesia includes: (1) decreased oxygen in inspired air, which arises only from anesthetic error or accident; (2) decreased oxygen tension in arterial blood, secondary to airway obstruction, hypoventilation, increased physiological shunting and, particularly, anemia; (3) decreased cardiac output; and (4) abnormal tissue metabolism, as in response to fever (Bendixen and Laver, 1965). Age, obesity, pre-existing cardiopulmonary disease, and trauma to the respiratory or circulatory systems may contribute to hypoxia before anesthesia. In addition, age, pulmonary and cardiac disease, anemia, position, respiratory binders, and such drugs as reserpine, phenothiazines, morphine, and barbiturates can all contribute to a decreased ability to compensate for hypoxia (Bendixen and Laver, 1965).

Cyclopropane, halothane, and methoxyflurane are all potent respiratory depressants and hence potential causes of hypoxia. Nitrous oxide may act similarly, especially if used following barbiturates and opiates. A fall in arterial oxygen tension appears to take place regardless of the anesthetic used, or whether ventilation is controlled or spontaneous. This effect which appears to be due to atelectasis can be minimized by periodic large tidal volumes (Bendixen and Laver, 1965).

Without exception, anesthetics are myocardial depressants. This effect becomes more evident if the compensatory sympathetic response is impaired, possibly causing hypoxia. Interfering with central autonomic control or efferent autonomic pathways can also modify the circulatory response. Thus, adrenergic block, such as that caused by the preanesthetic use of reserpine or chlorpromazine will impair the response to sympathetic discharge and thus interfere with the redistribution of blood to vital centers.

ARRHYTHMIAS OBSERVED DURING SURGERY

General (Nonthoracic) Surgery. The incidence of serious arrhythmias in general surgery is small, particularly when compared with that in cardiac surgery. They tend to occur most often in patients of the older age group and in those with previous cardiac damage and other predisposing factors. Much depends on the presence or absence of heart disease, the age of the patient, a history of previous arrhythmias, the type of anesthesia and surgery, and previous cardiac medication, especially digitalis.

In a series of 154 consecutive patients ranging in age from six weeks to 86 years the use of special monitoring equipment revealed the overall incidence of arrhythmias to be 61.7 per cent; the surgical procedures involved the following: abdomen (47 patients), extremities (34), head and neck (18), thorax excluding the heart (14), the urologic area (6), the neurologic system (4), and others (31) (Kuner et al., 1967). The most frequent disturbances were wandering pacemaker, A-V dissociation, junctional rhythms, and premature ventricular systoles. Although more serious arrhythmias do occur, however, they are uncommon. The principal factors responsible for the onset of these disturbances were the type of anesthetic, intubation, hyperventilation, and duration of the surgery.

Noncardiac Thoracic Surgery. The incidence of arrhythmias associated with noncardiac thoracic surgery ranges from 10 to 20 per cent, occurring in greatest number after pneumonectomy and mediastinal exploration and biopsy for neoplastic disease (Cerney, 1957). A majority of the arrhythmias occur within two weeks postoperatively and respond to conventional therapy. The highest proportion of cases appears in patients over 50 years of age.

Factors operative in the production of these arrhythmias in addition to the general aforementioned factors are: infection, pre-existing paroxysmal fibrillation, conduction defects of unknown cause, coronary artery disease, right heart failure, pericardial effusion, or localized pericarditis.

The arrhythmias are predominantly atrial in origin and consist of multiple atrial ectopic beats occurring in groups, supraventricular tachycardia, atrial flutter, and atrial fibrillation (Cerney, 1957). A retrospective study of 574 patients who had undergone resectional lung surgery revealed that atrial fibrillation or flutter was precipitated in 3.1 per cent of lobectomies and 19.4 per cent of pneumonectomies. The incidence and type of arrhythmias in similar studies may be revised as data from continuous monitoring become available.

Cardiac Surgery. Continuous electrocardiographic recording during cardiac surgery is important in recognizing serious disturbances of rhythm, particularly during the time of intracardiac manipulations. Atrial fibrillation is the most common arrhythmia occurring after mitral valvulotomy. The incidence may range from 20 to 47 per cent (Heinz and Hultgren, 1957; MacCuish, 1958; Kittle and Crockett, 1959). This postoperative complication was more frequent in older patients, especially in those with previous episodes of atrial fibrillation and in those with some degree of associated mitral insufficiency. Local trauma to the left atrium incident to the atriotomy was the most important etiologic factor (Kittle and Crockett, 1959).

The Postoperative Period. During the postoperative period, conditions can exist which may directly or indirectly predispose to the development of arrhythmias. Included are hypotension, shock, hemorrhage, electrolyte imbalance (especially involving potassium and sodium), reflexes from the gastrointestinal tract and other viscera, and anxiety. These conditions may lead to further postoperative complications, such as pulmonary embolism and pneumonia.

TREATMENT

The treatment of arrhythmias occurring as a result of anesthesia and surgery begins with the prophylactic therapy: (1) avoid factors which predispose to arrhythmias; (2) equipment, drugs, and electrolyte solutions for treatment of possible complications; (3) special preparation of those patients with pre-existing cardiac abnormality or history of arrhythmias to avoid hypoxia and shock by providing an adequate airway, proper positioning, prompt correction of blood loss and fluid and electrolyte imbalance, and avoidance of myocardial irritation, anxiety, and anesthetic agents that may lead to arrhythmias; (4) prophylactic administration of drugs: (a) preoperative digitalis, chiefly to patients subject to development of ectopic rhythms or with congestive failure, (b) atropine to block vagal reflexes, and (c) barbiturates to allay apprehension. During surgery, continuous monitoring of the electrocardiogram and pulse rate, blood pressure, respiration, oxygen and carbon dioxide tensions, and blood pH identify potentially dangerous situations. During the postoperative period, one should be on the alert for the development of arrhythmias and their warning signals—precordial pain, dyspnea, hypotensive state, and shock.

When an arrhythmia complicating anesthesia and surgery does occur, the treatment is based upon the same principles that govern the therapy under ordinary circumstances. The only differences are that during anesthesia and surgery it is necessary to rely upon parenteral medication and electrical devices and the institution of measures to control the abnormalities as quickly as possible.

References

Bendixen, H. H., and Laver, M. B.: Hypoxia in anesthesia: a review. Clin. Pharmacol. Ther., 6:510, 1965.

Cerney, C. I.: The prophylaxis of cardiac arrhythmias complicating pulmonary surgery. J. Thorac. Surg., 34:105, 1957.

Cullen, D. J., Eger, E. I., and Gregory, G. A.: The cardiovascular effects of cyclopropane in man. Anesthesiology, 3:398, 1969.

Heinz, R., and Hultgren, H.: Atrial fibrillation following mitral valvulotomy. Arch. Intern. Med., 99:896, 1957.

Katz, R. L., and Epstein, R. A.: The interaction of anesthetic agents and adrenergic drugs to produce cardiac arrhythmias. Anesthesiology, 29:763, 1968.

Kittle, F. C., and Crockett, J. E.: The etiology and prevention of atrial fibrillation after mitral valvulotomy. J. Thorac. Surg., 38:353, 1959.

Kuner, J., et al.: Cardiac arrhythmias during anesthesia. Dis. Chest, 52:580, 1967.

MacCuish, R. K.: Cardiac arrhythmias following mitral valvulotomy and their management. Acta. Med. Scand., 161:125, 1958.

Ngai, S. H., Neff, N. H., and Costa, E.: The effect of cyclopropane and halothane on the biosynthesis of norepinephrine in vivo. Anesthesiology, 31:53, 1969.

Price, H. L., Warden, J. C., Cooperman, L. H., and Miller, R. A.: Central sympathetic excitation caused by cyclopropane. Anesthesiology, 30:426, 1969.

Reid, J. M., and Stevenson, J. C.: Cardiac arrhythmias following successful surgical closure of atrial septal defect. Brit. Heart J., 29:742, 1967.

Vanik, P. E., and Davis, H. S.: Cardiac arrhythmias during halothane anesthesia. Anesth. Analg., 47:299, 1968.

Chapter 26 *Cardiac Catheterization and Angiocardiography*

CARDIAC CATHETERIZATION
   Etiology of Arrhythmias During Cardiac Catheterization
   Arrhythmias
   Therapy

ANGIOCARDIOGRAPHY
   Cineangiography
   Untoward Effects
      Arrhythmias Produced by Angiocardiography
   Coronary Arteriography

CARDIAC CATHETERIZATION

Cardiac catheterization occupies an important niche in the diagnosis of cardiac abnormalities, both congenital and acquired. The most important complication of this procedure consists in the occasional development of arrhythmias, some of which may be serious and may, in rare instances, lead to a fatality (Fig. 26–1).

Etiology of Arrhythmias During Cardiac Catheterization. Arrhythmias encountered during cardiac catheterization are due to a multiplicity of factors: (a) The presence of pre-existing heart disease, e.g., congenital heart disease, coronary artery lesions, and cardiopulmonary disease, which may be increased in frequency in the presence of cardiac arrhythmias prior to the cardiac catheterization. (b) The

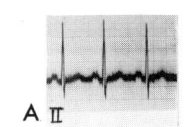

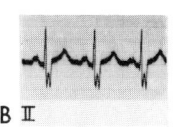

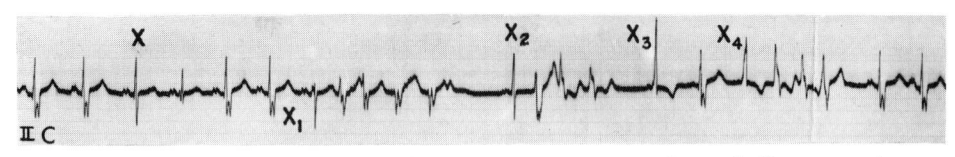

Figure 26–1. Effect of right heart catheterization on QRS complex and effect on production of premature beats. Ventricular premature beats occurring in various parts of the cardiac cycle showing fusion beats with narrow QRS complexes.
   (A) Control shows normal intraventricular conduction.
   (B) During right heart catheterization, note the presence of a right bundle branch block pattern.
   (C) X, X_1, X_2, and X_3 are fusion beats. X occurs at almost the completion of the P-R interval; X_1 occurs almost immediately after ventricular depolarization has started; X_2 occurs slightly before the normal depolarization begins. X_3 occurs somewhat closer to the beginning of atrial depolarization and resembles a W-P-W complex. X_4 and the three following QRS complexes represent ventricular premature beats without fusion.

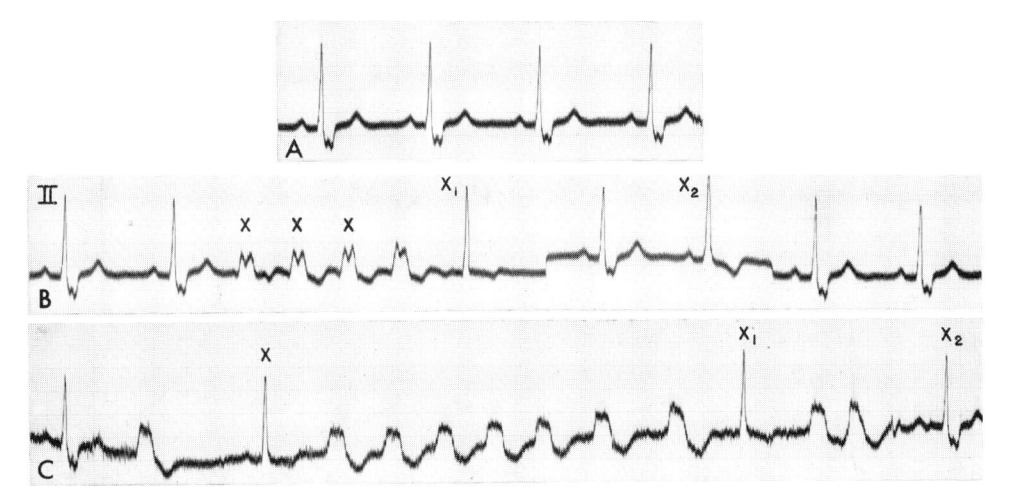

Figure 26-2. Right heart catheterization, showing premature beats, fusion beats, and short paroxysms of ventricular tachycardia.

(A) (Lead II). Control shows right bundle branch block; rate is 64 per minute.

(B) During right heart catheterization. Shows the development at X of premature ventricular beats with widened QRS of the left bundle branch type. X_1 is apparently a fusion beat representing a fusion between the premature beat and the widened QRS of sinus origin. A second fusion beat is observed at X_2.

(C) Note the appearance of fusion beats at X and X_1 (immediately following the short paroxysm of ventricular tachycardia—at X_1 "partial capture").

heart is highly sensitive to all stimuli. The direct mechanical impact of a catheter upon the endocardial lining, particularly that of the interatrial or interventricular septa, which contain the highly sensitive conduction tissue, may produce surface disturbances and alteration in de- and repolarization resulting in the production of ectopic rhythms or conduction defects. Occasionally, a small subendocardial hemorrhage may be produced which may lead to the persistence of the arrhythmia for several hours or days. (c) Reflex factors as a result of cardiac stimulation or other accidental manipulations. (d) Psychogenic factors, that is, anxiety of the patient during the period of cardiac catheterization, which may lead to increased secretion of catecholamines.

Arrhythmias. In a recent series of 12,367 catheterizations, 149 patients (1.2 per cent) experienced 153 major arrhythmias (Braunwald and Swan, 1968). Disorders of rhythm played a role in the deaths of 16 of these patients. Only potentially life-threatening arrhythmias were considered to be "major complications" in this study and were divided as follows: ventricular fibrillation (incidence, 0.48 per cent); asystole or marked bradycardia (0.30 per cent); supraventricular arrhythmias (0.28 per cent); ventricular tachycardia (0.10 per cent) (Fig. 26-2); complete heart block (0.06 per cent); bundle branch block (0.02 per cent); and bigeminy (0.01 per cent).

Ventricular fibrillation, the most frequent of the arrhythmias, occurred most commonly in infants less than 60 days old (2.8 per cent). These patients were all seriously ill with complex congenital cardiac malformations. In contrast to this age group, fibrillation, mostly from manipulation of the catheter, was experienced in less than 0.1 per cent of children between two months and 14 years of age, in 0.3 per cent of patients between 15 and 34 years of age, and in 0.55 per cent of patients above the age of 35 years exclusive of those studied by coronary arteriography (Braunwald and Swan, 1968). The 23 in this latter group make up the total of 50 subjects. The overall mortality from this arrhythmia was 13 per cent with one case (in 59) of irreversible brain damage.

Ventricular tachycardia that did not progress to fibrillation occurred in 12 patients; in three cases this arrhythmia developed after profound bradycardia. Five of the 12 patients were less than ten months of age; one was six years old; and six were 19 years old or older. Two of the infants and one adult reverted to normal sinus rhythm spontaneously; another adult did so after receiving procaine amide. The rest converted to sinus rhythm after countershock. One infant developed asystole and ultimately died.

The most common supraventricular arrhythmia was atrial tachycardia (16 patients), followed closely in frequency by atrial fibrillation (11 patients), with atrial flutter, nodal rhythm, and sinus tachycardia making up the total of 35 patients. All 11 cases of atrial fibrillation occurred in 20 patients, six to 61 years of age. Five of the 29 had Ebstein's anomaly; three had the Wolff-Parkinson-White syndrome.

It is not uncommon to observe a persistent right bundle branch block due to injury of the right bundle by the catheter tip; usually, this is transient. Stein et al. (1966) have described this phenomenon in four patients with preexisting left bundle branch block which resulted in complete A-V heart block; this is usually transient. Similar instances have been observed by others, including our laboratory.

Complete A-V heart block does not commonly appear during catheterization. It developed in four infants, four days to 14 months old, in two 13-year-old girls, and in one adult.

Fowler et al. (1951) report nine cases in a series of 106 catheterizations complicated by the appearance of arrhythmias in which the abnormal rhythm persisted after the catheter was withdrawn. They believed that the cause of their persistence was probably a small subendocardial hemorrhage.

Therapy. As a rule, prophylactic therapy is not ordinarily employed except in certain specific cases where it is known that the patient is subject to the development of arrhythmias or manifests ectopic rhythms prior to catheterization. The use of digitalis or the antiarrhythmic drugs such as quinidine and procaine amide may be efficacious under these conditions. Often, only mild to moderate sedation will suffice. Because of the possibility of the patient developing cardiac arrest or ventricular fibrillation, equipment should be available for external cardiac resuscitation (see p. 217).

ANGIOCARDIOGRAPHY

This procedure involves injection of a contrast material either proximal to or directly into the central circulation within a very short period of time. Within 10 to 15 seconds (or longer) following the injection, serial x-ray or cinematographic studies are made as the contrast material passes through the heart and great vessels. In this way, valuable information usually unobtainable otherwise may be secured with particular reference to lesions in congenital or acquired heart disease, aortic and other types of valvular disease, diseases of the coronary arteries, and (indirectly) various types of mediastinal and pulmonary diseases. In addition, many congenital vascular defects such as coarctation of the aorta and anomalous pulmonary veins are readily demonstrated by contrast visualization. Angiocardiography is the diagnostic method of choice in delineating aortic aneurysm and differentiating between the common and dissecting types. Accurate diagnosis may now be made in about 90 per cent of patients with congenital cardiovascular malformations.

The major difficulties of the procedure lie in the fact that most untoward effects of angiocardiography are observed in those conditions in which this technique is most valuable e.g., in subjects with either congenital or advanced forms of acquired heart disease.

Cineangiography. The introduction of the image amplifier has made possible the introduction and widespread use of cineangiography. This enables the physician to observe the procedure from start to finish and to elicit data regarding the dynamic state of the heart. The techniques employed in cineangiography of the heart are basically those employed with serial angiography. The procedure can be observed on a television monitor. The speed is usually set at 60 frames per second. Film can be developed in less than an hour and studied with the aid of a projector that may be stopped or reversed as needed to thoroughly study the coronary circulation.

Untoward Effects. The untoward effects of angiocardiography depend upon many factors: the type and amount of contrast material employed; the type of angiocardiographic procedure for visualization of the right atrium or ventricle, left atrium or ventricle, or coronary arteries; and the previous condition of the cardiovascular system.

Studies of the effect of different radiopaque contrast media injected into the experimental animal indicate that the peripheral blood pressure generally falls. Furthermore, studies in both the experimental animal and the human subject have revealed that (a) radiopaque materials lower peripheral resistance; (b) the simultaneous pulmonary artery and venous pressure increase suggests a compensatory adrenergic release; (c) a more dangerous reaction is the obstruction of the blood flow through the lungs; (d) the increase in cardiac output found during angiocardiography merely emphasizes that this test per se causes some degree of cardiovascular stress. Patients with mitral valvular and other types of heart disease are incapable of increasing the output beyond normal or even subnormal levels and many manifest evidence of cardiac abnormality in the form of myocardial ischemia or ectopic rhythms.

Arrhythmias Produced by Angiocardiography. Arrhythmias occur rather frequently following angiocardiography. Fortunately, the more serious types are rare. Nevertheless, evidence is accumulating that angiocardiography may produce direct and sometimes fatal cardiac disturbances. Some of the rare serious reactions reported have been thought to result primarily from respiratory collapse.

The type of arrhythmia that appears during an angiocardiographic procedure depends upon the technique used, the location of the catheter tip, the contrast material employed, and the presence of any pre-existing myocardial damage.

Supraventricular and ventricular premature beats are a common occurrence. Atrial tachycardia and bigeminy also frequently appear. Bundle branch block and prolonged ventricular ectopic rhythms are encountered only rarely but must be recognized and guarded against carefully.

In a National Heart Institute sponsored study (Braunwald and Swan, 1968), of 9482 patients in whom angiocardiography was performed, the following arrhythmias were encountered: ventricular fibrillation (10 cases), ventricular tachycardia (2 cases), marked bradycardia or asystole (8 cases), complete heart block (1 case), and supraventricular arrhythmias (3 cases).

With five of the patients experiencing ventricular fibrillation, a defect was found in the injector causing the discharge of a significant electrical current of brief duration. Rowe and Zarnstorff (1965) similarly reported ventricular fibrillation due to a transient electrical discharge from several different types of injectors. While other factors may contribute to ventricular fibrillation, this nevertheless remains a simple and readily correctable source of difficulty.

The etiologic factors precipitating arrhythmias and occasional death after angiocardiography include the following: (a) hemodynamic effects (noted previously); (b) toxic effect on the myocardium, especially on the A-V node and other portions of the conduction system; (c) vascular effects such as coronary spasm and coronary damage (the contrast substance may effect a change in the coronary circulation, thus inducing myocardial hypoxia and electrocardiographic changes, including an abnormal rhythm); (d) hypoxia secondary to respiratory depression or pulmonary vascular damage and replacement of oxygen-bearing blood by the dye; (e) "speed shock" leading to sudden death following rapid intravenous injection; (f) allergic manifestations to the dye; (g) an obstruction of the blood flow through the lungs; and (h) improper grounding of the injector with consequent production of transient electric currents.

In view of the untoward effects previously noted, it is suggested that angiocardiography be performed only when it is definitely indicated and that care be taken in its performance in poor-risk patients.

The therapy of arrhythmias arising during angiocardiographic procedures is similar to that mentioned for cardiac catheterization (see page 286). These procedures should be carried out in a setting in which continuous monitoring is available so that immediate therapy may be instituted.

Coronary Arteriography. Although coronary arteriography allows us to study deviations from normal anatomy and pathology of the coronary arteries in the living subject, it may also present certain complications. A cooperative study organized under the auspices of the National Heart Institute (Braunwald and Swan, 1968) reported an overall complication rate of 1.9 per cent in a patient sample of 3312 coronary arteriographic procedures performed on 3264 patients. However, if the data from Sones' laboratory, where 81 per cent of all procedures were performed, is excluded, the complication rate becomes 6.1 per cent.

The most common complication of coronary arteriography is a major arrhythmia which in the aforementioned study occurred in 27 patients (0.82 per cent). Most frequent was ventricular fibrillation (including one episode of ventricular tachycardia), which occurred in 24 patients—18 women and six men. Thus, while women constituted only 31 per cent of the population undergoing coronary arteriography, they accounted for 75 per cent of the subjects who developed ventricular fibrillation. Fifteen of the 24 who experienced fibrillation or tachycardia had received injections into the right coronary artery; nine, into the left. No serious sequelae followed in any patient. The only other arrhythmia connected with coronary arteriography in this study was asystole, which was encountered in only three patients in the study group, one of whom could not be resuscitated. The conclusion from these studies is that these procedures involve a definite risk. Care must be taken in the choice of patients to be submitted to the manipulations that must be undergone with coronary arteriography.

References

Abrams, H. L., and Adams, D. F.: The coronary arteriogram. New Eng. J. Med., 281:1276, 1969.

Begg, F. R., et al.: Hemodynamic and coronary arteriography patterns during acute myocardial infarction. J. Thorac. Cardiov. Surg., 58:647, 1969.

Benchimol, A., and McNally, E. M.: Hemodynamic and electrocardiographic effects of selective coronary arteriography in man. New Eng. J. Med., 274:1217, 1966.

Braunwald, E., and Swan, J. H. C. (eds.): Cooperative Study on Catheterization. American Heart Association Monograph Association, Inc., 1968. Circulation, 37–38:III–1, 1968.

Fowler, N. O., Westcott, R. N., and Scott, R. C.: Disturbances in cardiac mechanism of several hours' duration complicating cardiac venous catheterization. Amer. Heart J. 42:652, 1951.

Fraser, R. S., Macaulay, W. D., and Rossall, R. E.: Arrhythmias induced during intracardiac catheterization. Amer. Heart J., 64:439, 1962.

Hultgren, H. N., and Abrams, H. L.: Coronary arteriography. Amer. Heart J., 72:737, 1967.

Krovetz, L. J., Shanklin, D. R., and Schiebler, G. L.: Serious and fatal complications of catheterization and angiocardiography in infants and children. Amer. Heart J., 76:39, 1968.

Levy, M. J., and Lillehei, C. W.: Percutaneous direct cardiac catheterization. New Eng. J. Med., 271:273, 1964.

Mody, S. M., and Richings, M.: Ventricular fibrillation resulting from electrocution during cardiac catheterization. Lancet, 2:698, 1962.

Rowe, G. G., and Zarnstorff, W. C.: Ventricular fibrillation during selective angiocardiography. JAMA, 192:105, 1965.

Spaum, J. F., Jr., Mason, D. T., Beiser, G. D., and Gold, H. K.: Myocardial effects of angiographic dye. Amer. J. Cardiol., 23:140, 1969.

Stein, P. P., Mathur, V. S., Herman, M. V., and Levine, H. D.: Complete heart block induced during cardiac catheterization of patients with pre-existent bundle branch block. Circulation, 34:783, 1966.

Chapter 27 Brain and Heart Relationships

GENERAL CONSIDERATIONS
ECG EFFECTS AND ARRHYTHMIAS RESULTING FROM EXPERIMENTAL STIMULATION OF VARIOUS PARTS OF THE BRAIN
  Hypothalamus
  Reticular Formation
THE EFFECT OF ARRHYTHMIAS IN ALTERING CEREBRAL FUNCTION

THE EFFECT OF BRAIN DAMAGE OR DYSFUNCTION ON THE HEART AND CIRCULATION
PSYCHOSOMATIC DISORDERS
  General Considerations
  Etiologic Factors
  Pathophysiology

GENERAL CONSIDERATIONS

It has been known for many years that the central nervous system, particularly the higher centers, plays a significant role in cardiovascular regulation. The older concepts about localization of regulatory centers in the medulla have given way to new ideas about the complex interrelationships existing among the higher centers of the brain and the peripheral effector cells. The result has been the establishment of a cause-and-effect relationship between functional and organic disturbances in the brain and the cardiac manifestations that often accompany them. Some of these interrelationships have been discussed in Chapter 2, page 24. Additional experimental, pathologic, and clinical data relative to specific areas of cardiovascular control are discussed here in terms of structural, humoral, and psychological factors.

Electrical stimulation of the hypothalamus, thalamus, or amygdala causes an increase in plasma lipid levels. Furthermore, Redding and Schally (1970) have shown that the hypothalamus of experimental animals as well as man contains substances that stimulate lipolysis in fat cells. These substances may mediate the plasma lipid response observed following electrical stimulation. Hypothalamic stimulation also affects blood pressure and fright and rage reactions. These various effects of hypothalamic stimulation play a role in the development of stress-related cardiac disease.

Just as the hypothalamus can exert an influence over the medullary level of cardiovascular control, it in turn is influenced by higher centers in the cerebral cortex and limbic systems (Bard, 1960). The proper role of the hypothalamus in cardiovascular regulation is thus one of many links in a complex, integrated neural chain of control.

ELECTROCARDIOGRAPHIC EFFECTS AND ARRHYTHMIAS RESULTING FROM EXPERIMENTAL STIMULATION OF VARIOUS PARTS OF THE BRAIN

Profound electrocardiographic effects result from electrical and chemical stimulation of various parts of the brain, namely, the hypothalamus, reticular formation, and portions of the cerebral cortex.

Hypothalamus. Stimulation of various portions of the hypothalamus produce ischemic-like electrocardiographic changes and serious arrhythmias through sympathetic and parasympathetic effects. The alterations noted include T wave inversion, S-T interval changes, widening of the QRS complex, ectopic beats, A-V dissociation, and bouts of paroxysmal tachycardia (Attar et al., 1963). Depressor effects may be accompanied by no change in rate, bradycardia, or tachycardia (Smith et al., 1960). Some of the effects are due to an increase in catecholamine response which tends to increase the cardiac output and to increase atrial and ventricular contractility (Fig. 27–1). Intense, prolonged, and repeated lateral stimulation enhances the development and persistence of the electrocardiographic changes. Bilateral stimulation can produce the pathologic picture of acute myocardial infarction.

Reticular Formation. Stimulation of the reticular formation, central gray substance of the midbrain, or the ventromedial region of the thalamus causes sinus tachycardia, followed by ventricular fusion beats, ventricular premature contractions (frequently multifocal and coupled to the preceding normal sinus complex, in bigeminal and trigeminal patterns), ventricular tachycardia, and sometimes ventricular fibrillation, always in that order, as the intensity of stimulation increases. Bilateral vagotomy does not affect the response but propranolol completely abolishes it. Thus, the action of norepinephrine at sympathetic neuroeffector sites in the myocardium may be responsible for these arrhythmias.

THE EFFECT OF ARRHYTHMIAS IN ALTERING CEREBRAL FUNCTION

While we have discussed the effect of alterations in the brain on the pro-

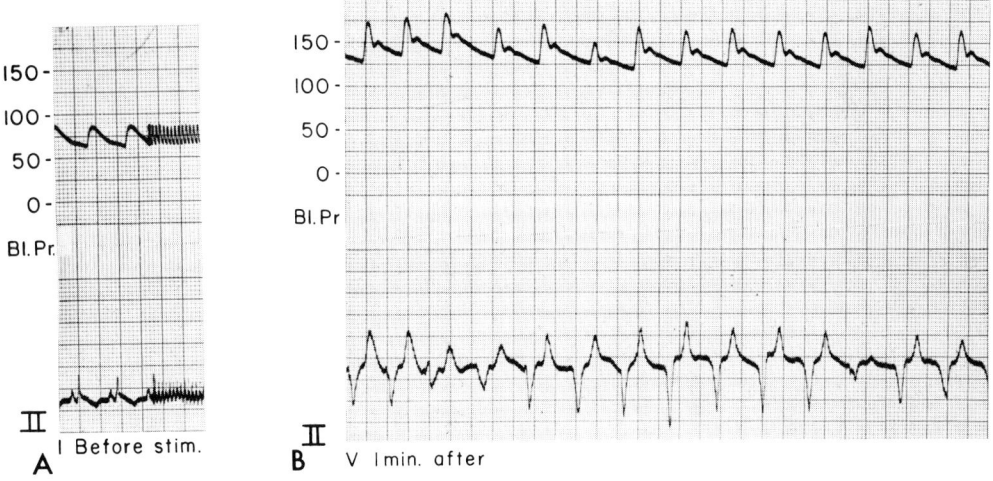

Figure 27–1. Effect of hypothalamic stimulation on the production of arrhythmias (experiment in the cat).
(A) Control before stimulation. Blood pressure is 85/60, and electrocardiogram shows normal sinus rhythm.
(B) 1 minute after stimulation. Note rise in blood pressure to 175/135. An idioventricular pacemaker now controls the heart rhythm. Note the widened QRS complexes and the irregularity in rhythm. Normal rhythm returned after cessation of the stimulation. (From Attar, H. J., Gutierrez, M. T., Bellet, S., and Ravens, J. R.: Circ. Res., *12:*14, 1963.)

duction of arrhythmias, it is also known that certain arrhythmias may produce a decrease in the cerebral blood flow, resulting in cerebral ischemia (Walter et al., 1970). This may occur in the bradycardia accompanied by hypotension, with extremely rapid ventricular rates, or during Stokes-Adams attacks. We have observed patients, particularly in the older age groups, who, following the development of atrial fibrillation with rapid ventricular rate or ventricular tachycardia, developed syncopal attacks or psychotic seizures. These episodes ceased as the heart rate returned to normal. Walter et al. (1970), employing continuously recorded ten-hour electrocardiograms, observed periods of supraventricular tachycardia or high grades of A-V heart block in ten of 39 patients manifesting symptoms of cerebral ischemia who previously had not been noted to have any arrhythmias by routine electrocardiographic examination.

THE EFFECT OF BRAIN DAMAGE OR DYSFUNCTION ON THE HEART AND CIRCULATION

The effect of certain types of brain damage or trauma has been correlated with various disturbances in circulatory function, including the production of arrhythmias. These include head trauma, subarachnoid and cerebral hemorrhage, cerebrovascular accidents, pneumoencephalography, and intracranial surgery.

It has been known for some time that severe head trauma may precipitate arrhythmias, particularly paroxysmal atrial fibrillation and premature beats. In experimental animals, moderate to severe concussion produces bradycardia, A-V junctional rhythm, and a shortening of the $Q-T_c$ (up to 38 per cent reduction).

Following cerebrovascular accidents, a characteristic electrocardiographic pattern has been observed (Burch et al., 1954; Wasserman et al., 1956; and Kreus et al., 1969). This consists of deep T wave inversion and lengthening of the Q-T segment. The most frequent changes occurred in subjects with subarachnoid hemorrhage (71.5 per cent), followed by those with cerebral hemorrhage (57.1 per cent) (Kreus et al., 1969). In contrast, only 41.1 per cent of patients with unclassified cerebrovascular accident demonstrated electrocardiographic alterations; these consisted predominantly of prominent U waves. Alteration in brain function may indirectly produce functional alterations in the heart muscle by various mechanisms, which, in turn, produce electrocardiographic changes.

PSYCHOSOMATIC DISORDERS

General Considerations. The effect of the mind and emotions on the circulation has been recognized for many years. The heart is one of the most sensitive targets for stimuli of psychic origin. When such stimuli recur frequently over a period of time, the heart becomes sensitized and a point is reached at which the individual may be conscious of the slightest cardiac irregularity.

Psychogenic factors may precipitate ectopic rhythms in normal hearts as well as in those with structural disease. While similar factors are operative in both groups, patients with cardiac abnormalities are more vulnerable to their development. Cardiac irregularities often accompany or follow an emotional episode. The patient may complain of heart consciousness, of his heart "jumping out of his throat," of dizziness, or syncopal attacks. In the sensitive individual, awareness of premature beats or other arrhythmias may be quite disturbing.

Etiologic Factors. Arrhythmias associated with psychosomatic disorders

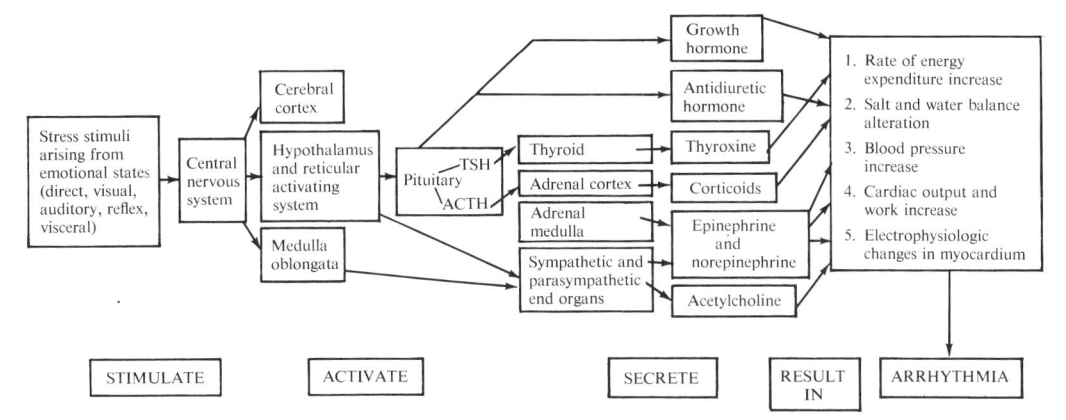

Figure 27-2. Effect of central nervous system on the production of cardiac arrhythmias.

result from the interaction of many factors. Basic is the personality pattern and the life situation of those patients who tend to develop disturbances in cardiac rhythm. Studies in these subjects have shown the following as the most commonly observed emotional traits: chronic anxiety, excessive hostility, inadequate expression of hostility, compulsiveness, and a ready susceptibility to depression. While the chronic stress of the individual's life situation is considered the basic underlying etiologic factor, an acute exacerbation may precipitate an added degree of tension, with the resultant production of arrhythmias in susceptible subjects. The stress or tension may result from a variety of factors: sudden fear, anger, loss of sleep with excessive fatigue, or the excitement of watching a football game, a prize fight, or any other sport event.

Pathophysiology. The precipitation of ectopic rhythms by psychogenic factors may result from many causes. Among the most important are stimuli from the central nervous system affecting both the autonomic nervous system and the endocrine systems, especially the thyroid and adrenal. These factors, acting alone or in combination, result in increased cardiac excitability.

The important centers involved include the cortex, the hypothalamus, pituitary, and medulla. The subsidiary centers may coordinate with or act independently of the central nervous system. Hypothalamic stimulation may exert both sympathetic and parasympathetic effects (see p. 291). Parasympathetic effects may occur almost simultaneously with or independently of sympathetic activity; indeed, there may be a vagal outflow at the very height of sympathetic activity. It appears that simultaneous intense sympathetic and parasympathetic activity is a very potent arrhythmogenic stimulus and may well account for the disturbances which are observed under these conditions (Fig. 27-2).

References

Abildskov, J. S.: Electrocardiographic wave form and the nervous system. Circulation, 41:371, 1970.

Attar, H. J., Gutierrez, M. T., Bellet, S., and Ravens, J. R.: The hypothalamus and the reticular activating system in the control of cardiac rhythm. Circ. Res., 12:14, 1963.

Bard, P.: Anatomical organization of the central nervous system in relation to control of the heart and blood vessels. Physiol. Rev., 40:3, 1960.

Benedict, R. B., and Evans, J. M.: Second degree heart block and Wenckebach phenomena associated with anxiety. Amer. Heart J., 43:626, 1952.

Burch, G. E., Colcolough, H., and Giles, T.: Intracranial lesions and the heart. Amer. Heart J., 80:574, 1970.

Burch, G. E., Meyers, R., and Abildskov, J. A.: A new electrocardiographic pattern observed in cerebrovascular accidents. Circulation, 9:719, 1954.

Combs, J. J., Jr., Bryant, G. N., Bodgonoff, M. D., and Warren, J. V.: The effect of induced anxiety and hostility on cardiovascular functions. J. Clin. Invest., 37:885, 1958.

Connor, R. C. R.: Myocardial damage secondary to brain lesions. Amer. Heart J., 78:145, 1969.

Corday, E., and Irving, D. W.: Effect of cardiac arrhythmias on the cerebral circulation. Amer. J. Cardiol., 6:803, 1960.

Kreus, K. E., Kemila, S. J., and Takala, J. K.: Electrocardiographic changes in cerebrovascular accidents. Acta Med. Scand., 185:327, 1969.

Redding, T. W., and Schally, A. U.: Lipid mobilizing factor from the hypothalamus. Metabolism, 19:641, 1970.

Selye, H.: The Physiology and Pathology of Exposure to Stress. Montreal, Acta, Inc., 1950.

Smith, O. A., Jr., Suhayi, J., Rushmer, R. F., and Lasher, E. P.: Role of hypothalamic structures in cardiac control. Physiol. Rev., 136:40, 1960.

Walter, P. F., Reid, S. O., and Wenger, N. K.: Transient cerebral ischemia due to arrhythmia. Ann. Intern. Med., 72:471, 1970.

Wasserman, F., Choquette, G., Cassinelli, R., and Bellet, S.: Electrocardiographic observations in patients with cerebrovascular accidents. Amer. J. Med. Sci., 231:502, 1956.

Chapter 28: Coronary Artery Disease and Myocardial Infarction

ARRHYTHMIAS IN ACUTE MYOCARDIAL INFARCTION

GENERAL CONSIDERATIONS
PATHOPHYSIOLOGY
INVOLVEMENT OF SPECIALIZED TISSUES
  Internodal Pathways
  A-V Junction
  Bundle of His
ELECTROPHYSIOLOGICAL FACTORS
HEMODYNAMICS
EFFECT OF ARRHYTHMIAS ON THE ECG DIAGNOSIS OF ACUTE MYOCARDIAL INFARCTION

CORONARY CARE UNITS

GENERAL CONSIDERATIONS AND HISTORY
PERSONNEL
  Nursing Personnel
  Physicians
PHYSICAL DESIGN AND INSTRUMENTATION
INCIDENCE OF ARRHYTHMIAS FOLLOWING ACUTE MYOCARDIAL INFARCTION
PREMONITORY ARRHYTHMIAS
PROPHYLAXIS
TREATMENT OF CIRCULATORY ARREST
TREATMENT OF SPECIFIC ARRHYTHMIAS
  Supraventricular Arrhythmias
  Ventricular Arrhythmias

  Antiarrhythmic Prophylaxis in Acute Myocardial Infarction
Bradyarrhythmias
  First Degree A-V Heart Block
  Second Degree A-V Heart Block
  Complete A-V Heart Block
  Slow Idioventricular Rhythm
MORTALITY
INTERMEDIATE CORONARY CARE UNIT
PREHOSPITAL MANAGEMENT OF ACUTE MYOCARDIAL INFARCTION
  Immediate Coronary Care
    Mobile Coronary Care Units

ARRHYTHMIAS IN CHRONIC CORONARY ARTERY DISEASE AND HEALED MYOCARDIAL INFARCTION

GENERAL CONSIDERATIONS
MECHANISMS OF ARRHYTHMIA PRODUCTION IN HEALED INFARCTION AND CHRONIC CORONARY ARTERY DISEASE

SUDDEN DEATH

GENERAL CONSIDERATIONS
ETIOLOGY
PREDISPOSING FACTORS
  Detection of the Coronary-Prone Individual
FACTORS PRECIPITATING SUDDEN CARDIAC DEATH
TREATMENT OF RISK FACTORS

More than one-half million people die annually following a myocardial infarction in the United States. Many of these deaths are caused by potentially reversible arrhythmias. Coronary care units have enabled monitoring and early treatment of these arrhythmias; however, many occur in the immediate postinfarction period, and the patients often die before arriving at the hospital. This chapter will consider: (1) arrhythmias complicating acute myocardial infarction; (2) arrhythmias occurring in chronic coronary artery disease; and (3) sudden death.

ARRHYTHMIAS IN ACUTE MYOCARDIAL INFARCTION

GENERAL CONSIDERATIONS

Myocardial infarction occurs commonly in the natural course of coronary artery disease. Many aspects of cardiac function are deranged in acute myocardial infarction. An important result is the frequent occurrence of relatively benign as well as life-threatening arrhythmias. It has been well documented that patients who collapse suddenly outside the hospital within the first few hours following a myocardial infarction almost invariably manifest either ventricular fibrillation or asystole. Frequently, it is difficult to determine in such cases whether the clinical state is due primarily to the arrhythmia, to the underlying myocardial infarction, or to a combination of both factors. However, one can be certain that prolonged tachyarrhythmias or bradyarrhythmias associated with hypotension may cause extension and aggravation of the underlying ischemic process.

PATHOPHYSIOLOGY

Correlating the extent and type of myocardial damage with the occurrence of arrhythmias is difficult; however, one may make certain generalizations: (1) There is usually a correlation between the size of the infarct and gravity of the clinical state, on the one hand, and the incidence and severity of arrhythmias on the other. (2) Sinus rhythm is transiently or permanently abolished by infarcts involving the S-A node. (3) Atrial fibrillation and other atrial arrhythmias are often associated with atrial infarction. (4) A-V heart block of variable degree and duration is produced by hypoxia or occlusion of the artery supplying the A-V junction and the bundle of His (see Chapters 1 and 10).

Often, a fairly accurate diagnosis of the site of the occlusion can be made from the electrocardiogram in conjunction with a knowledge of the anatomy of the coronary arteries. However, many arrhythmias that occur in acute infarction can be produced by derangements in various portions of the heart, and there may be no direct relationship between the site and size of the infarct and the resultant arrhythmia.

The initial ischemic damage to the myocardium causes a loss of excitability and conduction in the area of the infarct. As organization and repair take place, the electrical function of the damaged area returns at least partially to normal. Recovery of excitability may take place at different times in ischemic areas and adjacent normally perfused areas, thereby predisposing to re-entry phenomena and repetitive responses.

Acute myocardial infarction causes the release of large amounts of epinephrine and norepinephrine from sympathetic nerve endings and from the adrenal medulla. The latter begins to secrete epinephrine into the blood within minutes of the infarction, and the rate of secretion continues to rise for 30 minutes or more. Blood levels of epinephrine return to normal 24 hours after the infarction. However, circulating norepinephrine levels are elevated within 24 hours and remain elevated until about 72 hours after the infarction. This elevation may be associated with the occurrence of certain arrhythmias (Griffiths and Leung, 1971). A relationship has been shown in humans between serum free fatty acid (FFA) levels immediately following myocardial infarction and vulnerability to arrhythmias detected by continuous monitoring of the electrocardiogram during several days following the infarction (Oliver et al., 1968). A consistent positive correlation is found between FFA levels and ectopic activity with a time lag of a few minutes between peak fatty acid levels and the greatest incidence of arrhythmias. Recently, Rutenberg et al. (1969) observed that the serum FFA tends to be elevated at the time various complications developed during the hospital course, such as various arrhythmias, chest pain, and congestive heart failure. Although the FFA values were elevated, they were unable to definitely correlate the occurrence of arrhythmias with a relative increase in FFA. Apparently, many other factors may be operative in the production of arrhythmias.

Slowing of the heart occurs frequently in the postinfarction period. Most instances of bradyarrhythmias are thought to be due to either: (1) direct damage to the S-A node or A-V junction, or (2) activation of vagal reflexes. Increased vagal tone has been attributed to impaired blood flow to the S-A node, to direct stimulation of vagal nerve endings, and to an additional depressor reflex that is initiated from receptors in the injured myocardial tissue or in the coronary vasculature. The slow heart rate per se may predispose to the development of other arrhythmias. Ectopic beats occur earlier and in a larger proportion of the animals when they are paced at slow heart rates (Han et al., 1966). The probable mechanism by which bradycardia hastens the onset of ectopic activity in acute myocardial infarction has been shown to be a significant increase in the temporal dispersion of the refractory period duration at slow rates.

Furthermore, many patients with acute myocardial infarction receive one or more drugs that predispose to arrhythmia production under certain circumstances. Such drugs include various antiarrhythmic agents (digitalis, quinidine, procaine amide, lidocaine, diphenylhydantoin) and other drugs that have effects on the cardiovascular or autonomic nervous systems, such as antidepressants and phenothiazine tranquilizers.

INVOLVEMENT OF SPECIALIZED TISSUES

Internodal Pathways. Those lesions that disrupt the normal function of the S-A node may also derange transmission across the right atrium. Experiments have shown that disruption of the atrial specialized pathways has a profound influence on the sequence of A-V junctional conduction.

A-V Junction. Occlusion of either the main right coronary artery or the penetrating vessels from the posterior descending branch of the right coronary arteries, which in 90 per cent of hearts supplies the A-V junction, is usually associated with high-grade partial or complete A-V heart block (see Fig. 28–1). Because collateral circulation usually is adequate to avoid complete necrosis of the A-V junction in myocardial infarction, the A-V heart block accompanying inferior myocardial infarction is frequently transient (see Chapter 10). Although much less common than with inferior infarction, advanced A-V heart block may be associated with anterior infarction. Only about 5 to 10 per cent of cases of anterior infarction are associated with high grade or complete A-V heart block. When this is the case, one of the following occurs: (1) the A-V junction is supplied by the left circumflex artery (a pattern seen in approximately 10 per cent of hearts); or more commonly, (2) there is associated abnormality, occlusion, stenosis, or hypoplasia of the right coronary artery or its branches; or (3) there is diffuse, extensive disease of the interventricular septum as a result of massive infarction or preexisting disease.

Bundle of His. The bundle of His receives its vascular supply in part from the A-V nodal artery and in part from perforating branches that usually stem from the left coronary artery. Rarely does the bundle of His undergo necrosis because of occlusion of the

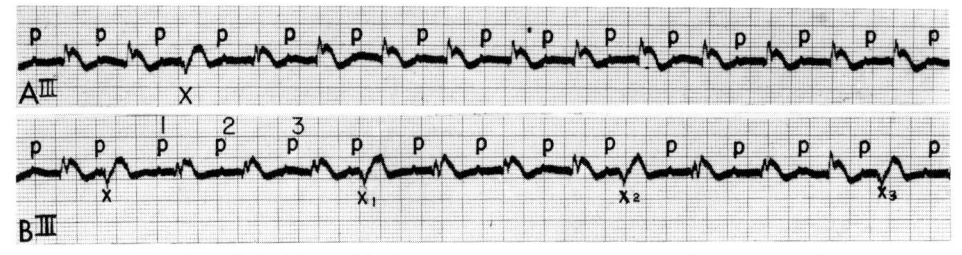

Figure 28-1. Partial A-V heart block occurring in the presence of an acute inferior infarction, showing Wenckebach period and a parasystolic ventricular rhythm (patient 60 years of age).

(A) (Lead III) Note prolonged P-R intervals (0.32 second) and the premature aberrant beat at X. The elevated R-ST segment is due to the acute inferior infarction.

(B) (Lead III) Wenckebach periods showing increasing length of the P-R interval in cycles 1, 2, and 3 followed by the occurrence of ventricular premature beat at X. Following this, the P-R interval becomes prolonged again until X_1; this recurs at X_3. The beats X, X_1, X_2, and X_3 represent ventricular parasystolic beats.

A-V nodal artery. On the other hand, left bundle branch block and, less commonly, complete A-V heart block, associated with acute myocardial infarction, may result from necrosis of the bundle of His due to occlusion of the perforating branches from the left coronary artery. These A-V conduction disturbances, however, are less common than those due to involvement of the A-V nodal artery (see Chapter 10). It should be emphasized at this point that coronary artery disease is not as common a cause of complete A-V heart block as idiopathic fibrosis of the distal portion of the A-V junction and bundle of His (see Chapter 10).

ELECTROPHYSIOLOGIC FACTORS

Acute myocardial infarction is associated with many factors known to produce arrhythmias. The proarrhythmic derangements in acute myocardial infarction include: (1) myocardial injury, encompassing both necrosis and inflammation which cause alterations in the electrophysiology of the pacemaker tissues, the conduction system, and the undifferentiated myocardium; (2) hypoxia, caused by impairment of the coronary circulation, shock-like state, and depressed respiration; (3) release of potassium from injured cells; (4) increased levels of circulating catecholamines; (5) elevation of plasma-free fatty acids; (6) activation of both vagal and sympathetic reflexes due to a multiplicity of causes (e.g., hemodynamic alterations, pain, and fear); (7) electrolyte alterations, acidosis, and alkalosis; (8) the effect of certain cardioactive drugs often used in patients with acute infarction; and (9) altered myocardial hemodynamics.

These derangements which occur in subjects with acute myocardial infarction produce brady- or tachyarrhythmias by means of the following mechanisms: (1) enhancement of or decrease in automaticity of certain pacemakers and potential pacemakers; (2) factors leading to a decrease in the threshold for repetitive responses and fibrillation; (3) the occurrence of either gross or microre-entry leading to varying grades of electrophysiologic inhomogeneity of the myocardium; and (4) injury causing loss of automatic function or block of conduction in the S-A node, the A-V junction, or the His Purkinje system. Factors that commonly enhance automaticity in the presence of myocardial infarction include: (1) inflammation, (2) increased catecholamines, (3) acidosis, (4) hypokalemia, (5) hypercapnia, (6) hypoxia, and (7) mechanical stretch (see Chapter 2).

Myocardial ischemia causes a significant increase in the usual temporal dispersion of refractoriness (Han, 1969). The existence of adjacent cells and regions that differ with respect to their excitability at the moment when an impulse arrives underlies microreentry and even circus movement. In addition, metabolic derangements and electrophysiologic inhomogeneity cause a decrease in the threshold for repetitive responses to a single stimulus and for ventricular fibrillation. Myocardial ischemia has this effect, as shown by the marked decrease in the number of successive premature beats required to initiate ventricular fibrillation in the experimental animal following coronary ligation (see Chapter 15) (Bellet and Kostis, 1971; Bellet et al., 1972). This state persists until stability is restored to the infarcted area in the healed stage.

HEMODYNAMICS

The hemodynamic consequences of acute myocardial infarction are quite variable, depending in part on the previous cardiovascular state and circulatory function and on the severity of the infarction. Left ventricular failure is often considered an intrinsic feature of the disease. The cardiac output and stroke volume are usually decreased in patients with recent myocardial infarction and the degree of subnormality is very roughly correlated with the gravity of the manifest clinical state (Broch et al., 1959). Serious arrhythmias occur more frequently and are often refractory to treatment in patients with cardiogenic shock complicating acute infarction.

Tachyarrhythmias cause hemodynamic changes in patients with acute myocardial infarction that range from a momentary change in stroke volume due to a ventricular premature beat to complete cessation of circulation due to ventricular fibrillation. Rapid but coordinated contraction of the atria (PAT and supraventricular tachycardia) with a rapid ventricular rate usually, but not always, causes a decrease in cardiac output because the rapid rate is unable to compensate for the decrease in stroke volume. Supraventricular tachycardias depress the circulation to an intermediate degree. Ventricular tachycardia impairs stroke volume even further. Occasionally, patients with acute myocardial infarction may for brief periods tolerate episodes of tachyarrhythmias rather well; in others, the arrhythmia encroaches upon the remaining cardiac reserve, leading to rapid deterioration, shock, and eventual death.

Complete A-V heart block occurring during acute myocardial infarction manifests an especially deleterious effect on the circulation because myocardial impairment limits the maximal stroke volume. The infarction often causes acute myocardial failure, and as a result, arterial pressure may fall markedly when complete A-V heart block occurs. Other serious arrhythmias often superimposed may be fatal. Artificial pacing is often mandatory as an emergency measure (see Chapter 37). In one study, cardiac output was increased by pacing in all but two patients from a mean CI of 2.22 L./minute/M^2 to 2.85 L./minute/M^2. The tension-time index was low in complete heart block (1308 mm. Hg second/minute) and increased markedly with pacing (6782 mm. Hg second/minute), suggesting a marked increase in myocardial oxygen requirements (Lassers et al., 1968).

EFFECT OF ARRHYTHMIAS ON THE ELECTROCARDIOGRAPHIC DIAGNOSIS OF ACUTE MYOCARDIAL INFARCTION

Arrhythmias, particularly frequent premature beats, atrial fibrillation and flutter, may obscure the electrocardiographic diagnosis of acute infarction. Moreover, QRST patterns in ventric-

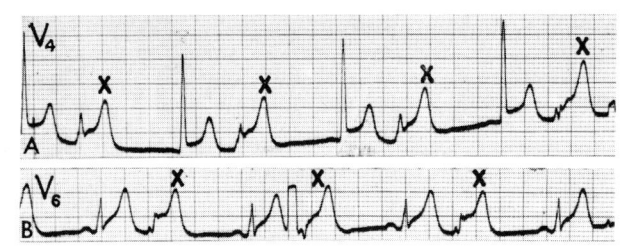

Figure 28-2. Shows the effect of myocardial infarction on the ST configuration of premature beats.

(A) (V$_2$) Note the elevation of the ST segments in the premature beats (X). Note that the ST segment elevations are particularly marked in the premature beats and they are only slightly in evidence in the normal complexes.

(B) (V$_6$) Note elevation of ST segment in premature atrial beats at X.

ular premature beats may resemble those of acute myocardial infarction and may lead to a misdiagnosis. Occasionally, however, infarction may be diagnosed only by the patterns of the ectopic beats and not by those of the sinus beats (Bisteni et al., 1961) (Fig. 28-2). The diagnosis may be made on the basis of the deep Q wave, elevated RS-T junction, and coved negative T wave in ectopic beats in leads II, III, and aVF.

CORONARY CARE UNITS (CCU)

GENERAL CONSIDERATIONS AND HISTORY

In recent years, the high mortality rate (30 to 40 per cent) associated with acute myocardial infarction has become the object of widespread study. The main objectives have been the prevention, effective management, and immediate treatment of cardiac arrhythmias, immediate resuscitation in the event of cardiac arrest or ventricular fibrillation, and investigation of specific causes of death. From this research has come the concept of the intensive coronary care unit as the ideal location for the treatment and study of patients suffering from acute myocardial infarction.

The effectiveness of the coronary care unit is based on constant observation by a team of physicians and nurses well trained in the diagnosis and treatment of the various complications of myocardial infarction. The unit contains electronic equipment for constant monitoring of the electrocardiogram, heart rate and rhythm, and physiological parameters and provides immediate availability of resuscitative equipment, such as the defibrillator, pacemaker, and positive pressure breathing respirators and apparatus, for closed-chest cardiac compression. Modern electronic equipment can be used most effectively in specific diagnoses and treatment to support the patient through the first few critical days. Complications can be quickly detected and appropriate therapy immediately instituted.

A constantly available, highly trained nursing service is reassuring to the patient and contributes substantially to his recovery. The coronary care unit requires constant attendance by the house physician, who is on standby alert for an unusual occurrence, to resolve a diagnostic problem or to handle any catastrophic episode. The incidence of successful resuscitation of the acute coronary patient in ventricular fibrillation or cardiac arrest is much higher in the coronary care unit than on the general floors of the hospital.

PERSONNEL

Smooth operation of the coronary care unit requires a team approach to patient care by the medical and nursing staff.

Nursing Personnel. A focus on preventing cardiac arrest requires highly trained nursing personnel, competent in recognizing electrocardiographic patterns and capable of knowing when to alert the physician of significant changes in the clinical state of the patient and in the electrocardiogram. The trained cardiac nurse must be a specialist in the management of myocardial infarction and must be prepared to institute life-sustaining measures, such as administering intravenous drugs, closed-chest heart massage, positive-pressure breathing, defibrillation, and external pacemaking in the event of cardiac arrest. The coronary care nurse must also handle the emotional responses of patients to their heart attacks, which may be manifested as hostility, depression, anxiety, and fear of death (Killip and Kimball, 1968).

Physicians. At least one member of the house staff should be present in the CCU or on the same floor at all times. Alarm facilities should be arranged so that the responsible physician can be alerted to an emergency with no undue loss of time.

PHYSICAL DESIGN AND INSTRUMENTATION

The area is an air-conditioned, noise-free, tranquil environment. The rooms are distributed around a central nurses' station which permits direct patient observation. Each room is provided with an oscilloscope, cardiotachometer, multiple lead selector, demand pacemaker, and rate-activated alarm. At the head of each bed are outlets for oxygen, suction, an intercom system, and a clock that is activated by an episode of cardiac arrest.

The nurses' station contains a large slave oscilloscope which simultaneously displays the electrocardiographic traces from each of the patients with an automatic recorder that is activated by any deviation from rate limits preset for each patient. Equipment for long-term (6 to 12 hour) monitoring on tape is desirable, although not essential. Recently, the computer has been employed in long-term monitoring of the electrocardiogram of patients in the CCU.

There is a cardioversion room in the area with immediately available defibrillation equipment. An alternative is a central cart that contains a defibrillator, pacemaking and pulmonary ventilation equipment, airways, minor auxiliary equipment, and emergency drugs. A direct-writing electrocardiograph for continuous and rapid electrocardiographic diagnosis should also be available.

INCIDENCE OF ARRHYTHMIAS FOLLOWING ACUTE MYOCARDIAL INFARCTION

Long-term monitoring reveals the incidence of arrhythmias in myocardial infarction to be about 90 per cent. Most supraventricular arrhythmias associated with acute myocardial infarction are benign. However, the more serious arrhythmias of this group include marked slowing of the primary pacemaker, producing sustained bradycardia. This is much more prevalent in shock patients. Sinus arrest or bradycardia is observed in 13 per cent of patients with acute infarction (Day, 1965; Kimball and Killip, 1968). Atrial fibrillation is observed in 9 per cent, atrial tachycardia in 1.6 per cent, atrial flutter in 4 per cent, and junctional tachycardia in 3 per cent of patients (Kimball and Killip, 1968).

The most common arrhythmia in a representative series (Kimball and Killip, 1968) was ventricular premature beats (78 per cent). Intermittent or sustained ventricular tachycardia is encountered in 30 per cent of the patients, while primary ventricular fibrillation (ventricular fibrillation not preceded by ventricular tachycardia) occurred in only 2 per cent of patients without shock and 9 per cent of patients with shock. First degree A-V block occurred in 13 per cent; second degree block, in 7 per cent; third degree (complete) A-V block, in 5 per cent of patients in the absence of shock but in 60 per cent of the patients with shock.

Care must be used in interpreting the oscilloscope tracing. Most electrocardiographic monitoring oscilloscopes produce artefacts that render correct interpretations difficult (Arbeit et al., 1970). These include widening and an increase in the amplitude of the QRS complexes and a change from a normal to an elevated or depressed R-T segment. Abnormalities due to arrhythmias are usually not disturbed, however. For more exact evaluation, the oscilloscopic findings should be compared with the conventional electrocardiographic tracing taken directly from the patient.

PREMONITORY ARRHYTHMIAS

During the first few days after a myocardial infarction, the premonitory changes in rhythm that must be treated promptly are ventricular ectopic beats, bradycardia, and A-V heart block. Recent observations in coronary care units suggest that mortality is correlated with the incidence of ventricular arrhythmias. Unexpected cardiac arrest due to ventricular fibrillation is observed in about 10 per cent of patients with myocardial infarction; but because ventricular fibrillation is preceded by ventricular premature beats and ventricular tachycardia in about 15 to 20 per cent of cases, the institution of vigorous treatment of ectopic beats will reduce the incidence of fibrillation. Occasionally, ventricular fibrillation may appear suddenly without a preceding period of premature beats or ventricular tachycardia. This complication often occurs within the first few hours after infarction and is almost always fatal if not detected and immediately treated. Asystole associated with myocardial infarction is difficult to manage and has a poor prognosis; the incidence is about 5 per cent, with a mortality of more than 80 per cent. Prolonged A-V conduction may be premonitory to complete A-V heart block or asystole.

PROPHYLAXIS

The prophylactic therapy of arrhythmias following acute myocardial infarction may be considered in two phases: (1) therapy prior to the appearance of any arrhythmia, and (2) therapy following the onset of the mild premonitory arrhythmias. The therapy prior to the appearance of arrhythmias consists of general supportive measures. Prophylactic treatment of arrhythmias with procaine amide, quinidine, lidocaine, and recently, propranolol should be instituted as soon as premonitory arrhythmias appear. Factors predisposing to the production of arrhythmias should be controlled: chest pain, anxiety, hypotension, hypoxia, and pH disturbances which are quite common. Ayres and Grace (1969) have reported hypoxemia and alkalemia in more than 40 per cent of their patients in the coronary care unit.

Metabolic acidosis and the combination of hypoxia, alkalemia, and hypokalemia may become manifest by arrhythmias that cannot be terminated until the derangement is corrected. The following arrhythmias have been documented in such patients: atrial fibrillation and flutter, supraventricular tachycardia and ventricular premature beats, ventricular tachycardia and fibrillation (Gunnar et al., 1966). These metabolic abnormalities should be treated immediately by administration of oxygen and adjustment of ventilatory rate to prevent either acidosis or alkalosis, as well as by correction of electrolyte imbalance (Ayres and Grace, 1969).

Left heart failure occurs in many patients with acute infarction and may lead to certain arrhythmias. The presence of basilar rales, hepatomegaly, and edema of the lower extremities suggests the institution of treatment with diuretics and digitalis.

Procaine amide, quinidine, and lidocaine have been used as prophylactic agents in the coronary care unit following acute myocardial infarction. Lidocaine has been employed for the treatment of ventricular arrhythmias following acute myocardial infarction. Adequate doses of lidocaine (50 to 100 mg. in an intravenous bolus followed by an intravenous drip at 1 to 4 mg. per minute) prevent ventricular arrhythmias in 80 per cent or more of patients with acute myocardial infarction who are monitored in a coronary care unit. Diphenylhydantoin and bretylium, relatively new agents, have not been sufficiently studied to assess their therapeutic potential except in specific states.

In summary, the major goals of prophylactic care in the coronary care unit should be: (1) to abolish ventricular ectopic beats during the first 48 to 72 hours after the onset of acute myocardial infarction; (2) to increase the ventricular rate in bradyarrhythmias that are associated with ectopic beats or hemodynamic deterioration; (3) early detection of left ventricular failure and prompt therapy; and (4) correction of hypoxemia and electrolyte imbalance. When these have been accomplished, it may be possible to reduce the incidence of ventricular fibrillation to less than 1 per cent (Ayres and Grace, 1969).

TREATMENT OF CIRCULATORY ARREST

Circulatory arrest may be recognized by evidence of asystole or ventricular fibrillation in the electrocardiogram or by the absence of a palpable pulse (cardiovascular collapse). Immediate treatment should begin with a blow on the precordium, followed by electrical defibrillation if necessary. If asystole or profound cardiovascular collapse is present, artificial ventilation and external cardiac compression should be instituted by the nurse, and the physician called. Treatment includes external electrical defibrillation, use of appropriate drugs for arrhythmias and hypotension, maintenance of cardiac output by external cardiac compression, provision of an open airway, pulmonary ventilation, and artificial pacing if needed. The regimen of emergency treatment of cardiac arrest is discussed in detail in Chapter 16.

TREATMENT OF SPECIFIC ARRHYTHMIAS

The specific therapy for each individual arrhythmia encountered in the coronary care unit is discussed in detail in the appropriate chapter. The factors relating particularly to acute myocardial infarction are summarized in the following paragraphs.

Supraventricular Arrhythmias. The therapeutic approach to each type of supraventricular arrhythmia should be based on their frequency, tolerance by the patient, and rapidity of the ventricular rate. In general, no treatment is necessary for occasional premature contractions. However, if the beats assume trigeminal or bigeminal form or if short runs of atrial tachycardia are noted, quinidine sulfate (200 to 400 mg. every 6 hours, by mouth) or procaine amide (500 to 750 mg. every 4 to

6 hours, intramuscularly or by mouth) should be given.

In atrial fibrillation, digitalis should be administered in sufficient dosage to effectively slow the heart rate. If atrial fibrillation with rapid ventricular response persists for several hours in spite of therapy, electric countershock should be employed and quinidine maintenance initiated (see p. 77).

Digitalis is indicated in the treatment of atrial flutter to slow the ventricular rate and to convert flutter to fibrillation; if large doses are required, if the reaction of the patient is not prompt, and if the ventricular rate is unduly rapid, electrical conversion is the method of choice.

Ventricular Arrhythmias. Premature ventricular contractions are the most common arrhythmia observed in patients with acute myocardial infarction. Prompt antiarrhythmic therapy is necessary if the contractions occur more often than five per minute, occur in groups, are multifocal, or fall near the apex of the T wave of conducted beats. Treatment consists of 25 to 50 mg. of 2 per cent lidocaine in one intravenous injection. This may be repeated if the arrhythmia persists. Lidocaine can then be given as a constant intravenous drip at the rate of 1 to 4 mg. per minute. Recurrence or persistence of frequent premature ventricular contractions warrants additional therapy. If lidocaine controlled the arrhythmia earlier, the effective dose may be administered again as a single intravenous bolus. Once the premature ventricular contractions have been controlled, maintenance therapy is instituted by the administration of procaine amide, intramuscularly or orally, or quinidine sulfate, orally. Generally, ectopic activity diminishes or disappears by the third day, at which point antiarrhythmic therapy can be tapered off (Kimball and Killip, 1968).

Drug therapy for intermittent, nonsustained ventricular tachycardia is essentially the same as the treatment for premature ventricular contractions. On the other hand, sustained ventricular tachycardia is associated with an immediate and severe compromise of systemic pressure and cardiac output. Prompt termination is necessary. If no response occurs after administering a 60-mg. bolus and then a 100-mg. bolus of lidocaine, immediate electrical conversion is indicated. Ventricular tachycardia associated with circulatory collapse should be treated immediately with electric countershock. Time should not be wasted on manual cardiopulmonary resuscitation, drug administration, or even attempts at synchronizing the electrical discharge with the R wave. Immediately following a successful resuscitation from ventricular tachycardia, a dose of lidocaine may be given and maintenance therapy started with lidocaine in a continuous intravenous drip (Grace and Haywood, 1968; Kimball and Killip, 1968).

Because of its effect of sharply reducing the susceptibility of the ventricle to fibrillation, bretylium tosylate may be indicated in the treatment of ventricular tachycardias that prove refractory to lidocaine (Bacaner, 1968). (This drug is discussed in detail in Chapter 33.)

Antiarrhythmic Prophylaxis in Acute Myocardial Infarction. Recently, studies have been performed relative to the effect of the prophylactic administration of procaine amide, lidocaine and quinidine in subjects with acute myocardial infarction. Careful monitoring during the administration of these drugs in therapeutic doses has shown a significant decrease in the number of premature ventricular beats as compared to a control group, a decrease ranging from 43 to 60 per cent (Koch-Weser et al., 1969; Mogensen, 1970). Bloomfield et al. (1971) reported on a carefully controlled study using quinidine with continuous monitoring over a period of 24 hours for a period of five days. After a loading procedure, 300 mg. of quinidine sulfate or placebo was administered orally every six hours for five days under random, double-blind conditions. Although there was no decrease in mortality in the treated and untreated variety in the CCU, these studies suggest that where the control group is not being continually monitored under conditions where immediate antiarrhythmic therapy may be administrated such prophylactic therapy could be extremely beneficial in preventing various complications due to arrhythmias and even sudden death.

Bradyarrhythmias. A bradyarrhythmia is defined as a heart rate below 50 to 60 per minute; however, the rate may drop to 30 per minute or less. The cardiac mechanism may be sinus bradycardia, sinoatrial block, slow A-V junctional rhythm, or the various degrees of A-V heart block. The possible underlying causes of the bradycardia and the associated hypotension include disease in pacemaker tissue, local ischemia from low coronary perfusion, and poor brain perfusion with overactive vagal tone.

Atropine is the drug of choice for the treatment of sudden episodes of sinus bradycardia, particularly in the presence of cardiogenic shock. Atropine, 0.6 mg. administered intravenously in two to three doses within a two- to three-hour period, has beneficial effects in 90 per cent of patients. The duration of action often is several hours. Atropine is advised for acute sinus bradycardia but not recommended for maintenance.

The occasional patient who does not respond to atropine may be treated by the intravenous administration of isoproterenol (1 mg. in 250 to 500 cc. of dextrose in water). The rate of infusion is adjusted to maintain a normal cardiac rate.

The safest method for treating recurrent bradycardia is by pervenous intracardiac pacing of the right atrium or ventricle. This has the following advantages: (a) it negates the need for atropine or isoproterenol; (b) in the presence of A-V block, it permits proper synchronization of atrial and ventricular contractions; and (c) it avoids the hazard of inducing ventricular tachycardia or fibrillation. The indications for therapeutic pacing are based on the patient's clinical state. In the presence of bradycardia, the following factors favor the use of this procedure: (1) poor or inadequate response to drugs, (2) concomitant presence of frequent premature contractions, (3) hypotension, (4) progressive cardiac decompensation, and (5) frank shock (Kimball and Killip, 1968).

First Degree A-V Heart Block. In first degree A-V heart block (P-R interval measuring greater than 0.22 second) treatment is not usually required for the heart block per se. However, the patient should be carefully monitored, and should a more advanced degree of A-V heart block develop, a transvenous pacemaking electrode should be inserted and the patient prepared for artificial pacemaking in order to ensure immediate control of the heart rate if the degree of block increases still further.

Second Degree A-V Heart Block. Although atropine and isoproterenol may be used, it is preferable to pace these patients. A demand pacemaker is usually recommended.

Complete A-V Heart Block. An immediate attempt should be made to increase the ventricular rate by atropine or isoproterenol; whether effective or not, transvenous pacing should be instituted. Demand pacing at a rate of between 60 and 80 per minute is indicated.

Slow Idioventricular Rhythm. This is observed in shock-like states and occasionally results from drug toxicity (potassium or digitalis).

MORTALITY

Mortality from myocardial infarction treated in a general care facility is usually higher than in the coronary care unit; it usually approximates 30 per cent. The coronary care unit has markedly improved the prognosis of myocardial infarction by reducing the mortality to an average of 20 per cent (with a range of 10 to 25 per cent) (Killip and Kimball, 1968; Kimball and Killip, 1968). The important causes are shock-like state, cardiac arrest, pump failure, and congestive heart failure.

Arrhythmias account for about 40 per cent of deaths.* Of these, two thirds are due to ventricular fibrillation and one third to bradycardia, heart block, asystole or factors associated with the severity of infarction, its location, and associated hemodynamic deterioration. The length of time after the infarction occurs and before the patient is admitted influences survival. Mortality reaches its peak at the onset of myocardial infarction and decreases almost exponentially thereafter. Sixty-five per cent of the deaths occur in the first three days and 85 per cent occur in the first week.

Complete A-V heart block is associated with a high mortality. The onset of complete heart block is usually accompanied by cardiac arrest, particularly in patients with cardiogenic shock. In one series, 32 of 39 patients with complete heart block died (Kimball and Killip, 1968).

Long-term prognosis apparently is also affected by the site of the infarction. Several studies have confirmed the fact that when complete heart block is present long-term survival rates are lower in patients with anterior infarction than in those with posterior infarction. One-year survival of 67 per cent (22 patients) with inferior infarction and complete A-V heart block was observed in one series, whereas no patient in a series of 19 patients with anterior infarction and complete A-V heart block survived one year (Julian et al., 1969).

INTERMEDIATE CORONARY CARE UNIT

Because the period of care in the CCU is relatively short, it has been estimated that as many as 30 per cent of hospital deaths from acute myocardial infarction occur after the sixth day or after discharge from the coronary care unit. In a large proportion of this group, death is sudden and unexpected (Grace and Yarvote, 1970). In some institutions an intermediate coronary care unit has been established which is equipped with the usual life-saving measures in the event of serious arrhythmias or other complications and with nurses and personnel trained in ECG techniques and resuscitation (Grace and Yarvote, 1970). The reduction in deaths in this unit has been impressive. The data so far obtained suggest that such a unit is of considerable help for the care of the patient with acute myocardial infarction and is an essential intermediate step prior to admission to the general hospital facility (Grace and Yarvote, 1970).

PREHOSPITAL MANAGEMENT OF ACUTE MYOCARDIAL INFARCTION

The prehospital management of the acute coronary suspect assumes special importance because roughly 60 per

---

* This statement as applied to some cases may be misleading. Although in many series death followed the development of arrhythmias, an important question is whether death was due to the arrhythmia or to the extensive infarction. Under these conditions, the arrhythmia is a manifestation of the disease process but cannot be regarded as the primary cause of death.

cent of deaths from acute infarction occur before the patient reaches the hospital and because many of the deaths are due to causes, such as arrhythmias, that are often reversible with proper treatment. Optimal prehospital care for the patient who has suffered acute myocardial infarction depends on several factors: (1) patients must be educated to recognize and respond to the early symptoms of infarction; (2) a tentative diagnosis must be made promptly on the basis of a telephone description of the symptoms to a personal physician or hospital or by self-referral to nearby medical facilities; (3) treatment must be instituted at the first signs of significant arrhythmia or shock; and (4) the patient must be transported without delay to a hospital setting.

Many episodes of acute myocardial infarction go unrecognized for crucial minutes or hours of the immediate postinfarction period. It has been suggested recently that patients with an exacerbation of previous symptoms of coronary heart disease or with the onset of new cardiac symptoms might benefit from evaluation in an organized coronary outpatient study unit (Levine, 1969). In this unit, each patient could be thoroughly evaluated; those with clear evidence of myocardial infarction would be transferred immediately to the coronary care unit; other subjects would be evaluated carefully over a four- to six-hour period. Such a unit would be of clinical benefit because more patients with myocardial infarction would reach the hospital quickly.

Immediate Coronary Care

Mobile Coronary Care Units. In view of the large number of deaths that occur prior to hospitalization, considerable effort has recently been devoted to developing better systems of prehospital care. Chief among these is the mobile coronary care unit. Many of these deaths are attributed to potentially correctable arrhythmias, including ventricular fibrillation. A special ambulance equipped and staffed to cope with this problem was introduced by Pantridge and Geddes (1967) and has now been employed by many groups (Barber et al., 1970; Pantridge and Adgey, 1969). The ambulance is equipped with a battery-operated electrocardiogram monitor and direct writer, a D.C. defibrillator, and a pacemaker. The patient is monitored with no attempt to transfer him to the ambulance until any evidence of ventricular irritability (e.g., the R-on-T pattern in the electrocardiogram) has been treated by antiarrhythmic drugs. Of 312 patients encountered over a 15-month period when this mobile unit was in use, no deaths occurred in transit, as compared to a one-year study of coronary deaths at the same hospital in which 102 of 414 patients were dead on arrival.

St. Vincent's Hospital in New York City has recently instituted a mobile coronary care unit. Grace (Grace and Chadburn, 1969) has reported on its inception and the problems they face, such as traffic congestion, false alarms, and cancelled calls, many of which are peculiar to a large metropolitan area. Although the existing mobile coronary care units have been shown to be relatively effective, their impact has not been as great as had been anticipated. The yield of successful resuscitations varies with the equipment of the unit and the environmental setting in which the unit operates. In addition, the initial investment in personnel and equipment required to establish the unit is high, as are operating and upkeep costs. Despite the problems in organization, communication, staffing, and financing posed by the mobile coronary care unit, its usefulness appears beyond question as a life-preserving extension of the hospital intensive care concept.

ARRHYTHMIAS IN CHRONIC CORONARY ARTERY DISEASE AND HEALED MYOCARDIAL INFARCTION

GENERAL CONSIDERATIONS

Coronary artery disease is widespread in the adult population. From 30 to 50 per cent of both men and women in all age groups over the age of 50 manifest electrocardiographic evidence of coronary artery disease. Chronic coronary artery disease, with or without healed previous myocardial infarction, is an important etiologic factor in many arrhythmias, especially atrial fibrillation and flutter, frequent ventricular premature beats, A-V heart block, and intraventricular block. Their occurrence is important because: (1) they may cause symptoms or disability; (2) they may predispose to sudden cardiac death; and (3) prophylactic treatment may be beneficial in their prevention.

MECHANISMS OF ARRHYTHMIA PRODUCTION IN HEALED INFARCTION AND CHRONIC CORONARY ARTERY DISEASE

Subjects with coronary artery disease frequently manifest a number of abnormalities that predispose to arrhythmias. Localized ischemic damage to areas of the myocardium enable the development of action potential differences between normal and ischemic tissue, leading to the development of microre-entry circuits, which is an important mechanism in the production of atrial and ventricular premature beats. In the presence of an elevated heart rate, electrophysiologic inhomogeneity due to moderate degrees of organic damage may cause premature beats and occasionally ventricular fibrillation.

Some additional mechanisms leading to arrhythmias in patients with chronic coronary artery disease deserve brief mention: (1) sympathetic tone is elevated in many patients with coronary artery disease because of their emotional make-up, lack of exercise, or other factors; (2) metabolic disturbance in areas of localized ischemia, especially hypoxia, predispose to enhanced pacemaker activity (Ayres and Grace, 1969); (3) sclerotic damage to the A-V transmission system is a frequent cause of A-V heart block, which may progress suddenly from partial to complete A-V heart block and eventuate in Stokes-Adams seizures (see Chapter 10); (4) arrhythmias may result from permanent cardiac damage which, coupled with chronic coronary artery insufficiency, drastically reduces the coronary blood flow; (5) the frequent occurrence of congestive heart failure in these patients is an additional factor tending to precipitate ectopic rhythms; (6) damage to or destruction of the S-A node underlies the so-called "sick sinus syndrome"; and (7) the stress of exercise or emotion in the presence of coronary artery disease would produce hypoxia and metabolic disturbances that could lead to abnormalities which may result in premature beats, paroxysmal tachycardia, or ventricular fibrillation.

The most common arrhythmias in healed infarction are atrial and ventricular premature beats and atrial fibrillation, although almost any type of ectopic rhythm may occur. Sudden death from ventricular fibrillation or ventricular standstill is also a possible threat to the patient.

SUDDEN DEATH

GENERAL CONSIDERATIONS

Sudden death has been defined as demise due to natural causes occurring within 24 hours of the beginning of the fatal event in an apparently previously well patient. Despite the relatively wide latitude of the definition, it should be emphasized that most of the sudden fatalities due to coronary artery disease occur within minutes to hours of the onset of the terminal infarction or arrhythmia. The exact mechanism in most instances of sudden death is unknown. However, many patients are observed to die suddenly without evidence of cardiac pain, suggesting that the mechanism of death in these patients is the abrupt onset of ventricular fibrillation or asystole. The precipitating factors, which are often difficult to determine, will be discussed shortly. Even though many of these events could be reversed by the immediate application of appropriate therapeutic measures, their unpredictability generally precludes successful treatment.

In a large necropsy study from Westchester County, New York, Spain et al. (1960) reported that 90 per cent of sudden fatalities resulted from coronary artery disease. In an epidemiologic study in Tecumseh, Michigan, of those who died suddenly from coronary heart disease, 50 per cent had a history of clinical heart disease, 27.8 per cent, a history of hypertension, and 11.4 per cent, a history of diabetes (Chiang et al., 1969a).

ETIOLOGY

The etiology of sudden death may be divided into two categories (1) the time and increase the risk of sudden death (see next section), and presence of predisposing factors that exist over a considerable period of (2) precipitating factors that initiate the coronary failure or potentially fatal arrhythmia.

PREDISPOSING FACTORS

Detection of the Coronary-Prone Individual. Numerous risk factors that predispose to coronary artery disease have been delineated, including the following: (1) elevated serum cholesterol (over 260 mg./100 ml.); (2) diabetes mellitus; (3) hypertension (systolic blood pressure over 180 mm. Hg); (4) cigarette smoking, especially more than one pack per day; (5) lack of physical exercise; (6) hyperreactive personality type; (7) familial history of coronary artery disease; and (8) electrocardiographic abnormalities, especially nonspecific ST-T changes and evidence of left ventricular hypertrophy. The coexistence of two or more risk factors for coronary artery disease (CAD) in the same subject is quite common; this results in a cumulative risk for the development of CAD. Individuals with many of the risk factors are almost certain to develop serious manifestations of coronary artery disease (Gertler et al., 1964).

FACTORS PRECIPITATING SUDDEN CARDIAC DEATH

Sudden death may be precipitated by any of the following acute derangements in cardiac function: (1) increased sympathetic tone due to emotional stress, fear, or reflexes which lead to acute cardiac overload or fatal arrhythmias; (2) acute arrhythmias, such as ventricular tachycardia or complete A-V heart block, which progress to ventricular fibrillation or asystole; (3) acute myocardial infarction, especially the massive type or occlusion of the vessels supplying the A-V node; and (4) certain agents that lower the fibrillation threshold and disturb cardiac function in other ways as well, including drugs that release catecholamines (amphetamines and similar drugs, model airplane glue, nicotine, and possibly caffeine).

Prevention of sudden cardiac death involves the following principles: (1) detection of the coronary-prone individual; (2) treatment of the underlying disease state; (3) institution of a regimen to minimize existing or potential risk factors; (4) planning the management from the development of the initial symptoms of myocardial infarction until the patient reaches the coronary care unit; and (5) early detection of significant arrhythmias and institution of prophylactic therapy. A wider spectrum of indications for the implantation of permanent pacemakers should be considered. Antiarrhythmic medication should be considered in selected patients who appear to have a high risk of developing serious arrhythmias.

TREATMENT OF RISK FACTORS

Myocardial infarction may be postponed or prevented in many individuals by the reduction of risk factors. This requires the cooperation of the patient which is often difficult to obtain because of psychologic or economic factors. Appropriate measures include: (1) loss of excess weight; (2) diet low in saturated fats; (3) minimizing emotional and physical stress; (4) avoiding the use of nicotine, caffeine, amphetamines, and the like in selected individuals; (5) participation in appropriately supervised exercise; and (6) education of the public to have frequent examinations and to seek medical attention at the initial appearance of cardiac symptoms.

References

Anttonen, V. M., et al.: The diagnostic value of unipolar precordial patterns of ventricular premature beats in myocardial infarction. Acta Med. Scand., Suppl. 387, 1962.

Arbeit, S. R., Rubin, I. L., and Gross, H.: Dangers in interpreting the electrocardiogram from the oscilloscope monitor. JAMA, *211:*453, 1970.

Ayres, S. M., and Grace, W. J.: Inappropriate ventilation and hypoxemia as causes of cardiac arrhythmias. Amer. J. Med., *46:*495, 1969.

Bacaner, M. B.: Treatment of ventricular fibrillation and other acute arrhythmias with bretylium tosylate. Amer. J. Cardiol., *21:* 530, 1968.

Barber, J. M., et al.: Mobile coronary care. Lancet, *2:*133, 1970.

Bellet, S., DeGuzman, N., Kostis, J., Roman, L., and Fleischmann, D.: Effect of cigarette smoke inhalation on ventricular fibrillation threshold in normal dogs and dogs with acute myocardial infarction. Amer. Heart J., 83:67, 1972.

Bellet, S., and Kostis, J.: Effect of caffeine on ventricular fibrillation threshold in dogs, 1971 (In press).

Bellet, S., Roman, K., Nichols, G. J., and Muller, O. F.: Detection of coronary-prone subjects in a normal population by radioelectrocardiographic exercise test. Follow-up studies. Amer. J. Cardiol., *19:*783, 1970.

Bisteni, A., Medrano, G., and Sodi-Pallares, D.: Ventricular premature beats in the diagnosis of myocardial infarction. Brit. Heart J., *23:* 521, 1961.

Bloomfield, S. S., Romhilt, D. W., Chou, T-C., and Fowler, N. O.: Quinidine for prophylaxis of arrhythmias in acute myocardial infarction. New Eng. J. Med., *285:*979, 1971.

Broch, O. J., Humerfelt, S., Haarstad, J., and Myhre, J. R.: Hemodynamic studies in acute myocardial infarction. Amer. Heart J., *57:* 522, 1959.

Chapman, J. M., and Massey, F. J.: The interrelationship of serum cholesterol, hypertension, body weight, and risk of coronary disease. Results of the first ten years' follow-up in the Los Angeles heart study. J. Chronic Dis., *17:*933, 1964.

Chiang, B. N., et al.: Predisposing factors in sudden cardiac death in Tecumseh, Michigan. A prospective study. Circulation, *41:*31, 1969a.

Chiang, B. N., Perlman, L. V., Ostrander, L. D., and Epstein, F. H.: Relationship of premature systoles to coronary heart disease and sudden death in the Tecumseh epidemiological study. Ann. Intern. Med., *70:*1109, 1969b.

Day, H. W.: Effectiveness of an intensive coronary care area. Amer. J. Cardiol., *15:*51, 1965.

Gertler, M. M., White, P. D., Cady, L. D., and Whiter, H. H.: Coronary heart disease—a prospective study. Amer. J. Med. Sci., *248:* 377, 1964.

Grace, W. J., and Chadburn, J. A.: The mobile

coronary care unit. Dis. Chest, 65:452, 1969.
Grace, W. J., and Haywood, L. J.: Prevention and treatment of arrhythmias and principles of resuscitation. p. 18. Proceedings National Conference on Coronary Care Units, Mar. 1968.
Grace, W. J., and Yarvote, P. M.: The intermediate coronary care unit (ICCU). Amer. J. Cardiol., 26:635, 1970.
Griffiths, J., and Leung, F.: The sequential estimation of plasma catecholamines and whole blood histamine in myocardial infarction. Amer. Heart J., 82:171, 1971.
Gunnar, R. M., et al.: Myocardial infarction with shock. Hemodynamic studies and results of therapy. Circulation, 33:753, 1966.
Han, J.: Mechanisms of ventricular arrhythmias associated with myocardial infarction. Amer. J. Cardiol., 24:800, 1969.
Han, J., Millet, D., Chizzonitti, B., and Moe, G. K.: Temporal dispersion of recovery of excitability in atrium and ventricle as a function of heart rate. Amer. Heart J., 71:481, 1966.
Hinkle, L. E., Jr., Carver, S. T., and Stevens, M.: The frequency of asymptomatic disturbances of cardiac rhythm and conduction in middle-aged men. Amer. J. Cardiol., 24:629, 1969.
Julian, D. G., Lassers, B. W., and Godman, M. J.: Pacing for heart block in acute myocardial infarction. Ann. N.Y. Acad. Sci., 167:911, 1969.
Killip, T., and Kimball, J. T.: A survey of the coronary care unit: concept and results. Prog. Cardiov. Dis., 11:45, 1968.
Kimball, J. T., and Killip, T.: Aggressive treatment of arrhythmias in acute myocardial infarction: procedures and results. Prog. Cardiov. Dis., 10:483, 1968.
Koch-Weser, J.: Antiarrhythmic prophylaxis in acute myocardial infarction. New Eng. J. Med., 285:1024, 1971.
Koch-Weser, J., Klein, S. W., Foo-Canto, L. L., et al.: Antiarrhythmic prophylaxis with procainamide in acute myocardial infarction. New Eng. J. Med., 281:1253, 1969.
Kurien, V. A., and Oliver, M. F.: A cause for arrhythmias during acute myocardial hypoxia. Lancet, 1:813, 1970.
Lassers, B. W., et al.: Hemodynamic effects of artificial pacing in complete heart block complicating acute myocardial infarction. Circulation, 38:308, 1968.
Levine, H. J.: Pre-hospital management of acute myocardial infarction. Amer. J. Cardiol., 24:826, 1969.
Lown, B.: Approaches to sudden death from coronary heart disease. (Lewis A. Conner Memorial Lecture, Amer. Heart Assoc. 43rd Scientific Sessions, presented Nov. 12, 1970). Circulation, 41–42:III-37, 1970.
Mogensen, L.: Ventricular tachyarrhythmias and lignocaine prophylaxis in acute myocardial infarction: A clinical and therapeutic study. Acta Med. Scand. (Suppl.), 513:1, 1970.
Norris, R. M.: Heart block in posterior and anterior myocardial infarction. Ann. N.Y. Acad. Sci., 167:911, 1969.
Oliver, M. F., Kurien, V. A., and Greenwood, T. A.: Relation between serum free fatty acids and arrhythmias and death after acute myocardial infarction. Lancet, 1:710, 1968.
Pantridge, J. F., and Adgey, A. A. J.: Pre-hospital coronary care: Mobile coronary care unit. Amer. J. Cardiol., 24:666, 1969.
Pantridge, J. F., and Geddes, J. S.: A mobile intensive care unit in the management of myocardial infarction. Lancet, 2:271, 1967.
Rutenberg, H. L., Pamintuan, J. C., and Soloff, L. A.: Serum free fatty acids and their relation to complications after acute myocardial infarction. Lancet, 2:559, 1969.
Spain, D. M., Bradess, V. A., and Mohr, C.: Coronary atherosclerosis as a cause of unexpected and unexplained death: An autopsy study from 1949–1959. JAMA, 174:384, 1960.
Wallace, A. G., and Klein, R. F.: Role of catecholamines in acute myocardial infarction. Amer. J. Med. Sci., 258:139, 1969.

Chapter 29   *Disturbances of Electrolyte Balance*

GENERAL CONSIDERATIONS
POTASSIUM
   Hypopotassemia
      Etiology
      Electrophysiology
      Therapy
   Hyperpotassemia
      Etiology
      Clinical Manifestations
      Effect on ECG and Production of Arrhythmias
      Diagnosis
      Factors Modifying Tolerance to Potassium
      Treatment
CALCIUM
   Hypocalcemia
   Hypercalcemia
      Cardiac Effects
      ECG Alterations
MAGNESIUM
   Hypomagnesemia
   Hypermagnesemia

GENERAL CONSIDERATIONS

The tissues of the body are bathed in a nutrient medium containing various electrolytes which remain within rather stable limits. Deviation from the normal concentration of one or more of the electrolytes may result in a variety of disease states. Changes in electrolyte concentrations may have a marked effect on the cardiac rate and rhythm.

The electrolytes that are particularly implicated in the production of arrhythmias include potassium, calcium, and magnesium. The effects of alterations in sodium and phosphates may have indirect effects and are of lesser importance. Electrolyte disturbances may result from disturbances within the body endogenously, chiefly involving the gastrointestinal, cerebral, renal, or endocrine systems, or exogenously through the introduction of electrolytes from outside the body. Usually, electrolyte disturbances are easily recognized, and in many instances normal levels may be restored with relative rapidity.

POTASSIUM

Hypopotassemia. The term "hypopotassemia" is used to denote potassium depletion that may be manifested by a decrease of potassium in the tissues, the plasma, or both. A decrease in plasma potassium usually, but not invariably, indicates some decrease in tissue potassium; nevertheless, a low plasma potassium may be associated with no decrease in body or tissue potassium, as occurs in familial periodic paralysis. In most instances, however, a low plasma potassium indicates body potassium depletion. The plasma potassium level usually gives a rough gauge of body potassium levels and can be dependably relied upon with some limitations to determine the effect of therapy (Bellet, 1955). Since the extracellular fluid contains only 3 gm. of potassium, a decrease of only 1 gm. would have a definite clinical effect and would be indicated by chemical analysis and probably by the electrocardiogram.

Etiology. Hypopotassemia is usually, but not invariably, observed in the presence of alkalosis. The following conditions produce a depletion of potassium that is manifested in the plasma, in the intracellular compartment, or both: (a) a lack of intake of potassium (normal intake is 50 to 100 mEq. or 2 to 4 gm.) as occurs in starvation and malnutrition; (b) a loss from the gastrointestinal tract during vomiting, diarrhea, intestinal drainage by Wangensteen suction, ileostomy, or biliary fistula; (c) urinary loss during salt-losing nephritis, diuretic phase of renal shutdown, or diuretic therapy; (d) hormone administration (corticoids); (e) the use of alkalinizing agents, sodium bicarbonate, and molar sodium lactate, resulting in alkalosis and a shift of potassium into the cells, as well as an increase in potassium elimination through the kidneys; and (f) the use of insulin and glucose, which shifts potassium from the serum to the cells, especially in the muscles and liver.

Electrophysiology. With low potassium levels, the action potentials of nonautomatic cells show increased amplitude and duration. The higher amplitude can be attributed to an augmented resting potential that increases the amount of change needed to reach the threshold potential. In automatic cells, a decrease in potassium concentration increases the slope of diastolic depolarization (phase 4) and decreases the threshold and maximal diastolic resting potential of automatic cells (Trautwein, 1963). These effects would tend to increase automaticity.

The alterations in the electrocardiogram in this state are confined chiefly to the S-T segment, the T wave, and the T-U interval. The presence of a prominent U wave has additional diagnostic import. A definite relationship exists between the severity of the changes observed and the decrease in serum potassium.

Therapy. Treatment consists of the administration of potassium to compensate for the deficit. In a patient unable to take food by mouth, parenteral administration of potassium may be accomplished at a fast or slow rate, depending upon the urgency in the individual case. The preparations usually employed are potassium chloride, potassium phosphate, or other potassium salts; however, potassium chloride is preferred.

Treatment should also be directed to the correction of the underlying clinical state and other electrolyte alterations.

Hyperpotassemia. Hyperpotassemia is not uncommon; it is observed in many clinical states, especially those accompanied by acidosis, renal insufficiency, and a shock-like state. The diagnosis is simply made from the history of a predisposing factor and by electrocardiographic findings and is finally established by chemical studies. The importance of hyperpotassemia lies in the fact that it is accompanied by serious cardiotoxic effects that might be fatal; it is easily diagnosed; it is usually reversible in the initial stage and frequently in the advanced stages. Prompt therapy may be life-saving.

Etiology. Excess potassium can be derived from two sources: (a) endogenously, from a shift of potassium from the cells to the extracellular fluid, or (b) exogenously, from administration of this cation. A shift of potassium from the cells to the extracellular fluid may result from: (1) increased tissue destruction, e.g., gangrene, crush syndrome, intravascular hemolytic reactions; (2) acidosis, which is associated with increased tissue metabolism and a shift of potassium from the intracellular to the extracellular phase; (3) hypoxia, which leads to a similar shift of potassium; and (4) dehydration and shock.

Clinical Manifestations. The syndrome of hyperpotassemia involves various systems, particularly the cardiovascular, voluntary muscle and nervous systems. It is characterized by manifestations of general weakness and paralysis of the skeletal muscle. These manifestations are frequently accompanied by listlessness, mental confusion, numbness, tingling in the extremities, a sense of weakness and heaviness in the legs, coldness, pallor, bradycardia with totally irregular rhythm, peripheral vascular collapse, poor heart sounds, low blood pressure, and descending flaccid paralysis.

The effects of an excess of potassium on the heart are in many ways similar to those of quinidine and procaine amide. They consist of a decrease in excitability, an increase of the refractory period of the heart muscle, and a slowing of conduction. In a later stage of toxicity the blood pressure falls, owing to a direct depressing effect of potassium on heart muscle contraction, accompanied by peripheral vasodilatation.

Effect on Electrocardiogram and Production of Arrhythmias. In general, the effects of hyperpotassemia on the electrocardiogram may be divided into four stages. These may be followed rather clearly in dogs when potassium is infused slowly but are less clearly defined in the human subject. The first stage consists of an increase in the amplitude of the T wave with narrowing of the base (at a serum level of about 6 to 9 mEq./L.); the second stage is characterized by the development of sinus pauses, accompanied by slight irregularity of the heart rate (at a serum level of 7 to 10 mEq./L.). Stage 1 merges imperceptibly into Stage 2. Often, the characteristic T-wave changes in hyperpotassemia are more apparent at this latter state than in the initial phase (see Figs. 29–1; 29–2). In Stage 3 (at a serum level of 10 to 13 mEq./L.), the ventricular complexes are widened and the ventricular rhythm is irregular. Marked depression of atrial activity is seen at this point. The ventricular rate tends to slow (50 to 70 per minute); occasionally it is rapid (90 to 110 per minute). Stage 4 (at a serum level of 14 to 18 mEq./L.) is characterized by a slow idioventricular rhythm and increased widening of the ventricular complexes. Between Stage 3 and Stage 4, a sinoventricular rhythm is frequently present (Fig. 29–1). In the normal dog, death usually occurs with cardiac asystole with a serum potassium concentration about four times that of normal (16 to 18 mEq./L.). If the potassium is infused rapidly, ventricular fibrillation is the usual terminal event.

In the human subject, similar stages occur but they are not as clearly defined and toxic effects are observed at lower concentrations of potassium. The T waves become tall and peaked when the potassium concentration ranges from 5.5 to 6.5 mEq./L. The P wave decreases in amplitude and both the P wave and the QRS complex widen as the serum concentration is increased, until the P waves disappear at a serum concentration of 7 to 9 mEq./L. The impulse from the S-A node may still reach the ventricle through special conducting pathways despite the absence of atrial depolarization, resulting in a sinoventricular rhythm (see following discussion). The ventricular rhythm in humans becomes irregular when the potassium concentration becomes greater than 8 to 10 mEq./L. A slow idioventricular rhythm is rarely observed in humans unless the patient is continuously monitored.

Vassalle and Hoffman (1965), in an investigation of the spread of sinus impulses through the atria, have demonstrated that sinus activity propagates to the ventricles even though the atrial muscle fibers have been made unexcitable by induced hyperpotassemia. This sinoventricular rhythm rules out the possibility that sinus impulses propagate only through nonspecialized atrial muscle fibers and supports the existence of a specialized conduction pathway between the

DISTURBANCES OF ELECTROLYTE BALANCE

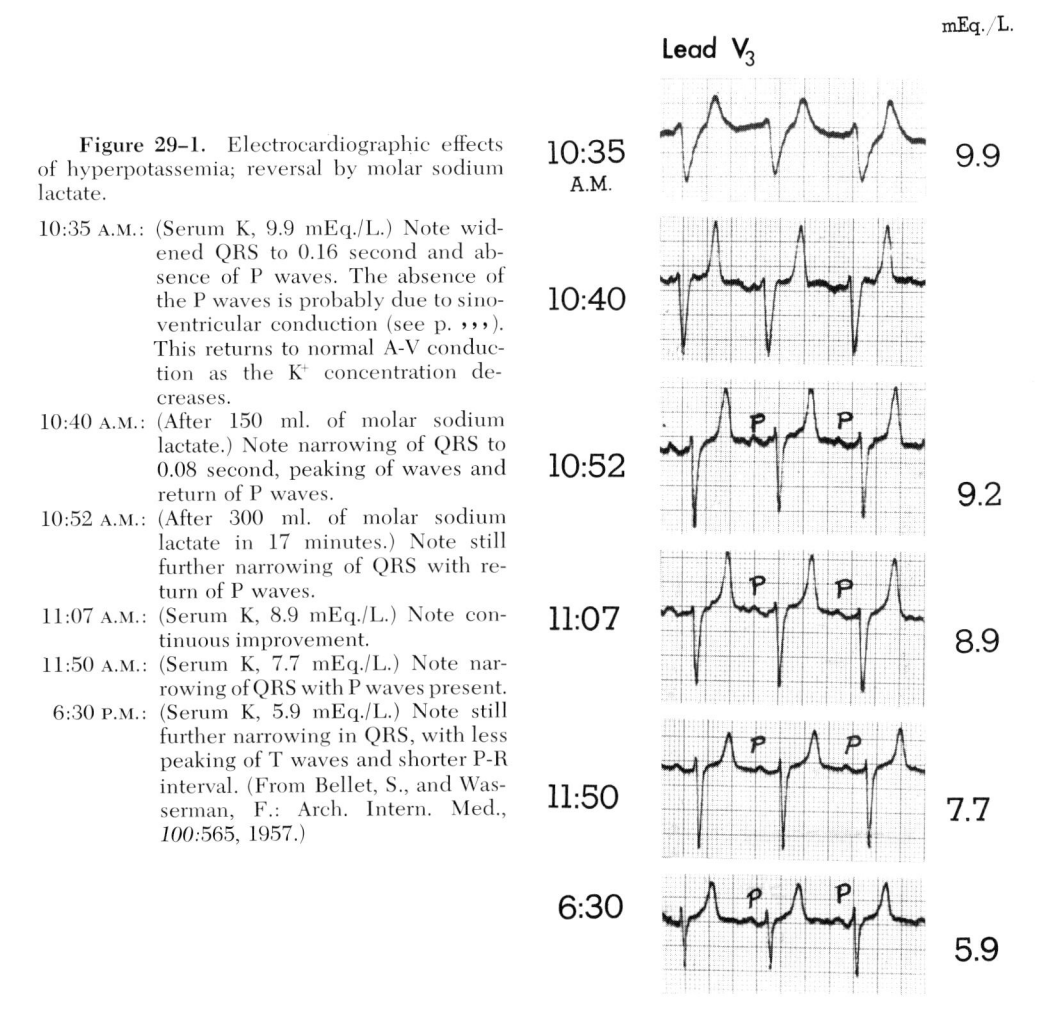

Figure 29–1. Electrocardiographic effects of hyperpotassemia; reversal by molar sodium lactate.

10:35 A.M.: (Serum K, 9.9 mEq./L.) Note widened QRS to 0.16 second and absence of P waves. The absence of the P waves is probably due to sinoventricular conduction (see p. ,,,). This returns to normal A-V conduction as the K⁺ concentration decreases.

10:40 A.M.: (After 150 ml. of molar sodium lactate.) Note narrowing of QRS to 0.08 second, peaking of waves and return of P waves.

10:52 A.M.: (After 300 ml. of molar sodium lactate in 17 minutes.) Note still further narrowing of QRS with return of P waves.

11:07 A.M.: (Serum K, 8.9 mEq./L.) Note continuous improvement.

11:50 A.M.: (Serum K, 7.7 mEq./L.) Note narrowing of QRS with P waves present.

6:30 P.M.: (Serum K, 5.9 mEq./L.) Note still further narrowing in QRS, with less peaking of T waves and shorter P-R interval. (From Bellet, S., and Wasserman, F.: Arch. Intern. Med., *100*:565, 1957.)

sinus node and the atrioventricular junction that is especially resistant to depolarization by increased potassium concentrations (Fig. 29–3) (Vassalle and Hoffman, 1965).

Diagnosis. The diagnosis of hyperpotassemia may be made from the following data: (a) history of a condition leading to hyperpotassemia—azotemia, oliguria, anuria, tissue destruction, shock-like state, and the like; (b) symptoms suggesting the presence of hyperpotassemia; (c) typical electrocardiographic pattern; and (d) blood studies which usually show azotemia, acidosis, increased serum potassium, and, frequently, low sodium and calcium levels.

Factors Modifying Tolerance to Potassium. The tolerance of the heart to potassium varies considerably in different patients. The electrocardiographic pattern is often a more important indicator of cardiotoxicity than is the serum potassium level. The effect of potassium on the heart depends on the degree of myocardial damage, the age of the patient (patients in the older age groups are more sensitive to potassium), and the serum levels of

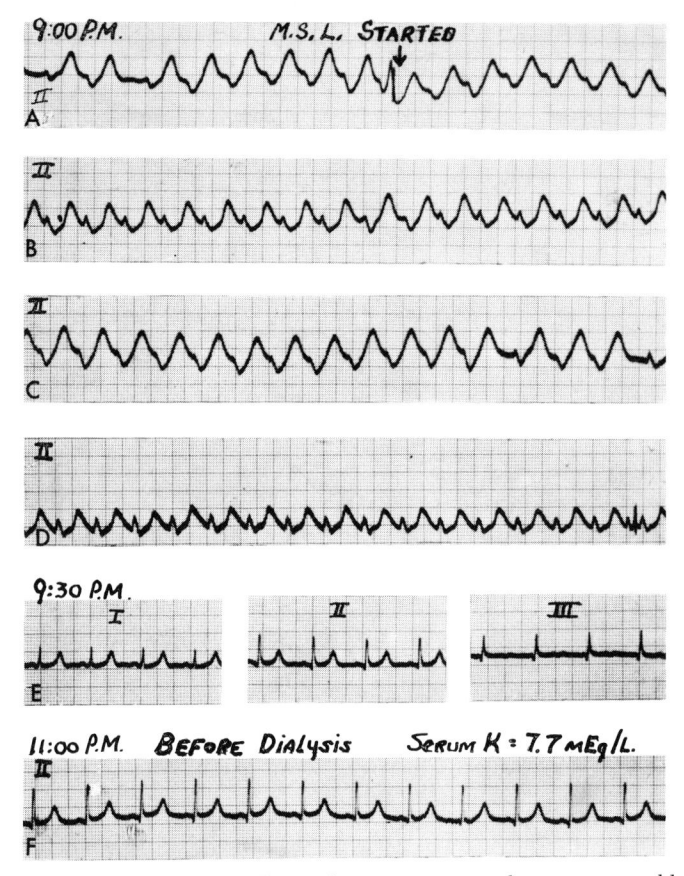

Figure 29-2. Electrocardiographic effect in hyperpotassemia showing reversal by molar sodium lactate.

(A) (Lead II) Taken at 9:00 P.M., when the patient was in coma and circulatory collapse. Bizarre ventricular beats resembling ventricular flutter are present. The serum potassium was 10.7 mEq./L. Molar sodium lactate was started slowly as indicated.

(B) (Lead II) Taken at 9:10 P.M. after 60 mEq. of molar sodium lactate was given intravenously in ten minutes. The rhythm still appears to be ventricular flutter but is somewhat less bizarre.

(C) (Lead II) Taken at 9:14 P.M. after 50 ml. of 50 per cent dextrose with 80 units of regular insulin had been given intravenously two minutes previously. No additional lactate was given. Note further deterioration of the complexes compared to strip B above.

(D) (Lead II) Taken at 9:25 P.M., five minutes after an additional 110 ml. of molar sodium lactate was given rapidly in two minutes. The QRS complexes have narrowed significantly; the ventricular rate is regular at 137 per minute. No P waves are discernible.

(E) (Leads I, II, and III) Taken at 9:30 P.M. Sinus rhythm has been restored. The rate has slowed to 100 per minute. The QRS complexes have narrowed to approximately 0.06 sec.

(F) (Lead II) Taken at 11:00 P.M., shows a relatively normal electrocardiogram. The Q-T interval (0.36 second) is slightly prolonged for the heart rate. (From Bellet, S., and Wasserman, F.: Arch. Intern. Med., *100*:565, 1957.)

other electrolytes, particularly calcium and sodium. These two electrolytes act as pharmacologic antagonists to potassium, so that when their levels are low there is a relative increase in the effect of the potassium.

Treatment. The treatment consists of two categories: prophylactic and active. Prophylactic treatment includes early recognition and careful management of patients with renal insufficiency and close observation of patients during anesthesia and in the postoperative period. The active treatment is comprised of: (a) dietary regimen low in potassium; (b) a decrease in serum potassium by use of alkalinizing agents; (c) calcium infusion; (d) glucose and insulin; (e) cation exchange resins or dialysis (renal or peritoneal); and (f) with slow heart rates (Stage 3) due to a slow idioventricular rhythm, the temporary insertion of an artificial pacemaker may be indicated.

CALCIUM

Calcium is primarily an extracellular electrolyte, although cells contain a small quantity of this cation.

Hypocalcemia. The clinical conditions in which hypocalcemia is most common are: (a) low calcium intake; (b) postoperatively, following partial parathyroidectomy; (c) idiopathic hypoparathyroidism (decreased parathyroid activity occasionally parallels a decrease in thyroid activity); (d) chronic renal failure associated with retention of phosphorus; (e) high intestinal fluid loss (vitamin D deficiency, diarrhea); (f) high urinary calcium loss (essential hypercalciuria and renal tubular acidosis); (g) respiratory and metabolic alkalosis; and (h) pseudohypoparathyroidism. Occasionally, hypopotassemia and hypocalcemia occur simultaneously during alkalosis, e.g., in association with upper intestinal obstruction.

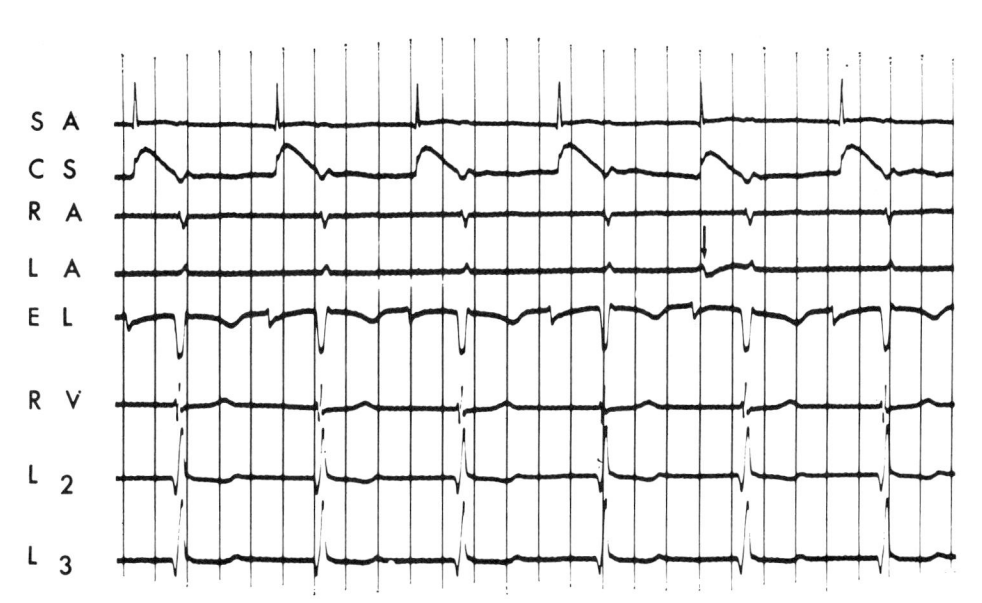

Figure 29-3. Sinoventricular conduction. Sinus impulses propagate regularly to the coronary sinus and the ventricles in absence of activity in the other atrial leads and with complete absence of the P wave. The arrow shows a single activation of the left appendage. SA trace retouched to show rapid deflections. Paper speed 100 mm./sec.; time lines at intervals of 100 msec. (SA: sinus node; CS: coronary sinus; RA: right atrial musculature; LA: left atrial musculature; EL: unipolar record obtained through the catheter lead in right atrium; RV: epicardial surface of right ventricle; L_2: standard Lead II; L_3: standard Lead III.) (From Vassalle, M., and Hoffman, B. F.: Circ. Res., 17:285, 1965.)

Effects of Hypocalcemia. In this condition, the symptoms include increased nervous excitability, tetany, and convulsions. The more marked grades are associated with a hypotensive state. The variations in the electrocardiographic pattern depend to a degree on whether the subject has pure hypocalcemia or if other electrolyte alterations, particularly potassium, are also present. The degree of Q-T prolongation parallels closely the lowering of the serum calcium. This prolongation disappears immediately with an increase in serum calcium level.

Hypercalcemia. Hypercalcemia is observed in primary hyperparathyroidism, hypervitaminosis D, multiple myeloma, sarcoidosis, and metastatic carcinoma, and transiently following the intravenous administration of calcium.

Cardiac Effects. In man, spontaneous (usually gradual) elevation of serum calcium rarely imperils the heart. However, following the therapeutic administration of calcium salts by intravenous injections, sudden transient increases in concentration may attain a level of 10 to 15 mEq./L. Occasionally, deaths result from such rapid elevation in calcium concentrations, most often with previously damaged hearts. In a fully digitalized patient, the danger of ventricular fibrillation seems to increase with a rise in calcium levels, either because of some synergism of digitalis with calcium or because of the effect of the increased calcium level in association with underlying heart disease in these patients.

Electrocardiographic Alterations. During hypercalcemia, the Q-T interval is shortened, usually followed by a prominent U wave; this returns to normal with restitution of a normal serum calcium level. This effect appears after the administration of 10 to 20 ml. of a 10 per cent solution of calcium gluconate; the serum calcium level may acutely increase to about 20 mg./100 ml. of blood. Occasionally, particularly in diseased hearts, premature beats, paroxysmal tachycardia, and even death may result from hypercalcemia.

MAGNESIUM

The effect of magnesium on the heart has been noted and investigated for many years, but interest in this field has recently increased. Magnesium is important because it is, next to potassium, the major intracellular electrolyte.

Magnesium depresses the conduction and spontaneous rhythm of the heart independently of vagal effects. Increasing the serum level of magnesium through intravenous infusion of magnesium salts lengthens the P-R interval. Intraventricular conduction is delayed if administration is continued (Seller and Moyer, 1969).

Hypomagnesemia. There are several clinical conditions in which low serum magnesium is found. These include malignancy, during recovery from diabetic acidosis, hyperthyroidism, and eclampsia. Its occurrence has been reported during the polyuric phase of recovery from renal failure and during the period of diuresis secondary to ammonium chloride and mercurial therapy in congestive heart failure. Magnesium levels are also decreased in the malabsorption syndrome, chronic alcoholism, prolonged or severe loss of body fluids, hyperparathyroidism, primary aldosteronism, and hepatic cirrhosis (Seller and Moyer, 1969). Of clinical significance is the fact that many diuretics lower not only potassium levels but magnesium levels as well.

Hypomagnesemia seems to predispose to digitalis toxicity. Only 70 per cent of the dose of acetylstrophanthidin necessary to establish a toxic arrhythmia in an adult mongrel dog with normal serum magnesium concentration is needed for arrhythmia production if the dog is made hypomagnesemic by dialysis (Seller and Moyer, 1969). Hypomagnesemia, which leads to intracellular potassium loss, may compound the digitalis-induced potassium efflux and thereby potentiate the toxic effects of digitalis. The arrhythmias can usually be corrected immediately by the infusion of 2 to 6 ml. of 25 per cent $MgSO_4$.

Hypermagnesemia. Hypermagnesemia is usually due to renal retention, injection of magnesium, or dehydration. Serum levels over 6 mEq./L. are associated with progressive depression of cardiac conduction and neuromuscular activity. As with hypomagnesemia, direct cardiovascular effects of hypermagnesemia have not been found clinically in man.

Cardiac Manifestations. When intravenous magnesium salts are given to man, an initial bradycardia is followed by a tachycardia. The P-R interval is prolonged, intraventricular conduction is slowed, and some T wave changes occur. Large amounts cause hypotension, which is less marked in hypertensive patients.

References

Bellet, S.: The electrocardiogram in electrolyte imbalance. Arch. Intern. Med., 96:618, 1955.

Brown, H., Tanner, G. L., and Hecht, H. H.: Effects of potassium salts in subjects with heart disease. J. Lab. Clin. Med., 37:506, 1951.

Davidson, S., and Surawicz, B.: Ectopic beats and atrioventricular conduction disturbances in patients with hypopotassemia. Arch. Intern. Med., 120:280, 1967.

Fisch, C., Knoebel, S. B., Feigenbaum, H., and Greenspan, K.: Potassium and the monophasic action potential, electrocardiogram, conduction and arrhythmias. Prog. Cardiov. Dis., 8:387, 1966.

Gettes, L., and Surawicz, B.: Effects of low and high concentrations of potassium on the simultaneously recorded Purkinje and ventricular action potentials of the perfused pig moderator band. Circ. Res., 23:717, 1968.

Holley, H. L., and Carlson, W. W.: Potassium Metabolism in Health and Disease. New York, Grune and Stratton, 1955.

Kahil, M. E., Parrish, J. E., Simons, E. L., and Brown, H.: Magnesium deficiency and carbohydrate metabolism. Diabetes, 15:734, 1966.

Seller, R. H., and Moyer, J. H.: Magnesium and digitalis toxicity. Heart Bull., 18:32, 1969.

Shanahan, E. A., Anderson, S. T., and Morris, K. N.: Preoperative, intraoperative and postoperative potassium supplementation of the incidence of postoperative ventricular arrhythmias. J. Thorac. Cardiov. Surg., 47:413, 1969.

Surawicz, B.: Relationship between electrocardiogram and electrolytes. Amer. Heart J., 73:814, 1967.

Trautwein, W.: Generation and conduction of impulses in the heart as affected by drugs. Pharm. Rev., 15(2), June 1963.

Vassalle, M., and Hoffman, B. F.: The spread of sinus activation during potassium administration. Circ. Res., 17:285, 1965.

Chapter 30 Infectious Diseases and Other Disease States

INFECTIOUS DISEASES
INFILTRATIVE DISEASES
NEUROMUSCULAR DISEASES
NEOPLASTIC DISEASE
COR PULMONALE
ARRHYTHMIAS ASSOCIATED WITH VARIOUS RESPIRATORY MANEUVERS
  Breath-Holding
  Valsalva Maneuver

Hyperventilation
Cheyne-Stokes Respiration
EFFECT OF CHANGES IN POSTURE ON HEART RATE, A-V CONDUCTION, AND THE PRODUCTION OF CERTAIN ECTOPIC RHYTHMS
  Orthostatic Paroxysmal Acceleration of the Heart

INFECTIOUS DISEASES

The heart is involved in varying degrees by the infectious process. The degree and severity of involvement depend on the etiologic agent, its predilection for the heart, and the susceptibility of the cardiac tissue to the organism. The involvement of the heart is usually diffuse and may include the atria, ventricles, and the conduction system. In addition to direct toxic effects, infectious processes often cause disturbances in cardiac metabolism.

Certain bacterial and rickettsial infections show a marked predilection for the heart, affecting it by means of either direct involvement or toxic factors. Subacute bacterial endocarditis (staphylococcal, streptococcal, pneumococcal, meningococcal), tuberculosis, typhoid fever, typhus, Q fever, and diphtheria may be accompanied by myocarditis.

Cardiac involvement in myocarditis, though sometimes mild, is severe in the majority of cases. Occasionally, the patient may go into a state of congestive failure. Even upon subsidence of the infection, several months may pass before the cardiovascular state returns to normal.

Serial electrocardiograms frequently reveal marked changes. Tachycardia, bradycardia, T wave inversion, and R-ST segment deviations may be recorded; Q-T interval prolongation and varied arrhythmias are not uncommon.

The arrhythmias most commonly associated with these diseases are premature beats; however, sinus tachycardia (or bradycardia especially in diphtheria), paroxysmal atrial or ventricular tachycardia, and varying degrees of A-V conduction disturbance are encountered. A-V junctional rhythm, atrial fibrillation, and ventricular fibrillation are less common. These electrocardiographic alterations, particularly the arrhythmias, may be due to one or a combination of the following: (a) infection; (b) impaired nutrition; (c) alteration in myocardial metabolism; (d) anemia; (e) electrolyte alteration; (f) vitamin deficiency; and (g) strain resulting from increased cardiac work. These factors may lead to persistent arrhythmias that usually respond poorly to therapy, particularly digitalis.

Syphilitic heart disease rarely if ever

produces a diffuse myocarditis and thus is usually associated with arrhythmias arising from myocardial dysfunction associated with aortic insufficiency, narrowing of the orifices of the coronary arteries, cardiomegaly, and congestive heart failure, or rarely gummatous involvement of the A-V conduction system.

Viral diseases have only recently been recognized as a significant cause of cardiovascular disease. Pathologic changes in the heart, especially myocarditis, have been observed in viral hepatitis, infectious mononucleosis, poliomyelitis, roseola (measles), influenza, and particularly coxsackie infections. This cardiac involvement produces various electrocardiographic changes (e.g., elevation or depression of the S-T segment, T wave flattening and inversion) and is occasionally associated with arrhythmias. These include premature beats, sinus tachycardia, and, very commonly, A-V conduction disturbances.

Certain parasitic diseases, including trichinosis, schistosomiasis, echinococcus disease, and particularly Chagas' disease (trypanosomiasis), are associated with myocardial pathology which leads to arrhythmias. Direct cardiac involvement underlies the pathology of these diseases. Various electrocardiographic alterations and arrhythmias, commonly, premature beats, are observed; however, the most striking are the A-V conduction disturbances caused by Chagas' disease. This disease causes progressive A-V heart block, and all stages of bundle branch block leading to trifascicular heart block may be seen.

INFILTRATIVE DISEASES

Cardiac involvement in primary amyloidosis and hemochromatosis is relatively common. These diseases may be the cause of heart disease of obscure etiology, particularly in the older age group. The most common electrocardiographic alteration is low voltage in all leads. Paroxysmal tachyarrhythmias may occur, but varying degrees of A-V conduction disturbance are the most commonly encountered arrhythmias.

NEUROMUSCULAR DISEASES

Involvement of cardiac muscle in progressive muscular dystrophy and Friedreich's ataxia is not uncommon. The degenerative myocardial lesions which are observed may be the cause of the atrial and ventricular premature beats and A-V conduction delays which are encountered.

NEOPLASTIC DISEASE

Tumors involving the heart may be primary or metastatic; the latter are more common. The primary tumors are usually myxomata which commonly produce atrial arrhythmias and only rarely A-V conduction delays. The less frequently seen primary tumors, sarcomata, most commonly cause A-V heart block. The manifestations of metastatic tumors of the heart depend largely upon the location of the tumors; however, they generally produce ectopic rhythms. Atrial fibrillation is a common arrhythmia in this situation. The sudden appearance of arrhythmias in a patient with a primary neoplasm outside the heart is highly suggestive of cardiac metastasis.

COR PULMONALE

Cor pulmonale is characterized by predominantly right-sided heart enlargement due to disease of the pulmonary parenchyma or vascular bed. The involvement of the heart may be acute or chronic. The arrhythmias which accompany acute cor pulmonale are usually of atrial origin, sinus tachycardia, and rarely, S-A block and atrial fibrillation. Chronic cor pulmonale is associated with arrhythmias in one-third to one-half of cases. These include predominantly atrial rhythm disturbances (i.e., frequent atrial premature beats, paroxysmal atrial tachycardia, atrial flutter, and fibrillation) and only rarely junctional rhythms or conduction disturbances.

ARRHYTHMIAS ASSOCIATED WITH VARIOUS RESPIRATORY MANEUVERS

Normal respiration and certain simple respiratory maneuvers affect the rhythm of the heart in various ways: (a) Vagal reflexes may be initiated by stimulation of stretch receptors in the visceral pleura or the lung parenchyma. From these receptors the impulse is transmitted via vagal afferent fibers and then vagal efferent (cardiac) fibers to complete the reflex arc. The normal variation of the cardiac rate between inspiration and expiration may represent the most common manifestation of this reflex. However, this phenomenon may be due to other factors, including (b) the effect of changing intrathoracic pressure and venous filling of the heart. Arrhythmias may also result from (c) alterations in blood gases, hypoxia, and hemodynamic events resulting from the marked changes in respiration.

Breath-Holding. A deep breath held in maximal inspiration results in significant slowing of the heart rate as a result of the vagal reflex previously described. Vagal slowing is probably a more important cause of this syncope. Other arrhythmias seen with breath-holding include transient cardiac arrest with ventricular escape, transitory A-V block without ventricular response, and changes in bundle branch conduction. It is of interest that this maneuver may at times convert W-P-W conduction to normal (Lamb et al., 1958). At the height of inspiration certain subjects may develop premature ventricular systoles. These may occur regularly and without evidence of other cardiac arrhythmias. Following prolonged inspiration, releasing the breath may result in premature ventricular beats and occasionally bigeminal rhythm (Lamb et al., 1958); occasionally, a rapid ectopic rhythm may be abolished.

Valsalva Maneuver. This respiratory maneuver consists of a forced expiration against a closed glottis. The hemodynamic changes in the Valsalva maneuver are due in part to the trapping of blood outside the thorax, thus impeding venous return to the right side of the heart.

One might expect cardio-inhibition during the Valsalva maneuver as a result of powerful vagal reflexes. However, this is balanced by the "need" for a tachycardia (to compensate for the decreased venous return and decreased cardiac output) that outweighs the influence of pulmonary vagal reflexes. Upon release, the pressure overshoot is associated with a bradycardia. Bradycardia and frequent premature beats have been noted with the Valsalva maneuver; occasionally, the maneuver may abolish a supraventricular tachycardia (Fig. 30–1).

Hyperventilation. Hyperventilation is characterized by excessive breathing due to an increased rate or volume of respiration. In a normal subject the biochemical result of hyperventilation is a decrease in the arterial pCO_2 (the arterial carbon dioxide tension). If sufficiently prolonged, respiratory alkalosis will ensue. The following arrhythmias may be observed: bigeminal or trigeminal rhythm following hyperventilation; transitory A-V dissociation with junctional tachycardia; irregular multifocal atrial complexes with rates up to 220 per minute, occasional transient episodes of atrial fibrillation, and ventricular fibrillation.

INFECTIOUS DISEASES AND OTHER DISEASE STATES

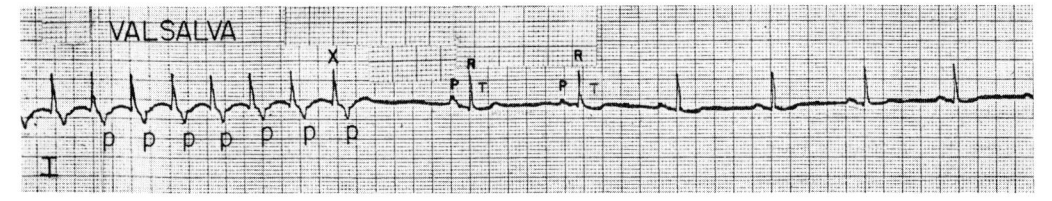

Figure 30-1. Shows the effect of the Valsalva maneuver in terminating supraventricular tachycardia (junctional). Note the tachycardia rate of 140 per minute with the QRS followed by an inverted P wave. Following the Valsalva maneuver at X, note the pre-automatic pause and the restoration of normal sinus rhythm (with a "warming-up" effect).

Cheyne-Stokes Respiration. Cheyne-Stokes respiration is a form of periodic breathing in which periods of hyperpnea alternate with periods of apnea. The apnea results from cerebral hypocapnea, which depresses the respiratory centers. Various arrhythmias are associated with this respiratory pattern. Bradycardia may be due to sinus slowing, A-V junctional rhythm, or partial or complete A-V heart block. Other arrhythmias reported include premature beats, prolonged P-R interval, idioventricular rhythm, ventricular tachycardia, and electrical alternation of the heart (Scherf and Schott,

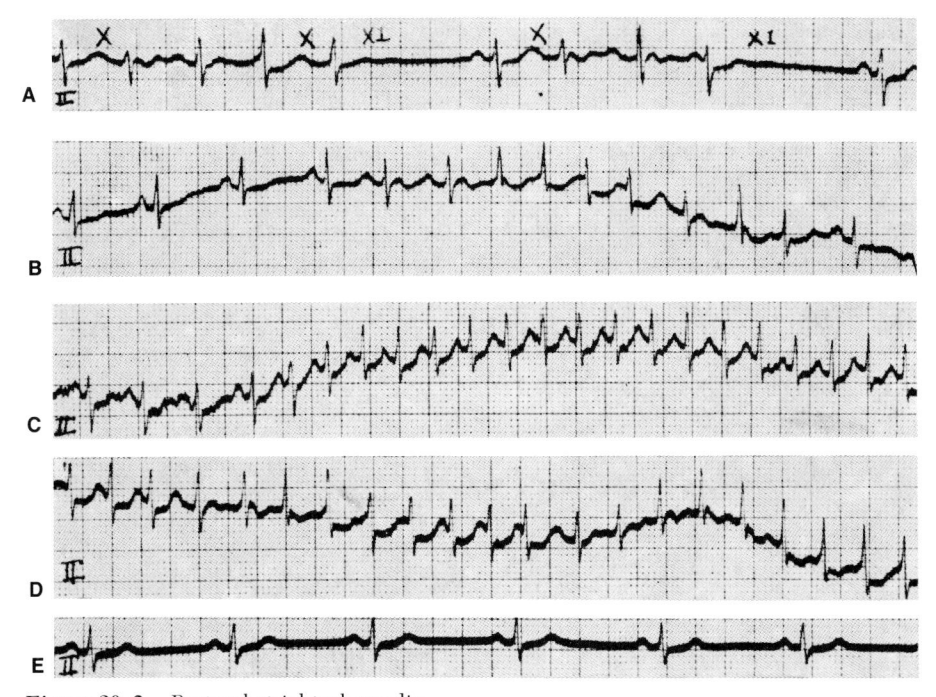

Figure 30-2. Postural atrial tachycardia.
(A) Control—supine. Note the presence of a normal sinus rhythm with occasional atrial premature beats at X and cycles of sinoatrial heart block at X_1.
(B) One minute after standing. Note frequent atrial premature beats and short paroxysms of supraventricular tachycardia.
(C) Three minutes after standing. Note the presence of supraventricular tachycardia.
(D) After 0.5 mg. neostigmine intramuscularly. It took seven minutes after standing for the tachycardia to appear.
(E) When maintained on neostigmine, no tachycardia resulted even on prolonged standing.

1953). Several instances have been reported in which A-V heart block appeared during hyperpnea and disappeared during apnea.

EFFECT OF CHANGES IN POSTURE ON HEART RATE, A-V CONDUCTION, AND THE PRODUCTION OF CERTAIN ECTOPIC RHYTHMS

Of 31 cases of partial A-V block, 26 revealed a shortening of the P-R interval when the patients changed from the recumbent to the upright position (Scherf and Dix, 1952). An increase in sympathetic tone and a reciprocal decrease of the vagal tone are assumed to be responsible for the shortening of the P-R interval in normal subjects and in patients with A-V block in standing positions.

Orthostatic Paroxysmal Acceleration of the Heart. Patients are occasionally encountered in whom the assumption of the upright position results in the production of a rapid ectopic rhythm (atrial tachycardia, atrial flutter, or ventricular tachycardia). This may be the result of the following factors: (a) increased sympathetic tone in the upright position manifesting cardiac effects in those hearts that are vulnerable, and (b) fall in blood pressure and "inadequate venous return" to the right atrium due to pooling of abnormally large quantities of blood in the lower extremities with a decrease in coronary flow in addition to the compensatory increase in sympathetic tone.

Elastic stockings and sympathomimetic drugs (ephedrine, hydroxyamphetamine, or amphetamines) might also help in such instances. In a recent case under our observation, parasympathetic drugs, e.g., prostigmine and digitalis, prevented the recurrence of orthostatic tachycardia (Fig. 30–2).

References

Barkve, T., and Stavem, P.: Cardiac arrhythmia associated with Cheyne-Stokes breathing. Acta Med. Scand., *180*:395, 1966.

Benson, R., and Smith, J. F.: Cardiac amyloidosis. Brit. Heart J., *18*:529, 1956.

Fletcher, E., and Brennan, C. F.: Cardiac complications of Coxsackie-virus infection. Lancet, *1*:913, 1957.

Holmes, J. H., and Weill, D. R., Jr.: Incomplete heart block produced by changes in posture. Amer. Heart J., *30*:291, 1945.

James, T. N., and Carrera, G. M.: Pathogenesis of arrhythmias associated with metastatic tumors of the heart. New Eng. J. Med., *260*:869, 1959.

Lamb, L. E., Dermksian, G., and Sarnoff, C. A.: Significant cardiac arrhythmias induced by common respiratory maneuvers. Amer. J. Cardiol., *2*:563, 1958.

McIntosh, H. D., Burnum, J. F., Hickam, J. B., and Warren, J. V.: Circulatory changes produced by the Valsalva maneuver in normal subjects, patients with mitral stenosis, and autonomic nervous system alterations. Circulation, *9*:511, 1957.

Massumi, R. A., and Nutter, D. O.: Arrhythmias with Cheyne-Stokes respiration. Bull. Johns Hopkins Hosp., *66*:335, 1940.

Reich, N. E.: The Uncommon Heart Diseases. Springfield, Ill., Charles C Thomas, 1954.

Scherf, D., and Dix, J. H.: Effects of posture on A-V conduction. Amer. Heart J., *43*:494, 1952.

Scherf, D., and Schott, A.: Extrasystoles and Allied Arrhythmias. New York, Grune & Stratton, 1953.

Wessler, S., and Freedberg, A. S.: Cardiac amyloidosis. Electrocardiographic and pathologic observations. Arch. Intern. Med., *82*:63, 1948.

Wildenthal, K., Fuller, D. S., and Shapiro, W.: Paroxysmal atrial arrhythmias induced by hyperventilation. Amer. J. Cardiol., *21*:436, 1968.

Woodward, T. E., McCrumb, F. R., Jr., Carey, T. N., and Togo, Y.: Viral and rickettsial causes of cardiac disease, including the Coxsackie virus etiology of pericarditis and myocarditis. Ann. Intern. Med., *53*:1130, 1960.

Chapter 31: General Methods Available in Therapy

GENERAL PROBLEMS IN THERAPY
APPROACH TO THERAPY
  Choice of Specific Therapeutic Agent
METHODS EMPLOYED IN THERAPY
  Removal of Precipitating Factors
  Drugs Which Increase Cardiac Automaticity
  Drugs Which Decrease Automaticity
  Vasopressor Drugs

  Electrolytes and Restoration of Acid-Base Balance
  Omission of Proarrhythmic Drugs
OTHER METHODS AVAILABLE IN THERAPY
  Respiratory and Mechanical Procedures
  Surgical Procedures
  Electrical Devices

GENERAL PROBLEMS IN THERAPY

Having once determined the presence of a specific arrhythmia, one should endeavor to determine the cause, the effect on cardiovascular dynamics, and the ideal method of therapy among the numerous agents available, and the urgency of its implementation. The therapy of cardiac arrhythmias consists of the use of drugs, certain mechanical and electrical devices, and, often, psychotherapy.

The purpose of this section is to briefly discuss the various drugs and procedures available in therapy. These are considered in more detail in the remaining sections of this chapter and in Chapters 32 to 38.

APPROACH TO THERAPY

In a systematic approach to therapy, one should consider: (a) the factors involved in the pathologic physiology; (b) the common disturbances tending to produce arrhythmias (i.e., infections, toxic and degenerative states, coronary artery disease, hypoxia, metabolic, endocrine, and electrolyte disturbances, drugs, especially digitalis, and functional conditions); (c) the results of physical examination (i.e., the presence and type of heart disease); (d) the pertinent facts in the history (i.e., a history of previous attacks, their duration, the heart rate and rhythm during their continuance, the presence of precordial pain or congestive failure during the arrhythmia, the previous response to therapeutic measures, previous digitalization or administration of other drugs with a cardiac action, or electric countershock); (e) pertinent laboratory data, including the electrolyte status, with special attention to serum potassium and acid-base balance; and (f) the treatment of the underlying factor of a given disturbance (i.e., congestive heart failure, thyrotoxicosis), if it can be ascertained.

Choice of the Specific Therapeutic Agent. Since the pharmacologic armamentarium for the treatment of arrhythmias is ever increasing, it is not surprising that the physician is perplexed by the choice of a specific agent that will be most effective in a particular patient. Although many agents are available, the therapeutic modality to be used in a specific case depends on the type of arrhythmia, the etiology, the clinical status of the patient, and the potential hemodynamic effects of the agent to be employed. By approaching each case individually and systematically, the maximal benefit and the optimal therapeutic regimen can be achieved.

METHODS EMPLOYED IN THERAPY

The following methods are available in therapy: (a) removal of factors precipitating arrhythmias; (b) drugs; (c) electrical devices; (d) surgical procedures; (e) respiratory maneuvers (i.e., Valsalva maneuver, breath-holding); (f) mechanical maneuvers (e.g., carotid sinus pressure); and (g) various combinations of these modalities. The effects of these methods are discussed only briefly in this section; a more detailed discussion appears under the individual subjects.

Removal of Precipitating Factors. Considerable attention should be paid to the treatment of factors that might be operative in precipitating arrhythmias (Gettes, 1971). These include hypoxia, acidosis, and electrolyte disturbances, bradycardia, and abnormal sympathetic stimulation. The modalities that may be employed in suppressing the precipitating factors include the following: (a) Hypoxia, ischemia, and the presence of a dilated heart with low cardiac output may be treated by oxygen, digitalis, and diuretic agents and, in selected cases, by isoproterenol. These measures may lead to an increase in contractility and coronary blood flow, thus leading to a decrease in inhomogeneity and areas of refractoriness. (b) Metabolic acidosis may be treated by sodium bicarbonate; specific electrolyte disturbances require appropriate therapy. (c) Those arrhythmias that may be due to increased circulatory catecholamines, i.e., those associated with hyperexcitability, exercise, and general anesthesia, may be treated by beta-sympathetic blocking agents. (d) Since bradycardia contributes to the development of arrhythmias, agents that increase the heart rate may prevent or reverse this process. This may be accomplished by atropine, beta-stimulating agents and cardiac pacing.

Drugs Which Increase Cardiac Automaticity. These agents are indicated in the presence of symptomatic slow heart rates (bradyarrhythmias). They may be associated with syncopal attacks (especially those of Stokes-Adams syndrome) or marked hypotension, sinus pauses, and periods of cardiac arrest. The administration of these drugs alone may suffice to increase the heart rate; in the presence of coexistent hypotension, vasopressor agents are also indicated. Frequently, artificial pacemakers are indicated (see Chapter 37).

The preparations that increase cardiac automaticity consist of: (a) sympathomimetic amines (isoproterenol, epinephrine), (b) parasympathetic blocking agents (e.g., atropine), and (c) alkalinizing agents (molar sodium lactate or sodium bicarbonate).

The sympathomimetic amines include isoproterenol, epinephrine, and others. The indications, method of administration, and dose are discussed in Chapters 32 and 36.

The parasympathetic blocking agents include atropine and methantheline, which act by diminishing or abolishing parasympathetic tone. These preparations are discussed in Chapter 32.

The alkalinizing agents are discussed in Chapter 32. Molar sodium lactate and sodium bicarbonate are powerful agents for increasing cardiac automaticity under certain conditions; the principles underlying their action differ from those of sympathomimetic amines. They are particularly efficacious in the treatment of slow heart rates due to hyperpotassemia and in states accompanied by hypoxia or acidosis, in repeated Stokes-Adams attacks, and in cardiac arrest during anesthesia and surgery.

In most instances where the bradycardia persists in spite of drug administration or where this is only partially effective, it is best to insert an artificial pacemaker which is the only dependable procedure for its correction.

Drugs Which Decrease Automaticity. These agents are indicated in the treatment of premature beats and especially in tachyarrhythmias. This category may be divided into two groups.

Parasympathetic stimulation is effective in the abolition of supraventricular tachycardias (atrial and junctional) and will often transiently slow the ventricular rate in atrial flutter, and, rarely, convert the flutter to atrial fibrillation or normal sinus rhythm. Parasympathetic stimulation may be accomplished by drugs, mechanical means (carotid sinus or ocular pressure), or a combination of both.

Of the parasympathomimetic drugs, prostigmine and digitalis are commonly used. Recently, edrophonium (Tensilon), a short-acting drug producing its parasympathetic effect by a brief reversible inhibition of cholinesterase, has been employed with beneficial effects.

The most important drugs which slow tachyarrhythmias are quinidine, procaine amide, lidocaine, bretylium, diphenylhydantoin, potassium salts, propranolol and alprenolol, and antihistamines (e.g., antazoline). These drugs are discussed in Chapters 33 to 36.

Vasopressor Drugs. Vasopressor drugs are frequently indicated in the treatment of ectopic rhythms because of a concomitant hypotensive state. They increase the blood pressure and thus help to maintain coronary blood flow while efforts are being made to control the arrhythmias by other means. In addition, they may prevent the hypotensive effect of certain antiarrhythmic drugs, e.g., quinidine or procaine amide.

Electrolytes and Restoration of Acid-Base Balance. Some arrhythmias may result from electrolyte imbalance. Electrolytes, especially potassium, calcium, and magnesium, have occasionally been used for the therapy of certain arrhythmias, particularly those arising from depletion or excess of one or more of these cations. The effect of electrolytes in the therapy of arrhythmias is discussed in Chapter 35.

Omission of Proarrhythmic Drugs. Many drugs possess proarrhythmic qualities. This should be kept in mind when determining the cause of a specific arrhythmia prior to the institution of therapy. Withdrawal of the drugs may itself abolish an arrhythmia. Some of the more common drugs in this category include digitalis, sympathomimetic amines, chlorothiazide and similar compounds, molar sodium lactate and other alkalinizing agents, quinidine and procaine amide, caffeine, nicotine, meperidine and veratrine. These are discussed in more detail in Chapter 36.

OTHER METHODS AVAILABLE IN THERAPY

Respiratory and Mechanical Procedures. The Valsalva and breath-holding maneuvers act through increasing vagal effects on the myocardium. They have a limited use in the treatment of paroxysmal atrial tachycardia, and are of primary interest as a diagnostic stress test in producing arrhythmias (see Chapter 20).

Carotid sinus pressure is efficacious in converting a paroxysmal atrial tachycardia or a junctional tachycardia to normal sinus rhythm through vagal stimulation. Other effects of carotid sinus pressure are discussed in more detail in Chapter 33.

Other common mechanical maneuvers are those used in the treatment of cardiac arrest and ventricular fibrillation (see Chapters 15 and 16). These include thumping on the precordium, closed-chest cardiac massage, and open-chest resuscitation. Following cessation of the heart beat or during periods of ventricular tachycardia, a vigorous thump over the precordium occasionally restores effective cardiac beating at least temporarily and permits time for the institution of other more effective procedures. Closed-chest resuscitation, which involves manual sternal compression, has successfully restored cardiac beating during cardiac arrest. It should be accompanied by respiratory support and appropriate drug therapy.

Surgical Procedures. Thoracotomy with manual cardiac systole is rarely employed except for specific indications or during surgery. See Chapter 16 on cardiac arrest.

Sympathectomy has been used with beneficial results in certain refractory cases of paroxysmal atrial and ventricular tachycardia. This is based on recent data which have disclosed a definite physiologic basis, namely, a marked increase in sympathetic tone, for the frequent recurrence of episodes of paroxysmal atrial tachycardia and other arrhythmias. Surgical interruption of accessory pathways in refractory PAT associated with W-P-W is discussed elsewhere.

Electrical Devices. Therapeutic methods employing electrical devices have proven invaluable in the treatment of various cardiac arrhythmias. The following are of particular significance: (a) artificial pacing, (b) overdrive suppression, (c) right atrial stimulation, (d) defibrillation, (e) direct current electrical countershock, and (f) carotid sinus stimulation.

References

Damato, A. N., and Lau, S. H.: Clinical value of the electrogram of the conduction system. Prog. Cardiov. Dis., *13*:119, 1970.

Escher, D. J., and Furman, S.: Emergency treatment of cardiac arrhythmias. Emphasis on use of electrical pacing. JAMA, *214*:2028, 1970.

Gettes, L. S.: The electrophysiologic effects of antiarrhythmic drugs. Amer. J. Cardiol., *28*: 526, 1971.

Rosen, K. M., Lau, S. H., Stein, E., and Damato, A. N.: The effects of lidocaine on atrioventricular and intraventricular conduction in man. Amer. J. Cardiol., *25*:1, 1970.

Chapter 32 *Drugs Which Increase Cardiac Automaticity*

SYMPATHOMIMETIC AMINES
CLASSIFICATION OF SYMPATHOMIMETIC DRUGS
EPINEPHRINE
  Mechanism of Action
  Hemodynamic Effects
  Indications
  Dose and Method of Administration
NOREPINEPHRINE
  Mechanism of Action
  Hemodynamic Effect
  Effect on Electrocardiogram
  Indications
  Dose and Method of Administration
  Untoward and Toxic Effects
ISOPROTERENOL (ISUPREL)
  Mechanism of Action
  Hemodynamic Effects
  Indications
  Dose and Method of Administration
  Untoward and Toxic Effects

PARASYMPATHETIC BLOCKING AGENTS

GENERAL CONSIDERATIONS
ATROPINE
  Mechanism of Cardiac Action
  Effect of Atropine in Arrhythmias
  Indications
  Untoward and Toxic Effects
  Place of Atropine in the Therapy of Bradycardiac States
METHANTHELINE (BANTHINE)
  Indications
  Dose and Method of Administration

ALKALINIZING AGENTS

SODIUM LACTATE AND BICARBONATE
  Mechanism of Cardiac Effects
  Relationship to Sympathomimetic Amines
  Indications
  Toxic Effects and Contraindications
TROMETHAMINE (THAM)
  Cardiac Effects
  Indications
  Untoward and Toxic Effects

The drugs which increase automaticity in general act by increasing the heart rate and the speed of conduction through the A-V junction. They are indicated in the therapy of symptomatic bradyarrhythmias. Included in this category are: (1) sympathomimetic amines, (2) parasympathetic blocking drugs, and (3) alkalinizing agents.

SYMPATHOMIMETIC AMINES

It has long been known that adrenergic mediators manifest both excitatory and inhibitory actions on various target organs. Two patterns emerge: (1) epinephrine is most effective and isoproterenol least effective in producing peripheral vasoconstriction; and (2) isoproterenol is most potent and norepinephrine least so in producing cardiac stimulation, coronary vasodilation, and bronchodilation. These patterns are attributed to the existence of two separate types of adrenergic receptors, termed *alpha* and *beta* receptors. A large number of adrenergic blocking agents with specific alpha or beta antagonism have been developed (see Chapter 33).

The cardiovascular system possesses both alpha and beta receptors. Alpha receptors predominate in most of the peripheral vascular system, where their stimulation causes arteriolar constriction that leads, in turn, to a decrease in blood flow and an increase in blood pressure. Adrenergic influences on the myocardium are thought to be mediated solely by beta receptors. Stimulation of myocardial beta receptors causes: (1) enhancement of cardiac contractility; (2) enhancement of cardiac rate, acceleration of A-V conduction, and the restoration of excitability and conductivity in severely diseased or hypoxic hearts; and (3) a variety of metabolic effects, including glycogenolysis. In the following discussion, we consider the effects of beta-receptor stimulation on (1) cardiac automaticity, which determines the rate of impulse formation, (2) the excitability and conduction of the cardiac impulse, and (3) the duration and temporal dispersion of the repolarization process, which are important factors in the production of certain arrhythmias.

CLASSIFICATION OF SYMPATHOMIMETIC DRUGS

The sympathomimetic drugs vary in their relative potency of alpha- and beta-stimulation and as to whether they predominantly affect the heart or the peripheral vasculature. The drugs which act directly on beta receptors are principally employed for their stimulating actions of the heart. Isoproterenol, originally introduced as a bronchodilator, is the chief drug in this class and is discussed in detail on page 333. The sympathomimetic amines that act principally on alpha receptors are characterized predominantly as vasoconstrictors. Phenylephrine and methoxamine, when administered parenterally, cause a significant degree of peripheral vasoconstriction. An important component of the action of certain sympathomimetic drugs occurs indirectly by the release of catecholamines from adrenergic terminals. In addition, some of these agents have direct actions on both alpha and beta receptors. Of these drugs, ephedrine, metaraminol, and mephentermine are the most useful clinically.

EPINEPHRINE

Mechanism of Action. Epinephrine acts directly on effector organs supplied by the autonomic nervous system, causing stimulation of both alpha and beta receptors. In moderate doses, the cardiostimulatory effects of epinephrine are marked, indicating that beta receptors are highly sensitive to epinephrine.

The positive inotropic effects of epinephrine and other catecholamines may result from an augmentation of the sarcotubular calcium pool, mediated, in part at least, by an elevation of cyclic $3', 5'$-AMP levels produced by activation of an adenyl cyclase localized to the sarcoplasmic reticulum. Furthermore, it has been postulated that catecholamines augment calcium influx by increasing the depolarization spike and thereby increasing the electrical gradient acting upon calcium movement.

One of the most important actions of epinephrine is its ability to increase pacemaker activity by increasing automaticity. In addition, when tested directly on the isolated papillary muscle of the cat heart, epinephrine causes an increase in contractile force, excitability, and oxygen consumption. In accelerating the intact heart, epinephrine causes: (1) shortening of systole more than diastole; (2) abbreviation of the refractory period of atrial and ventricular muscle; and (3) acceleration of A-V conduction and reduction of the degree of A-V block occurring as a result of disease, drugs, or vagal stimulation.

Hemodynamic Effects. The cardiovascular effects of epinephrine result in a significant increase in cardiac output, accomplished by a slight increase in heart rate and a greater increase in stroke volume. The cardiac actions of epinephrine are not of major importance in raising blood pressure, since the pulse rate, at first elevated, may be slowed markedly at the height of the pressor response by compensatory vagal discharge elicited by carotid sinus reflexes.

In normal subjects, injection of epinephrine results in a rise in the pulse rate, systolic blood pressure, cardiac output, stroke volume, respiratory rate, and respiratory volume. Coronary blood flow also increases in proportion to the increased cardiac work. Total peripheral resistance decreases due to the predominance of beta-stimulating effects on the blood vessels. The hemodynamic responses to epinephrine, it must be noted, depend on the rate and route of administration (Fig. 32-1).

Indications. At present, epinephrine is not frequently used to stimulate cardiac pacemaker activity because of its transient action and frequent production of untoward effects (i.e., ventricular fibrillation). It has been replaced by more efficacious and safer methods of treatment, especially isoproterenol and the artificial pacemaker (see Chapter 37). Epinephrine is infrequently employed in the treatment of A-V heart block for the aforementioned reasons.

Epinephrine administered during resuscitative efforts for cardiac arrest has the beneficial effects of increasing cardiac contractility and restoring membrane potential to normal if it has been decreased by hypoxia. However, since it lacks the strong vasoconstrictor effect of norepinephrine, epinephrine is not the drug of choice.

Dose and Method of Administration. The dose and method of administration depend upon the gravity of the clinical state. Intravenous infusion is

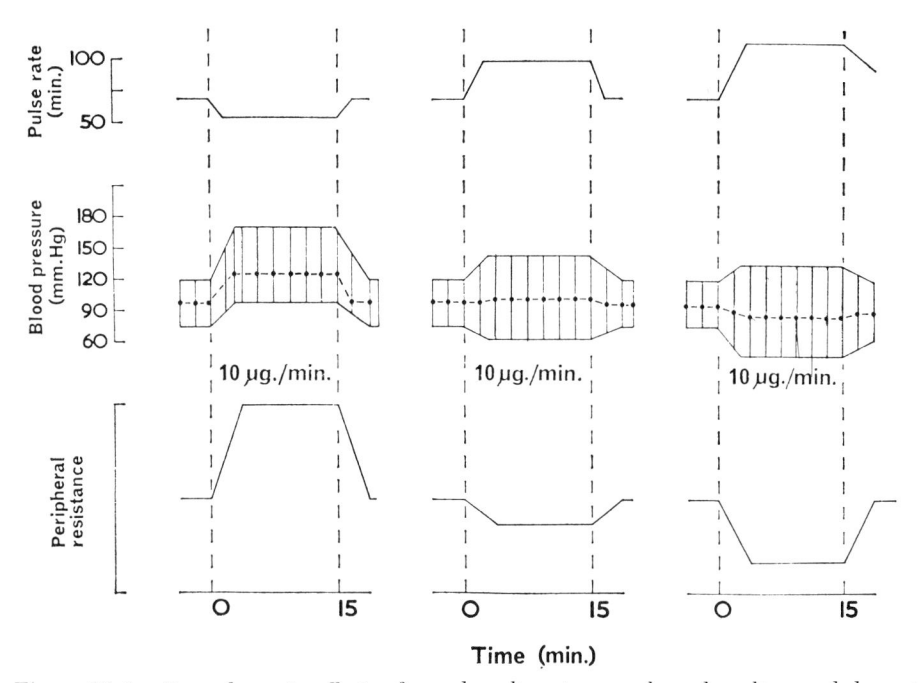

Figure 32-1. Hemodynamic effects of noradrenaline, isopropylnoradrenaline, and dopamine. (From Allwood, M. J., Cobbold, A. F., and Ginsburg, J.: Brit. Med. Bull., 19:132, 1963.)

no longer commonly used, because other agents are more beneficial in situations that would indicate this method of administration (e.g., during cardiac resuscitation procedures). When intravenous infusion is employed, epinephrine should be injected slowly in a dose of 0.25 ml. of a 1:1000 solution (0.25 mg.). This dose may be most conveniently administered by diluting 1 ml. of the 1:1000 solution with 10 ml. of saline (making a 1:10,000 solution) and administering 2.5 ml. This may be repeated two to three times within a period of 15 to 20 minutes as indicated. A total dose of 1 mg. may be injected in this way without untoward effects. For intracardiac injection during cardiopulmonary resuscitation, 0.5 to 1.0 mg. (1 ml. of 1:1000 epinephrine diluted to 10 ml. with saline contains 0.1 mg./ml.) may be administered.

NOREPINEPHRINE

Mechanism of Action. Norepinephrine acts principally on alpha receptors, except in the heart, where its actions are mediated by beta receptors. The direct effect of norepinephrine on cardiac beta receptors leads to an increase in heart rate, stroke volume, and cardiac output. However, the positive chronotropic effects of the drug are masked by reflex vagal tone, elicited by an increase in arterial blood pressure (Fig. 32–1).

Hemodynamic Effect. During infusion of norepinephrine the blood flow to most organs is maintained by the increase in mean arterial pressure despite the increase in arteriolar tone. However, blood flow is decreased to the kidney, brain, and liver and sometimes to skeletal muscle and the splanchnic vascular bed. The net effect in normotensive human subjects is ordinarily to decrease the cardiac output. However, when the blood pressure is low, infusion of norepinephrine may actually increase diuresis, indicating that the rise in blood pressure overcompensates the local renal efferent arteriolar vasoconstriction. Renal blood flow may actually be improved appreciably by norepinephrine administration during hemorrhagic hypotension.

Effect on the Electrocardiogram. Abnormal S-T segment or T wave changes are observed in leads reflecting the potential of the left ventricle, a decrease in height or inversion of T waves in right chest leads, and increases in the height of R waves in one or more of the left precordial leads.

Indications. Norepinephrine is generally employed as a vasopressor agent in the therapy of shock-like states. However, its role in treating shock is not universally accepted, and, in fact, the proper therapy in this clinical state has been the subject of intense controversy in recent years. The use of norepinephrine in cardiogenic shock is based on its ability to sustain peripheral perfusion by maintaining systemic blood pressure. Favorable results have been observed in operative and postoperative hypotension and in shock associated with myocardial infarction, trauma, septicemia, and overdosages of procaine amide, veratrum alkaloids, and hexamethonium. It is used in arrhythmias associated with hypotensive states and to reverse the hypotensive effects of other antiarrhythmic agents.

Dose and Method of Administration. Norepinephrine is usually administered by continuous intravenous infusion. Four ml. of the commercially available solution (4 mg.) are diluted in 1000 ml. of 5 per cent dextrose or 0.9 per cent sodium chloride solution to a final concentration of 4 μg. of norepinephrine base per milliliter. After testing the pressor response to a test dose (1 to 2 μg. of base per 10 Kg. of body weight), the infusion rate is adjusted to obtain the desired pressor response. An infusion at the rate of 2 to 4 μg. of base per minute (0.5 to 1.0 ml./min.) is normally adequate.

Untoward and Toxic Effects. There are few untoward effects of norepinephrine when the drug is administered in proper dosage; however, hyperthyroid patients may be particularly sensitive to the drug. Subjective symptoms of anxiety, respiratory difficulties, awareness of the slow, forceful heart beat, and transient headaches are often noted. It sometimes produces transient ventricular arrhythmias, and intravenous infusion of quantities of 4 to 26 μg. per minute has been found to precipitate ventricular arrhythmias in patients anesthesized with cyclopropane.

Norepinephrine, as well as epinephrine, can cause severe cardiac lesions even when used in therapeutic doses. These consist of extensive hemorrhagic myocarditis and severe edema of the cardiac valves. The mechanical influence on the heart caused by the rise in arterial pressure probably does not entirely explain the injurious effect on the heart muscle. The one serious deleterious effect incident to norepinephrine infusion is necrosis of the overlying skin when the solution accidentally extravasates.

ISOPROTERENOL (ISUPREL)

Mechanism of Action. Isoproterenol is a potent stimulator of beta-adrenergic receptors, with only slight effects on alpha-adrenergic receptors. Its cardiovascular effects, therefore, consist of potent cardiac stimulation and peripheral vasodilation, especially in the skeletal muscle beds. In addition, it causes relaxation of bronchial and gastrointestinal smooth muscle.

As would be expected of a potent beta-adrenergic stimulator, the cardiac effect of isoproterenol resembles that of epinephrine, but its positive chronotropic and inotropic actions are more marked. It increases the sinus rate and may produce sinus tachycardia; it abolishes induced cardiac standstill and increases the ventricular rate in partial A-V heart block by enhancing A-V conduction.

The pattern of cardiac acceleration produced by isoproterenol is similar to that of epinephrine; however, it is five times as potent as epinephrine in stimulating cardiac pacemakers, especially the S-A and A-V nodes. Epinephrine tends to produce ventricular fibrillation, particularly when previous cardiac damage exists. Isoproterenol, on the other hand, administered under similar conditions, produces this arrhythmia less frequently, probably because it does not elevate the arterial blood pressure.

Isoproterenol increases the ventricular rate in bradycardia and may stimulate the basic pacemaker to resume automaticity during episodes of asystole. It may also restore pacemaker activity during Stokes-Adams seizures, even in the presence of transient periods of ventricular tachycardia or ventricular fibrillation. Its greater potency in these respects, together with the absence of pressor action, renders isoproterenol preferable to epinephrine in the therapy and prevention of certain types of cardiac arrhythmias.

Hemodynamic Effects. Isoproterenol increases coronary blood flow and myocardial contractility. Contractility is increased so that normal or increased stroke volume is delivered in a greatly shortened ejection time. The direct cardiac action of isoproterenol combined with its peripheral vasodilator action produces a marked increase in cardiac output, a variable effect on systolic pressure, and an increase in pulse pressure.

Indications. Of the various sympathomimetic agents that have been used through the years to stimulate cardiac automaticity, isoproterenol has proved to be the most effective and the most direct in its action. In addition its action is not accompanied by a significant rise in blood pressure.

Isoproterenol may be employed: (a) to stimulate cardiac automaticity during Stokes-Adams seizures; (b) to maintain the heart rate and cardiac output during acute episodes of high-grade A-V heart block, occurring either spontaneously or secondary to acute myocardial infarction; (c) for the active treatment and prophylaxis of transient periods of cardiac standstill due to cardioinhibitory type of carotid sinus syncope; and (d) to increase the heart rate in other forms of bradycardia. In addition, intravenous infusion of isoproterenol is often used during the active implantation of a catheter-pacing electrode, and it has been observed to enhance the cardiac output in paced subjects both at rest and during exercise.

Dose and Method of Administration. The drug may be administered by one of the following methods: (a) sublingually in a dose of 10 to 20 mg. every three or four hours, or as required; (b) subcutaneously, 0.2 mg. every six hours, or as indicated; (c) intravenously, as a continuous infusion of 1 mg. of isoproterenol in 200 ml. of 5 per cent glucose in distilled water, or 5 μg. per ml. at a rate of 9 to 20 drops per minute. The cardiovascular action of isoproterenol appears immediately following its intravenous administration.

Untoward and Toxic Effects. Isoproterenol has proved less toxic than epinephrine because it lacks a significant pressor effect. Few side effects are observed with sublingual administration. However, isoproterenol should be infused with caution by the intravenous route, particularly in the presence of acute coronary occlusion and in heart failure. In the early stage of acute myocardial infarction when catecholamine secretion has already increased, isoproterenol may produce additional untoward effects by further increasing the sympathetic effects. This could increase the automaticity of cardiac pacemakers sufficient to produce a refractory, even irreversible, tachyarrhythmia in susceptible patients. Recent data has indicated that isoproterenol may increase the oxygen demand of the heart which in the presence of coronary insufficiency and especially in acute infarction could have a deleterious effect. In patients with heart damage, it may at times produce ventricular tachycardia and ventricular fibrillation, although such an occurrence is much less likely than with epinephrine. It should not be administered with epinephrine; however, the two drugs may be used alternately.

The tendency of isoproterenol to produce untoward effects has led to a significant reduction of its use in increasing the heart rate in bradyarrhythmias.

As with epinephrine and norepinephrine, hemorrhagic lesions and necrosis of the myocardium has occurred following large doses of isoproterenol.

PARASYMPATHETIC BLOCKING AGENTS

GENERAL CONSIDERATIONS

Parasympathetic blocking agents are used in cases in which parasympathetic effects play a role in the precipitation of arrhythmias (e.g., slow heart rate and bradyarrhythmias). The parasympatholytic drugs discussed in this chapter are atropine and methantheline.

ATROPINE

Alkaloids of the belladonna plants are known to block vagal effects on various organs, including the heart. Atropine and scopolamine are naturally occurring alkaloids.

Mechanism of Cardiac Action. The fundamental action of atropine is the competitive blockade of the effects of acetylcholine. The cardiac action of atropine is exerted directly on the receptor sites located on the effector cells of the conduction system and the atrial muscle.

The increase of the sinoatrial rate caused by atropine is due not only to blockade of the direct effect of acetylcholine upon the S-A nodal fibers but also to blockade of the interaction between acetylcholine and norepinephrine present in the S-A node. Thus, atropine not only increases the sinus rate by blocking the direct chronotropic effects of acetylcholine, but it also releases the inhibited sympathetic effects.

The effect of atropine on the heart rate depends on the total dose, the route and rapidity of administration, and the age and physiologic state (anesthetized or not) of the patient. Although the parasympathetic blocking action of atropine is fairly well known and commonly recognized, the early parasympathomimetic effects have received little attention. The degree and duration of the bradycardiac response decrease as the rapidity of injection is increased. The initial drop in heart rate may last from 15 seconds to 15 minutes, depending on the route and rate of administration; the tachycardia then follows. The heart rate gradually returns to normal over a period of 90 to 150 minutes as the atropine level in the blood falls. These changes are usually greater and more rapid after intravenous administration and relatively slower and less intense after subcutaneous injection.

The dosage of atropine required to produce complete vagal paralysis or the maximal increase in heart rate has been found to vary. The peak response occurs at an intravenous dose between 1.8 to 3.0 mg., usually in a dose closer to the latter figure (Chamberlain et al., 1967).

Complete autonomic blockade can be accomplished in healthy and diseased hearts by the intravenous injection of propranolol (0.2 mg./kg.) and atropine (0.04 mg./kg.). The most obvious feature of cardiac function following blockade of autonomic activity is a fixed heart rate (intrinsic heart rate), which is usually higher in normal than in diseased hearts.

Effect of Atropine in Arrhythmias. Arrhythmias due to vagal hyperactivity can usually be partially or entirely abolished by atropine. The dose administered is important; to produce complete vagal paralysis, 1.8 mg. to 3.0 mg. is required intravenously; however, it must be kept in mind that cardiac slowing may be due to direct depressant effects of hypoxia, drugs, or other factors not of vagal origin.

Atropine is often effective in treating patients with acute bradycardia that is frequently observed in association with a low cardiac output. This may occur in the presence of acute myocardial infarction, atrial fibrillation with a slow ventricular rate, and other situations. The mechanisms involved may be hypoxia, particularly involving the S-A and A-V nodes, increased parasympathetic tone, markedly diminished sympathetic tone, and administration of certain drugs with parasympathomimetic activity, e.g., morphine and digitalis. The rapid intravenous administration of atropine (0.4 to 0.6 mg.) in these situations may markedly increase the heart rate and raise the blood pressure, but this effect is usually temporary.

Indications. Atropine may be administered in: (1) sinus bradycardia (rate below 50 per minute) due to increased vagal tone; (2) sinus (respiratory) arrhythmia; (3) sinoatrial block; (4) atrial flutter and fibrillation associated with slow ventricular response; (5) partial A-V heart block due to increased vagal tone; (6) digitalis intoxication to combat the manifestations due to vagal stimulation. It may be employed diagnostically to evaluate the degree of vagal tone in: (1) complete A-V heart block, (2) A-V junctional rhythm, and (3) the differential diagnosis of supraventricular arrhythmias accompanied by slow ventricular rates.

Untoward and Toxic Effects. Although side effects are uncommon when the recommended therapeutic doses are administered, toxic symptoms may result with larger doses. Symptoms associated with moderate dosage (1 to 2 mg.) include: (1) difficulty in swallowing, (2) disturbed speech, (3) headache, (4) weak pulse, (5) marked pupillary dilatation, (6) hallucinations, and (7) coma. Atropine toxicity can be treated with neostigmine. It will effectively counteract both peripheral and central nervous system manifestations of toxicity.

Place of Atropine in the Therapy of Bradycardiac States. Atropine is a safe drug to use and it effectively controls certain bradyarrhythmias; however, its effects are transient and certain unpleasant side effects must be accepted to achieve the cardiovascular actions required. In certain situations (e.g., slow idioventricular rhythm), it is not effective. Atropine should therefore be used in those situations in which fast but temporary therapy is indicated or as a temporary measure which will be replaced by a more long-acting agent.

METHANTHELINE (BANTHINE)

This drug has an atropine-like effect on parasympathetic receptors and a curare-like effect on the neuromuscular junction. With respect to cholinergic neuro-effector blockage, methantheline has about two-thirds the potency of atropine.

Indications. The indications for the use of methantheline are similar to those of atropine. The drug has advantages over atropine in that it manifests a more prolonged action and possesses fewer side effects with doses producing comparable vagal release, although side effects are similar qualitatively.

Dose and Method of Administration. The usual route of administration is oral. This requires a dose four to five times larger than that administered by the intravenous route. The average dose of methantheline in gastrointestinal diseases is 50 to 100 mg., while that of Pro-Banthine is 20 to 40 mg., administered every six hours. However, for cardiac action, larger doses are often necessary to maintain the desired vagolytic effect.

ALKALINIZING AGENTS

Much evidence indicates that alkalosis has a profound effect on maintaining and accelerating the heart beat. In addition, acidosis tends to retard and alkalosis tends to accelerate conduction. Among the more important alkalinizing agents are sodium lactate, sodium bicarbonate, and tromethamine (THAM).

SODIUM LACTATE AND BICARBONATE

Mechanism of Cardiac Effects. One major effect of molar sodium lactate or sodium bicarbonate is a relative decrease of potassium in the extracellular fluid; this is accomplished by expansion of the extracellular space and movement of potassium intracellularly. A low serum potassium causes increased automaticity of cardiac pacemakers.

The effects of these alkalinizing agents depend upon the underlying clinical state, the dose, and the method and rapidity of administration. When administered in the absence of acidosis or hyperpotassemia, the effects may not be as dramatic or clearcut.

Relationship to Sympathomimetic Amines. The effectiveness of the sympathomimetic amines in increasing the idioventricular rate is markedly impaired in metabolic or respiratory acidosis, hyperpotassemia, and hypoxia. This decreasing effectiveness is proportional to the decrease in the blood pH. Correction of the acidosis with alkalinizing agents (molar sodium lactate or sodium bicarbonate) restores the effectiveness of the sympathomimetic amines (Guzman et al., 1959).

Indications. The experience to date suggests that alkalinizing agents—molar sodium lactate or sodium bicarbonate—are efficacious in the treatment of Stokes-Adams attacks, in cardiac arrest during surgery and in sudden cardiac arrest due to other causes and are especially indicated in those states associated with acidosis or hyperpotassemia, particularly if associated with slow heart rates. Because its action is based on a different principle from that of the vagolytic and sympathomimetic drugs, it may supplement these agents and has been shown to be effective under conditions in which they have proved to be partially effective or useless. In clinical hyperpotassemia and in hyperpotassemia experimentally produced in the dog, molar sodium lactate and sodium bicarbonate almost always reversed the cardiotoxic effects, at least temporarily.

Toxic Effects and Contraindications. The following circumstances either contraindicate the use of molar sodium lactate or indicate extreme caution in its use: (a) the appearance or increased frequency of premature beats following its administration; (b) severe heart damage, particularly in association with overt or impending congestive heart failure; (c) hypopotassemia; or (d) alkalosis.

TROMETHAMINE (THAM)

Cardiac Effects. Intravenous THAM is able to increase the low ventricular contractile force that accompanies acidosis in experimental animals. Moreover, the drug is effective in slightly augmenting the contractile force in the dog with normal acid-base balance. Tromethamine enhances conduction through the A-V node but slows conduction in Purkinje tissue and ventricular muscle. Excitability of the ventricle is decreased and the threshold for ventricular fibrillation is elevated (Cline et al., 1968).

Indications. The effective buffering capacity of tromethamine suggests its use in: (a) acidosis resulting from chronic pulmonary disease such as emphysema, carcinoma, bronchiectasis, and fibrosis; (b) correction of respiratory and mixed acidosis that might occur following prolonged surgery (particularly endotracheal); (c) shock syndrome with acidosis that is resistant to the pressor amines; (d) management of acidosis occurring with cardiopulmonary bypass procedures and hypothermia; (e) metabolic acidosis; (f) acidosis resulting from chronic cardiac disorders; and (g) salicylate intoxication.

Untoward and Toxic Effects. The development of hypoglycemia and the side effects of hypotension, periodic breathing, retching, and vomiting following the administration of tromethamine have been reported.

The tendency for hypoglycemia to occur is more marked as the blood pH is shifted to the alkaline side. It must be remembered that tromethamine depresses the respiratory center either directly or through a change in pH. Because of these effects, caution should be used in the treatment of patients suffering from chronic hypoventilation or in subjects in whom drugs which depress respiration have been administered.

References

Ahlquist, R. P.: A study of adrenotropic receptors. Amer. J. Physiol., 153:586, 1948.

Allwood, M. J., Cobbold, A. F., and Ginsburg, J.: Peripheral vascular effects of noradrenaline, isopropylnoradrenaline, and dopamine. Brit. Med. Bull., 19:132, 1963.

Aviado, D. M., Jr.: Sympathomimetic Drugs. Springfield, Ill., Charles C Thomas, 1970.

Bellet, S., Hamdan, G., Somlyo, A., and Lara, R.: The reversal of cardiotoxic effects of quinidine by molar sodium lactate: an experimental study. Amer. J. Med. Sci., 237:165, 1959.

Bellet, S., Wasserman, F., and Brody, J. I.: Treatment of cardiac arrest and slow ventricular rates in complete A-V heart block: use of molar and half molar sodium lactate: a clinical study. Circulation, 11:685, 1955.

Burn, J. H.: The relation of the autonomic nervous system to cardiac arrhythmias. Prog. Cardiov. Dis., 2:334, 1960.

Chamberlain, D. A., Turner, P., and Snedon, J. M.: Effects of atropine on heart rate in healthy man. Lancet, 2:12, 1967.

Cline, R. E., Wallace, A. G., Sealy, W. C., and Young, G. Y.: Antiarrhythmic properties of tris (hydroxymethyl) aminomethane. Amer. J. Cardiol., 21:38, 1968.

Cooper, J. A., and Frieden, J.: Atropine in the treatment of cardiac disease. Amer. Heart J., 78:124, 1969.

Corday, E., Williams, J. H., Gold, H., and Fields, J.: Vasopressor therapy of the cardiac arrhythmias. Circulation, 18:707, 1958.

Entman, M. L., Levey, G. S., and Epstein, S. E.: Mechanism of action of epinephrine and glucagon on the canine heart. Evidence for increase in sarcotubular calcium stores mediated by cyclic 3', 5'-AMP. Circ. Res., 25:429, 1969.

Fielder, D. L., Nelson, D. C., Anderson, T. W., and Gravenstein, J. S.: Cardiovascular effects of atropine and neostigmine in man. Anesthesiology, 30:637, 1969.

Gorten, R., Gunnells, J. C., Weissler, A. M., and Stead, E. A., Jr.: Effects of atropine and isoproterenol on cardiac output, central venous pressure, and mean transit time of indicators placed at three different sites in the venous system. Circ. Res., 9:979, 1961.

Greenstein, S., Goldburgh, W. P., Guzman, S. V., and Bellet, S.: A comparative analysis of molar sodium lactate and other agents in the treatment of induced hyperkalemia in nephrectomized dogs. Circ. Res., 8:223, 1960.

Guzman, S. V., DeLeon, A. C., Jr., West, J. W., and Bellet, S.: Cardiac effects of isoproterenol, norepinephrine, and epinephrine in complete A-V heart block during experimental acidosis and hyperkalemia. Circ. Res., 7:666, 1959.

Han, J., Garcia de Jalon, P., and Moe, G. K.: Adrenergic effects on ventricular vulnerability. Circ. Res., 14:516, 1964.

Hayes, A. H., and Katz, R. A.: Homatropine bradycardia in man. Clin. Pharmacol. Ther., 11:558, 1970.

Hoffman, B. F., and Singer, D. H.: Appraisal of the effects of catecholamines on cardiac electrical activity. Ann. N.Y. Acad. Sci., 139:914, 1967.

Hoffman, S. A., et al.: Postoperative ventricular arrhythmias caused by isoproterenol: conversion with insulin. J. Thorac. Cardiov. Surg., 58:664, 1969.

Kaiser, S. C., and McLain, P. L.: Atropine metabolism in man. Clin. Pharmacol. Ther., 11:214, 1970.

Kassebaum, D. G., and Van Dyke, A. R.: Electrophysiological effects of isoproterenol on Purkinje fibers of the heart. Circ. Res., 19:940, 1966.

Maling, H. M., and Highman, B.: Exaggerated ventricular arrhythmias and myocardial fatty changes after large doses of norepinephrine and epinephrine in unanesthetized dogs. Amer. J. Physiol., 194:590, 1958.

Chapter 33 — Agents Which Decrease Cardiac Automaticity

CAROTID SINUS PRESSURE
FACTORS MODIFYING RESPONSE TO CAROTID SINUS PRESSURE
INDICATIONS
  Treatment of Arrhythmias
  Diagnosis of Arrhythmias
TECHNIQUE OF APPLICATION OF CAROTID SINUS PRESSURE IN HUMAN SUBJECT
  Causes of Failure
OTHER METHODS OF INCREASING VAGAL TONE
CONTRAINDICATIONS
COMPLICATIONS AND UNTOWARD EFFECTS
SUMMARY

DRUGS THAT DECREASE CARDIAC AUTOMATICITY

PARASYMPATHOMIMETIC DRUGS
  Neostigmine
  Edrophonium
QUINIDINE
  Electrophysiologic Effects
  Pharmacologic Effects
  Absorption and Metabolism
    Plasma Levels
  Effects on the Electrocardiogram
  Indications
  Dose and Method of Administration
    Oral Quinidine Preparations
    Maintenance Doses
    Use in Conjunction with Propranolol
  Toxicity of Quinidine
  Contraindications
PROCAINE AMIDE
  Electrophysiology
  Pharmacologic Effects
  Hemodynamic Effects
  Absorption and Metabolism

  Indications
  Dose and Method of Administration
  Toxic Effects
  Contraindications
LIDOCAINE
  Electrophysiology
  Hemodynamic Effects
  Indications and Place in Therapy
  Dose and Method of Administration
    Intravenous Administration
    Intramuscular Administration
  Toxicity
  Contraindications
SYMPATHETIC BLOCKING AGENTS
  Mode of Action of Sympathetic Antagonists
  Beta-Adrenergic Blocking Agents
    Beta-Blocking Agents with Selective Action
    Beta-Blocking Effects
    Direct Effects
    Indications
    Dose and Method of Administration
    Toxicity
  Agents That Act at Adrenergic Nerve Endings
  Other Antiadrenergic Agents
    Chlorpromazine (Thorazine, Largactil)
DIPHENYLHYDANTOIN (DPH)
  Introduction
  Pharmacologic Effects
  Hemodynamics
  Absorption and Metabolism
  Use in Arrhythmias
  Dose and Method of Administration
  Toxic Effects
  Contraindications
    Drug Interactions
BRETYLIUM
  Electrophysiologic Effects
  Pharmacologic Effects
  Clinical Arrhythmias
  Dose and Route of Administration
  Place in Therapy
  Contraindications

There are a number of agents, drugs,* and mechanical maneuvers which decrease cardiac automaticity. These include: (1) vagal stimulation by drugs or mechanical means; (2) quinidine; (3) procaine amide; (4) lidocaine; (5) beta-adrenergic blocking agents; (6) diphenylhydantoin; (7) bretylium; (8) antazoline and other antihistaminic drugs; and (9) digitalis, which will be

---

* It should be noted that some of these drugs (e.g., quinidine and procaine amide), in toxic doses or in subjects with severe myocardial disease who manifest marked depression of fiber activity, may increase cardiac automaticity by their effects on Stage 4 depolarization.

discussed in detail in Chapter 34. These agents decrease automaticity by: (1) increasing parasympathetic tone; (2) decreasing parasympathetic tone; (3) direct depressant effects on automatic fibers; or (4) a combination of these mechanisms. The drugs which decrease the automaticity of myocardial fibers tend to slow or abolish tachyarrhythmias and abolish premature beats; these are their principal indications. In addition, tachyarrhythmias may be slowed or abolished by over-drive suppression, by artificial pacemakers, or by the use of right atrial stimulation.

CAROTID SINUS PRESSURE

In its physiologic role, the carotid sinus plays an important part in the regulation of the cardiac rate and arterial blood pressure. Compression of the carotid sinus at its bifurcation (which raises the pressure within the sinus) causes a marked slowing of the heart rate, vasodilatation, and a fall in blood pressure. This procedure is often used therapeutically to terminate certain supraventricular tachycardias. It is quite simple to apply carotid sinus pressure; this procedure with certain precautions is quite safe. The cardiac effects appear quickly and any untoward effects are usually transitory.

FACTORS MODIFYING RESPONSE TO CAROTID SINUS PRESSURE

The factors that modify the response to carotid sinus pressure are: (1) Age. Approximately 10 per cent of the individuals present hyperactivity of the carotid sinus mechanism; this increases with age, so much so that in the older age groups with advanced grades of arteriosclerosis, even slight stroking in the region of the carotid artery or sinus may be sufficient to slow or even stop the heart. (2) Presence of atherosclerosis, coronary artery disease, myocardial infarction, and congestive failure (i.e., myocardial hypoxia). (3) Hypertension. It has been suggested that in hypertension, increased carotid sinus sensitivity is caused by an impaired nervous mechanism due to dilatation in the region of the carotid artery bifurcation, abnormal relaxation, decreased pulsatile expansion, or loss of elasticity of the narrow sensitive arterial walls. (4) Gall-bladder disease and biliary obstruction. Following surgery, carotid sinus sensitivity disappears in many patients with liver disease. Bradycardia that accompanies jaundice may be due to increased baroreceptor activity resulting from receptor sensitization by the retained bile pigments. (5) Alterations in pH, particularly towards the acidotic side, increase carotid sinus sensitivity. (6) Drugs. The following drugs increase carotid sinus sensitivity: cholinergic drugs (neostigmine, acetylcholine), digitalis (by increasing sensitivity of pressoreceptors in the carotid sinuses and, in addition, by increasing the refractory period of the S-A node), potassium, reserpine, and insulin.

INDICATIONS

Treatment of Arrhythmias. Carotid sinus pressure is effective in the therapy of paroxysmal supraventricular tachycardia (i.e., atrial and junctional). This procedure, employed either alone or combined with parasympathomimetic drugs, will frequently abolish these ectopic tachycardias (Fig. 33-1). Their termination

AGENTS WHICH DECREASE CARDIAC AUTOMATICITY

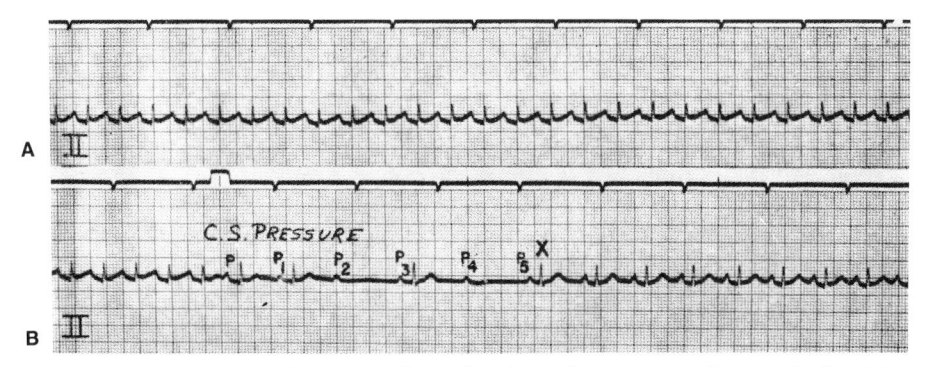

Figure 33-1. Reversion of paroxysmal atrial tachycardia to a normal sinus rhythm following carotid sinus pressure.
(A) Note the presence of atrial tachycardia with the P wave superimposed on the T wave. The heart rate is 150 per minute.
(B) Following carotid sinus pressure, note the occurrence of a normal sinus beat at P_1. P_2 and P_4 represent dropped beats with a 2:1 A-V heart block. Note the restoration of normal sinus rhythm in the cycles following X.

is often accompanied by the occurrence of atrial or junctional premature beats, followed by a long postparoxysmal pause. The change to normal sinus rhythm is usually abrupt—rarely is it accompanied by a gradual slowing of the rapid ventricular rate before the resumption of a normal sinus rhythm. Once the normal sinus rhythm is restored, it usually persists. The simplicity and relative safety of carotid sinus pressure make it the initial procedure of choice in the therapy of these arrhythmias.

Carotid sinus pressure has the following effects on other supraventricular arrhythmias: (1) *Paroxysmal atrial tachycardia with A-V block.* Carotid sinus pressure is usually effective only during the period of its application. Once the pressure is removed, the original rhythm returns. However, in some instances, the ventricular rate may be slowed for relatively long periods of time by this procedure. Its action resembles that in atrial flutter.

(2) *Atrial flutter.* Carotid sinus pressure, if effective, will merely slow the ventricular rate and increase the degree of A-V block. This slowing is enhanced by a digitalis effect or that of other parasympathomimetic drugs (e.g., neostigmine).

(3) *Premature beats.* Carotid sinus pressure will frequently abolish premature beats during the period of pressure; this abolition may be maintained for relatively long periods of time (Fig. 33-2). Slowing of the heart rate usually accompanies or follows this suppression.

(4) *Bidirectional type of junctional tachycardia due to digitalis toxicity.* Carotid sinus pressure slows the heart rate by abolishing the series of junctional beats, leaving the others unaffected (Fig. 34-6). This suggests that, under these conditions, the tachycardia is due to the focus under vagal control probably junctional in origin.

(5) *Sinus tachycardia.* Sinus tachycardia is not ordinarily slowed by carotid sinus pressure. Slight or conspicuous degrees of slowing may occasionally occur in patients with overactive vagal tone or in those receiving full doses of digitalis. However, the tachycardia usually returns immediately upon removal of the carotid sinus pressure.

Diagnosis of Arrhythmias. The atrial mechanism is often difficult to determine in many tachyarrhythmias with the routine electrocardiogram. Carotid sinus pressure (CSP) may be employed in the differential diagnosis of various supraventricular arrhythmias in which the atrial mechanism is obscured by the rapid heart rate (Fig. 33–3). By slowing the ventricular rate, CSP reveals the character of the supraventricular activity. Those rhythms which may be clarified include: (1) sinus tachycardia; (2) supraventricular tachycardia with aberration; (3) paroxysmal atrial tachycardia; (4) PAT with block; and (5) atrial flutter (Fig. 33–2).

Carotid sinus pressure is occasionally helpful in the diagnosis of digitalis intoxication which may not be apparent otherwise; it may result in advanced grades of A-V heart block, and with the slow ventricular rate, ectopic activity may become evident (Fig. 33–2).

The diagnosis of acute myocardial infarction may be obscured by disturbances in rhythm (e.g., supraventricular or ventricular tachyarrhythmias or premature beats). Carotid sinus pressure by restoring normal sinus rhythm even transiently in the supraventricular type may help to clarify the diagnosis by showing characteristic S-T segment changes.

TECHNIQUE OF THE APPLICATION OF CAROTID SINUS PRESSURE IN THE HUMAN SUBJECT

The pressure should usually be applied with the patient in the recumbent or semirecumbent position. The sitting position is less satisfactory because of the increased likelihood of precipitating episodes of unconsciousness and convulsive seizures. When carotid sinus pressure has repeatedly failed in the recumbent position, it may be attempted in the sitting position. The head is tilted backward to one side; the carotid artery is then palpated as high up in the neck as

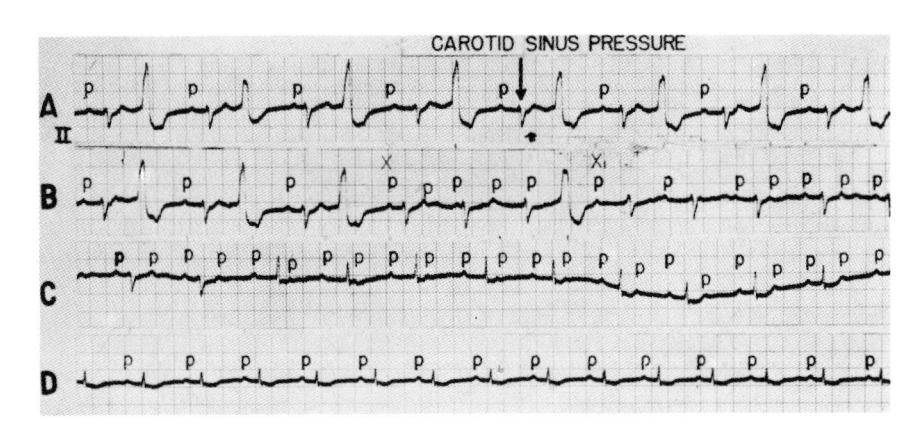

Figure 33–2. Effect of carotid sinus pressure in clarifying the presence of digitalis toxicity in the presence of paroxysmal atrial tachycardia, A-V dissociation, and coupled ventricular premature beats.

(A) (Lead II) Note prolonged P-R interval and coupled ventricular premature beats. Carotid sinus pressure is applied at the arrow.

(B) Note the decrease in the incidence of the premature beats at X, followed by their abolition at X_1, and the presence of complete A-V dissociation with unchanged QRS.

(C) Note paroxysmal atrial tachycardia with an atrial rate of 140 per minute and a ventricular rate of 72 per minute. Complete A-V dissociation. Starting with the third QRS the ventricular complexes are narrow (disappearance of aberration).

(D) Two days later, with cessation of digitalis, note the return to normal sinus rhythm; P-R interval is shortened towards the end of the strip.

In summary, carotid sinus pressure abolished the ventricular premature beats but disclosed other evidence of digitalis toxicity, namely, atrial tachycardia and A-V dissociation, which is not discernible in strip A.

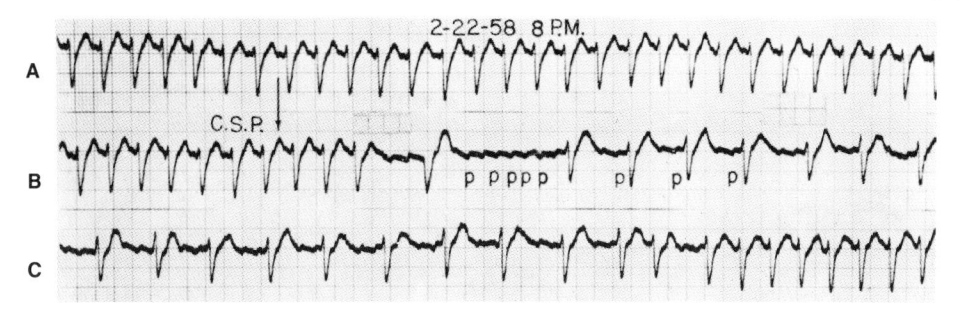

Figure 33–3. Effect of carotid sinus pressure in clarifying atrial mechanism in the presence of atrial flutter (lead II).

(A) Atrial flutter with 2:1 A-V block. Note that the diagnosis remains unclear until after carotid sinus pressure in B.

(B) At the arrow carotid sinus pressure results in a higher degree of A-V heart block where the flutter waves can be distinctly observed.

(C) Note that the ventricular rate is about 88 per minute for nine cycles (4 to 1 response) and atrial flutter with 2 to 1 response returns at the end of the strip.

This tracing is instructive by showing the value of carotid sinus pressure in determining the atrial mechanism and ruling out the possibility of atrial or ventricular tachycardia. It also shows a characteristic feature of atrial flutter, namely, the resumption of the rapid ventricular rate soon after the carotid sinus pressure is removed.

possible and pressed firmly against the vertebral column. This vessel is frequently an elusive structure and one must make certain that the carotid artery and not the soft tissue of the neck is pressed upon. Lateral retraction of the carotid artery may prevent its slipping. During the maintenance of pressure, a stethoscope should be continually applied to the precordium or the heart should be monitored by the electrocardiogram, or both procedures should be carried out. As the heart rate slows, the pressing finger should be immediately removed. By so doing, one may avoid prolonged bradycardia or cardiac standstill and thereby the possibility of cerebrovascular complications.

First the right and then the left carotid sinus may alternately be pressed upon. Although both the right and left vagus supply both the S-A node and A-V junction, the right vagus supplies a greater number of fibers to the S-A node, and the left a preponderant number to the A-V junction. Some observers have reported different results from right and left carotid sinus pressure, but there is no unanimity of opinion on this subject.

One should be extremely careful in pressing on the carotid sinus when the contralateral carotid artery is partially or totally occluded, since untoward effects are likely to occur.

Simultaneous bilateral carotid sinus pressure should never be applied, since such pressure results in a severe grade of cerebral hypoxia and may precipitate serious ectopic rhythms or other complications.

Causes of Failure. The following are some of the common causes for failure of carotid sinus pressure: (a) application of the pressure on soft tissue and not on the carotid artery; (b) the presence of marked increase in sympathetic tone, as in highly nervous states, thyrotoxicosis, and fever; (c) the prior administration of sympathomimetic drugs (e.g., benzedrine, ephedrine, paradrine, phenylephrine); (d) the previous use of quinidine which, in full doses, tends to inhibit the carotid sinus reflex by reducing vagal tone; (e) the presence of ectopic rhythms other than those of supraventricular origin; and (f) marked resistance to the effect of increased parasympathetic tone (e.g., occasionally in atrial flutter or certain junctional tachycardias).

OCULOCARDIAC REFLEX

Parasympathetic stimulation may also be produced by the oculocardiac reflex, which is excited by pressure over the closed eyes, applied just below the supraorbital ridge, not over the cornea. Because of the untoward effects occasionally observed (e.g., retinal detachment), however, we feel that this is not the preferred method of producing parasympathetic stimulation.

OTHER METHODS OF INCREASING VAGAL TONE

There are several other techniques which may be used to increase vagal tone. These include: (1) respiratory maneuvers (e.g., Valsalva maneuver, Müller maneuver, breath-holding, blowing into a balloon), or (2) induced vomiting either by emetics (e.g., ipecac, apomorphine) or a finger placed in the throat. The principal advantage of these maneuvers is that they may be easily performed by the patient immediately upon the onset of the arrhythmia. A recent innovation which may allow patients suffering from frequent and repeated attacks is the carotid sinus stimulator which was first introduced for the control of angina pectoris (Braunwald et al., 1969). This latter device, however, has not gained wide acceptance for the treatment of tachyarrhythmias.

CONTRAINDICATIONS

Carotid sinus pressure is generally not attempted in patients older than 75 years. Similarly, in the presence of cerebrovascular disease, this maneuver should be avoided, unless there are very definite indications. In such individuals, there is not only the hazard of sclerosed and narrow cerebral vessels, but the reflex may be unduly sensitive with resultant prolonged asystole. Except for diagnostic purposes, this procedure is also contraindicated in the presence of occlusion of a carotid artery. Caution should be exercised in the presence of coronary disease, high grades of A-V heart block, bundle branch block, and other conditions associated with slow rates.

COMPLICATIONS AND UNTOWARD EFFECTS

Occasional serious reactions have been reported, chiefly resulting from improper technique or the application of pressure prolonged beyond the onset of cardiac standstill. These complications consist of syncope and convulsions, especially in patients with pre-existing cerebrovascular disease. Occasionally, during the period of conversion to normal sinus rhythm, ectopic rhythms and, rarely, dangerous arrhythmias are observed. Ventricular premature beats followed by normal sinus rhythm, ventricular tachycardia, and prefibrillatory ventricular arrhythmias, lasting up to several seconds, may be observed. Rarely, ventricular fibrillation or prolonged asystole occurs.

Carotid sinus pressure may present a greater risk in the presence of certain conduction abnormalities. In the presence of bundle branch block, vagal stimulation may inhibit conduction in the remaining bundle, resulting in complete A-V heart block, accompanied by an intervening Stokes-Adams seizure.

Because of the occasional development of untoward effects, it is suggested, when carotid sinus pressure is indicated, particularly in patients with heart disease, that it be performed in a setting in which monitoring is continuous and a defibrillator and other resuscitative equipment are available.

SUMMARY

As a result of fairly extensive experience, the author feels that although minor complications occasionally occur, carotid sinus pressure, properly employed, is a relatively safe procedure. However, it is important to observe the aforementioned precautions.

DRUGS WHICH DECREASE CARDIAC AUTOMATICITY

PARASYMPATHOMIMETIC DRUGS

The important parasympathomimetic agents that manifest antiarrhythmic action include acetylcholine, methacholine, neostigmine, and edrophonium. Of those drugs that manifest primarily parasympathomimetic effects, neostigmine and, more recently, edrophonium are the most frequently used because they produce the least side effects. Parasympathomimetic drugs are indicated, particularly in the treatment of supraventricular tachycardias.

Neostigmine

Mechanism of Action. Neostigmine (Prostigmin) is a synthetic compound and a potent specific inhibitor of cholinesterase activity. Because neostigmine acts by competitively inhibiting the action of cholinesterase, normal amounts of acetylcholine that have been released by nerve stimulation are able to exert their effects for a longer period of time before enzymatic inactivation occurs. Indirectly, therefore, it is a cholinergic drug. The effects of neostigmine are the same as acetylcholine and will be manifest wherever the parasympathetic system is a functional component. Use of the drug results in a diminution in cardiac rate and contractile force. While moderate doses slow the pulse rate, the blood pressure is increased. Higher doses cause a further slowing of the rate, but the blood pressure drops. The terminal vagal fibers in the heart are preferentially affected, so that stimulation of the vagi in the presence of neostigmine results in a summation of the parasympathetic effect.

Indications. There are several indications for neostigmine. (a) Neostigmine is indicated in supraventricular tachycardia (either alone or in conjunction with carotid sinus pressure). (b) In certain supraventricular tachyarrhythmias, by slowing the ventricular rate at least temporarily, it clarifies the atrial mechanism and may be of help in the differential diagnosis between paroxysmal atrial tachycardia, paroxysmal atrial tachycardia with A-V block, and atrial flutter. (c) In the presence of atrial fibrillation and flutter, neostigmine will usually slow the ventricular rate and renders it more sensitive to carotid sinus stimulation. (d) In the postural type of paroxysmal tachycardia oral administration of neostigmine may be of value in reducing undue sympathetic overactivity that occurs when an upright posture is assumed

Untoward and Toxic Effects. "Alarming" reactions to neostigmine have occasionally occurred, but severe toxic effects are relatively uncommon. Unpleasant but transient side effects after oral administration include nausea, salivation, perspiration, dizziness, loose bowel movements, occasional muscular aches and pains, abdominal cramps, and vomiting. Usually these reactions subside after 15 or 30 minutes, but the large doses required for effective oral treatment may lead to actual toxicity, particularly in patients with enhanced intestinal absorption.

Contraindications. Neostigmine and other cholinesterase inhibitors are contraindicated in the presence of coronary occlusion, bronchial asthma, hyperthyroidism, intestinal obstruction, and peptic ulcer.

Dose and Method of Administration. Neostigmine, given as the methylsulfate or bromide salt, is administered orally, subcutaneously, or intramuscularly. It is best given by the parenteral route because therapeutic effects from oral administration are unpredictable. Intramuscular administration is the method of choice (0.25 to 0.5 mg. every three or four hours if necessary). In paroxysmal atrial tachycardia, the drug is usually injected in doses of 0.5 to 2 mg. (1 to 4 ml. of a 1:2000 solution). The therapeutic effect of neostigmine is temporary. The onset of action occurs in about 20 minutes, reaching a peak at one hour and subsiding in three to five hours. The intravenous route is rarely used because of the dangerous side effects.

Edrophonium (Tensilon). Edrophonium, or 3-hydroxyphenyldimethylethylammonium chloride, chemically resembles neostigmine. The mechanism of action of edrophonium is similar to that of neostigmine; however, its duration of action is shorter. While edrophonium has been employed chiefly as a diagnostic agent in myasthenia gravis and for its anticurare effects, it does have limited use in the therapy of arrhythmias. This drug has proven to be an effective agent in the abolition of supraventricular tachycardias. In addition, it is efficacious in slowing the ventricular rate in patients with supraventricular tachycardia. An effective dose as an antiarrhythmic agent is 5 to 10 mg. given intravenously. Experimentally, no adverse effects with edrophonium have been found in the heart, except for an increase in atrioventricular conduction time, which can be partially controlled with propranolol (Grossman et al., 1969b).

The toxic side effects of edrophonium resemble those of other parasympathomimetic drugs. Rapid administration of the drug may cause transient slowing of the heart, transient hypotension, and increased bronchial secretion, all of which can be abolished by atropine. Suggested contraindications include acute myocardial infarction, peptic ulcer, asthma, or any condition in which it is not desirable to augment parasympathetic activity.

QUINIDINE

Quinidine, a stereoisomer of quinine and a natural product of the cinchona bark, is one of the most effective antiarrhythmic drugs. Although newer drugs and electric countershock have supplanted it for certain indications, quinidine remains the primary maintenance drug for the control of many arrhythmias.

Electrophysiologic Effects. Quinidine has many complex and interrelated pharmacologic effects. Its cardiac electrophysiologic effects can be summarized as follows: (1) the sinus rate is unaffected; (2) atrial automaticity, excitability, and conductivity are all depressed, and the refractory period is prolonged; (3) therapeutic concentrations have little or no effect on conduction velocity through the A-V junction; (4) automaticity is depressed, conduction velocity slowed, and the refractory period prolonged in the His-Purkinje system; and (5) ventricular excitability and conductivity are depressed. All of these electrophysiologic effects are more pronounced at rapid than at relatively slow heart rates.

Pharmacologic Effects. In addition to its electrophysiologic effects, quinidine exerts several direct pharmacologic effects upon the heart.

Myocardial Contractility. Quinidine manifests variable effects on myocardial contractility which depend upon several factors: (1) the cardiac state, (2) the dose of the drug, and (3) its effect on cardiac excitability and conductivity. It may depress contractility when given in high doses or when administered to aged patients or patients with organic myocardial derangement or hemodynamic depression due to arrhythmia. A negative inotropic effect is commonly observed in patients with severe myocardial disease, in subjects with arrhythmias that cause hypotension, and in older patients. Whereas quinidine may have a positive inotropic effect in low concentrations, it clearly depresses contractility in toxic doses, even in normal hearts.

Electrolyte Flux. Quinidine exerts a powerful effect in depressing the outward flux of potassium across the cell membrane. In addition, it stimulates the movement of extracellular potassium into the cells. In this way it results in a buildup of intracellular potassium and inhibits the generation and maintenance of the action potential. This action which appears to be the opposite of the digitalis effect on sodium-potassium flux may not only explain the electrophysiologic effects of quinidine but also the myocardial depressant action. These depressant effects are due to alteration in calcium metabolism which excludes calcium from the active region of the actin-myosin molecules (cf. with mechanism of action of digitalis, p. 375).

Vagolytic Action. Although it has been proposed that quinidine either blocks the release of or competes with acetylcholine, little evidence exists that therapeutic doses administered to human subjects produce a vagolytic effect.

Absorption and Metabolism. Quinidine is rapidly absorbed following either oral or intramuscular administration, reaching peak serum levels in one to three hours and in 30 to 90 minutes respectively. Peak plasma levels are attained almost immediately after intravenous infusion, compared with the delays noted previously following administration by other routes.

The peak concentration attained in skeletal muscle, liver, kidney, and the heart may be 20 or more times that found simultaneously in the plasma. Myocardial activity of the drug does not reach its peak until four to six hours after administration, although the concentration of quinidine in the serum decreases linearly from its peak level after oral administration. The cardiac concentration of quinidine probably determines its effectiveness, but only the serum level can be measured clinically.

Following concentration in the tissues, quinidine is degraded and has a half-life of approximately two hours. This process, which occurs principally in the liver, produces two different hydroxylated metabolites of quinidine. Their excretion seems to be a function of the glomerular filtration rate.

Plasma Levels. The plasma level of quinidine at any given time depends upon the dose administered, the time elapsed since the last dose, and the rapidity with which quinidine is metabolized and excreted by the individual patient. Certain correlations can be made between the plasma levels of quinidine and the therapeutic and toxic effects of the drug. Although the ideal is to give quinidine in doses that keep plasma levels of the drug within the usual therapeutic range, monitoring the electrocardiogram is often an excellent method of assessing the effect of the drug in the individual patient (see p. 229).

The relationship between serum quinidine levels and the therapeutic effects of the drug is indirect, since the latter probably depends upon cardiac concentrations or the ratio of the tissue to plasma levels; nevertheless, a rough correlation can generally be established: (1) antiarrhythmic actions are rare with serum concentrations below 2 mg./L.; (2) a therapeutic effect is generally associated with plasma levels in the range of 4 to 8 mg./L., with the chance of toxic effects increasing at the higher end of this range; and

(3) toxic effects are commonly noted at concentrations greater than 10 mg./L. Plasma levels within the therapeutic range do not guarantee that toxic effects will not occur. In certain cases, the doses of quinidine required to convert an ectopic rhythm resulting from massive infarction or toxic digitalis effects may be so high that they evoke depressive effects—the therapeutic dose may approach or exceed the toxic dose. Indeed, instances occasionally occur in which quinidine administered up to the toxic dose does not effect conversion.

Unusually high plasma levels of quinidine often result when standard doses are given to patients with conditions that predispose to quinidine retention, especially congestive heart failure and renal insufficiency. The higher serum quinidine levels in patients with congestive heart failure and renal insufficiency are due to decreased urinary excretion caused by a decrease in the glomerular filtration rate (Fig. 33–4). The higher serum quinidine levels attained in such patients when treated with quinidine probably explain the more frequent occurrence of quinidine toxicity and ventricular arrhythmias observed in this group.

Effects on the Electrocardiogram. The changes in the electrocardiogram caused by quinidine are related to its electrophysiologic effects. Slowing of A-V conduction velocity causes lengthening of the P-R interval, while

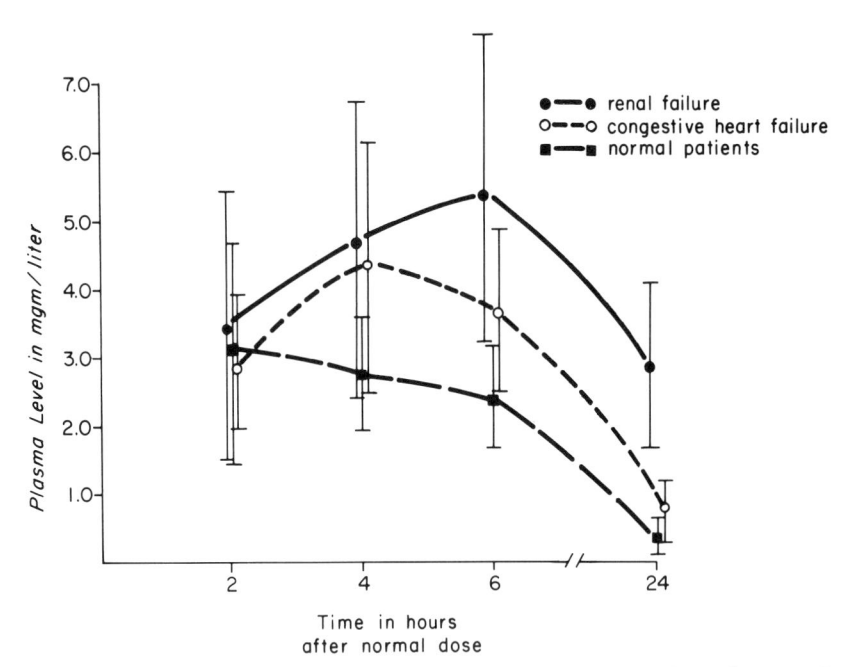

Figure 33–4. Relation between serum quinidine levels in normals and in subjects with congestive heart failure and renal insufficiency.

Note the variation in the plasma levels in the three groups. In normal subjects, the maximal concentration occurred in about two hours and gradually decreased. In the presence of congestive failure, the maximal concentration occurred in about four hours and decreased much more gradually. Note also that the concentration exceeded that in the normal group and the high level was maintained for a longer period of time.

In the group with renal failure, note that the maximal concentration occurred in about six hours and was much higher than that in the previous two groups and declined much more slowly (see text). (From Bellet, S., Roman, L., and Boza, A.: Amer. J. Cardiol., 27:368, 1971.)

prolongation of the ventricular action potential is reflected by prolongation of the Q-T$_c$ interval. The QRS duration is also increased. These effects are related to the plasma concentration; however, the increase in QRS duration occurs at lower plasma levels and is an earlier indication of quinidine effects than alteration of the Q-T$_c$ (Heissenbuttel and Bigger, 1970).

Quinidine can produce changes in the other components of the electrocardiogram. There may be notching of the T wave due to the superimposition of a U wave in its terminal portion, decrease in amplitude of the T waves, S-T segment depression and the T wave inversion.

In late stages of toxicity, the P waves are somewhat widened and often notched. Conspicuous slowing of the atrial rate with the development of intra-atrial block and atrial standstill occurs. With very high blood concentrations, the QRS complex may widen progressively to that of typical bundle branch block with a QRS approaching 0.16 to 0.18 second, accompanied by T wave and S-T segment changes. This marked widening of the ventricular complexes may precede development of ventricular tachycardia and ventricular fibrillation.

In a patient with a normal intraventricular conduction time, a 50 per cent increase in QRS complex width is dangerous; if possible, such widening should not be increased above 25 per cent of the control value. The practice of withholding quinidine after the QRS complex is prolonged 25 to 50 per cent (or above 0.11 to 0.13 second) appears desirable. An extra hazard appears when an already prolonged intraventricular conduction time exists, since further widening may induce serious ectopic rhythms, particularly ventricular fibrillation.

Indications. Quinidine is primarily indicated for the following conditions: (1) Premature beats of atrial, A-V junctional, and ventricular origin. (2) Conversion of atrial flutter and fibrillation to normal sinus rhythm. (However, digitalis is the drug of choice for the initial treatment of these arrhythmias because of its ability to slow the ventricular rate.) (3) Maintenance of normal sinus rhythm in subjects converted from atrial fibrillation or flutter, and for the continued suppression of frequent premature beats. (Quinidine is the drug of choice in these situations.) (4) Prophylaxis of arrhythmias associated with countershock. (5) Termination of ventricular tachycardia and in suppression of repetitive episodes of tachyarrhythmias associated with W-P-W syndrome (see Chapter 13).

The following indications for the use of quinidine remain in doubt, despite the enthusiasm of proponents who have long used quinidine in these instances: (1) Quinidine is not primarily indicated for either prophylaxis or active treatment of ventricular flutter and fibrillation since both lidocaine and bretylium are probably more effective. Furthermore, quinidine increases the energy required to achieve defibrillation. (2) Quinidine has been employed at various times as a prophylactic antiarrhythmic agent in acute myocardial infarction; however, this point has as yet not been finally settled. In the coronary care unit, it may be more properly administered as specific arrhythmias appear.

Dose and Method of Administration. Quinidine may be administered orally, intramuscularly or intravenously; the oral route is the method of choice. Because of its possible toxic effects, the administration of quinidine in large doses and in the initial stages of therapy should be correlated with frequent electrocardiographic records. A test dose of 200 mg. (3 gr.) of quinidine may be administered; however, unfortunately, this "test dose" is sometimes administered in the confidence that a patient who tolerates that dose can tolerate average therapeutic levels of the drug. This interpretation is incorrect; one has simply demonstrated that the patient is able to tolerate the specific dose administered. There is no substitute for careful attention to the clinical signs of quinidine intolerance as they develop. Plasma levels are quite valuable in judging the effect of therapy. Unfortunately, however, they are often not available.

Oral Quinidine Preparations. Although quinidine sulfate is the oral preparation most commonly used, other salts, including quinidine gluconate and quinidine lactate, are available. These preparations differ only slightly from quinidine sulfate in gastrointestinal absorption. Furthermore, the gluconate is effective when incorporated into a long-acting preparation of quinidine (Quinaglute). This is probably due to its high solubility in water (10 times greater than the sulfate). The long-acting preparation tends to maintain the plasma concentration at a relatively constant level, avoiding the valleys and peaks often obtained with short-acting medications. It is often possible to maintain therapeutic levels of the drug through the night without administration of a night dose.

Effect of Multiple Doses. Since the peak level is reached in about two hours, a frequently used regimen is that of administering 0.3- to 0.4-gm. doses five times per day at two-hour intervals. By this regimen, a plasma level of 40 per cent of the peak is observed 12 hours after the last dose. Therefore, maintenance of this dose schedule for two or three days progressively increases the blood level. A blood level of 4 to 8 mg./L. may then be reached in about three days (Fig. 33–5).

Another accepted regimen is to give a 0.4-gm. dose, four times a day for three days. If conversion does not occur, this may be increased, in the absence of toxicity, by 0.2 gm. per dose, i.e., 0.5 or 0.6 gm., four times a day. In refractory cases, a total of 3 gm. per day is given for three days; if no conversion results, one may increase the dose cautiously unless evidence of toxicity appears or the blood level exceeds 9 or 10 mg./L. (Fig. 33–6).

The daily dose necessary for effective conversion has been shown to be

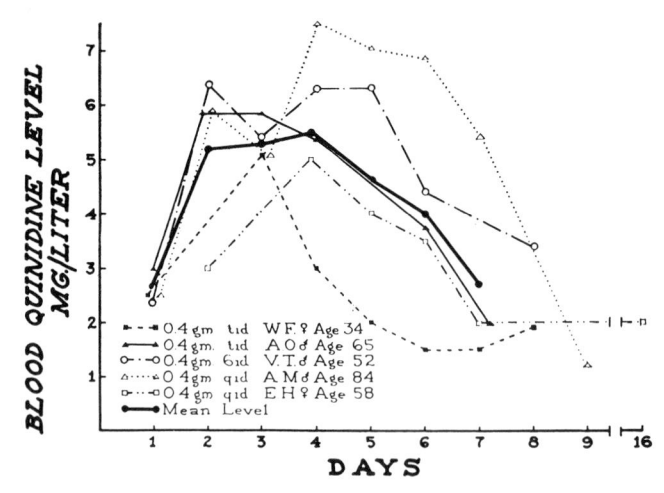

Figure 33–5. Parabolic curve obtained with fixed daily doses of quinidine. By observing the *mean level* (dark black line) it can be seen that a peak blood level is attained within two to five days when patients are given a fixed daily dose of quinidine. After the peak there is a gradual decline in the level, despite continued medication at the fixed dosage. (From Sokolow, M., and Edgar, A. L.: Circulation, *1*:576, 1950.)

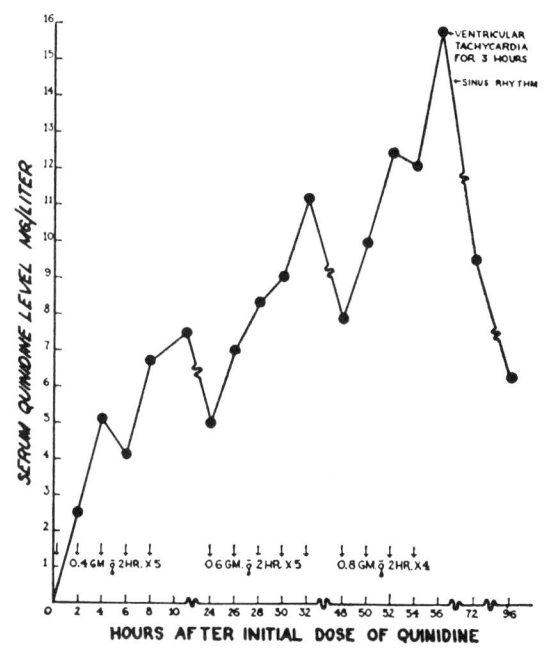

Figure 33–6. (Patient, age 39; atrial fibrillation.) A graph illustrating the progressive rise in blood quinidine level that occurs with the five-dose daily schedule when the individual dose is increased from 0.4 to 0.8 gm. Note the high percentage of quinidine remaining in the blood 12 hours after the peak evening level. (From Sokolow, M., and Edgar, A. L.: Circulation, 1:576, 1950.)

3 gm. or less in 80 per cent of those cases which convert. On a dose schedule of 3 gm. daily, peak serum concentrations vary from patient to patient. This variation of serum concentration is important, because the majority of successful conversions occur at levels below 8 mg./ml., while toxicity increases sharply when this level is exceeded.

Maintenance Doses. Following conversion to normal sinus rhythm, quinidine is administered in maintenance doses to prevent recurrent attacks. Failure to control the ectopic rhythm frequently results from inadequate maintenance dosage. Upon return to normal rhythm, patients are subject to various influences which are conducive to the resumption of the ectopic rhythm unless adequate doses are administered. Among these are exercise, emotional states, and any other factors that might increase cardiac work or metabolism. It is difficult to determine the exact maintenance dose in a given case. One may start with 0.3 gm., four times a day; if the ectopic rhythm recurs, the daily dose is increased by 0.3 gm. per day until a dose that controls attacks is reached. It has been stated that if a given dose produces no toxic effects after four or five days, there is little risk of further accumulation and toxicity. However, in ambulatory cases, it may be unwise to continue patients on excessive doses, because the depressant effect may be as harmful as the arrhythmia.

Quinidine sulfate often gives disappointing results in preventing recurrences of ectopic rhythms, because maintenance doses of quinidine, given three to four times a day, produce valleys in plasma levels during which the ectopic rhythm may recur. The maintenance of a uniform plasma level would appear very desirable. Quinidine gluconate (Quinaglute), because of its greater solubility (1:9) in water as compared to quinidine sulfate (1:90), is preferable. Long-acting quinidine, in the form of quinidine gluconate, gives effective and sustained plasma levels and is usually well tolerated. Because of these factors, it appears to be a drug of choice for maintenance therapy.

Use in Conjunction with Propranolol. Propranolol has been considered to be a beneficial adjunct to quinidine in both active and maintenance therapy for atrial fibrillation. The value of such a combination would appear to be restricted by the possible additive effects of adrenergic blockade and cardiovascular depression; however, combined therapy may avoid the need to use large doses of quinidine (Oravetz and Slodki, 1968).

Toxicity of Quinidine. The toxic effects of quinidine constitute a major deterrent to the use of this drug in situations in which other equally effective agents are available. In most patients, toxicity can be controlled by proper adjustment of the dose or discontinuance of the drug if necessary. However, the possible danger is emphasized by the fact that a mortality of 2 to 4 per cent is attributed to quinidine when it is employed in chronic treatment.

Patients given quinidine, especially those with underlying heart failure, renal insufficiency, or a history of allergic reactions to other drugs, should be watched carefully. Careful observation is especially important during the first one to two weeks of administration. Extreme caution should be exercised in patients with severe heart disease and congestive heart failure, with digitalis intoxication or renal insufficiency (Bellet et al., 1971a). Quinidine should be administered cautiously, if at all, to senile patients. Hospitalization for close clinical observation, electrocardiographic monitoring and possibly the determination of plasma quinidine levels is indicated when large doses are given and when the patient presents an increased risk. All patients should be checked for signs of hypersensitivity to quinidine. Signs of idiosyncrasy include febrile reactions, skin eruptions, thrombocytopenic purpura, and respiratory embarrassment.

Factors Influencing Toxicity. The determinants of the toxic effects of quinidine include: (a) the type and severity of underlying heart disease; (b) the age of the patient; (c) the dose and method of administration; (d) the plasma level and its probable relationship to tissue level; (e) the concentration of electrolytes, particularly calcium, sodium, and potassium; (f) the pH; (g) the presence of congestive heart failure; and (h) renal insufficiency.

Clinical Toxic Manifestations. Allergic reactions are rare. Skin rashes have been reported, but the best documented case reports concern the occurrence of fever and thrombocytopenic purpura. Nausea, vomiting, and diarrhea may occur even with small doses. Under the term "cinchonism" may be grouped impairment of hearing, ringing in the ears, blurred vision, lightheadedness, giddiness, and tremor. Convulsions may result from a direct effect of quinidine on the central nervous system or from hypoxia due to cardiac asystole in the course of restoring the normal rhythm. Atrial embolism and sudden death are unpredictable hazards of quinidine therapy and have acted as deterrents to its effective use. The incidence of embolism has been reported at about 4 per cent and that of sudden death at 1.8 per cent. Respiratory failure following quinidine has been described as a rare complication; the site where this occurs has not been definitely established.

Quinidine may precipitate heart failure in patients with atrial fibrillation if they had not been previously digitalized. The electrocardiographic effects of cardiotoxicity have been noted previously; the most important

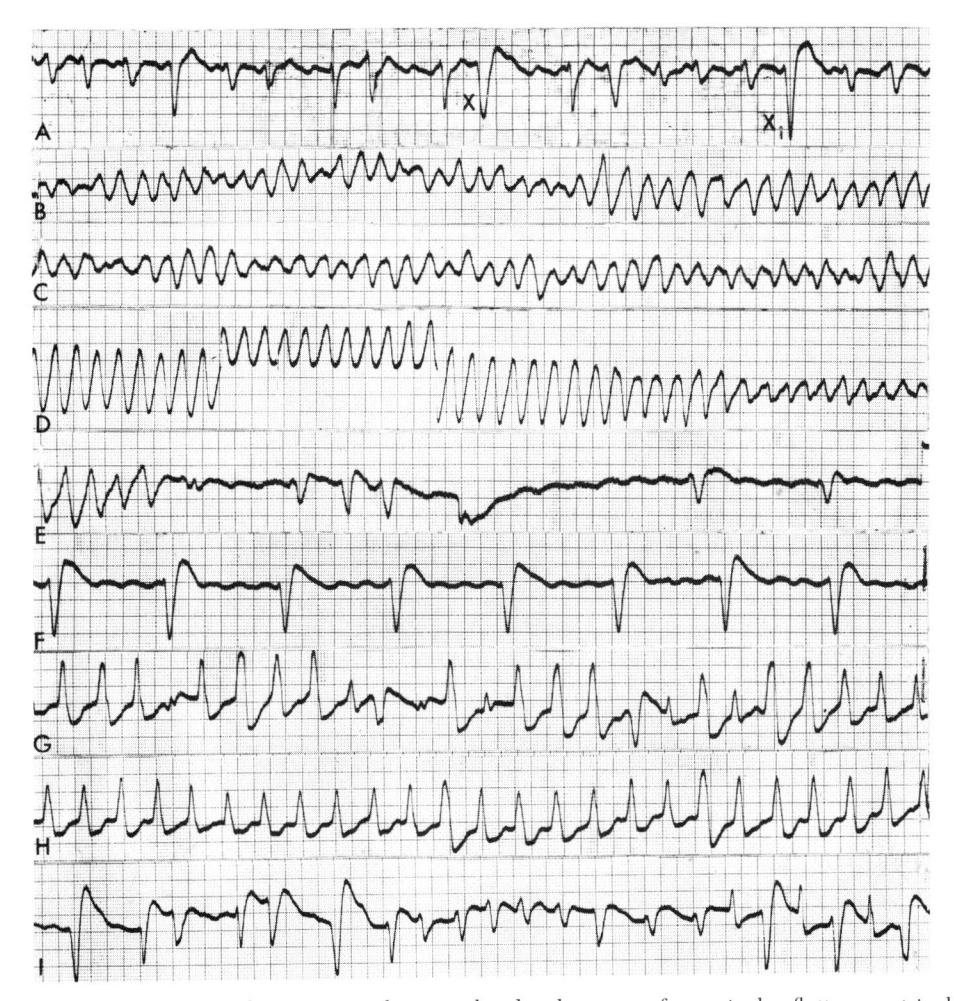

Figure 33–7. Quinidine toxicity showing the development of ventricular flutter, ventricular fibrillation, and a chaotic rhythm.

This patient was a 47-year-old male with a diagnosis of acute myocarditis and atrial fibrillation. Quinidine was administered for the purpose of conversion to a normal sinus rhythm. He received 0.2 gm. of quinidine every two hours for four doses the first day; 0.3 gm. every two hours for five doses on the second day; and 0.4 gm. for five doses on the third day, following which he developed a sudden episode of syncope and shock.

(A) Control shows the presence of atrial fibrillation with aberrant beats at X and X_1.

(B) and (C) Represent the occurrence of ventricular fibrillation and flutter.

(D) Shows ventricular flutter.

(E) Shows termination of ventricular fibrillation with the presence of a slow idioventricular rhythm.

(F) Shows the return of control complexes of the aberrant type. The rate is regular at 44 per minute.

(G) Note the return to a chaotic rhythm.

(H) Shows the supraventricular tachycardia with an almost regular rate with variation in the configuration of the ventricular complexes. Heart rate is 136 per minute.

(I) Shows the persistence of the chaotic rhythm with bidirectional ventricular complexes towards the end of the strip.

Following this, the rhythm reverted to atrial fibrillation, similar to the control, A. The patient was thereafter put on digitalis, which adequately controlled the ventricular rate.

consist of depression of atrial activity, which may ultimately lead to atrial standstill, widening of the QRS complexes, which may precipitate ventricular flutter or fibrillation, and occasional instances of paroxysmal ventricular tachycardia and ventricular fibrillation (Fig. 33–7).

Contraindications. Quinidine is contraindicated in the presence of the following conditions: (a) partial or complete A-V heart block; (b) intraventricular conduction disturbances and bundle branch block; (c) serious hypotensive states, unless they are caused by an arrhythmia that might be correctable by administration of quinidine; (d) when relatively low doses of quinidine result in accumulation of toxic plasma levels (which is especially likely in renal tubular acidosis and in older patients); and (e) in subjects manifesting either clinical signs or a history of hypersensitivity to the drug. Signs of sensitivity to quinidine include febrile reactions, thrombocytopenia, and skin reactions.

Quinidine should be administered with caution in the following conditions, and further administration is contraindicated should quinidine aggravate the basic defect: (a) congestive heart failure; (b) digitalis intoxication (since quinidine may accentuate existing conduction defects); and (c) hyperpotassemia, since the effect of potassium to depress conduction is additive to the effect of quinidine.

PROCAINE AMIDE

In 1951, Mark et al. (1951) reported that procaine amide was an effective antiarrhythmic agent in man and had less central nervous system effects than procaine. Subsequently, procaine amide was subjected to extensive investigation which led to its widespread clinical use.

Electrophysiology. The effects of procaine amide on the specialized tissue of the heart are, in general, similar to those of quinidine. The most beneficial and best established action of the drug is to reduce the automaticity of fibers in the His-Purkinje system; however, procaine amide also manifests effects on conduction and excitability.

Atrium. Procaine amide causes a reduction in the excitability of the atrium and raises the threshold to electrical stimulation. High doses of the drug also slow conduction through the atrium. It has no significant effect on the heart rate.

A-V Junction. In the majority of patients given therapeutic doses of procaine amide, no slowing of the A-V conduction can be demonstrated. However, when higher doses are administered or a more sensitive method is employed (i.e., by recording the His-bundle electrogram), the A-V conduction time is found to be generally prolonged.

His-Purkinje System. In doses within the therapeutic range, procaine amide depresses automaticity and conductivity in the His-Purkinje system. However, conduction defects caused by diastolic depolarization in the conduction system may be improved by procaine amide.

In toxic doses, procaine amide causes: (1) enhancement of automaticity, (2) severe depression of excitability and conduction, and (3) prolongation of the action potential and the effective refractory period.

Pharmacologic Effects. The pharmacologic effects of procaine amide include: (1) an anticholinergic action, (2) depression of myocardial metabolism, and (3) effects on the electrocardiogram. Electrocardiographic alterations are quite similar to those of quinidine. The P-R interval is occasionally slightly prolonged. The Q-T interval or electrical systole is prolonged; however, this is not an invariable effect of procaine amide and cannot be used as a gauge of its action, as with quinidine. The T wave amplitude may be decreased, and occasionally, with large doses, T wave inversion may appear. These effects are not necessarily toxic, since they may occur within the therapeutic range.

Widening of the QRS complexes is a characteristic toxic effect and requires precautions similar to those following the administration of quinidine. If there is widening of the QRS over 25 per cent, or if the QRS width exceeds 0.14 second, further administration should be avoided or one should proceed with great caution; the drug should probably not be given if the QRS width exceeds 0.16 second. In the presence of tachyarrhythmias, conversion to normal sinus rhythm occasionally occurs soon after this width is reached.

Hemodynamic Effects. The alterations in circulatory dynamics depend on the cardiovascular state of the patient and on the rate and route of administration of the drug. Thus, full doses of procaine amide administered rapidly by the intravenous route to patients with severe heart disease may produce marked hemodynamic impairment (i.e., decrease in cardiac output and arterial pressure); however, smaller doses infused slowly or given intramuscularly or orally may not impair circulatory function.

Absorption and Metabolism. Procaine amide is rapidly and almost completely absorbed from the gastrointestinal tract following oral administration; plasma levels reach a peak in 60 to 90 minutes and then fall by 10 to 20 per cent each hour. Identical oral and intravenous doses of procaine amide produce identical peak levels after an hour, followed by a similar rate of decline. After intramuscular administration, peak levels are reached in 30 to 60 minutes (Bellet et al., 1952).

Indications. Data obtained during nearly 30 years of clinical use indicate that procaine amide is an effective antiarrhythmic agent, and its major uses are similar to those of quinidine.

Supraventricular Arrhythmias. Procaine amide is efficacious in treating atrial and junctional tachycardia, including those associated with the W-P-W syndrome. Quinidine is, however, usually more satisfactory than procaine amide for long-term prophylaxis of arrhythmias, because quinidine has greater efficacy and produces allergic reactions less frequently. Procaine amide is of little efficacy for the conversion of atrial fibrillation or flutter to normal sinus rhythm and is of little help in maintenance after normal rhythm has been restored.

Ventricular Arrhythmias. Procaine amide has been successful in decreasing the frequency of ventricular premature beats and converting ventricular tachycardia to normal sinus rhythm. An analysis of the experience of 279 cases of clinical arrhythmias treated with procaine amide shows that ventricular tachycardia is terminated in 69 per cent of the cases, ventricular premature beats in 91 per cent, and supraventricular tachycardia in 68 per cent (Bellet et al., 1952). Nevertheless, at present it has a lower priority than other methods, especially lidocaine and electric countershock.

The place of procaine amide vis-a-vis quinidine in the treatment of arrhythmias is often a matter of personal preference. However, a suggested procedure is somewhat as follows: (a) For oral medication, quinidine is the drug of choice except in those instances in which the patient manifests allergy to quinidine and its group of drugs. (b) For short-term parenteral medication (intramuscular and rarely intravenous use) in selected cases, I prefer procaine amide because it is somewhat better tolerated. The intramuscular route is preferred for parenteral medication not only because its effect may be attained in a relatively short period, but also because it produces a minimal degree of hypotension. The intravenous route is used when the patient is in a shock-like state and absorption following intramuscular administration is apt to be slow or uncertain.

Digitalis Toxicity. Procaine amide successfully abolishes ventricular premature beats, usually without significant degrees of atrioventricular or intraventricular block (unless large doses are used), and controls ventricular tachycardia due to toxic doses of digitalis. The use of procaine amide should be reserved for those patients in whom it can be used in moderate doses with relatively slight side effects.

During Anesthesia and Surgery. Procaine amide has been successfully employed as a prophylactic measure to prevent arrhythmias during anesthesia, especially in patients undergoing thoracic surgery. It diminishes the incidence and severity of cardiac arrhythmias attributable to the increased sensitization of the cardiac conducting mechanism occasioned by various inhalant anesthetic agents. However, it does not prevent the development of cardiac arrhythmias due to inadequate ventilation or respiratory obstruction. Procaine amide may be given prophylactically prior to surgery in patients who either have ectopic rhythms or who are known to be subject to their development. However, the dose should be relatively small, i.e., 500 mg. intramuscularly for one or two doses. The routine administration of procaine amide in doses large enough to produce an effective therapeutic level is accompanied by alterations in the hemodynamics and enzymatic changes in the heart muscle, which, when added to the various hazards of anesthesia (hypoxia, vagal effects, hypotension), might actually be additive in producing various ectopic rhythms and even cardiac arrest.

In addition, excellent results have been obtained with the use of procaine amide for the active treatment of arrhythmias occurring during anesthesia. The drug is given by slow intravenous infusion in small doses (100 to 300 mg.) under constant electrocardiographic monitoring. The minimal dose required to suppress the arrhythmia should be given.

Prophylaxis of Arrhythmias in Acute Myocardial Infarction. Procaine amide administered prophylactically considerably reduces the incidence of serious arrhythmias in patients with acute myocardial infarction (Koch-Weser et al., 1969). However, this drug should not be used unless arrhythmias are actually observed.

Dose and Method of Administration

Oral Administration. Following administration of a 1-gm. dose of procaine amide, the plasma level reaches a peak in one hour. This declines slowly during the second hour at a rate of about 20 per cent per hour, and at the end of four hours, the plasma concentration ranges from 0.1 to 0.3 mg. per cent (see Fig. 33–8). The decline in plasma level following an oral dose of procaine amide is somewhat less rapid in patients who have been receiving procaine amide regularly for 24 hours or more.

The dose to be administered varies with the urgency of the clinical situation and the rapidity with which therapeutic plasma levels of the drug must be attained. (1) To restore normal sinus rhythm in a severely ill patient suffering from an ectopic rhythm, the suggested dose ranges from 0.5 to 1.0 gm. every two hours. (2) If there is no urgency, the suggested dose is 250 to 500 mg. administered every four hours. (3) For the prophylaxis of recurrent ectopic rhythms, for the suppression of occasional ectopic beats, and for the prevention of arrhythmias in acute myocardial infarction, 0.25 to 0.5 gm. may be given four times daily. If larger total doses are required for a therapeutic effect, four-hour intervals are desirable to maintain a relatively stable plasma level (see Fig. 33–9).

AGENTS WHICH DECREASE CARDIAC AUTOMATICITY

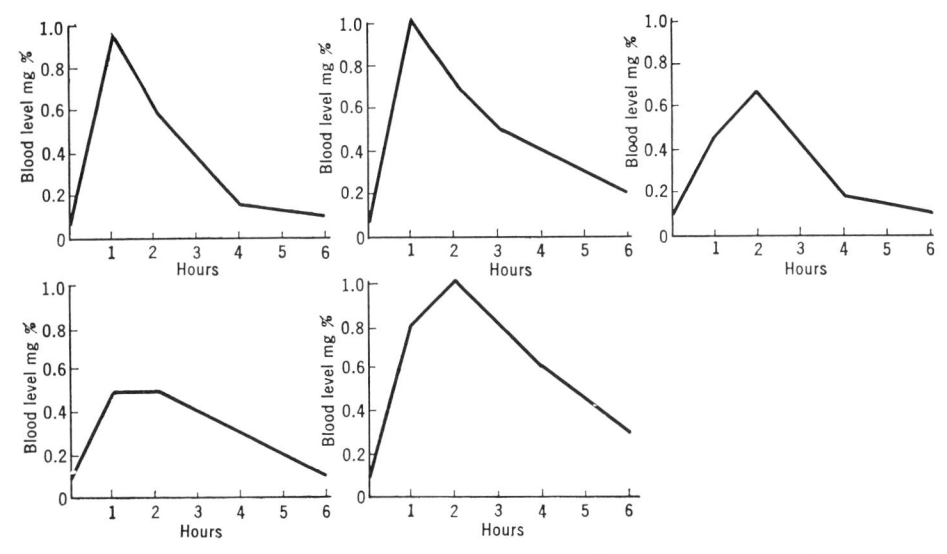

Figure 33–8. Blood levels following oral administration of 1.0 gm. procaine amide hydrochloride (850 mg. Pronestyl base) in five normal subjects. Note that the blood level increases to a range of 0.6 to 1.0 mg. per cent within the first hour, the peak level is attained in one to 1½ hours, following which a gradual decline occurs. At the end of six hours, very little is seen in the blood. (From Berry, K., Garlett, E. L., Bellet, S., and Gefter, W. I.: Am. J. Med., *11*:231, 1951.)

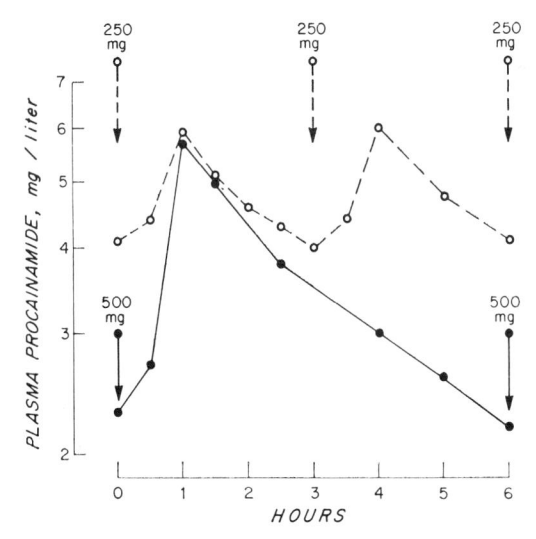

Figure 33–9. Fluctuation of plasma procaine amide concentration in the same patient on two dosage schedules. Note that when procaine amide (500 mg.) was given every 6 hours p.o., the patient did not maintain plasma procaine amide levels within the therapeutic antiarrhythmic range (4 to 6 mg./L.) for three to four hours during each six-hour interval. On the other hand, when procaine amide (250 mg.) was given every three hours p.o., the plasma procaine amide concentration fluctuates but remains within the therapeutic range. (Koch-Weser, J., et al.: New Eng. J. Med., *281*:1253, 1969.)

Intramuscular Administration. Intramuscular administration is preferred when procaine amide must be given parenterally (e.g., in the presence of nausea, vomiting, and shock-like states, or to patients under anesthesia). Although the onset of action is slower by the intramuscular than by the intravenous route, it is simpler and entails less risk of toxic effects. Peak plasma levels of the drug are attained within 15 to 60 minutes following intramuscular injection, followed by decline at the same rate as with oral administration. The gluconate and the hydrochloride are available for intramuscular use. Because the hydrochloride contains a higher percentage of the procaine amide base, it is the preferred preparation. About 0.5 to 1.0 gm. (5 to 10 ml.) may be used for a single injection and repeated every four to six hours.

Although intramuscular procaine amide may result in a fall in blood pressure, this occurs less frequently than following intravenous administration. In general, the toxic effects of intramuscular procaine amide are minimal and no more marked than those following oral medication. No nausea or vomiting occurs.

Intravenous Administration. Intravenous administration of procaine amide is only rarely indicated. It is used when there is manifest urgency for conversion to a normal sinus rhythm, in the presence of a shock-like state, and during anesthesia. Lidocaine is usually the preferred drug for the active therapy of ventricular arrhythmias that require urgent treatment (see p. 361). When given intravenously, procaine amide must be infused slowly (e.g., 100 mg. over four minutes), with constant monitoring of the electrocardiogram and the blood pressure.

Intravenous medication is occasionally accompanied by serious toxic effects, and fatalities have occurred. Most instances of serious hypotension due to this drug have followed administration by this route.

Serum Levels of Procaine Amide. The serum levels after oral and intramuscular administration run somewhat parallel, but with the intramuscular route, the levels are slightly higher and are attained more rapidly (see Figs. 33–8, 33–10). We are not certain as to the optimal serum level for the abolition of an ectopic rhythm. The figure apparently varies considerably and depends upon many factors. The available data suggest that procaine amide exerts therapeutic effects when its plasma levels are between 4 and 10 μg./ml. (Bigger and Heissenbuttel, 1969; Koch-Weser, 1969). In some patients, however, the beneficial effect on the ectopic rhythm occurs after relatively small doses and at lower serum levels.

Toxic Effects. The toxicity of procaine amide is in many respects similar to that of quinidine. The factors influencing toxicity include the dose and method of administration, age, previous cardiovascular state, and the presence of congestive heart failure, and renal insufficiency (Fig. 33–11). In addition, chronic administration may often lead to allergic reactions.

Cardiotoxicity. The most commonly encountered cardiotoxic effect of procaine amide is hypotension which in certain patients may precipitate anginal attacks or convulsive seizures. It depresses pacemaker automaticity and is contraindicated in cases of high-grade partial or complete A-V heart block. In toxic doses, procaine amide enhances automaticity of ventricular pacemakers leading to ventricular tachycardia or fibrillation.

In patients with hypotension resulting from tachycardia, vasopressor agents should be administered. These agents will often sustain the coronary blood flow until the antiarrhythmic agents act. They also tend to reverse the depressant effect of procaine am-

AGENTS WHICH DECREASE CARDIAC AUTOMATICITY

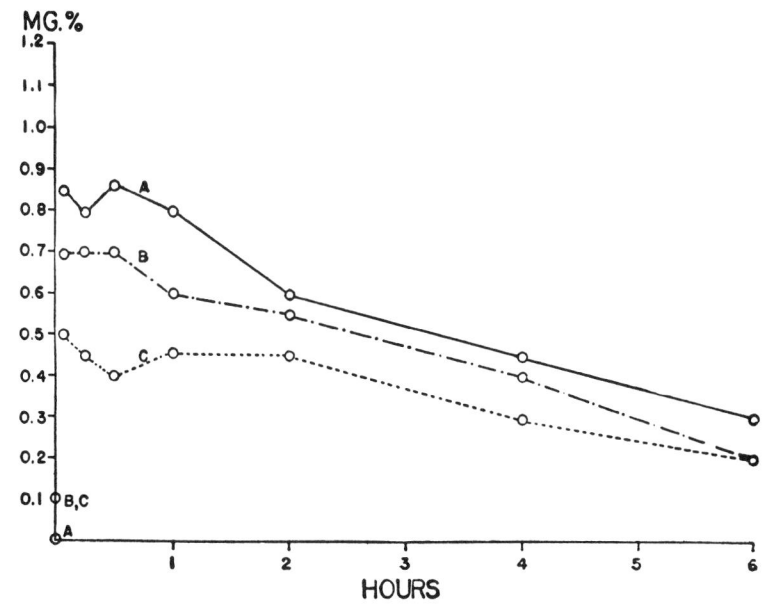

Figure 33-10. Serum levels after 1.0 gm. procaine amide hydrochloride (850 mg. base) in three normal subjects. Each graph represents a subject (intramuscular injection). Note the presence of a significant serum level in 15 minutes after injection; this is increased at 30 minutes and attains a peak at about one hour. The peak level is maintained for about another hour, after which the serum level gradually declines. A significant level is still observed at the end of five to six hours. (From Bellet, S., Zeeman, S. E., and Hirsch, S. A.: Am. J. Med., *13*:145, 1952.)

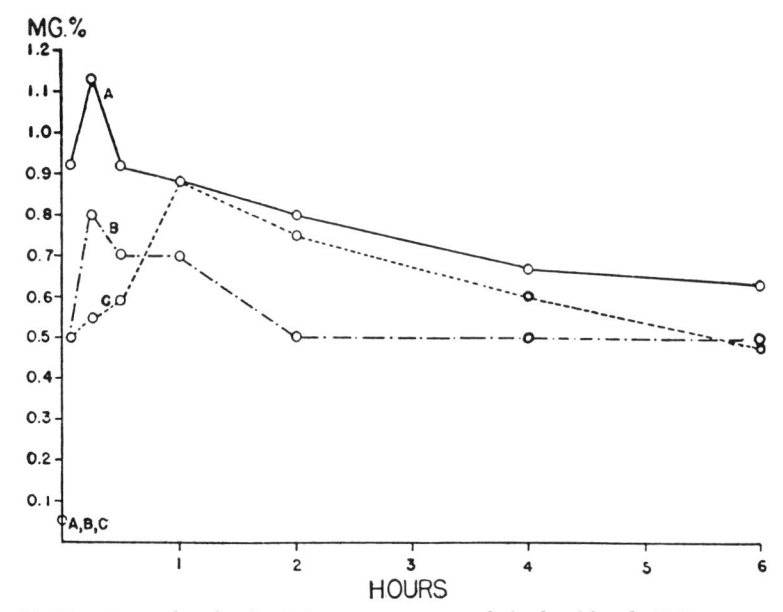

Figure 33-11. Serum levels after 1.0 gm. procaine amide hydrochloride (850 mg. procaine amide base) in patients with congestive heart failure and relatively mild renal insufficiency (intramuscular injection). Note the high serum levels attained 15 to 30 minutes after injection and the extremely gradual decline. Significant levels are still found after six hours. (From Bellet, S., Zeeman, S. E., and Hirsch, S. A.: Am. J. Med., *13*:145, 1952.)

ide. Hypotensive effects can be minimized by using intramuscular instead of intravenous administration, by using small doses, and in instances where the blood pressure is low, by using other agents and approaches, especially countershock.

Therapy depends on the degree and type of toxicity. Molar sodium lactate and other alkalinizing agents tend to reverse the depressed automaticity and conductivity and tend to decrease the QRS widening.

A number of fatalities have been reported following the use of procaine amide; however, these patients were often in extremis when treated. Fatalities have been reported with a dose as little as 300 mg. given intravenously, but most have occurred with much larger doses. The fatal outcome usually follows intravenous medication and often occurs when administration is relatively rapid (Fig. 33–12).

Gastrointestinal System. Anorexia, nausea, and vomiting are not infrequently observed in patients receiving large doses of procaine amide orally (e.g., 4 to 6 gm. per day). Nausea and vomiting are rarely observed with smaller doses, except when they are given over a prolonged period. These symptoms were observed by Berry et al. (1951) in six of 57 patients.

Central Nervous System Effects. Procaine amide, unlike procaine, produces minimal central stimulatory effects. Transient psychoses due to procaine amide may develop.

Allergic Manifestations. One of the most important developments with respect to procaine amide is the growing realization that an apparently reversible clinical syndrome resembling

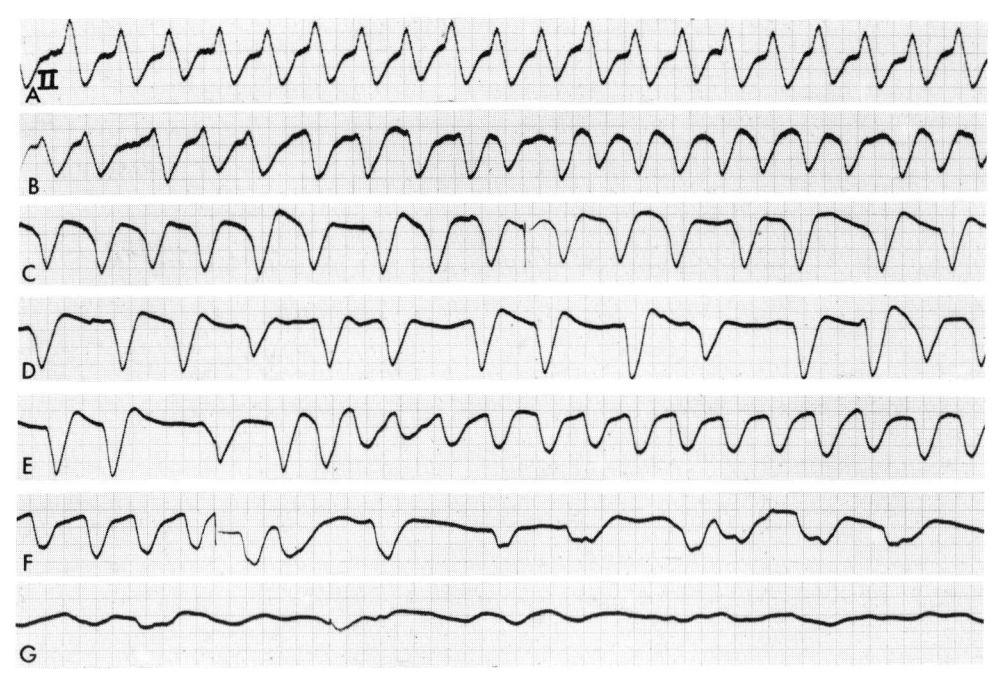

Figure 33–12. Cardiotoxic effect of intravenous procaine amide infusion in a patient with ventricular tachycardia and an idioventricular rhythm. (Illustrates the value of monitoring.)
(A) (Lead II). Following the infusion of procaine amide, note widening of the QRS complexes with a marked degree of aberration. (B) Note still further deterioration of the ventricular complexes with marked widening of the QRS complexes and irregularity. (C, D, and E) Show further deterioration, which approaches a chaotic rhythm and the slow type ventricular fibrillation. (F) Shows a still further type of ventricular fibrillation. (G) Ventricular fibrillation associated with cardiac arrest.

systemic lupus erythematosus occurs in a substantial proportion of patients receiving maintenance doses of procaine amide. This side effect appears to be related to the chronicity of therapy rather than to dose levels. The incidence varies, but is probably about 20 per cent. An incidence as high as 70 per cent of patients on long-term procaine amide treatment has been reported.

The most frequent clinical findings include arthralgia, pleuropneumonic complaints, fever, hepatomegaly, and myalgia. A considerable number of these patients have a history of hypersensitivity reactions. The most characteristic laboratory findings are the presence of antinuclear antibody (100 per cent of patients studied) and of LE cells (94 per cent). In the majority of patients the symptoms are abolished within a few weeks to months after discontinuance of the drug. In all the remaining patients, the administration of steroids following discontinuance of the drug abolishes the symptoms (Dubois, 1969).

Other Allergic Manifestations. Urticaria and a skin rash are occasionally observed. Several instances of fatal agranulocytosis have been reported due to procaine amide. These occurred only after prolonged oral medication.

Contraindications. The contraindications for the use of procaine amide are similar to those of quinidine. Procaine amide should be administered with caution in the presence of bundle branch block or hypotension. It is contraindicated in the presence of complete A-V heart block with Stokes-Adams seizures because it depresses pacemaker automaticity.

Procaine amide should be avoided, if possible, in patients with a susceptibility to allergic responses because of the likelihood of producing a systemic lupus erythematosus-like syndrome. It should be used with caution in patients with a history of bronchial asthma and myasthenia gravis since serious side effects are more likely to occur. Prolonged administration should warrant frequent clinical and hematologic observation.

LIDOCAINE

Widespread use of lidocaine began about 1960 when it attained great popularity for the treatment of ventricular arrhythmias associated with cardiac surgery, digitalis intoxication, and acute myocardial infarction. Extensive experience has shown lidocaine to be an effective and relatively safe drug for the termination of ventricular arrhythmias. In most instances it is preferable to quinidine or procaine amide.

Electrophysiology. The electrophysiologic effects of lidocaine are closely related to its therapeutic usefulness. In general, it has a far greater effect on the ventricles than the atria and its actions on them differ somewhat from those of quinidine and procaine amide. In therapeutic doses, lidocaine has a minimal effect on atrioventricular and intraventricular conduction; however, it causes a dose-related depression of automaticity in His-Purkinje fibers and the excitability of both atria and ventricles. Lidocaine causes a dose-related increase in the minimal transmembrane potential at which an action potential can be elicited (diastolic threshold), without a concomitant shift in the Weidmann curve. Furthermore, it results in a marked decrease in the capacity of ventricular fibers to follow very rapid stimulation and causes suppression of repetitive responses elicited by a premature beat.

Lidocaine has been found to have either no effect or only a slight negative inotropic effect in therapeutic doses. However, doses in excess of the therapeutic range may depress myocardial contractility. In addition, large doses have caused peripheral vasodilation and a significant decrease in arterial pressure in experimental animals. This has little clinical importance, except in the event of serious overdosage.

Hemodynamic Effects. In therapeutic doses, lidocaine does not cause significant alterations in cardiac output, stroke volume, or mean arterial pressure in human subjects with normal hearts, in subjects with various forms of heart disease, in the presence of acute myocardial infarction, or in anesthetized human subjects during cardiac surgery.

Indications and Place in Therapy. Lidocaine is indicated for the abolition of ventricular premature beats and tachycardia; it is especially effective in the termination or continued suppression of frequent ventricular premature beats, ventricular bigeminy, and ventricular tachycardia. Although mostly used for these arrhythmias when they occur in acute myocardial infarction, lidocaine is equally effective for severe ventricular arrhythmias caused by other types of cardiac involvement, including atherosclerosis, hypertension, rheumatic heart disease, and digitalis intoxication, and during recovery from cardiac surgery. In addition, it may be used to prevent arrhythmias which develop following countershock.

Despite lidocaine's considerable efficacy, its use is largely restricted to selected patients in a hospital setting because of several features: (1) it is almost always given intravenously; (2) the infusion rate must be carefully controlled; (3) the patient's response to the drug must be monitored; and (4) many patients who suffer from arrhythmias that require lidocaine are, as a result, seriously ill and also suffer from hypotension and frequently renal and cardiac insufficiency. In addition to the usual serious clinical situation that prevails under these circumstances, lidocaine metabolism is depressed by heart and kidney failure so that toxic plasma levels may be produced by the usually employed doses. Plasma levels of lidocaine should be determined frequently during its administration, particularly in this group of subjects.

Dose and Method of Administration

Intravenous Administration. In the majority of patients, lidocaine is administered intravenously in a bolus which may be followed by a continuous infusion. The effective antiarrhythmic dose is 1 to 2 mg./Kg. infused rapidly over 30 seconds. A second dose may be given soon; however, a total dose given over a short period should not exceed 5 mg./Kg. or 300 mg. Constant drip infusion should be given at a rate of 15 to 45 μg./Kg./min. Long-term infusion should be monitored by frequent clinical observations and plasma levels.

Intramuscular Administration. Lidocaine may also be administered by the intramuscular route. This has been the subject of recent interest because of the difficulty of intravenous administration under certain conditions (i.e., at the home of a patient with acute myocardial infarction, before the arrival of a physician or during transport of the patient to a hospital). Plasma levels within the range of 1 to 4 mg./L. (1 to 4 μg./ml.) are attained within 15 minutes and maintained for 60 to 90 minutes following intramuscular injection of 300 mg. of the drug (Fig. 33–13). A significant antiarrhythmic effect is observed in patients with various forms of heart disease who received 300 mg. of the drug. By 120 minutes, the antiarrhythmic effect of the drug completely subsides. Intramuscular injections of lidocaine are usually given in a 2 to 4 per cent solution (Fig. 33–14). Recently, 10 per cent solutions have proved to be free of local or systemic complications. A plasma level of 2 μg./cc. can be maintained by a combination of 50 mg. of lidocaine intravenously, accompanied by 200 mg. intramuscularly. A mean plasma level is attained in two minutes and levels are well maintained at 60 minutes.

AGENTS WHICH DECREASE CARDIAC AUTOMATICITY

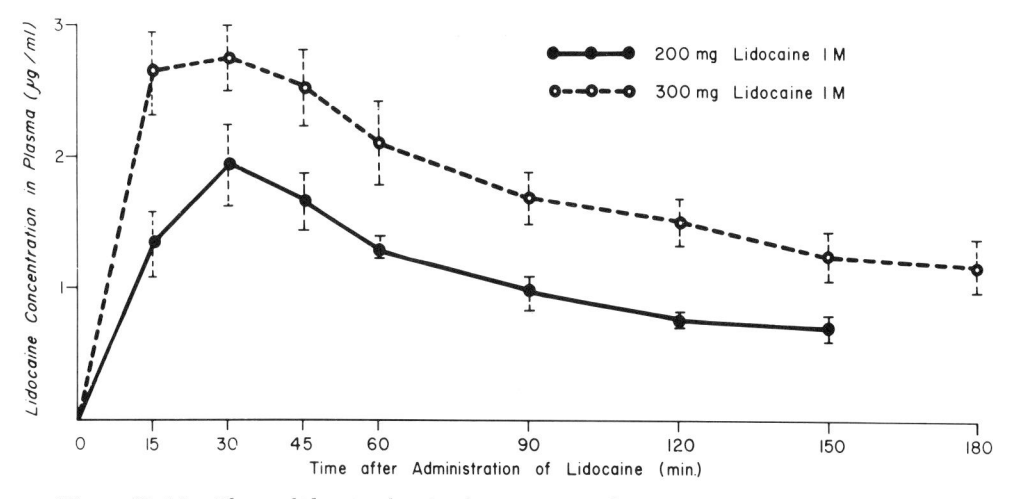

Figure 33-13. Plasma lidocaine levels after intramuscular injection. Mean levels as well as the standard level of the mean are indicated.

After 300 mg. of lidocaine, an average concentration of 2.4 to 2.8 μg./cc. was maintained for the first 45 minutes. This reached its maximum between 15 to 30 minutes and gradually declined thereafter. With a dose of 200 mg. during the same period, significantly lower levels were obtained, ranging in an average of 1.3 to 1.9 μg. (From Bellet, S., Roman, L., Kostis, J. B., and Fleischmann, D.: Amer. J. Cardiol., 27:291, 1971.)

Toxicity. Constant electrocardiographic monitoring is required during the intravenous infusion of lidocaine. The infusion should be promptly terminated at the first signs of depression of cardiac conductivity, such as prolongation of the P-R interval or the QRS complex, the appearance or aggravation of arrhythmias, and the appearance of cerebral manifestations. It is mandatory to have emergency resuscitative equipment and drugs immediately available to manage possible adverse reactions involving the cardiovascular, respiratory, or central nervous systems. Toxicity is more likely to occur in patients with severe cardiac, renal, or hepatic insufficiency. Lidocaine should be used with caution in patients suffering from hypovolemia because of decreased plasma clearance (Thomson et al., 1969).

Cardiovascular System. Lidocaine may produce clinically significant hypotension, but this is relatively uncommon when given in nontoxic doses. Massive doses may cause medullary depression and cardiovascular

Figure 33-14. Intramuscular lignocaine in 13 patients — maximal blood concentrations related to dose. From this figure, it can be seen that doses greater than 13 mg./Kg. body weight are likely to produce blood concentrations in excess of 10 μg./ml., an amount associated with toxic manifestations in the intravenous series. Bromage, P. R., and Robson, J. G.: Anaesthesia 16:461, 1961.)

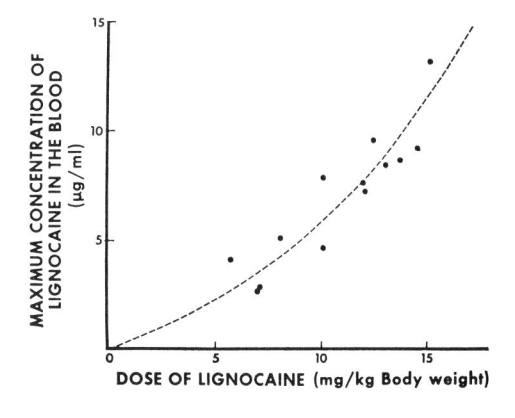

collapse. The frequency of premature beats may be increased immediately following infusion of lidocaine, followed by the usual decrease in their frequency. Similarly, premature beats may become more frequent in patients with sinus bradycardia in whom lidocaine is used without prior acceleration of the heart rate (e.g., by isoproterenol or artificial pacing).

Contraindications. Lidocaine is contraindicated: (1) in patients with a history of hypersensitivity to local anesthetics of the amide type; (2) in the presence of complete A-V heart block, because of the drug's action of reducing the automaticity of ventricular pacemakers; (3) in Stokes-Adams attacks; or (4) in severe grades of sinoatrial, atrioventricular or intraventricular block. It should be employed with caution in patients with lesser grades of A-V conduction disturbances and hypotension.

SYMPATHETIC BLOCKING AGENTS

The reduction of sympathetic tone and the antagonism of the effects of circulating catecholamines have a place in the therapy of certain arrhythmias and hypertension. Numerous agents are available that have sympathetic blocking activity; however, their mechanisms of action differ considerably. It is important to understand these differences when choosing the drugs most useful for a particular situation.

Mode of Action of Sympathetic Antagonists. The sympathetic blocking agents may be divided into four general groups, depending on their mechanisms of action: (1) the beta-adrenergic receptor antagonists, which have considerable importance in the treatment of certain arrhythmias; (2) the alpha-adrenergic receptor antagonists, which are most often used to combat hypertension; (3) drugs that prevent the release of norepinephrine from peripheral nerve endings; and (4) drugs that deplete the norepinephrine stores in adrenergic nerve terminals and cause a proportionate decrease in the amount of the transmitter released.

Beta-Adrenergic Blocking Agents. In addition to propranolol, the most commonly employed beta-blocking drugs that have been introduced include: (1) Sotalol (MJ 1999), (2) Alprenolol (H56/28), and (3) Practolol (ICI 50, 172).

The electrophysiologic effects of the beta-adrenergic blocking agents may be considered under two principal headings: (a) their specific beta-blocking actions, which consist of the antagonism of the cardiac effects of sympathetic stimulation and sympathomimetic drugs; and (b) their direct effects, which occur independently of the level of adrenergic tone.

The dose administered and the level of endogenous adrenergic tone determine which actions will predominate. Beta-adrenergic blockade is responsible for virtually all the alterations observed when small doses of these drugs are given to subjects with elevated sympathetic tone. Conversely, the direct effects predominate when large doses are given to subjects with little or no resting adrenergic tone.

Beta-Blocking Agents with Selective Action. At present, the agents in this class may be divided into three groups on the basis of their actions. The first group consists of drugs that possess both beta-blocking and quinidine-like effects: L-propanolol, L-alprenolol, ICI 45, 763, or Kö-592 (Somani, 1969), Trasicor, and Butidrine. The second group possesses quinidine-like actions without beta-blocking potency: D-propranolol and D-alprenolol. Finally, the third group consists of beta-blocking agents that lack quinidine-like effects: Sotalol (MJ 1999), INPEA

(Gibson and Sowton, 1969), and practolol. These agents are still experimental in this country and have not been widely employed.

Beta-Blocking Effects. Beta-blockade causes a reversal of the sympathetic effects that may be present, resulting in alterations in various regions of the heart, as follows:

S-A NODE. The catecholamine-induced increase in the slope of Stage 4 and acceleration of the sinus rate is prevented.

ATRIAL MUSCLE. Beta-blockade reverses the increase in automaticity of atrial foci, the increase in conduction velocity, and the shortening of the refractory period.

A-V TRANSMISSION. The enhancement in automaticity, the increase in conduction velocity, and the shortening of the A-V junctional refractory period are all reversed.

HIS-PURKINJE SYSTEM. The increase in automaticity, shortening of the refractory period, and variable effects on conduction velocity are prevented.

VENTRICULAR MUSCLE. The increase in conduction velocity and the shortening of the refractory period due to adrenergic stimulation are reversed.

Direct Effects. In addition to beta-blockade, many of the beta-adrenergic antagonists manifest direct actions on cardiac cells that resemble those of the more traditional antiarrhythmic agents. These actions are independent of the level of adrenergic tone or of circulating catecholamines. They are probably responsible for much of the antiarrhythmic potency of these agents, which was originally ascribed to beta-blockade.

S-A NODE. Propranolol causes a dose-related reduction in the rate of firing of the denervated S-A node (which is thus free of adrenergic influences) owing to a decreased slope of Stage 4 depolarization in the individual cells.

A-V TRANSMISSION. Propranolol (0.1 mg./Kg.) administered intravenously to human subjects during fixed-rate atrial pacing causes a 12 to 14 per cent increase in A-V conduction time (as reflected by the P-H interval in the electrogram).

HIS-PURKINJE SYSTEM. Presently, no evidence exists that beta blockers have any direct effect on automaticity or conductivity in this tissue.

Pharmacologic Actions. Most of the studies on the pharmacology of beta-adrenergic agents have been performed with propranolol. These studies have revealed significant actions on hemodynamics, the electrocardiogram, respiratory function, and certain metabolic processes normally under adrenergic control. While other beta-blocking agents have generally similar actions, some have been found to differ significantly from propranolol, both qualitatively and quantitatively.

HEMODYNAMIC PROPERTIES. Both the beta-blocking and direct actions of these drugs tend to exert a *negative inotropic effect*. The magnitude of this effect depends on the dose employed, the method of administration, whether the agent used manifests direct effects, and the degree to which adrenergic tone is supporting cardiac functions. The effect of practolol, which has minimal direct action on contractility, is relatively slight.

In patients without clinically evident heart disease, usual therapeutic doses of propranolol and other beta blockers prolong systolic ejection time and produce a fall in velocity of shortening of myocardial fibers, heart rate, dP/dt, stroke output, and left ventricular work. The usual result is a decrease in cardiac output. The direct negative inotropic effect of propranolol (and presumably of other beta blockers) probably results from its potent inhibition of calcium ion uptake by the sarcoplasmic reticulum.

Effect on hemodynamic response to exercise: In both normal subjects and patients with heart disease, the administration of propranolol in beta-blocking doses causes a roughly 40 per cent decrease in the ability to perform maximal exercise (Epstein et al., 1965). This is associated with decreases in cardiac output (22 per cent), mean arterial pressure (15 per cent), and left ventricular minute work (34 per cent); the arteriovenous oxygen difference was increased (12 per cent), as was the central venous pressure (2.8 mm. Hg). On the other hand, propranolol and practolol increase the exercise tolerance in those patients with angina pectoris (Wilson et al., 1969; Coltart, 1971).

EFFECTS ON THE ELECTROCARDIOGRAM. In all subjects propranolol causes bradycardia. It also causes Q-T interval shortening (corrected for cycle length) (95 per cent of cases), P-R interval prolongation (60 per cent of cases), and increased amplitude of the T wave (60 per cent of cases).

Indications. The well-established primary indications for propranolol are relatively few but important. Although a fair amount of clinical experience is available, propranolol is still a relatively new drug. Few of the other beta-blocking agents have received an extensive clinical trial. Since the indications and contraindications are not yet clearly defined or well established, the use of beta-blocking agents should be evaluated from the standpoint of their efficacy and safety in relation to the other available antiarrhythmic drugs, about which more is known. Although propranolol and (to a lesser extent) other beta blockers have been employed in a wide variety of atrial, junctional, and ventricular arrhythmias, we prefer to reserve propranolol for cases that would derive a particular benefit from its ability to block beta-adrenergic activity.

Propranolol is a useful agent in the treatment of the following conditions: (1) It may be used in selected cases of sinus tachycardia due to pheochromocytoma, thyrotoxicosis, or a strong anxiety factor, when the tachycardia is not an essential compensatory mechanism for an underlying disease process. (2) It may be used in conjunction with digitalis to maintain a satisfactorily slow ventricular rate in atrial flutter and fibrillation, but otherwise it is not indicated for use in these arrhythmias. By this action, the dose of digitalis is decreased and toxic effects avoided; however, this indication is not common. (3) Propranolol is often efficacious in the prevention of recurrent supraventricular tachyarrhythmias associated with the W-P-W syndrome. (4) It may be helpful in cases of repetitive tachycardias. (5) It has also been helpful in the tachycardias that occur with exercise.

Although some beta-blocking agents (e.g., alprenolol) have been shown to be efficacious in the therapy of atrial arrhythmias, they are not usually the drug of first choice for the treatment of supraventricular tachycardia; these agents are most commonly employed in recurrent cases or those that are refractory to the usual agents. Other agents, especially lidocaine and diphenylhydantoin, in addition to the traditional antiarrhythmic drugs, are generally more efficacious for junctional and ventricular tachycardia than propranolol.

Although propranolol has frequently been recommended for the therapy of digitalis toxicity (and indeed works quite well in this particular state), it is not the drug of choice because: (1) it produces a negative inotropic effect, and (2) it produces or accentuates A-V conduction disturbances. Diphenylhydantoin is often the preferred drug (see p. 368).

In ventricular tachycardia, propranolol is not usually the drug of choice; it may be employed if other drugs, especially lidocaine, have failed. It should be given with caution in the presence of hypotension and congestive failure. Electric countershock is preferred unless the tachycardia is of a recurrent type, in which case propranolol may help as a prophylactic measure.

Dose and Method of Administration. Propranolol (Inderal) is, at this writing, the only beta-adrenergic blocking agent approved for clinical use in the United States. Clinical experience has shown that oral administration is safe and reliable, and it is the route that is commonly employed. Intravenous administration is attended by a much greater risk of serious cardiac depression and should be reserved for instances that require a prompt effect.

The oral dosage for arrhythmias is 10 to 30 mg. three or four times daily. The usual intravenous dose is 1 to 3 mg. administered under electrocardiographic monitoring. The rate of administration should not exceed 1 mg. (1 cc.) per minute. Depending on the response, a second dose may be repeated after two minutes. Additional medication should not be given in less than four hours. Therapy with oral dosage is advisable as soon as possible. In children, the oral dose is 1 mg./Kg./day; the intravenous dose is 0.1 mg./Kg./day.

Should excessive bradycardia occur, atropine (0.6 mg. in one or two doses) should be administered intravenously. Propranolol is well absorbed by the oral route in human subjects, reaching peak levels from one to four hours following administration. The peak beta blockade usually coincides with the peak plasma level. The plasma half-life of propranolol is 2.3 hours following intravenous administration and 3.2 hours following oral administration.

Toxicity

CARDIOVASCULAR EFFECTS. Propranolol tends to slow the ventricular rate and should not be given in the presence of bradycardia or partial or complete A-V heart block. Since beta-adrenergic blockade manifests a negative inotropic effect, it may aggravate or precipitate congestive heart failure. However, in slight degrees of heart failure induced by rapid ectopic rhythms, propranolol, cautiously given, may result in improved hemodynamics. Other beta-blocking agents which lack a quinidine-like effect (e.g., practolol) may be better agents to use in this situation.

RESPIRATORY EFFECTS. Propranolol may tend to produce airway narrowing and cause a sudden decrease in ventilatory function. Certain cardio-selective beta-blocking agents (e.g., practolol and sotalol) may be used in obstructive airway disease because they do not affect the airways.

DRUG INTERACTIONS. The administration of propranolol should be instituted with great caution with patients receiving reserpine or reserpine-like drugs, because of the tendency of propranolol to produce an excessive reduction in sympathetic nervous activity. In addition, special care must be taken when using propranolol with hypoglycemic agents since the beta blockade will interfere with the homeostatic mechanisms which react to the hypoglycemia.

GENERAL EFFECTS. Propranolol should be administered cautiously in the presence of impaired renal or liver function.

Contraindications. The use of beta-adrenergic blocking agents is contraindicated in the following conditions: (1) slow heart rates (sinus bradycardia); (2) second-degree and complete A-V heart block; (3) cardiogenic shock; (4) in patients receiving anesthetics that produce myocardial depression, such as chloroform and ether; (5) heart failure; (6) bronchial asthma; (7) allergic rhinitis during the pollen season.

Agents That Act at Adrenergic Nerve Endings. The actions of the sympathetic nervous system may be effectively antagonized by reducing the amount of norepinephrine released from the adrenergic nerve endings in response to a stimulus proceeding along the nerve. Most of the drugs that exert an antiadrenergic action by reducing norepinephrine release are thought to act by depleting the amount of the neurotransmitter contained within the presynaptic terminal. Examples of drugs that act in this way are reserpine and guanethidine. In addition, bretylium decreases the release of norepinephrine from adrenergic terminals through a different mechanism—by reducing the proportion of stored norepinephrine that is released in response to a single nerve impulse (see p. 371).

Other Antiadrenergic Agents
Chlorpromazine (Thorazine, Largactil)

MECHANISM OF ACTION. Intravenous injections of chlorpromazine (25 to 50 mg.) usually produce systemic arterial hypotension and tachycardia. These effects are less pronounced after oral administration of the drug. The hypotension is due to a direct effect on musculature of the arteriolar walls.

INDICATIONS. The drug is sometimes used as an adjunct in the treatment of supraventricular arrhythmias, especially when the functional element is pronounced.

DOSE AND METHOD OF ADMINISTRATION. Chlorpromazine may be administered orally provided vomiting is absent, as well as by the parenteral route. The dose for adults is 25 to 50 mg., three or four times per day.

UNTOWARD AND TOXIC EFFECTS. Regular doses in normal patients may cause mild hypotension, compensatory tachycardia, nasal congestion, and dizziness. Larger doses can cause vascular syncope, unsteady gait, and Parkinsonian facies. Untoward effects also include nausea, anorexia and epigastric distress, and occasional allergic reaction. Jaundice, the most serious side effect, is due to a hypersensitivity reaction which induces cholestastis.

CONTRAINDICATIONS. Chlorpromazine should not be used when there is marked central depression, hypersensitivity to the drug, or liver disease. Older patients sometimes exhibit marked hypotensive reactions to the usual doses which may lead to cerebral and coronary thrombosis.

DIPHENYLHYDANTOIN

Introduction. The electrophysiologic actions of diphenylhydantoin (DPH) have made it particularly useful for the treatment of arrhythmias due to digitalis toxicity. Despite the considerable present enthusiasm for using DPH, many points have not yet been finally settled concerning its action, clinical effectiveness, and toxic effects.

Pharmacologic Effects. Diphenylhydantoin manifests important effects on transmembrane ion exchange at the cellular level; these actions are related to its antiarrhythmic as well as its antiepileptic effects. The cardiac electrophysiology and the hemodynamic effects of DPH are undergoing intensive study at the present time.

The actions of DPH on the heart have often been compared to those of quinidine, but several differences stand out. Quinidine-like drugs cause an increase in the diastolic threshold in the atria and ventricles, while DPH lowers the threshold for stimulation; furthermore, quinidine depresses the conduction velocity of Purkinje fibers, while DPH increases the conduction velocity. DPH manifests a less marked effect on automaticity than quinidine. Moreover, DPH does not prolong the QRS complex and in fact shortens the Q-T interval; both of these effects are opposite to that of quinidine.

There is some difference of opinion as to its effect on A-V conduction (Conn et al., 1967). In the opinion of some, it increases conductivity across the A-V junction. Experimentally, conduction of atrial premature beats is increased by DPH. On the other hand, some experimental evidence indicates that DPH prolongs the A-V conduction time. DPH slowed conduction in the A-V node of isolated hearts to a greater extent than in any other part of the heart, at all concentrations tested. At clinically effective concentrations, only conduction through the A-V node was slowed. Clinically, DPH increases the degree of block across the A-V junction (Rosen et al., 1967). These variations in results may be due in part to the heart rate, the animal studied, dose, and Na$^+$ or K$^+$ concentration.

Hemodynamics. The hemodynamic effects vary with the dose, method, and rapidity of administration and with the presence of myocardial abnormality. Immediately after rapid administration of 5 mg./Kg. DPH in dogs, systemic arterial blood pressure decreased, accompanied by vasodilation and an increase in cardiac output; however, massive doses lead to circulatory collapse. DPH directly depresses the myocardium and also produces a mild reflex depression of the heart through action on the peripheral vessels.

Absorption and Metabolism. When given orally, DPH is absorbed almost quantitatively from the gastrointestinal tract. For each mg./Kg. of body weight of DPH given orally, peak blood levels of approximately 3 μg./ml. are attained in about 8 to 12 hours. A rapid decline in plasma level occurs in the first hour after which the plasma half-life of DPH is 15 hours. DPH is metabolized by liver enzymes which are induced by various drugs, notably barbiturates. Concomitant use of these agents requires larger doses of DPH.

Use in Arrhythmias. Most instances in which DPH is efficacious are observed in arrhythmias produced by digitalis (Fig. 33–15); 60 per cent of all arrhythmias, atrial and ventricular, due to this drug, respond favorably to diphenylhydantoin. Only 41 per cent of all arrhythmias occurring in non-digitalized patients show a favorable response however. DPH has also been shown to be effective in prophylaxis against postcountershock arrhythmias.

Diphenylhydantoin is not effective in the conversion of atrial fibrillation or flutter to normal sinus rhythm. Indeed, it is of little efficacy in supraventricular arrhythmias, other than those related to digitalis excess.

Dose and Method of Administration. To rapidly obtain the antiarrhythmic

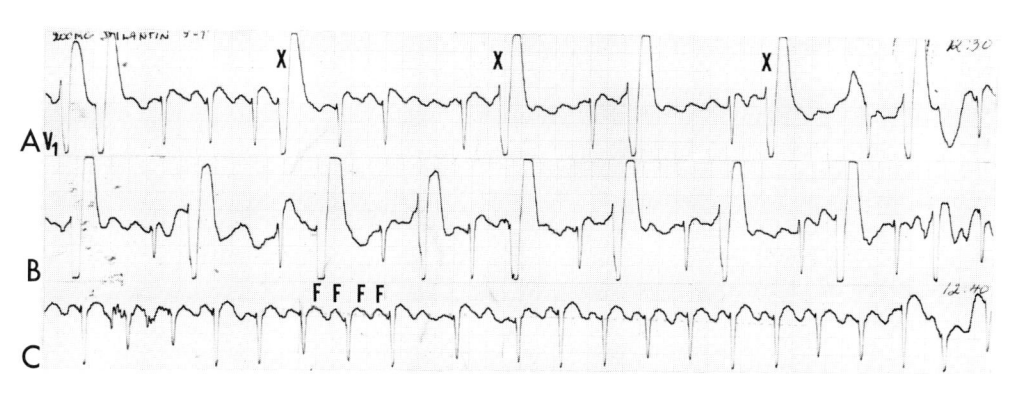

Figure 33–15. Effect of DPH in digitalis toxicity—abolition of ventricular premature beats. Patient with arteriosclerotic heart disease, age 62, showing atrial flutter with varying degrees of A-V heart block.

(A and B) (V$_1$) Show numerous ventricular premature beats; many of them are coupled, some occur in pairs.

(C) Following administration of 200 mg. of DPH, I.V., note the abolition of the ectopic beats within 10 minutes. The atrial flutter was unaffected.

plasma level, larger priming doses are required in order to maintain an antiarrhythmic blood level between 10 to 18 µg./ml. To obtain this level, a loading dose of 1000 mg. may be given on the first day, 500 to 600 mg. on the second and third days, and then maintenance doses of 400 to 500 mg. per day thereafter. Such a regimen usually provides adequate control of responsive arrhythmias within 24 hours (Bigger et al., 1968).

Intravenous therapy is given only as an emergency procedure and should be accompanied by constant electrocardiographic monitoring. Intravenous DPH is highly alkaline and usually causes pain at the site of injection. Local venous thrombosis may be avoided by inserting an intravenous catheter into one of the larger veins; this should be accompanied by repeated flushing of the catheter.

Three-fourths of responsive arrhythmias are abolished at plasma levels of DPH of 10 to 18 µg./ml. This result occurs following intravenous or oral dosage. Nystagmus, nausea, vomiting, drowsiness, or disorientation are encountered in 75 per cent of patients when the plasma DPH exceeded 20 µg./cc.

Toxic Effects. DPH manifests various types of untoward and toxic effects referable chiefly to the circulatory, central nervous, and hemopoietic systems. Circulatory effects include hypotension, bradycardia, transient A-V block and prolonged A-V conduction, ventricular standstill and death, and impaired myocardial contractility and peripheral vasodilatation. Respiratory effects consist of respiratory depression and arrest. The hematologic effects include such conditions as anemia and pancytopenia, reticuloendothelial disorders, including malignant lymphoma, infectious mononucleosis, and megaloblastic anemia (sometimes). Allergic effects include agranulocytosis with leukopenia or thrombocytopenia, jaundice and hepatitis, a morbilliform rash, or a fatal hemorrhagic erythema multiforme. Effects on the central nervous system include nystagmus, tremors, ataxia, cerebellar degeneration, giddiness, diplopia, blurring of vision, ptosis, or slurring of speech, fatigue and drowsiness, and insomnia and irritability. Other effects include gastric upset, hyperplasia of the gums, metabolic effects such as megaloblastic anemia, low protein-bound iodine, or depressed adrenal cortical function, and hypertrichosis.

Contraindications. Diphenylhydantoin is contraindicated in the following conditions: (1) hypotension, (2) severe bradycardia, (3) high-grade A-V heart block, (4) severe myocardial derangement, (5) congestive heart failure, and (6) hypersensitivity reactions.

Drug Interactions. Diphenylhydantoin is detoxified by parahydroxylation in the liver by the same microsomal enzyme system that detoxifies dicumarol, sulfaphenazole, and phenylbutazone. Therefore, administration of these drugs with DPH can cause an increase in the serum level of DPH and a considerable increase in its half-life in the blood. It is advisable that these drugs not be given concurrently with DPH; if an anticoagulant must be used, phenindione should be employed, because it does not interfere with DPH metabolism. On the other hand, phenobarbital, a powerful inducer of microsomal enzyme activity, increases the rate of metabolism of diphenylhydantoin and diminishes its pharmacologic effects.

BRETYLIUM

Introduction. Bretylium was introduced as an antihypertensive agent similar to guanethidine but has not been used for that purpose since tolerance to its antihypertensive properties develops rapidly. Its antiarrhythmic properties are being investigated but as yet it has not been introduced into general use.

Electrophysiologic Effects. In the intact subject, bretylium exerts electrophysiologic effects both through release of catecholamines from adrenergic terminals and directly through action of myocardial fibers. The catecholamine-mediated effects include increases in the resting membrane potential, the action potential amplitude, and the slope of phase 0. The direct actions of bretylium include prolongation of the action potential and the effective refractory period (Bigger and Jaffe, 1971). Bretylium does not, however, decrease automaticity or prolong the effective refractory period in relation to the action potential duration as do quinidine, procaine amide, diphenylhydantoin, propranolol, and lidocaine. The antiarrhythmic effects of bretylium thus probably result from hyperpolarization and enhanced conductivity which abolish re-entrant pathways.

Pharmacologic Effects. Bretylium causes slight hypotension following an initial tachycardia and hypertension. Unlike most antiarrhythmic agents, bretylium is a myocardial stimulant manifesting a predominant positive inotropic effect. It elevates the fibrillation threshold and therefore is useful in facilitating electrical defibrillation. Bretylium has another property that may prove to be useful in antiarrhythmic therapy — it increases cardiac automaticity. In dogs with heart block, bretylium significantly increased the idioventricular rate. This effect has not yet been fully investigated.

Clinical Arrhythmias. Bretylium has been found to be an effective therapeutic agent in the termination of ventricular fibrillation and the conversion to normal rhythm of other arrhythmias, especially those of ventricular origin. Bretylium abolishes premature ventricular contractions due to increased ventricular irritability caused by digitalis toxicity or hypokalemia or occurring as a sequel to open-heart surgery. However, other agents may be equally or more efficacious.

Side Effects. Hypotension (orthostatic and supine) is the only recognized significant side effect presently. It is easily treated. Since bretylium does not block myocardial response to catecholamines, a dilute catecholamine infusion (e.g., isoproterenol 1:50,000) and enough plasma to expand the circulating blood volume will immediately elevate the blood pressure.

Dose and Route of Administration. Bretylium is very soluble and rapidly absorbed after intramuscular injection. Nausea and vomiting are uncommon with intramuscular administration, and this should be the route of choice, except in emergencies such as ventricular fibrillation which indicate intravenous administration. If bretylium is given intravenously during cardiopulmonary resuscitation, effective circulation must be artificially maintained so that the drug is transported to the myocardium.

The consistently effective dose for intramuscular injection is 5 mg./Kg. After a satisfactory therapeutic response, this may be reduced to 2 or 3 mg./Kg. for maintenance therapy. Smaller doses have been effective in some cases, indicating that additional studies will be necessary to establish optimal as well as minimal effective dosage. For intravenous administration, the dose should be diluted in 50 ml. of 5 per cent dextrose in water and infused slowly over five minutes.

Place in Therapy. Bretylium originally showed great promise in the treatment of acute cardiac arrhythmias, particularly in patients who are resistant to more conventional drugs or cardioversion, episodes of ventricular tachycardia, and ventricular fibrillation. However, its use so far has been quite limited. It is not the drug of choice for the general treatment of arrhythmias; for occasional runs of premature beats, quinidine, procaine amide, and lidocaine are more frequently employed. The side effects of bretylium are not serious and are easily managed, and the positive inotropic effect that augments cardiac output is an advantage over other presently used antiarrhythmic agents, most of which are myocardial depressants. Therefore, in cases of ventricular premature beats or tachycardia refractory to all conventional therapy, bretylium may be given a clinical trial.

Contraindications. Bretylium would be contraindicated in those patients with hypotension which bretylium might exacerbate.

References

Abramson, E. A., Arky, R. A., and Woeber, K. A.: Effects of propranolol on the hormonal and metabolic responses to insulin-induced hypoglycaemia. Lancet, 2:1386, 1966.

Ahlquist, R. P.: Study of adrenotropic receptors. Amer. J. Physiol., 153:586, 1948.

Amsterdam, E. A., Spann, J. F., Jr., Mason, D. T., and Zelis, R. F.: Characterization of the positive inotropic effects of bretylium tosylate: A unique property of an antiarrhythmic agent. Amer. J. Cardiol., 25:81, 1970.

Anderssen, N., Erikssen, J., and Muller, C.: The prophylactic antiarrhythmic effect of quinidine in myocardial infarction. Acta Med. Scand., 184:171, 1968.

Angelakos, E. T., and Bloomquist, E.: Release of norepinephrine from isolated hearts by acetylcholine. Arch. Intern. Physiol., 73:397, 1965.

Angelakos, E. T., Daniels, J. B., and King, M.: Adrenergic mechanisms following treatment with quinidine. Circulation, 31–32: II-43, 1965.

Angelakos, E. T., and Hasting, E. P.: The influence of quinidine and procaine amide on myocardial contractility in vivo. Amer. J. Cardiol., 5:791, 1960.

Ariens, E. J.: The structure-activity relationships of beta-adrenergic drugs and beta-adrenergic blocking drugs. Ann. N. Y. Acad. Sci., 139:606, 1967.

Asokan, S. K., Beeson, C. W., and Frank, M. J.: Hemodynamic changes and survival rates in myocardial infarction with prophylactic lidocaine. Clin. Res., 17:227, 1969.

Austin, W. G., and Moran, J. M.: Cardiac and peripheral vascular effects of lidocaine and procainamide. Amer. J. Cardiol., 16:701, 1965.

Bacaner, M. B.: Bretylium tosylate for suppression of induced ventricular fibrillation. Amer. J. Cardiol., 17:528, 1966.

Batey, R. L., Guy, C. R., Lieberman, L. J., and Eliot, R. S.: Alprenolol—an effective beta-blocking antiarrhythmic agent. Circulation, 41–42:III-40, 1970.

Bellet, S., Hamdan, G., Somlyo, A., and Lara, R.: A reversal of the cardiotoxic effects of procaine amide by molar sodium lactate. Amer. J. Med. Sci., 237:177, 1959a.

Bellet, S., Hamdan, G., Somlyo, A., and Lara, R.: The reversal of cardiotoxic effects of quinidine by molar sodium lactate: an experimental study. Amer. J. Med. Sci., 237:165, 1959b.

Bellet, S., Roman, L., and Boza, A.: Relation between serum quinidine levels and renal function. Studies in normals, subjects with congestive failure and renal insufficiency. Amer. J. Cardiol., 27:368, 1971a.

Bellet, S., Roman, L., Kostis, J. B., and Fleischmann, D.: Intramuscular lidocaine in the therapy of ventricular arrhythmias. Amer. J. Cardiol., 27:291, 1971b.

Bellet, S., Zeeman, S. E., and Hirsch, S. A.: Intramuscular use of Pronestyl. Amer. J. Med., 13:145, 1952.

Bennett, A. M., and Cullum, V. A.: The biological properties of the optical isomers of propranolol and their effects on cardiac arrhythmias. Brit. J. Pharmacol., 34:43, 1968.

Bernstein, H., et al.: Sodium diphenylhydantoin in the treatment of recurrent cardiac arrhythmias. JAMA, 191:695, 1965.

Berry, K., Garlett, E. L., Bellet, S., and Gefter, W. I.: Pronestyl in treatment of ectopic rhythms. Amer. J. Med., 11:431, 1951.

Bigger, J. T., Jr., and Heissenbuttel, R. H.: The use of procaine amide and lidocaine in the treatment of cardiac arrhythmias. Prog. Cardiov. Dis., 11:515, 1969.

Bigger, J. T., Jr., and Jaffe, C. C.: The effect of bretylium tosylate on the electrophysiologic properties of ventricular muscle and Purkinje fibers. Amer. J. Cardiol., 27:82, 1971.

Bigger, J. T., Jr., and Mandel, W. J.: Effect of lidocaine on the electrophysiological properties of ventricular muscle and Purkinje fibers. J. Clin. Invest., 49:63, 1970.

Bigger, J. T., Jr., Schmidt, D. H., and Kutt, H.: Relationship between the plasma level of diphenylhydantoin sodium and its cardiac antiarrhythmic effects. Circulation, 38:363, 1968.

Bigger, J. T., Jr., Weinberg, D. I., et al.: Effects of diphenylhydantoin on excitability and automaticity in the canine heart. Circ. Res., 26:1, 1970.

Bolton, F. G., and Dameshek, W.: Thrombocytopenic purpura due to quinidine. Blood, 11:546, 1956.

Braunwald, E., Sobel, B. E., and Braunwald, N. S.: Treatment of supraventricular tachy-

cardia by electrical stimulation of carotid sinus nerve. New Eng. J. Med., 281:885, 1969.
Bromage, P. R., and Robson, J. G.: Concentrations of lignocaine in the blood after intravenous, intramuscular, epidural, and endotracheal administration. Anesthesia, 16:461, 1961.
Brooks, H., et al.: Sotalol-induced beta blockade in cardiac patients. Circulation, 42:99, 1970.
Burn, J. H.: The relation of the autonomic nervous system to cardiac arrhythmias. Prog. Cardiov. Dis., 2:334, 1960.
Colman, R. W., and Sturgill, B. C.: Lupus-like syndrome induced by procaine amide. Arch. Intern. Med., 115:214, 1965.
Coltart, D. J.: Comparison of effects of propranolol and practolol on exercise tolerance in angina pectoris. Brit. Heart J., 33:62, 1971.
Conn, H. L., Jr., and Luchi, R. J.: Some quantitative aspects of the binding of quinidine and related quinoline compounds by human serum albumin. J. Clin. Invest., 40:509, 1961.
Conn, R. D., Kennedy, J. W., and Blackman, J. R.: The hemodynamic effects of diphenylhydantoin. Amer. Heart J., 73:500, 1967.
Cullhed, I.: Hemodynamic effects of lidocaine. Acta Med. Scand., 186:53, 1969.
Damato, A. N.: Diphenylhydantoin: pharmacological and clinical use. Prog. Cardiov. Dis., 12:1, 1969.
Dollery, C. T., Paterson, J. W., and Conolly, M. E.: Clinical pharmacology of beta-receptor-blocking drugs. Clin. Pharmacol. Ther., 10:765, 1969.
Dubois, E. L.: Procaineamide induction of a systemic lupus erythematosus-like syndrome. Medicine, 48:217, 1969.
Eliakim, M., Bellet, S., Tawil, E., and Muller, O.: Effect of vagal stimulation and acetylcholine on the ventricle; studies in dogs with complete atrioventricular block. Circ. Res., 9:1372, 1961.
Epstein, S., Robinson, B. F., Kahler, R. C., and Braunwald, E.: Effects of beta adrenergic blockade on cardiac response to maximal exercise. J. Clin. Invest., 44:1745, 1965.
Finegan, R. E., Marlon, A. M., and Harrison, D. C.: Hemodynamic effects of practolol. Circulation, 41–42:III-40, 1970.
Freedman, A. L., Barr, P. S., and Brady, E. A.: Hemolytic anemia due to quinidine; observations on its mechanism. Amer. J. Med., 20:806, 1956.
Frieden, J.: Antiarrhythmic drugs. VII. Lidocaine as an antiarrhythmic agent. Amer. Heart J., 70:713, 1965.
Gent, G., Davis, T. C., and McDonald, A.: Practolol in treatment of supraventricular cardiac dysrhythmias. Brit. Med. J., 1:533, 1970.
Gianelly, R., Von der Groben, J. O., Spivack, A. P., and Harrison, D. C.: Effect of lidocaine on ventricular arrhythmia in patients with coronary artery disease. New Eng. J. Med., 277:1215, 1967.
Giardina, E., Heissenbuttel, R. H., and Bigger, J. T.: Antiarrhythmic plasma concentrations of procaine amide for ventricular arrhythmias. Circulation, 41–42:III-156, 1970.
Gibson, D., and Sowton, E.: The use of beta-adrenergic receptor blocking drugs in dysrhythmias. Prog. Cardiov. Res., 12:16, 1969.
Gibson, D. G., Balcon, R., and Sowton, E.: The clinical use of ICI 50, 172 as an antidysrhythmic agent in patients with heart failure. Brit. Med. J., 3:161, 1968.
Grossman, J. I., Cooper, J. A., and Frieden, J.: Cardiovascular effects of infusion of lidocaine on patients with heart disease. Amer. J. Cardiol., 24:191, 1969a.
Grossman, J. I., Cooper, J. A., and Frieden, J.: Hemodynamic and antiarrhythmic effects of edrophonium chloride (Tensilon). Circulation, 39–40:III-97, 1969b.
Hecht, H. H.: Cardiac transmembrane potentials. Ann. N.Y. Acad. Sci., 65:700, 1957.
Heissenbuttel, P. H., and Bigger, J. T.: The effect of oral quinidine on intraventricular conduction in man: correlation of plasma quinidine with changes in QRS duration. Amer. Heart J., 80:453, 1970.
Helfant, R. H., Scherlag, B. J., and Damato, A. N.: Protection from digitalis toxicity with the prophylactic use of diphenylhydantoin sodium. Circulation, 36:119, 1967.
Hurst, V. W., III, et al.: Increased survival with prophylactic quinidine after experimental myocardial infarction. Circulation, 36:294, 1967.
Jewitt, D. E., Koshon, Y., and Thomas, M.: Lignocaine in the management of arrhythmias after acute myocardial infarction. Lancet, 1:266, 1968.
Kaplan, J. M., Wachtel, H. L., Czarnecki, S. W., and Sampson, J. J.: Lupus-like illness precipitated by procaine amide hydrochloride. JAMA, 192:444, 1965.
Kennedy, B. L., and West, T. C.: Factors influencing quinidine-induced changes in excitability and contractility. J. Pharmacol. Exp. Ther., 168:47, 1969.
Kimball, J. T., and Killip, T.: Aggressive treatment of arrhythmias in acute myocardial infarction: Procedure and results. Prog. Cardiov. Dis., 10:483, 1968.
Klein, S. W., Sutherland, R. I. L., and Morch, J. E.: Hemodynamic effects of intravenous lidocaine in man. Can. Med. Assoc. J., 99:472, 1968.
Koch-Weser, J., et al.: Antiarrhythmic prophylaxis with procaine amide in acute myocardial infarction. New Eng. J. Med., 281:1253, 1969.
Koelle, G. B.: Parasympathomimetic agents. *In* Goodman, L., and Gilman, A. (eds.): The

Pharmacological Basis of Therapeutics. Ed. 2. New York, Macmillan, 1970, pp. 266–277.

LaRaia, P. J., and Sonnenblick, H.: Adrenergic and cholinergic control of adenyl cyclase and cyclic AMP in the myocardium. Circulation, 39–40:III-129, 1969.

Lieberson, A. D., et al.: Effect of diphenylhydantoin on left ventricular function in patients with heart disease. Circulation, 36:692, 1967.

Mansour, E., et al.: Clinical evaluation of antiarrhythmic and hemodynamic properties of bretylium. Circulation, 41–42:III-41, 1970.

Mark, L. C., et al.: The physiological disposition and cardiac effects of procaine amide. J. Pharmacol. Exp. Ther., 102:5, 1951.

Nagle, R. E., and Pilcher, J.: Lignocaine for arrhythmias. (Letter) Lancet, 1:1039, 1968.

Nayler, W. G., et al.: Some effects of diphenylhydantoin and propranolol on the cardiovascular system. Amer. Heart J., 75:83, 1968.

Oravetz, J., and Slodki, S. J.: Recurrent ventricular fibrillation precipitated by quinidine. Arch. Intern. Med., 122:63, 1968.

Pitt, D., and Ross, R. S.: Beta-adrenergic blockade in cardiovascular therapy. Mod. Conc. Cardiov. Dis., 38:47, 1969.

Rokseth, R., and Storsten, O.: Quinidine therapy of chronic atrial fibrillation. Arch. Intern. Med., 111:194, 1963.

Rosen, K. M., et al.: The effects of procaine amide on atrioventricular and intraventricular conduction in man. Circulation, 39–20:III-173, 1969.

Rosen, M. R., Lisak, R., and Rubin, I. L.: Diphenylhydantoin in cardiac arrhythmias. Amer. J. Cardiol., 20:674, 1967.

Rowe, G. G., et al.: Hemodynamic effects of quinidine; including studies of cardiac work and coronary blood flow. J. Clin. Invest., 36:844, 1957.

Shand, D. G., Nuckolls, E. M., and Oates, J. A.: Plasma propranolol levels in adults. Clin. Pharmacol. Ther., 11:112, 1970.

Shulman, N. R.: Immunoreactions involving platelets: I. A steric and kinetic model for formation of a complex from a human antibody, quinidine as a haptene, and platelets; and for fixation of complement by the complex; IV. Studies on the pathogenesis of thrombocytopenia in drug purpura using test doses of quinidine in sensitized individuals; their implications in idiopathic thrombocytopenic purpura. J. Exp. Med., 107:665–690, 711–730, 1968.

Sokolow, M., and Perloff, D. B.: The clinical pharmacology and use of quinidine in heart disease. Prog. Cardiov. Dis., 3:316, 1961.

Somani, P.: Antiarrhythmic activity of the beta-adrenergic blocking agent 1-isopropylamine-3-(3-tolylaxy)-2-propranol (ICI 25673). Amer. Heart J., 77:63, 1969.

Somani, P., and Lum, B. K. B.: Blockade of epinephrine and ouabain-induced cardiac arrhythmias in the dog heart-lung preparation. J. Pharmacol. Exp. Ther., 152:235, 1966.

Sowton, E.: Beta-adrenergic blockade in cardiac infarction. Prog. Cardiov. Dis., 10:561, 1968.

Stock, J. P. P.: Beta-adrenergic blocking drugs in the clinical management of cardiac arrhythmias. Amer. J. Cardiol., 18:444, 1966.

Strauss, H. C., Singer, D. H., and Hoffman, B. F.: Biphasic effects of procaine amide on cardiac conduction. Bull. N.Y. Acad. Med., 43:1194, 1967.

Swisher, W. P., et al.: Studies of quinidine plasma levels and rate of decline following cessation of quinidine administration. Amer. Heart J., 47:449, 1954.

Terry, G., Vallani, C. W., Higgins, M. R., and Doig, A.: Bretylium tosylate in treatment of refractory ventricular arrhythmias complicating myocardial infarction. Brit. Heart J., 32:21, 1970.

Thomson, G. W.: Quinidine as a cause of sudden death. Circulation, 14:757, 1956.

Thomson, P., et al.: The influence of heart failure and liver disease on plasma concentration and clearance of lidocaine in man. Circulation, 39–40:III-203, 1969.

Turner, J. R. B.: Propranolol in the treatment of digitalis-induced and digitalis-resistant tachycardias. Amer. J. Cardiol., 18:450, 1966.

Watanabe, Y., and Dreifus, L. S.: Interactions of quinidine and potassium on atrioventricular transmission. Circ. R s. 20:232, 1967. 1967.

Watt, D. A. L.: Sensitivity to propranolol after digoxin intoxication. Brit. Med. J., 3:413, 1968.

Wenckebach, K. F.: Die Unregelmassige Herztatigkeit und ihre Klinische Bedeutung. Leipzig and Berlin, W. Engelmann, 1912, p. 173.

Wilson, A. G., Brooke, O. G., Lloyd, H. J., and Robinson, B. F.: Mechanism of action of β-adrenergic receptor blocking agents in angina pectoris: comparison of action of propranolol with dexpropranolol and practolol. Brit. Med. J., 4:399, 1969.

Woolfolk, D. J., et al.: The effect of quinidine on electrical energy required for ventricular defibrillation. Amer. Heart J., 72:659, 1966.

Chapter 34 *Digitalis*

MECHANISM OF CARDIAC EFFECTS
  Onset of Action
ABSORPTION AND METABOLISM
  Factors Modifying Digitalis Tolerance
    Body Stores of Digitalis
    Physiologic and Myocardial Determinants of Digitalis Tolerance
    Electrolyte Alterations
    Drugs
USE IN ARRHYTHMIAS
  Indications
DOSE AND METHOD OF ADMINISTRATION
  Dosage Schedules
DIGITALIS TOXICITY
  Cardiac Manifestations of Toxicity
  Treatment of Digitalis Toxicity
    Potassium
    Beta-blocking Agents
    Diphenylhydantoin
    Electric Countershock
    Atrial Pacing
    Ventricular Pacing

Digitalis is a most important drug in the treatment of cardiac arrhythmias. It serves two main purposes in therapy: (a) to improve the efficiency of the heart in patients with congestive heart failure; and (b) to slow a rapid supraventricular ectopic rhythm and occasionally to restore the normal sinus mechanism. On the other hand, digitalis itself frequently causes ectopic rhythms of all types, so much so that their presence may be an important evidence of toxicity.

MECHANISM OF CARDIAC EFFECTS

The important direct and indirect cardiac actions of digitalis include: (a) increase in myocardial contractility, (b) increase in the cardiac output (in diseased hearts), (c) decrease in ventricular rate in certain arrhythmias, (d) increase in A-V conduction time, (e) variable effect on cardiac automaticity, and (f) decrease in central venous pressure.

Digitalis increases the cardiac output by three mechanisms: (1) increased venous return, (2) increased myocardial contractility, and (3) decreased peripheral resistance. Direct actions of digitalis cause an increase in all of these variables; in addition, when digitalis causes an improvement of circulatory dynamics, it causes (indirectly) a decrease in the "supernormal" sympathetic tone which maintains the failing circulation and which contributes to the occurrence of certain arrhythmias.

Onset of Action. The rate of development of cardiac action and the rapidity with which the maximal effect is attained vary markedly for the different digitalis glycosides. This point should be borne in mind when rapid digitalization is required. For instance, oral digitoxin may take six to ten hours for full development of effect; digoxin, three to five hours; ouabain (intravenously), approximately one half-hour; acetylstrophanthidin (intravenously), five to ten minutes (see Fig. 34–1).

ABSORPTION AND METABOLISM

Digitoxin and digoxin are well absorbed from the gastrointestinal tract.

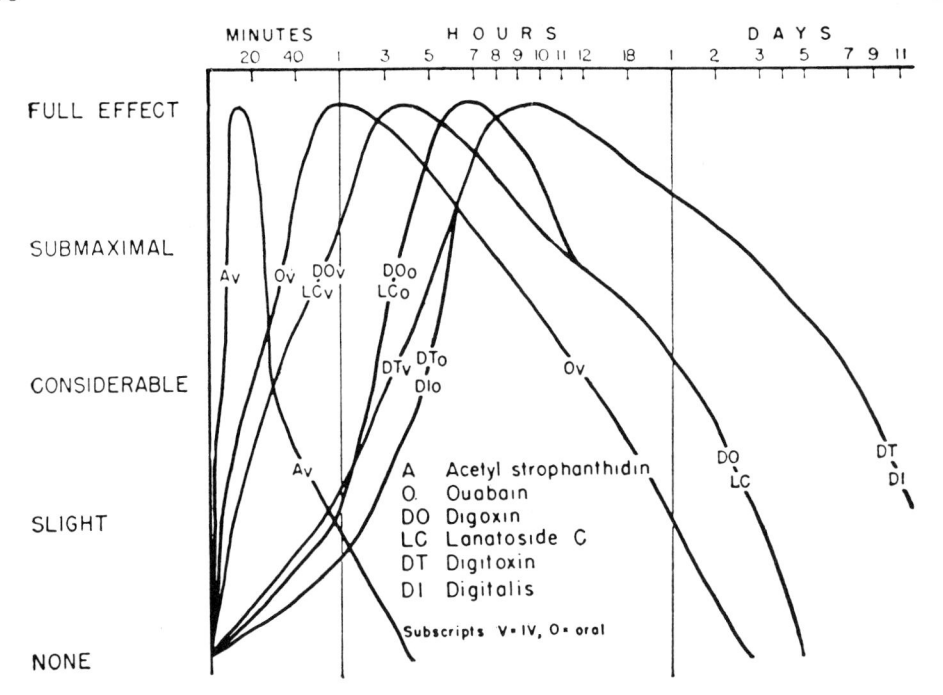

Figure 34-1. Approximate curves of accumulation and decline of the biological effects of single doses of cardioactive preparations in man. The curves of orally administered gitalin (amorphous) and of acetyl digitoxin, if plotted, would fall between those of oral digoxin and of oral digitoxin. (Kay, courtesy of Circulation.)

Digitalis is concentrated in the heart but not selectively and is found in many other tissues including the kidney and liver in high levels. Digitalis glycosides are transformed in the liver to a wide variety of metabolites which are excreted along with some unaltered glycosides by the kidney.

Factors Modifying Digitalis Tolerance. The tolerance to digitalis and the dose of digitalis required to produce a therapeutic effect depend upon several factors: (1) the amount of digitalis in the body, which may be estimated by plasma levels (the tissue levels must be extrapolated from this value); (2) physiologic modifications in patients with myocardial disease; (3) the effect of electrolyte alterations; and (4) alterations in sympathetic and parasympathetic tone and the effect of other drugs.

Body Stores of Digitalis. The amount of digitalis in the body is modified by variations in absorption, metabolism, and excretion (including acute loss by bleeding or cardiopulmonary bypass). The plasma levels of digitalis that are associated with optimal therapeutic and toxic effects are discussed on page 380. The following conditions alter the plasma concentration: (a) renal insufficiency, (b) alterations that occur with aging, (c) hypo- or hyperthyroidism, and (d) malabsorption syndromes.

When patients with renal failure are given a single intravenous dose of digoxin, the renal excretion is diminished in proportion to the elevation of the BUN. Digitalis toxicity is common when normal doses of a glycoside are administered to subjects with renal insufficiency. Even in the absence of overt renal disease, elderly patients frequently have decreased renal function, expressed by such variables as creatinine clearance, and may retain more digitalis than normal.

Patients with hyperthyroidism have serum concentrations lower than expected, while hypothyroid patients have elevated blood levels. Hence, patients with hypothyroidism may be unusually sensitive to accepted doses of digitalis.

Although the question of malabsorption syndrome and digitalis absorption has not been extensively studied, it appears that patients with malabsorption syndromes may have markedly decreased absorption of digitalis. Steady-state serum levels may average as little as 30 per cent of normal in patients with malabsorption syndromes.

Physiologic and Myocardial Determinants of Digitalis Tolerance. Certain physiologic and pathologic states alter the dose of digitalis required to produce a therapeutic effect. In children the dose required is increased. In patients in the older age groups and those with severe myocardial disease as well as in the presence of hypoxemia, the tolerance is decreased.

Electrolyte Alterations. Many digitalized patients develop hypopotassemia due to the potassium-wasting effect of a concurrently administered diuretic. Because hypokalemia enhances automaticity and frequently causes some depression of conduction in the heart, subjects with hypopotassemia are more sensitive to the effects of digitalis and often develop toxicity with smaller doses of the drug. On the other hand, increased extracellular potassium suppresses ectopic beats induced by digitalis. Hyperpotassemic subjects can tolerate larger doses of digitalis without developing ectopic activity.

Evidence indicates a synergism of calcium and digitalis on automaticity. At high serum calcium concentrations (15 mEq./L.) arrhythmias due to digitalis toxicity are produced with lower doses of digitalis (60 to 70 per cent of control) than when serum calcium levels are within normal limit. Thus, the combination of these drugs results in a summation effect; toxic effects may result from this combination (Nola et al., 1970).

Certain subjects with digitalis toxicity may have a decrease in plasma magnesium. In a survey of digitalized patients, 37 per cent of the toxic patients were hypomagnesemic (avg. <1.76 mEq./L.), whereas only 21 per cent of the nontoxic patients were hypomagnesemic (Beller et al., 1970).

Clinical states associated with heightened sympathetic tone may present an increased danger of digitalis-induced arrhythmias. However, on the basis of the available evidence, it is difficult to attribute this fact to a specific role of the sympathetic nervous system in the development of digitalis toxicity.

Drugs. Many of the drugs employed for antiarrhythmic effects (i.e., quinidine, procaine amide, lidocaine, diphenylhydantoin) tend to decrease the positive inotropic effects of digitalis and counteract the effect of digitalis on automaticity of ectopic pacemakers. The ectopic beats induced by digitalis may be suppressed by these antiarrhythmic drugs, both experimentally and clinically.

USE IN ARRHYTHMIAS

Digitalis exerts the following major effects in the therapy of arrhythmias: (a) direct depression of A-V conduction; (b) reflex increase in vagal tone and decrease in sympathetic tone; and (c) inotropic effects. The combination of these effects is seen in the action of digitalis on the S-A node, atrial muscle, and the A-V junction, but since few or no vagal fibers are present in the human ventricle, the ventricular effects are usually considered solely the result of a direct action.

Indications. Digitalis is indicated in the treatment of supraventricular ectopic rhythms accompanied by fast

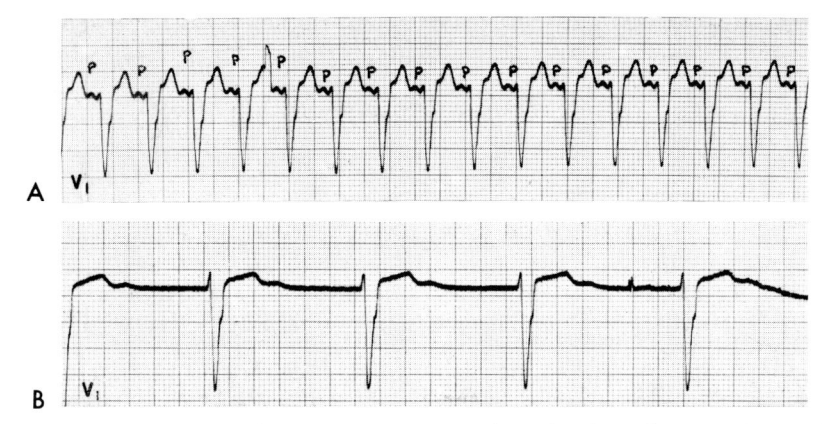

Figure 34-2. Effect of digitalis therapy in paroxysmal atrial tachycardia. (A) (V$_1$). Note the supraventricular tachycardia (rate 160 per minute). (B) *After digitalization,* note the presence of an A-V junctional rhythm with a rate of 47 per minute. The P waves are not observed; these may be buried in the QRS complexes(?). This probably denotes evidence of slight toxicity.

rates and, particularly, in the presence of atrial fibrillation, atrial flutter, and atrial or junctional tachycardia. It may also help in the treatment of ventricular premature contractions accompanied by, or resulting from, congestive heart failure. Digitalis therapy is not indicated and in some instances may prove fatal in the treatment of "true" ventricular tachycardia. The relative indications and contraindications for digitalis with respect to each arrhythmia are discussed in greater detail in the chapters on the individual arrhythmias (see Figs. 34-2, 34-3).

DOSE AND METHOD OF ADMINISTRATION

Administration of digitalis is performed in two stages. Initial "digitalization" establishes body stores of the drug that are associated with its therapeutic effect. Subsequently, doses are given at regular intervals, the amount of each dose being adjusted to increase, maintain, or decrease the body glycoside stores as indicated in each patient. Evidence is accumulating that a correlation exists between body glycoside stores and blood levels of digitalis and that under certain circumstances it may be possible to predict the levels that a given dosage schedule will produce.

In addition, the recent application of new laboratory methods has made it possible to determine the blood level of digitalis associated with therapeutic and toxic effects.

Dosage Schedules. Although the digitalizing dose varies considerably

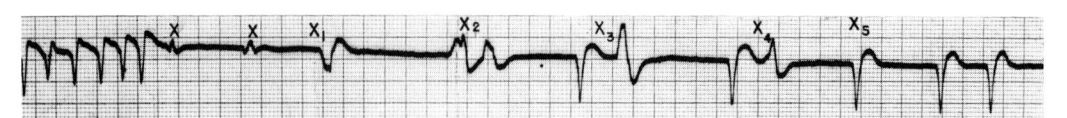

Figure 34-3. Atrial fibrillation with rapid ventricular rate (250 per minute): marked slowing after digitalis (lead III). Atrial fibrillation with a rapid ventricular rate is present in the initial part of the strip. Following the administration of Cedilanid (1.6 mg. in two divided doses given over a period of three hours), note the resumption of slow ventricular beating. Note the aberrant beats at X, X$_1$, and X$_2$ and the coupled beats at X$_3$ and X$_4$ as evidence of digitalis toxicity. Premature beats are absent at end of strip starting with X$_5$.

Table 34–1. DOSAGE SCHEDULES FOR DIGITALIS PREPARATIONS

DRUG	FULL DIGITALIZATION DOSE INTRAVENOUSLY (ORALLY)	DAILY MAINTENANCE DOSE
FOR ADULTS		
Digitalis Leaf	3 to 5 U.S.P. units (digalen)* (15 U.S.P. units; 1.3 gm.)	½ to 2 U.S.P. units (¾ to 3 gr.) (45 to 180 mg.)
Digitoxin	1.2 to 2.0 mg. (1.2 to 2.0 mg.)	0.05 to 0.2 mg.
Digoxin	1.25 mg. (2–5 mg.)	0.25 to 0.75 mg.
Desacetyl-lanatoside C (Cedilanid-D)	1.6 mg.	
Lanatoside C (Cedilanid)	1.6 mg. (5–10 mg.)	0.5 to 1.2 mg.
Gitalin	(5.5–6.0 mg.)	0.5 mg.
Ouabain	0.7 to 1.0 mg.	
FOR CHILDREN	DOSAGE FOR TOTAL DIGITALIZATION	
Digitoxin	Digitoxin group — 0.01 to 0.02 mg./lb. body weight, I.M., I.V. or orally.	
Digoxin	Orally: 0.02 to 0.03 mg./lb. I.M., or 0.01 to 0.02 mg./lb. I.V.	
Lanatoside A-B-C	0.01 to 0.02 mg./lb. I.M. or I.V.	
Strophanthin	.005 to .007 mg./lb. I.V.	
Ouabain	.003 to .006 mg./lb. I.V. (½ total dose) followed by ¹⁄₁₀ of total dose every ½ hr. for five doses.	

* Not usually given by vein.

in different individuals, most patients can be digitalized by doses within a well-established range for each preparation (see Table 34–1). For example, the initial oral digitalizing dose of digoxin in a 150-pound person is about 2 to 5 mg. Following initial digitalization, the patient is placed on a maintenance dose that will maintain roughly constant body stores of digitalis (Table 34–2) (Fig. 34–4).

There is no precise method of determining the proper digitalizing dose, except in patients with atrial fibrillation. When a glycoside is administered to control the ventricular rate in this arrhythmia, the maximal therapeutic effect is said to be attained when the apical rate drops to about 70 per minute with elimination of the pulse deficit. Determining the optimal digitalizing and maintenance doses in patients with normal sinus rhythm is much more difficult.

Intravenous digitalis administration is indicated only in cases of emergency when an almost immediate effect is desired and the effect by other routes is too slow and undependable. The preparations recommended for intravenous use include strophanthidin (0.6 mg., gr. ¹⁄₁₀₀), which may be repeated in three to four hours, depending on the effect of the initial dose; lanatoside C (Cedilanid), the total digitalizing dose of which is 1.6 mg.; and digoxin (Lanoxin), 1.25 mg. One-fourth to one-half of the total digitalizing dose is administered initially, and the remainder is given in two divided doses at four- to six-hour intervals, after noting the effect of the previous dose.

Table 34-2. DURATION OF ACTION OF DIGITALIS PREPARATIONS

DRUG	SPEED OF ACTION I.V.	Oral (hours)	ABSORPTION (PER CENT)	DURATION OF ACTION AFTER FULL DIGITALIZATION (DAYS)
Whole Leaf Digitalis	—	12–24	20	14–21
Digitoxin	—	12–24	75	14–21
Digoxin	¼–1 hr.	2–6	50	3–5
Lanatoside C	10–30 min.	1–4	40	3–5

In most arrhythmias, the rapidly acting forms, digoxin or lanatoside C, are used to bring the patient out of a critical state. The longer-acting preparations may be used for maintenance therapy.

These dosages should be reduced by one-third in cases of clinical renal insufficiency or laboratory evidence of abnormally low creatinine clearance.

DIGITALIS TOXICITY

Digitalis toxicity is normally manifested first by effects on the gastrointestinal system and slightly later by its action upon the heart. It should be emphasized, however, that this sequence may not pertain to all patients and that cardiotoxicity may represent the first adverse effect. The cardiotoxic effects are the most dangerous, since they may produce a marked alteration in cardiac function or cause a fatal arrhythmia. The neurologic, visual, and allergic effects are less frequent and have less importance. The numerous effects of digitalis are summarized in Table 34–3.

Cardiac Manifestations of Toxicity. The dose of digitalis required to produce an arrhythmia depends on many factors, the more important of which are: (1) the age of the patient, (2) the degree and type of heart disease, (3) the adequacy of renal function, (4) the manner and rapidity of administration, (5) the concentrations of serum electrolytes (especially potassium), and (6) the degree of vagal and sympathetic tone. These and other factors affecting tolerance to digitalis have been discussed previously (see p. 376). When the patient first comes under observation, it is often very difficult to determine whether an existent arrhythmia is due to the underlying heart disease, to the toxic effects of digitalis, or to both factors acting in combination.

The presence of an ectopic rhythm, or any sudden change in rhythm, in a patient receiving full doses of a glycoside is an important evidence of toxic-

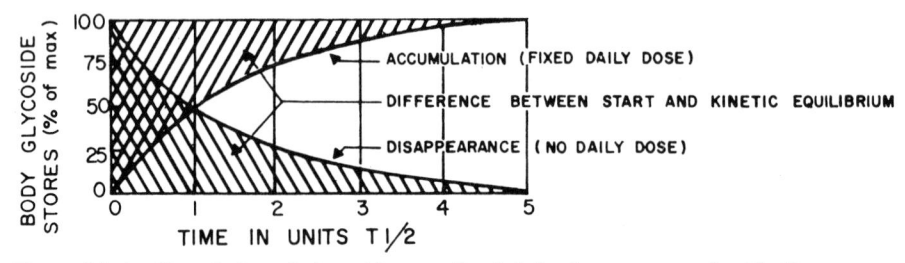

Figure 34-4. Cumulation of glycoside on a fixed daily dose, compared with disappearance of glycoside after therapy is stopped (1). Time is shown in units of drug half-life (T½). (From Jelliffe, R. W., et al., Ann. Intern. Med., 72:253, 1970.)

Table 34–3. MANIFESTATIONS OF DIGITALIS TOXICITY

	COMMON	UNCOMMON
Cardiac	Bradycardia, S-A block, sinus arrhythmias, all degrees A-V block (sometimes with paroxysmal tachycardia), A-V junctional rhythm (including premature beats, coupled ventricular premature beats, and paroxysmal tachycardia)	Atrial fibrillation, atrial flutter, ventricular tachycardia and fibrillation, complete A-V heart block
ARRHYTHMIAS THAT HAVE A HIGH PROBABILITY OF BEING CAUSED BY DIGITALIS TOXICITY	Multifocal ventricular premature beats, A-V junctional tachycardia, A-V dissociation, PAT with block	
Extracardiac		
GASTROINTESTINAL	Anorexia, nausea, vomiting	Diarrhea
VISUAL	Alterations in color perception, scotomata, blurring, shimmering, micropsia, macropsia	Amblyopia
NEUROLOGIC	Headache, fatigue, insomnia, depression	Convulsions, delirium
ALLERGIC	None	Urticaria, eosinophilia
ENDOCRINE	None	Gynecomastia

ity. Digitalis intoxication may cause virtually every known arrhythmia except cardiac asystole (Figs. 34–5, 34–6, 34–7). Alertness to this possibility is most important in the management of such arrhythmias.

Many instances of arrhythmias occurring in patients receiving digitalis present a problem in interpretation. Precise and rapid determination of plasma digitalis levels by radioimmunoassay or other methods may simplify this problem.

The use of radioimmunoassay to determine the concentration of digitalis glycoside in the blood has im-

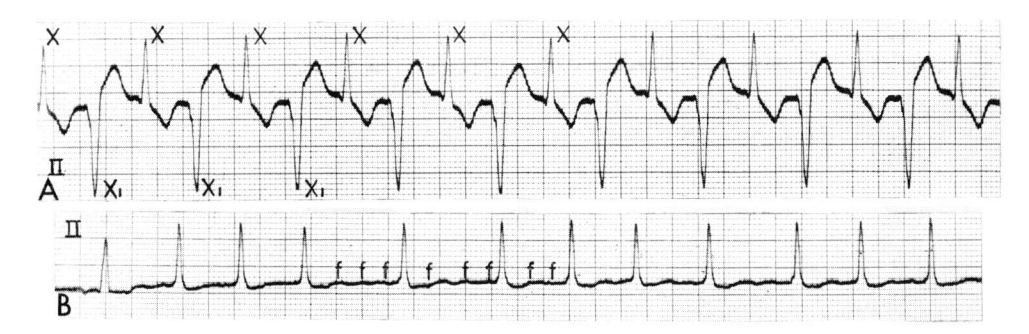

Figure 34–5. Junctional tachycardia (bidirectional type) resulting from toxic digitalis effects.
(A) Note that the upwardly directed deflection (X) has a relatively narrow QRS measuring 0.08 second. The downwardly directed complexes (X_1) have a slightly wider QRS width measuring 0.12 second. Note that the rhythm of the upwardly directed complexes is entirely regular at 75 per minute, and the same is true of the downwardly directed complexes, resulting in a regular ventricular rate, 150 per minute.
(B) After the omission of digitalis, note the presence of atrial fibrillation with the persistence of the upwardly directed complexes; the downwardly directed complexes have disappeared. These findings suggest that in A we are dealing with an A-V junctional rhythm with an ectopic focus occurring in some portion of the A-V node or bundle of His.

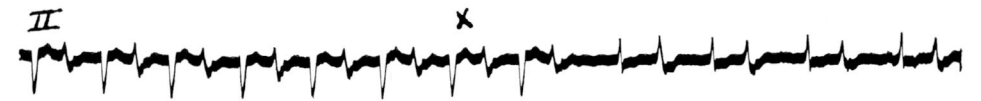

Figure 34-6. Bidirectional junctional tachycardia abolished by carotid sinus pressure (lead II).
The initial portion of the tracing shows a bidirectional junctional tachycardia that resulted from toxic digitalis effects. Following carotid sinus pressure at X, the rhythm is converted to atrial fibrillation, which was the original mechanism. It is of interest that the QRS complexes following the conversion possess a similar character and contour to those of the upright complexes of the paroxysm. The response to carotid sinus pressure suggests that the mechanism is junctional in origin.

proved considerably our ability to diagnose cardiotoxicity, but this method is still in the experimental stage.

Digoxin levels in the blood of patients on oral maintenance therapy with clinical evidence of therapeutic effects and no toxic complications fall into an area around 2.0 mg./ml. but with a scatter above and below this level (Smith and Haber, 1970). However, serum digoxin concentrations substantially above 2 mg./ml. are sometimes required to adequately control the ventricular response in atrial fibrillation and flutter without distinct evidence of toxicity (Smith, 1971). Plasma levels of digoxin or digitoxin are generally much higher in patients showing manifestations of toxicity, although there is considerable overlap between the distribution of plasma levels in patients with and without toxicity. Although this determination is of help in some patients, especially in those subjects with arrhythmias which may be due to its toxic effects,

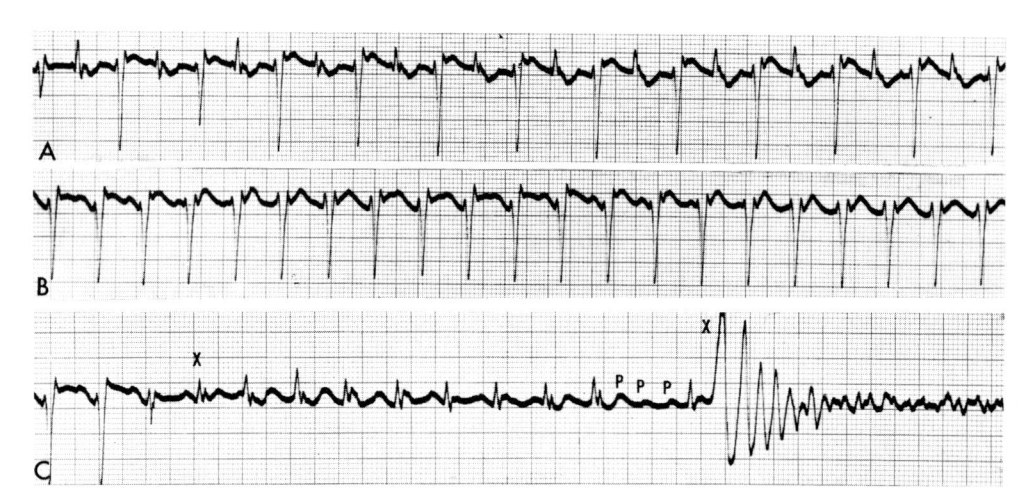

Figure 34-7. Male, age 60, with malignant hypertension, congestive failure, and renal insufficiency. BUN, 75 mgm. per cent.

(A) This patient had been receiving 0.1 mg. digitoxin for two months. In the week prior to this tracing, he had been receiving 0.5 mg. digoxin orally because of an irregular rhythm. After 0.4 mg. Cedilanid at 11:40 A.M., note the presence of a bidirectional junctional tachycardia.

(B) Probable ventricular tachycardia. The P waves occur at a slower rate and independently of the ventricular complexes.

(C) After 3 mg. of Pronestyl intravenously, note the occurrence of marked changes in the direction of the ventricular complexes, the appearance of atrial tachycardia in the cycle marked "X" with A-V block, probably due to toxic digitalis effects. Note the terminal ventricular flutter and ventricular fibrillation, illustrating that the initial beat of the terminal paroxysm occurs during the vulnerable period of the T wave.

the overall results in a larger series of patients often are not definitely informative as to whether or not the patient's plasma level is within toxic range. This is due to: (1) considerable overlapping of the limits of the therapeutic and toxic plasma levels, (2) observation of a number of false negatives and false positives, and (3) the fact that the most commonly used type of assay concerns digoxin, and this is of no help in determining levels of digitoxin, powdered leaf, or other preparations.

Recent studies have shown that differences of as much as 4 to 7 times in serum digoxin levels may be achieved in vivo after the oral administration of various preparations despite essentially equal digoxin tablet concentrations as measured in vitro (Lindenbaum et al., 1971). These variations were noted not only between preparations supplied by different companies but between different lots obtained from the same manufacturer. These differences are ascribed to variability in absorption due to differences in particle size, disintegration and dissolution rates, and the effects of various inert excipients and other additives (Linbenbaum et al., 1971). These features considerably complicate the values obtained by radioimmunoassay. The critical clinical evaluation of the patient with serial electrocardiographic findings is still probably the best single method for following such a patient.

Treatment of Digitalis Toxicity. Digitalis toxicity is usually easier to prevent than to treat. This is especially true of some digitalis glycosides because of their relatively slow onset of toxicity and long persistence of action. Many potential instances of digitalis toxicity can be avoided by strict observance of the following points: (1) Digitalization should be accomplished slowly, except in the presence of urgent clinical indications for rapid administration; (2) Special caution should be observed in subjects who excrete the drug slowly (e.g., subjects in the older age group, those with congestive heart failure and renal failure, and those with advanced heart disease, such as aortic stenosis); (3) Patients with a suspected low tolerance should be given a rapidly acting and rapidly eliminated digitalis preparation, i.e., digoxin (Lanoxin), rather than preparations with a marked cumulative effect (powdered leaf or digitoxin); and (2) Digitalized patients should be followed by frequent clinical observations, electrocardiograms, and electrolyte determinations (especially potassium). Any aspect of digitalis toxicity may be the first to appear in an individual patient; severe cardiotoxicity may occur in the absence of nausea, vomiting, or diarrhea.

One may encounter patients with atrial fibrillation who manifest sensitivity to digitalis by an increased degree of A-V block, so that the amount that can be administered does not produce a full therapeutic effect. With an artificial pacemaker, larger doses which may be closer to the therapeutic range can be given. In patients with atrial fibrillation who develop toxicity with small doses of digitalis, the use of propranolol combined with digitalis will result in satisfactory slowing of the ventricular rate with reduction in the digitalis dosage.

Three stages of digitalis cardiotoxicity may be observed:

(1) A mild grade of toxicity is characterized by intermittent S-A block, moderate grades of A-V heart block, and occasional premature beats. The initial step in the treatment of all grades of digitalis toxicity is to immediately stop administration of the drug. The electrolyte status, especially the concentration of potassium, and the pH should be determined. Further treatment depends on the severity of the toxic state. The conditions that characterize mild cardiac toxicity

usually disappear with no special treatment beyond termination of the drug.

(2) A more serious grade of digitalis toxicity is indicated by the occurrence of coupled rhythm and by ventricular premature beats that frequently occur in pairs or in runs of three or more, which may be premonitory to the development of ventricular tachycardia. Digitalis should be withdrawn from these patients and any abnormalities in serum electrolyte or acid-base status promptly corrected. The use of an antiarrhythmic drug such as lidocaine, diphenylhydantoin, procaine amide, or quinidine is indicated.

(3) Tachyarrhythmias due to digitalis constitute the most serious manifestations of toxicity: PAT with block, junctional, bidirectional, and ventricular tachycardias. These arrhythmias should be treated vigorously because of the likelihood that they will result in ventricular fibrillation and death. The following measures may be employed to treat digitalis toxicity in addition to stopping administration of the drug.

Potassium. In the presence of digitalis toxicity, it has frequently been suggested that potassium is the drug of choice. In our experience, the routine administration of potassium in patients with digitalis toxicity is often fraught with danger and, at times, may result in a fatality (see Fig. 34–8). During digitalis toxicity, the serum potassium level may be normal; however, it is frequently above normal levels. In the former instance, increments in serum potassium may occur subsequently, and in the latter instance, the administration of potassium may increase the degree of hyperpotassemia with resultant serious toxic effects.

Potassium may be given if the serum potassium level is below or at the lower level of the normal range. Potassium chloride may be administered orally in a dose of 1 to 2 gm. which may be repeated as needed; when the situation is more urgent, 40 mEq. of potassium dissolved in 500 ml. of normal saline may be given under continuous electrocardiographic con-

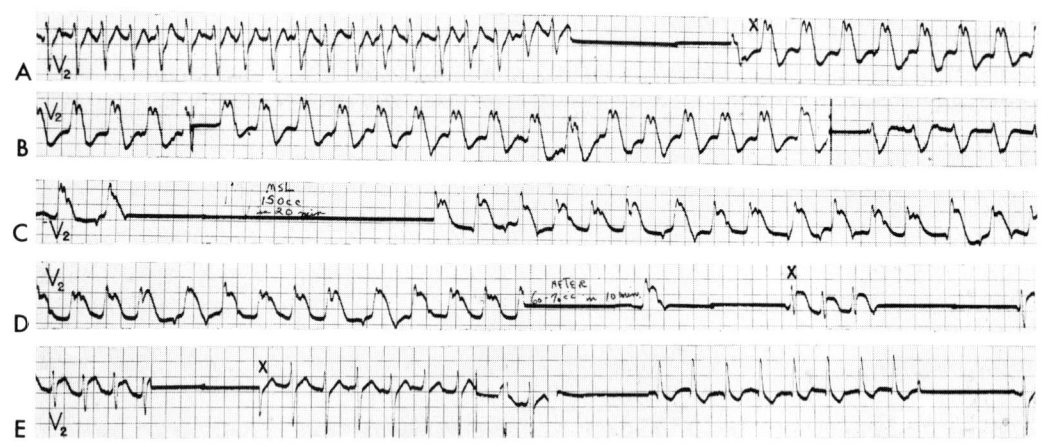

Figure 34–8. Shows the toxic effect of potassium chloride administration in a patient with digitalis toxicity. This patient was 64 years of age and received large doses of digitalis [195 mg. (gr. 3) per day for two weeks], following which he developed a heart rate of 150, probably A-V junctional in origin.

(*A*) Following the administration of potassium chloride, note the development of bizarre widened ventricular complexes starting at X. (*B*) Shows continuation of bizarre ventricular complexes. (*C*) 150 cc. of molar sodium lactate was given in 20 minutes. (*D*) After the additional administration of 70 cc. had been given in ten minutes, note the less bizarre shape of the QRS complexes at X. (*E*) Five minutes later, note the return of the control electrocardiographic pattern at X.

trol. This may be repeated as needed while the electrocardiogram and serum potassium level are monitored by frequent determinations to detect the early presence of hyperpotassemia. If hyperpotassemia does occur, it may be almost immediately reversed by the administration of 50 per cent glucose or molar sodium lactate. When the serum potassium level cannot be obtained or when continuous electrocardiographic monitoring is not expedient, lidocaine, diphenylhydantoin, quinidine, or procaine amide may be administered more safely.

Beta-blocking Agents. Beta-blocking agents, especially propranolol, have recently been used for the therapy of digitalis toxicity. The action depends chiefly on the beta-blocking and quinidine-like effects. Although beneficial effects may be obtained, the use of propranolol entails certain risk factors due to: (1) its negative inotropic effect, which may aggravate the patient's underlying heart failure; and (2) its tendency to slow A-V conduction, which may aggravate varying degrees of A-V heart block due to digitalis toxicity.

Diphenylhydantoin. Diphenylhydantoin may be administered intravenously in small doses (see Chapter 33). It occupies an important role in the therapy of digitalis toxicity since it has the advantage of decreasing automaticity of ectopic pacemakers, without, in most instances, causing impairment of A-V junctional or intraventricular conduction (see Fig. 33–15).

Quinidine or procaine amide may be employed alone or in combination with diphenylhydantoin. Lidocaine is especially useful in cases of ventricular tachycardia.

Electric countershock may be employed in the abolition of a rapid supraventricular or ventricular tachycardia under certain conditions. However, digitalis toxicity markedly increases the likelihood that countershock will induce serious arrhythmias, including ventricular fibrillation. Countershock should be employed for arrhythmias due to digitalis toxicity only after other measures have been attempted and after the patient has been prepared by the administration of other drugs (i.e., diphenylhydantoin or lidocaine) and certain precautions (e.g., use of low energy) have been taken (see Chapter 38).

Serious ventricular tachyarrhythmias produced by digitalis are often refractory to electric countershock. Although experimentally the average energy required to produce ventricular tachycardia is 400 watt sec., following recovery from digitalis-induced ventricular tachycardia, the electrical threshold for ventricular tachycardia is only 0.2 watt sec. About 80 per cent of the potentially toxic dose of ouabain has to be administered before the electrical threshold is lowered.

Atrial Pacing. Recently, rapid right atrial pacing has been shown to be effective in terminating supraventricular tachycardia in patients receiving digitalis. No complications have been encountered with this technique in contrast to the usually frequent occurrence of postcountershock arrhythmias in digitalis toxicity. This technique may prove to be safer and more reliable than countershock for supraventricular tachycardias due to digitalis toxicity.

Ventricular Pacing. In experimental animals glycoside-provoked junctional or ventricular tachycardias can be completely abolished by ventricular pacing at an appropriately rapid rate. The electrical stimulus is delivered at a more rapid rate than the frequency of the idiopathic ventricular focus, thereby suppressing the ectopic pacemaker. In addition, the faster electrical pacemaker is capable of depressing the slope of diastolic depolarization of the ectopic focus. It is emphasized that ventricular pacing should be employed only when standard measures fail; actually, this procedure is rarely required.

References

Balcon, R., Hoy, I., and Sowton, E.: Haemodynamic effects of rapid digitalization following acute myocardial infarction. Brit. Heart J., 30:373, 1968.

Beller, G. A., et al.: Prevalence of hypomagnesemia in a prospective clinical study of digitalis intoxication. Amer. J. Cardiol., 26:625, 1970.

Binnion, P. F., Morgan, L. M., Stevenson, H. M., and Fletcher, E.: Plasma and myocardial digoxin concentrations in patients on oral therapy. Brit. Heart J., 31:636, 1969.

Doherty, J. E., et al.: Tritiated digoxin XIV. Enterohepatic circulation, absorption, and excretion studies in human volunteers. Circulation, 42:867, 1970.

Evered, D. C., Chapman, C., and Hayter, C. J.: Measurement of plasma digoxin concentration by radioimmunoassay. Brit. Med. J., 3:427, 1970.

Fisch, C., Steinmetz, E. F., Fasola, A. F., and Martz, B. L.: Effect of potassium and "toxic" doses of digitalis on the myocardium. Circ. Res., 7:222, 1959.

Hecht, H. H.: The cellular action of digitalis compounds. Med. Clin. N. Amer., 54:221, 1970.

Koch-Weser, J.: Mechanism of digitalis action on the heart. New Eng. J. Med., 277:188, 1967.

Lindenbaum, J., Mellow, M. H., Blackstone, M. O., and Butler, V. P., Jr.: Variation in biologic availability of digoxin from four preparations. New Eng. J. Med., 285:1344, 1971.

Lister, J. W., Cohen, L. S., Bernstein, W. H., and Samet, P.: Treatment of supraventricular tachycardias by rapid atrial pacing. Circulation, 38:1044, 1968.

Mason, D. T., Jr., Spaun, J. F., Jr., and Zelis, R.: New developments in the understanding of the actions of the digitalis glycosides. Prog. Cardiov. Dis., 11:223, 1969.

Nola, G. T., Pole, S., and Harrison, D. C.: Assessment of the synergistic relationship between serum calcium and digitalis. Amer. Heart J., 79:499, 1970.

Oliver, G. C., Jr., Parker, B. M., Brasfield, D. L., and Parker, C. W.: The measurement of digitoxin in human serum by radioimmunoassay. J. Clin. Invest., 47:1035, 1968.

Seller, R. H., et al.: Digitalis toxicity and hypomagnesemia. Amer. Heart J., 78:57, 1970.

Smith, T. W.: The clinical use of serum cardiac glycoside concentration measurements. Amer. Heart J., 82:833, 1971.

Smith, T. W., Butler, V. P., and Haber, E.: Determination of therapeutic and toxic serum digoxin concentrations by radioimmunoassay. New Eng. J. Med., 281:1212, 1969.

Smith, T. W., and Haber, E.: Digoxin intoxication: The relationship of clinical presentation to serum digoxin concentration. J. Clin. Invest., 49:2, 377, 1970.

Surawicz, B., and Mortelmans, S.: Factors affecting individual tolerance to digitalis. *In* Fisch, C., and Surawicz, B. (eds.): Digitalis. New York, Grune & Stratton, 1969, pp. 127–147.

Weissler, A. M., and Schoenfeld, C. D.: Effect of digitalis on systolic time intervals in heart failure. Amer. J. Med. Sci., 259:4, 1970.

Chapter 35 Electrolytes Employed in Therapy

GENERAL CONSIDERATIONS
POTASSIUM
  Effects of Potassium in Certain Arrhythmias
  Dose and Duration of Effect
  Untoward and Toxic Effects
  Indication for Potassium Administration in the Therapy of Arrhythmias
CALCIUM
  Use of Calcium in Therapy
  Untoward and Toxic Effects
MAGNESIUM
  Use of Magnesium in Therapy

ALKALINIZING AGENTS: SODIUM LACTATE AND SODIUM BICARBONATE
  Indications
    Effects in Acidosis
    Hyperpotassemia
    Treatment of Quinidine and Procaine Amide Toxicity
    Use in Certain Cases of Complete A-V Heart Block
    Cardiac Arrest
  Toxic Effects and Contraindications

GENERAL CONSIDERATIONS

Electrolytes are particularly indicated for: (a) the restoration of acid-base balance and various types of electrolyte imbalance; and (b) the rather limited effects of treatment of ectopic rhythms independent of electrolyte alterations (e.g., atrial and ventricular premature beats and paroxysmal tachycardias). Potassium is important in the treatment of arrhythmias associated with digitalis toxicity (discussed on page 380). Magnesium has also been used in the therapy of ectopic rhythms, particularly atrial and ventricular tachycardia, but its effects (except for deficiency of this electrolyte) are inferior to those of other available drugs.

POTASSIUM

Effects of Potassium in Certain Arrhythmias. In general, the effect of potassium on arrhythmias qualitatively resembles that of quinidine and procaine amide; however, it differs from them in that it is extremely transient in its effect. Except for instances in which this electrolyte is deficient, quinidine, procaine amide, and other antiarrhythmic agents are generally superior in their antiarrhythmic effect. The beneficial effect of potassium salts in arrhythmias resulting from digitalis toxicity has been discussed (see p. 384).

Several effects of potassium on the various arrhythmias have been observed. Potassium is effective in abolishing or significantly decreasing the frequency of ectopic beats. For the most part (in approximately 80 per cent of instances), the ectopic beats disappear gradually within a period of 10 to 40 minutes after intravenous administration (Bettinger et al., 1956). Supraventricular ectopic beats are more easily controlled than ventricular ectopic beats. Similarly, potassium abolishes or significantly suppresses supraventricular tachycardia (77 per cent); however, it is ineffective in ventricular tachycardia.

No detectable change occurs in the atrial mechanism in atrial flutter or in atrial fibrillation treated with potassium. Generally, except for a slight decrease in the atrial rate, potassium has no effect on atrial fibrillation (Fig. 35-1).

Intravenous administration of potassium has a biphasic effect upon A-V conduction. Initially, mild hyperpotassemia accelerates A-V conduction by anticholinergic effects and a direct effect upon the action potential of the conduction fibers. Subsequently, continued elevation of potassium levels depresses A-V conduction by a potentiation of vagal effects and reduction of the resting potential and rate of rise of phase 0 of the action potential. Hyperpotassemia is known to potentiate the toxic effects of digitalis on the conduction system; however, the high levels of potassium required to produce this effect are far above the levels required to abolish ectopic beats. Potassium may transiently decrease the degree of partial A-V heart block in patients but the block soon returns to its pretreatment level.

Dose and Duration of Effect. The dose depends on the degree and severity of hypopotassemia and whether the patient can take food or potassium supplement orally. In slight grades of supplement orally. In slight grades of potassium depletion, the effective dose ranges from 20 to 60 mEq. given over a 10- to 120-minute period. The seven potassium levels at the time of disappearance or significant decrease in the arrhythmia are usually 1.0 to 1.5 mEq./L. higher than the levels before potassium administration.

There are wide variations in the persistence of the changes in heart rhythm produced by potassium infusion. The duration often persists for only a few minutes or a few hours.

Untoward and Toxic Effects. When

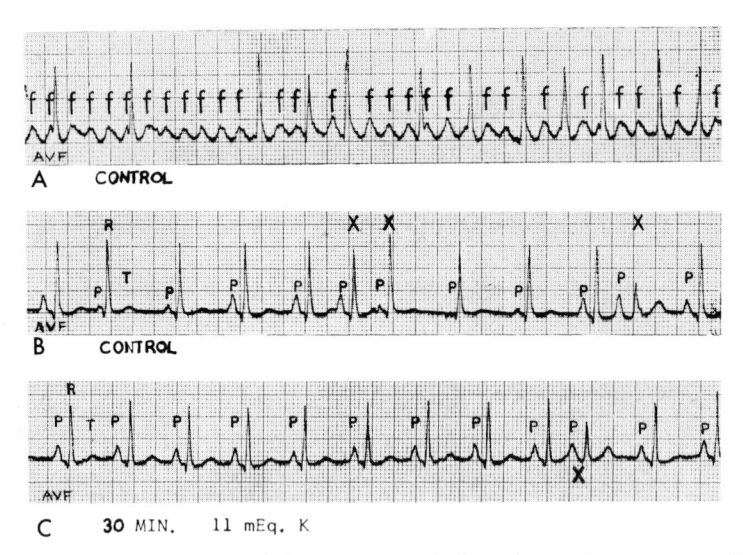

Figure 35-1. Conversion of atrial flutter to normal sinus rhythm by potassium. Electrocardiogram of a malnourished 51-year-old man with arteriosclerotic heart disease and bronchopneumonia. The patient had never received digitalis. (A) The upper strip is a portion of the control tracing which shows intermittent impure flutter and fibrillation. (B) Taken following the infusion of 11 mEq./L. of potassium in 30 minutes. The flutter and fibrillation mechanisms were abolished. Sinus beats are associated with frequent premature atrial contractions (at X). (C) Ectopic beats decreased in number. (Bettinger, J. C., et al.: Amer. J. Med., 21:521, 1956.)

administered with the appropriate safeguards, infusion of potassium salts produces few untoward or toxic effects. These effects consist of the development of hyperpotassemic T waves and at a later stage, widening of the QRS complexes. The intravenous administration of potassium is safe if the patient is carefully monitored; however, the margin between therapeutic and toxic effects is often very narrow. It should be pointed out that the role of potassium in the abolition of an arrhythmia in any patient is difficult to establish with certainty unless the intravenous route of administration is employed.

The ventricular pacemaker in complete A-V heart block is extremely sensitive to the effects of hyperpotassemia. This has been shown in the human subject and also experimentally in the dog (Guzman et al., 1959). Moreover, serious arrhythmias and cardiac arrest have been produced with increments of serum potassium that manifest little effect on the sinus node in the presence of normal sinus rhythm.

Indication for Potassium Administration in the Therapy of Arrhythmias. Potassium occupies an important but relatively minor role in the treatment of arrhythmias. It is indicated in those arrhythmias that are chiefly associated with hypopotassemia. Its effects are transient in normopotassemic subjects; in hypopotassemia the effects are also transient until the total body potassium depletion is corrected.

In the presence of digitalis toxicity, potassium may be employed when the plasma potassium level is below normal. If the serum potassium is normal, potassium either should not be given or should be given slowly by intravenous drip under continuous electrocardiographic monitoring. Aside from the aforementioned indications, quinidine, procaine amide, diphenylhydantoin, or lidocaine are the drugs preferred in the treatment of ectopic beats and paroxysmal tachycardias.

The rate at which potassium should be administered to correct potassium depletion is usually slower than the rate used for the treatment of arrhythmias. The following factors govern the rate of administration: (1) plasma potassium concentration or pretherapy electrocardiogram pattern; (2) renal function as related to the ability to excrete potassium; and (3) effects on the plasma K+ and the electrocardiogram during therapy (Surawicz, 1968).

CALCIUM

Use of Calcium in Therapy. Calcium is not often employed in the treatment of arrhythmias. However, it is of help under the following circumstances: (a) when hypocalcemia (under the conditions noted below) is associated with an ectopic rhythm, particularly in the presence of hyperpotassemia; (b) during resuscitative procedures in the therapy of cardiac arrest when the heart muscle manifests a loss of tone. In these instances, calcium may help to neutralize possible hyperpotassemic effects and increase contractility.

Untoward and Toxic Effects. Untoward and toxic effects involve the following factors: (a) Calcium should be used with caution in digitalized hearts since calcium and digitalis have an additive action on the heart which may result in severe cardiotoxicity or even a fatal outcome; (b) Hypercalcemia results in the production of premature beats, paroxysmal tachycardia, and other toxic rhythms, especially in the diseased heart.

MAGNESIUM

Use of Magnesium in Therapy. Magnesium salts have recently been used

390   ELECTROLYTES EMPLOYED IN THERAPY

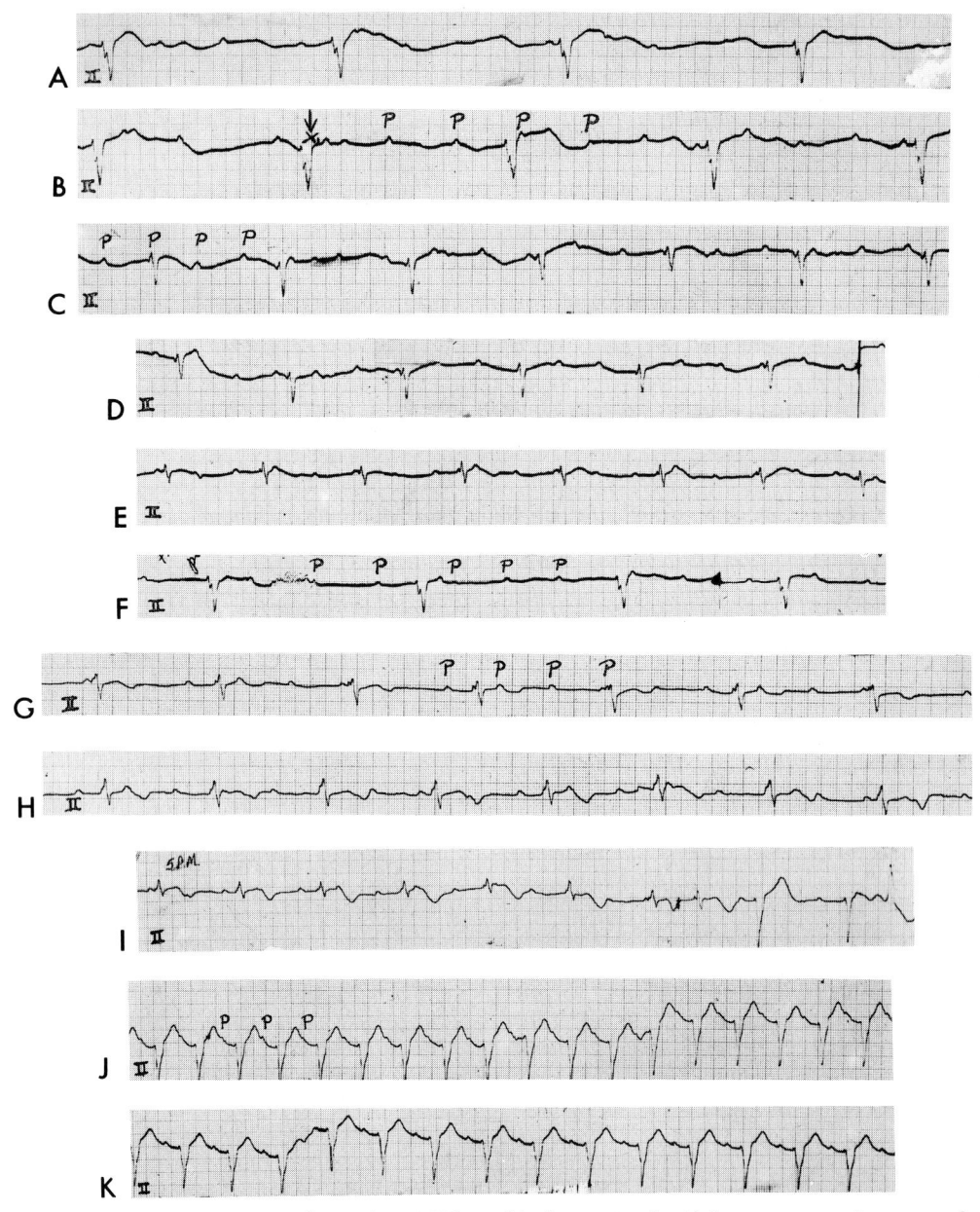

Figure 35-2. Reversion of complete A-V heart block associated with hyperpotassemia to normal sinus rhythm by sodium lactate in a male, 54 years of age.

(*A*) Control of electrocardiogram (Lead II). Ventricular rate is 19 per minute; atrial rate is 80 per minute. Complete A-V heart block is present. Note the width of the QRS complexes (0.18 second). The blood chemistry was as follows: BUN, 72 mg. per cent; blood sugar, 86 mg. per cent; Na, 137 mEq./L.; K, 7.5 mEq./L.; Cl, 90.0 mEq./L.; Ca, 7.2 mg. per cent; CO_2 vol., 25 per cent.

(*B*) Half molar sodium lactate started at X_1.

(*C*) Forty-eight seconds after sodium lactate infusion was begun. Note increase of ventricular rate to 33 per minute and the narrowing of the QRS complexes.

(*D*) One minute, 12 seconds after lactate infusion had been started. Ventricular rate is 38 per minute.

                                                                           (Legend continued on opposite page)

for the therapy of certain arrhythmias; however, except in occasional instances, their actions are inferior to the other available drugs described in this section. Knowledge of many of the effects of magnesium is still limited to the experimental animal.

Magnesium has been effectively used to abolish premature ventricular contractions and paroxysmal atrial tachycardias when due to digitalis toxicity. Recently, evidence has been presented that hypomagnesemia predisposes to digitalis toxicity. In the experimental animal, the digitalis toxicity arrhythmias usually are corrected rapidly by the infusion of 2 to 6 cc. of a 24 per cent solution of magnesium sulfate. A deficiency of magnesium, combined with the action of digitalis, may promote excessive loss of intracellular potassium. The presence of a normal concentration of magnesium might stimulate adenosinetriphosphatase, thus blocking the myocardial potassium loss induced by digitalis glycosides. This mechanism may explain the antiarrhythmic effect of magnesium sulfate in digitalis toxicity.

One disadvantage of magnesium salts, like most electrolyte solutions, is that their effect is quite transient. Furthermore, the use of magnesium in the presence of marked myocardial damage or intraventricular conduction disturbances is not without risk. In my experience, magnesium salts have not proven particularly effective in the treatment of arrhythmias, and I would rate this electrolyte low on a list of effective antiarrhythmic agents.

ALKALINIZING AGENTS: SODIUM LACTATE AND SODIUM BICARBONATE

Sodium lactate ($1/6$ molar and the molar solution) has been used for many years in the treatment of acidosis of various etiologies. More recently, sodium bicarbonate has replaced sodium lactate as the agent of choice in the treatment of acidotic states.

Indications. Experience to date suggests that alkalinizing agents are indicated in the treatment of hyperpotassemia, in states accompanied by acidosis, i.e., cardiac arrest, and in

---

Figure 35–2 (continued)

(*E*) Two minutes and 12 seconds after lactate infusion started. Ventricular rate remains 33 per minute; atrial rate, 94 per minute.

(*F*) Lactate infusion slowed to 20 drops per minute in attempt to titrate speed of administration against patient's heart rate. Note once again the return to slow ventricular rate (18 per minute) and widened QRS complexes (0.18 second).

(*G*) Subsequent to titration attempt, lactate was again speeded up. This tracing taken approximately three hours after continuous sodium lactate infusion. Note the more rapid ventricular rate and the narrowed QRS complexes; ventricular rate is 37 per minute.

(*H*) Three hours and five minutes after continuous sodium lactate administration. Ventricular rate is 43 per minute; atrial rate is 100 per minute.

(*I*) Five hours after lactate administration. Note more rapid ventricular rate, 46 per minute; atrial rate, 110 per minute.

(*J*) Five and one half hours after continuous sodium lactate administration. Patient now has sinus rhythm with a first degree A-V heart block. Sodium lactate was subsequently discontinued. The rate is 92 per minute. The QRS complexes have changed somewhat in configuration. The QRS width is 0.14 second; the P-R interval is 0.28 second.

(*K*) Two hours after cessation of sodium lactate infusion. The patient has normal sinus rhythm. The ventricular rate is 75 per minute; P-R is 0.28 second. (From Bellet, S., Wasserman, F., and Brody, J. I.: Circulation, *11*:685, 1955.)

selected cases of complete A-V heart block.

Effects in Acidosis. The acidotic state increases the tendency for arrhythmia production. The alkalinizing agents tend to either decrease or abolish the acidotic state. Since endogenous and exogenous catecholamines often fail to be effective during the acidosis of shock, hypoxia, or cardiac arrest, the restoration of a normal pH by alkalinizing agents may improve the vasopressor and chronotropic effects (Guzman et al., 1959).

Hyperpotassemia. Hyperpotassemia is commonly associated with acidosis. The decrease in serum potassium is accomplished by expansion of the extracellular space and the movement of the potassium intracellularly.

Treatment of Quinidine and Procaine Amide Toxicity. In our laboratory, quinidine cardiotoxicity treatment with molar sodium lactate was studied in both dogs and man (Bellet et al., 1959). Widened QRS complexes are frequently narrowed and may return to a normal width. This tends to occur characteristically in hyperpotassemia but may occur with quinidine and procaine amide toxicity.

Use in Certain Cases of Complete A-V Heart Block. Some instances of complete A-V heart block tend to be associated with hypoxia and acidosis, as well as hyperpotassemia. In both the experimental animal and in the human subject, alkalinizing solutions are particularly effective in increasing the automaticity of ventricular pacemakers in the presence of complete A-V heart block under these conditions (Fig. 35-2). However, they are usually ineffective in the usual type of complete block due to coronary artery disease.

Cardiac Arrest. Molar sodium lactate or sodium bicarbonate may be used in cases of cardiac arrest occurring during surgery. In some cases, it has been effective in restoring the heart beat after other measures, i.e., cardiac compression, electric defibrillation, and sympathomimetic drugs (epinephrine, phenylephrine and isoproterenol), employed over a period of ten to fifteen minutes, had failed.

When the cause of the arrest is a sudden process (independent of a chronic incurable disease), the administration of the alkalinizing agents is one of the modalities which, together with other resuscitative measures, might be efficacious in restoring the normal heart beat.

Toxic Effects and Contraindications. The following circumstances either contraindicate the use of molar sodium lactate or indicate extreme caution in its use: (a) the appearance or increased frequency of premature beats following the administration of sodium lactate; (b) severe heart damage, particularly in association with overt or impending congestive heart failure; (c) hypopotassemia; or (d) alkalosis.

References

Bellet, S.: Electrocardiogram in electrolyte imbalance. Arch. Intern. Med., 96:618, 1955.

Bellet, S., Hamdan, G., Somlyo, A., and Lara, R.: The reversal of cardiotoxic effects of quinidine by molar sodium lactate: an experimental study. Amer. J. Med. Sci., 237:165, 1959.

Bellet, S., Wasserman, F., and Brody, J. I.: Treatment of cardiac arrest and slow ventricular rates in complete A-V heart block: use of molar and half molar sodium lactate: a clinical study. Circulation, 11:685, 1955.

Bellet, S., Wasserman, F., and Brody, J. I.: Effect of molar sodium lactate in increasing cardiac rhythmicity. JAMA, 160:293, 1956.

Bettinger, J. C., et al.: The effect of intravenous administration of potassium chloride on ectopic rhythms, ectopic beats, and disturbances in A-V conduction. Amer. J. Med., 31:521, 1956.

Cline, R. E., Wallace, A. G., Sealy, W. C., and Young, G. Y.: Antiarrhythmic properties of tris (hydroxymethyl) aminomethane. Amer. J. Cardiol., 21:38, 1968.

Fisch, C.: Effect of potassium on A-V conduction. Circulation, 21:575, 1970.

Greenstein, S., Goldburgh, W. P., Guzman, S. V.,

and Bellet, S.: A comparative analysis of molar sodium lactate and other agents in the treatment of induced hyperkalemia in nephrectomized dogs. Circ. Res., 8:223, 1960.

Guzman, S. V., DeLeon, A. C., Jr., West, J. W., and Bellet, S.: Cardiac effects of isoproterenol, norepinephrine and epinephrine in complete A-V heart block during experimental acidosis and hyperkalemia. Circ. Res., 7:666, 1959.

Nola, G. T., Pole, S., and Harrison, D. C.: Assessment of the synergistic relationship between serum calcium and digitalis. Amer. Heart J., 79:499, 1970.

Surawicz, B.: The role of K in cardiovascular therapy. Med. Clin. N. Amer., 52:1103, 1968.

Chapter 36 *Other Drugs*

ANTITHYROID DRUGS AND ISOTOPES

GOITROGENS
RADIOACTIVE IODINE

ANTIHISTAMINIC DRUGS

ANTAZOLINE (ANTISTINE)

CORTICOIDS

VASOPRESSOR DRUGS

PHENYLEPHRINE (NEO-SYNEPHRINE)
METHOXAMINE (VASOXYL)
EPHEDRINE
METARAMINOL (ARAMINE)
MEPHENTERMINE (WYAMINE)

PROARRHYTHMIC DRUGS

DIGITALIS AND OTHER ANTIARRHYTHMIC AGENTS

DIURETIC AGENTS
 Chlorothiazide and Hydrochlorothiazide
 Furosemide (Lasix) and Ethacrynic Acid (Edecrin)
XANTHINES
 Aminophylline
 Caffeine
THYROID EXTRACT
SYMPATHOMIMETIC AMINES
ELECTROLYTE DISTURBANCES
ANESTHETIC AGENTS
MEPERIDINE (DEMEROL)
HEROIN
THIORIDAZINE (MELLARIL)
IMIPRAMINE HYDROCHLORIDE (TOFRANIL)
NICOTINE
FLUOROALKANE GASES

Occasionally, arrhythmias may occur in which the standard drugs (quinidine, procaine amide, lidocaine) are ineffective or are only partially effective in prohibitively high doses. These arrhythmias are often of the repetitive type. The following drugs warrant a trial: (1) antithyroid drugs; and (2) antihistaminic agents. The vasopressor drugs, which are useful in treating certain tachyarrhythmias (as a result of reflex increases in vagal tone) and the hypotension which accompanies many arrhythmias, are commonly employed drugs. Also important in the therapy of arrhythmias, particularly in resistant and repetitive cases, is the careful omission of proarrhythmic drugs.

ANTITHYROID DRUGS AND ISOTOPES

Antithyroid drugs are chemical agents that lower the basal metabolic rate by interfering with the synthesis, release, or peripheral action of thyroid hormone. They may be considered under the following two categories: (a) the goitrogens (propylthiouracil and methimazole), and (b) radioactive iodine.

GOITROGENS

Cardiovascular Effects. Propylthiouracil and methimazole administration leads to a reduction in basal oxygen consumption, a fall in venous pressure, augmentation of cardiac output, and an increase in exercise tolerance in patients with refractory heart failure. The discovery that a decrease in thyroid hormone led to improvement in cardiac metabolism and efficiency suggested the use of antithyroid drugs in the treatment of certain arrhythmias.

Indications. The use of goitrogens in cases of hyperthyroidism in which arrhythmias have developed as a result of increased thyroid activity is well known. They may bring about conversion of the arrhythmia to a normal sinus rhythm without the additional use of cardiac drugs. It is not so well recognized that, in many euthyroid patients with persistent or frequent bouts of premature beats and paroxysmal tachycardias resistant to other types of therapy, the administration of the goitrogens has been extremely helpful in controlling the arrhythmia. Although still used in occasional patients, these drugs have largely been replaced by other antiarrhythmic agents, particularly beta-blocking drugs (e.g., propranolol).

Untoward and Toxic Effects. Minor side effects, including skin rashes, pruritus, drug fever, lymphadenopathy, and nausea (overall incidence of about 10 per cent) have been encountered. More serious side effects including agranulocytosis (incidence of less than 1 per cent) and aplastic anemia (bone marrow aplasia) (incidence of less than 1 per cent) are seen occasionally.

RADIOACTIVE IODINE

The therapeutic action of radioactive iodine depends upon the destruction of thyroid tissue by internal radiation resulting from disintegration of the isotope. In the usual doses, the beta irradiation acts almost exclusively upon the parenchymal cells and causes little or no damage to the surrounding tissues.

Indications. The indications for ^{131}I in the therapy of arrhythmias are similar to those previously stated for the goitrogens.

However, because of the advent of recent antiarrhythmic agents, especially those with a beta-blocking effect (e.g., propranolol), fewer refractory cases are seen and this procedure is infrequently employed at present.

There are no immediate toxic effects of radioactive iodine; however, overdosage may lead to irreversible hypothyroidism, which cannot be controlled with small doses of thyroid extract. A late complication of radioactive ablation of the thyroid may be the development of carcinoma.

Recently, McDougall et al. (1971), following animal experiments, studied the use of ^{125}I for the treatment of thyrotoxicosis in humans. This isotope decreases thyroid cell function to a greater degree than ^{131}I. However, its use in the human subject is still in the experimental stage.

ANTIHISTAMINIC DRUGS

Recently, certain antihistaminic agents that have a chemical structure similar to that of quinidine have been found to possess antiarrhythmic qualities. Their role in the treatment of cardiac arrhythmias has been under investigation for a number of years.

ANTAZOLINE (ANTISTINE)

Effect on Arrhythmias. Antazoline has been efficacious in the therapy of certain supraventricular as well as ventricular arrhythmias. It has been successfully employed in occasional cases of atrial tachycardia; however, except for unusual instances, it has relatively little efficacy in the conversion of atrial flutter or fibrillation to normal sinus rhythm.

The best therapeutic results with this drug are obtained in the treatment of ventricular arrhythmias, premature ventricular beats, and ventricular tachycardia. However, the use of this drug is still in the experimental stage and has so far not attained an important role in the therapy of the arrhythmias. It may be employed in the treatment of atrial and ventricular premature contractions and paroxysmal tachycardias in those instances in which the patient manifests an intolerance to quinidine, procaine amide, or other antiarrhythmic drugs.

Dose and Method of Administration. The oral drug is generally well tolerated in dosages of 100 to 200 mg. three or four times daily for adults, and 50 to 100 mg. on the same schedule for children above the age of six. Administration with or just after meals probably will control any untoward gastrointestinal symptoms that may occur. Intravenous administration has been generally well tolerated in dosages up to 10 mg./Kg., for patients undergoing hypothermic procedures and for cardiac arrhythmias under other circumstances. Constant monitoring by electrocardiogram is desirable during intravenous administration, both to determine the nature of the changes and to show immediately the point at which improvement begins and drug injection can be stopped. Although oral medication may not be needed after reversion of the arrhythmia following intravenous antazoline, oral administration is suggested on a prophylactic basis. Further experience undoubtedly will serve to clarify this point.

Untoward and Toxic Effects. As with other antihistaminic drugs, drowsiness may be troublesome. Headache, nausea, vomiting, and diarrhea may occur at dosages of 300 mg. administered intravenously or 300 mg. administered orally three times a day. Other side effects include a diffuse sensation of heat, facial flushing, nausea and vomiting, dizziness, sedation, and occasional fall in blood pressure.

CORTICOIDS

Although the corticosteroids have attained widespread use in many other areas of medicine, their use remains limited in the therapy of arrhythmias. Furthermore, when administered simultaneously with other antiarrhythmic agents, corticoids may have toxic effects on the heart, or as a result of electrolyte alterations, may enhance the toxicity of other agents.

The only clinically established indication for the corticoids in the treatment of arrhythmias is in A-V heart block. The basis for their use in this situation has been their tendency to improve A-V conduction by lowering the serum potassium and reducing local inflammatory edema. Other indications for steroid therapy include rheumatic carditis and refractory heart failure (for diuretic effect).

VASOPRESSOR DRUGS

A vasopressor agent should have the following properties: it should elevate blood pressure, increase peripheral resistance, produce a proportionate increase in coronary blood flow, have minimal side effects, manifest a minimal effect on cardiac irritability, and should not decrease cardiac output. In addition, it should be possible to readily control the resulting pressor effect; reactive hypotension (secondary vasodilation) should be absent or minimal; the drug should be available for administration by convenient routes (subcutaneous, intramuscular and intravenous); it should be free from tachyphylactic activity (diminishing response with successive administration); it should cause minimal renal vascular constriction; and finally, it should not provoke local tissue damage at the sites of injection. Few drugs meet these ideal requirements.

Among the vasopressor agents to be discussed are the following: Phenylephrine (Neo-Synephrine), methoxamine (Vasoxyl), ephedrine, metaraminol (Aramine), and mephentermine (Wyamine).

PHENYLEPHRINE (NEO-SYNEPHRINE)

Mechanism of Action. Phenylephrine acts principally on alpha receptors, causing peripheral vasoconstriction. This results in a rise of diastolic and systolic pressure. Bradycardia of reflex vagal origin accompanies the rise in systemic arterial pressure.

Indications. Phenylephrine is used mainly in the following conditions: (a) to reverse hypotension in shock due to cardiovascular causes; (b) to sustain peripheral blood pressure during spinal anesthesia; and (c) in certain cases to terminate an attack of paroxysmal supraventricular tachycardia in normotensive subjects (by its reflex vagal effects). Although not a drug of choice for the therapy of this arrhythmia, phenylephrine is superior to other sympathomimetic amines because of its minimal side effects. However, it may occasionally produce runs of ventricular tachycardia and other tachyarrhythmias which are dangerous.

Dose and Method of Administration. Phenylephrine can be given parenterally or orally. The intravenous dose is 0.5 mg.; the subcutaneous, about 5 mg. Pressor effects are obtained after the oral administration of 20 to 50 mg.

Untoward and Toxic Effects. Minor toxic effects that may accompany the administration of phenylephrine are anxiety, tremor, palpitation, and headache. These are transient and not dangerous. Potential major toxic effects are subarachnoid hemorrhage, ventricular fibrillation, and acute pulmonary edema. However, these complications seldom occur.

METHOXAMINE (VASOXYL)

Mechanism of Action. The most marked action of methoxamine, like phenylephrine, is stimulation of alpha-adrenergic receptors, producing a significant rise in peripheral resistance and, hence, in blood pressure (Aviado, 1970). In addition, methoxamine is a weak beta-adrenergic blocking agent.

Indications. Methoxamine has been used primarily in the prevention of hypotension associated with spinal anesthesia. Attempts to use it in cardiogenic shock due to myocardial infarction have resulted in effective control of the blood pressure in only 20 per cent of cases.

Dose and Method of Administration. Methoxamine is usually administered intramuscularly in a single dose of 10 to 20 mg. It may be given intravenously, usually in a dose of 10 mg. The effects appear in 15 minutes following the intramuscular injection and persist for about 90 minutes. Intravenous injections produce an immediate effect that persists for about 60 minutes.

Untoward and Toxic Effects. Marked pilomotor stimulation and a desire to void may occur after the administration of methoxamine. In man, a tingling of the extremities and a sense of coldness may be noted; there is little effect on bronchial muscle or the central nervous system.

EPHEDRINE

Ephedrine possesses most of the cardiovascular actions of epinephrine; it causes stimulation of both alpha and beta receptors by direct actions and by release of norepinephrine from nerve terminals. It elevates the blood pressure, stimulates the myocardium, accelerates the heart rate, and increases the cardiac output. Adrenergic blockade decreases but does not readily reverse ephedrine-induced hypertension because of the weakness of its vasodilator action.

Cardiovascular Effects. The drug dilates the coronary arteries and increases the coronary blood flow, although at the expense of increasing cardiac work. Ephedrine, similar to epinephrine, may produce ventricular arrhythmias, such as premature beats, tachycardia, and fibrillation, particularly in the presence of myocardial abnormalities. However, this action is less marked after ephedrine than after epinephrine administration.

Indications. The indications for the use of ephedrine are similar to those for epinephrine. Both drugs are usually administered for their chronotropic or vasopressor effects. In complete A-V heart block with Stokes-Adams seizures, ephedrine accelerates the idioventricular rate, thereby preventing marked bradycardia and asystole. Because of these actions, it has been employed for long-term therapy in the intervals between Stokes-Adams attacks. However, with the advent of artificial pacemakers, its use for this purpose is rarely required.

Dose and Method of Administration. Ephedrine is administered orally for systemic effects in a dose of 15 to 50 mg. In A-V heart block, the minimal effective dose (15 mg. administered three times daily) should be exceeded only with caution because of possible untoward effects. The drug may also be given by injection, subcutaneously or intramuscularly, in doses similar to those for oral administration.

Untoward and Toxic Effects. The untoward effects of ephedrine vary in different patients; they include nervousness, insomnia, tremulousness, vertigo, headache, tachycardia, palpitation, sweating, and a sensation of warmth. There may be difficulty in urination due to vesical sphincter spasm. Most side effects are counteracted by sedatives, such as the barbiturates.

METARAMINOL (ARAMINE)

Mechanism of Action. Metaraminol is a vasopressor agent which, although less potent than norepinephrine, has a more prolonged duration of action. It combines the pressor effect of the aromatic hydroxysubstituted compounds with the prolonged duration of the isopropylamines.

The alpha-adrenergic stimulating properties of metaraminol are similar to but much more potent than those of ephedrine. Furthermore, metaraminol appears to have no vasodilator component and produces no primary or secondary fall in blood pressure, as noted with some of the other sympathomimetic amines. Experimental and clinical evidence to date indicates that metaraminol produces no detrimental alterations in cardiac rhythm.

Hemodynamic Effects. Following subcutaneous and intramuscular injections of metaraminol, a significant pressor effect, once obtained, usually persists for 30 minutes. Following the intravenous injection, a pressor response occurs within two minutes. While maximal pressor effect is manifested within five minutes, the response continues for an average of 25 minutes.

Atrial effects are reflected by a slight shortening of the P-R interval and flattening of the P waves. Junctional escape or rhythm is occasionally observed. No abnormality of ventricular rhythm or conduction is seen.

Indications. Metaraminol is usually effective in clinical shock due to various causes. It appears to have some advantage over norepinephrine in that its action is not so evanescent, thereby permitting maintenance of a more stable blood pressure. Compromised renal function is improved in that there is an increase in glomerular filtration rate, renal blood flow, and urinary output.

Dose and Method of Administration. Metaraminol may be effectively administered intravenously, intramuscularly, and subcutaneously without demonstrable injury to tissues at the site of injection. For intramuscular or subcutaneous injection, the suggested dose is 2 to 10 mg. (0.2 to 1 cc.); for intravenous infusion, 15 to 100 mg. (1.5 to 10 cc.) in 500 cc. of isotonic solution of sodium chloride or 5 per cent dextrose solution. The rate of infusion should be adjusted to maintain blood pressure at the desired level.

Untoward and Toxic Effects. Present indications are that metaraminol, like other β-hydroxy compounds, has a minimal toxic effect on the heart.

Place in Therapy. The results of therapy are as satisfactory as those reported for norepinephrine. The principal advantages of metaraminol are potent pressor action, its prolonged duration of action, the ease with which its administration can be controlled, and its availability for direct intravenous, intramuscular, and subcutaneous administration.

MEPHENTERMINE (WYAMINE)

Mechanism of Action. Mephentermine is efficacious in raising the systolic, diastolic, and pulse pressures, primarily by an increase in cardiac output. Mephentermine acts to increase the blood pressure principally by its beta-stimulating effects on the heart; however, it has sufficient potency on alpha receptors to cause an increase in total peripheral resistance.

Indications. Because of mephentermine's antifibrillatory and vasopressor actions, it has been advised for the prevention or treatment of the following conditions: (a) ventricular fibrillation induced by epinephrine in patients under cyclopropane anesthesia; (b) ventricular ectopic beats; (c) hypotensive states, such as those that accompany myocardial infarction; (d) pulsus alternans; (E) digitalis intoxication; and (f) shock. This drug's potential efficacy in treating shock is at present under investigation.

Dose and Method of Administration. The sulfate salt of mephentermine may be administered intravenously as a single dose of 15 to 30 mg., or as a continuous drip of about 1 mg. per minute (0.1 per cent solution in 5 per cent dextrose in water). The best method of administration is the intravenous route. Pressor effects last from 30 to 50 minutes after an intravenous injection, and up to four hours after an intramuscular injection.

Untoward and Toxic Effects. In cases of supraventricular tachycardia with second degree A-V block, mephentermine may have untoward effects leading to an increase in ventricular rate by facilitating conduction through the A-V node.

PROARRHYTHMIC DRUGS

Many drugs possess proarrhythmic qualities. When determining the cause of a specific arrhythmia, one should keep this point in mind before instituting therapy.

DIGITALIS AND OTHER ANTIARRHYTHMIC AGENTS

Digitalis is one of the most important proarrhythmic drugs because of its pharmacologic and electrophysiologic effects and its common use in patients with cardiac abnormalities. This drug can cause almost any type of arrhythmia when given in toxic doses or when administered to patients with electrolyte imbalance (see Chapter 34). Under certain conditions, quinidine procaine amide, lidocaine, potassium salts, and other antiarrhythmic agents cause an increase in automaticity and thus predispose to the development of ventricular tachycardia and fibrillation. These conditions are discussed fully in the chapters dealing with these drugs.

DIURETIC AGENTS

Chlorothiazide and Hydrochlorothiazide. The chlorothiazide group includes potent diuretic agents that are used extensively in the treatment of congestive heart failure, cirrhosis of the liver, renal disease, and hypertension. These drugs produce a marked increase in sodium and chloride excretion by inhibiting the tubular mechanism for electrolyte reabsorption; they also evoke a significant augmentation in potassium and magnesium excretion in amounts sufficient to produce severe hypopotassemia and hypomagnesemia. This factor is chiefly responsible for the production of cardiac arrhythmias. Furthermore, the indiscriminate use of thiazide diuretics in digitalized patients may provoke digitalis toxicity. To avoid electrolyte complications of thiazide therapy, potassium supplements are usually employed (see Chapter 35).

Furosemide (Lasix) and Ethacrynic Acid (Edecrin). These powerful diuretics promote sodium and chloride excretion as well as marked potassium excretion. They cause the same problems as the thiazide diuretics.

XANTHINES

Aminophylline. The intravenous administration of aminophylline in patients with severe myocardial damage, particularly if it is given rapidly, may occasionally produce rapid ectopic rhythms. Fatalities due to ventricular fibrillation have been reported. This is probably due to the fact that aminophylline increases cardiac contractility and increases the demands upon the coronary blood flow, which the diseased heart may not be able to meet.

Caffeine. Caffeine may produce ectopic rhythms by two mechanisms: (a) as a result of its direct stimulating effect on heart muscle (especially when given intravenously); and (b) as a result of its diuretic effects and loss of electrolytes, particularly potassium and calcium, in subjects who drink large quantities of coffee (six to ten cups per day).

THYROID EXTRACT

The thyroid extracts are employed in replacement therapy for hypothyroidism and various weight reduction regimens. Hyperthyroidism may result from the indiscriminate use of this class of drugs. Sinus tachycardia, atrial fibrillation, and other arrhythmias are not infrequently associated with the use of these drugs. (See Chapter 24 for further discussion of this topic.)

SYMPATHOMIMETIC AMINES

Sympathomimetic amines (e.g., epinephrine, isoproterenol, ephedrine, and amphetamine) may produce arrhythmias as a result of their initial sympathetic and subsequent parasympathetic effects, as well as their direct effect on the heart muscle. Norepinephrine manifests little tendency to produce arrhythmias except when given in large doses or to patients with serious myocardial abnormalities.

ELECTROLYTE DISTURBANCES

Electrolyte disturbances are often the underlying cause of ectopic rhythms. These are discussed in detail in Chapter 29.

ANESTHETIC AGENTS

Vagal effects are common during induction of anesthesia. Furthermore, various anesthetic agents, particularly halothane and cyclopropane, are arrhythmogenic because of an increase in the sympathetic effects. Elevated catecholamine levels may lead to an increase in the incidence of ectopic rhythms.

MEPERIDINE (DEMEROL)

Meperidine decreases the degree of A-V heart block with resultant increase in ventricular rate in atrial flutter and atrial fibrillation. This rapid heart action may manifest deleterious effects in patients with heart disease. On the other hand, it would appear to be the analgesic of choice in patients with slow heart rates, higher grades of A-V heart block, and complete A-V heart block without Stokes-Adams attacks.

HEROIN

Heroin and morphine, the metabolite to which heroin is converted in the body, produce various physiologic alterations that may predispose to the development of arrhythmias. Depression of respiration leads to hypoxia, and the inhibition of acetylcholinesterase and pseudocholinesterase produces increased vagal tone. The combined electrophysiologic effects of increased parasympathetic tone and hypoxia may lead to the evolution of various arrhythmias. Paroxysmal atrial fibrillation with a slow ventricular rate may occur in patients in heroin intoxication. The atrial fibrillation reverts to normal sinus rhythm following treatment of the heroin intoxication with nalorphine (Labi, 1969).

THIORIDAZINE (MELLARIL)

Premature ventricular contractions and ventricular tachycardia have been observed with this drug. First degree A-V heart block with intraventricular conduction delay, premature atrial beats, and atrial flutter have also been observed in patients on Mellaril therapy.

IMIPRAMINE HYDROCHLORIDE (TOFRANIL)

Imipramine in toxic doses causes Q-T prolongation and S-T segment changes which may be followed by the evolution of arrhythmias which may prove fatal.

NICOTINE

Except for a mild degree of bradycardia, nicotine infrequently produces arrhythmias under clinical conditions. The major action of nicotine is vagal stimulation followed by autonomic blockade. Nicotine has a stimulating as well as an inhibitory action on the heart through the release of epinephrine and norepinephrine from the heart stores.

Associated with this positive inotropic effect of nicotine is the development of automaticity in latent pacemakers. This was manifested by coupled premature ventricular contractions, A-V dissociation with an accelerated junctional pacemaker, and subsequent ventricular tachycardia.

Nicotine causes direct depression of conduction by decreasing the resting potential and maximal rising velocity of phase 0 in addition to the transient increased vagal tone it produces.

As a result of these actions, nicotine in the experimental animal depresses conductivity, which may lead to reentrant phenomena and temporal dispersion of repolarization, and lowers the fibrillation threshold, which may enhance the production of abnormal electrophysiologic mechanisms. Although these observations have not been extended to the human subject, the correlation of smoking with serious cardiac disease and sudden death coupled with the experimental results suggest that nicotine may be a very potent proarrhythmic agent.

FLUOROALKANE GASES

The fluoroalkane gases, which are used to propel various aerosols, including bronchodilators used by asthmatic patients, produce a wide spectrum of cardiotoxic reactions including sinus bradycardia, A-V heart block, and T-wave changes in experimental animals (Taylor and Harris, 1970). These effects are enhanced by hypoxia. It has been observed that the incidence of sudden death among asthmatic patients has risen steadily over the past ten years, as has the availability and use of the pressurized bronchodilators. Whether this increase is due to arrhythmias has not yet been determined.

References

Aber, C. P., and Jones, E. W.: Corticotrophin and corticosteroids in the management of acute and chronic heart block. Brit. Heart J., 27:916, 1965.

Alexander, C. S., and Nino, A.: Cardiovascular complications in young patients taking psychotropic drugs: preliminary report. Amer. Heart J., 78:757, 1969.

Anderson, G., et al.: Some observations on nicotine induced cardiac arrhythmias. Clin. Res., 17:509, 1969.

Aviado, D. M.: Sympathomimetic Drugs. Springfield, Ill., Charles C Thomas, 1970.

Bellet, S., et al.: Effect of exposure to cigarette smoke on the ventricular fibrillation threshold in normal dogs. Second Research Conference Committee for Research on Tobacco and Health, Scottsdale, Arizona. May 5–7, 1970.

Corday, E., Jaffe, H. L., and Irving, D. W.: Hypometabolic treatment of heart disease. Amer. J. Cardiol., 6:952, 1960.

Fleischbaker, H.: Cortisone und Digitalis. Wein. Klin. Wesche., 68:989, 1956.

Fletcher, G. F., Kazamias, T. M., and Wenger, N. K.: Cardiotoxic effects of Mellaril: Conduction disturbances and supraventricular arrhythmias. Amer. Heart J., 78:135, 1958.

Greenspan, K., Anderson, G., Bandura, J., and Edmands, R. E.: Arrhythmia induced by nicotine: electrophysiological mechanisms. Amer. J. Cardiol., 25:99, 1970.

Greenspan, K., Edmands, R. E., Knoebel, S. B., and Fisch, C.: Some effects of nicotine on cardiac automaticity, conduction, and inotropy. Arch. Intern. Med., 123:707, 1969.

Ingbar, S. H., and Woeber, K. A.: The thyroid gland. In Williams, R. H. (ed.): Textbook of Endocrinology. Philadelphia, W. B. Saunders, 1968.

Kurland, G. S., Schneckloth, R. E., and Friedberg, A. S.: The heart in I^{131} induced myxedema. New Eng. J. Med., 249:215, 1953.

Labi, M.: Paroxysmal atrial fibrillation in heroin intoxication. Ann. Intern. Med., 71:951, 1969.

Lefer, A. M.: Corticosteroid antagonism of the positive inotropic effect of ouabain. J. Pharmacol. Exp. Ther., 151:292, 1966.

McDougall, I. R., Greig, W. R., and Gillespie, F. C.: Radioactive iodine (^{125}I) therapy for thyrotoxicosis. Background and evaluation in 128 patients. New Eng. J. Med., 285:1099, 1971.

Mokler, C. M.: Antiarrhythmic activity of various steroidal spirolactones in dogs. Proc. Soc. Exp. Biol. Med., 105:257, 1960.

Muller, O. F., Goodman, N., and Bellet, S.: The hypotensive effect of imipramine hydrochloride in patients with cardiovascular disease. Clin. Pharmacol. Ther., 2:300, 1961.

Schoonmaker, F. W., Osteen, R. T., and Greenfield, J. C., Jr.: Thioridazine (Mellaril)-induced ventricular tachycardia controlled with an artificial pacemaker. Ann. Intern. Med., 65:1076, 1966.

Taylor, G. J., IV, and Harris, W. S.: Cardiac toxicity of aerosol propellants. JAMA, 214:81, 1970.

Chapter 37 Artificial Pacemakers

GENERAL CONSIDERATIONS
  Stimulation Threshold
    Determination of Threshold
TEMPORARY PACING
  Indications
    Overdrive Suppression
PERMANENT PACING
  Indications
  Sites of Electrode Placement
    Endocardial Placement
    Myocardial Electrode Placement
    Atrial Pacing
  Types of Implanted Pulse Generators
    Fixed-rate (Asynchronous) Pacemakers
    Atrial-triggered or "Synchronous" Pacemakers
    Ventricular-programmed ("Demand" and "Standby") Pacemakers
    Ventricular-inhibited ("Demand") Pacemaker
    Ventricular-triggered ("Standby") Pacemakers
    Bifocal Demand Pacing
    Atomic Power Supply
Hemodynamic Effects of Pacing
Problem of Competitive Rhythms
Cardioactive Drugs and Pacing
Clinical Results with Artificial Pacing
  The Prognosis of Triggered and Fixed-rate Pacemakers
Complications of Pacing
  Arrhythmias with Specific Types of Pacemakers
  Complications of Catheter Electrodes
  Pacing Failure
    Electrical Failure of Pulse Generators
    Detection of Incipient Pacemaker Failure
    Trans-telephonic Pacemaker Evaluation

GENERAL CONSIDERATIONS

The artificial cardiac pacemaker has been an important advance in the application of modern electronics to human biology and medicine. Its purpose is to initiate and maintain an acceptable heart rate when the natural pacemakers of the heart fail to initiate an impulse, produce too slow a heart rate, or fail periodically, causing Stokes-Adams attacks.

Artificial pacing depends upon the ability of the pacemaker to depolarize an area around its electrodes which will serve as the pacemaking focus of the heart. The pacemaker unit consists of a pulse generator, either temporary or permanent, which contains electrical circuitry and batteries which generate the pacing pulses and regulate their timing. Connected with the unit are electrodes which carry these pulses to the heart. A properly functioning cardiac pacemaker delivers to the heart electrical impulses of sufficient intensity to initiate orderly excitation and contraction.

Stimulation Threshold. The stimulation threshold may be defined as the minimal intensity of the stimulus that maintains continuous "capture" of the heart. It may be increased or decreased by various factors which may profoundly affect the result of pacemaker activity: the type of electrode, the site of stimulation, the period in the cardiac cycle within which the impulse falls, the polarity, duration, and wave form of the stimulus, the state of the myocardium (local inflammatory or fibrotic changes), electrolyte changes, and certain drugs. Following pacemaker implantation, threshold values may rise excessively as a result of infection or fibrosis around the electrode, causing an artificial "exit block" and consequent loss of an effective pacing impulse.

Determination of Threshold. Electrical analysis of threshold before permanent implantation of the pulse generator may obviate the need for additional surgery or revision and can prevent some of the deaths due to failure of pacing. Threshold values are expressed in milliamperes (mAmp.), assuming constant voltage and resistance, and a standardizing impulse duration at 2 msec. The pulse generator output should be matched to the stimulation threshold in the individual patient, and the impulse strength should be set at three to five times the threshold in order to provide a margin of safety. This will compensate for the increase in threshold with time as well as fluctuations due to drugs and physiologic factors. Since the fibrillation threshold generally ranges from 10 to 30 times the stimulation threshold, the stimulus intensity should not be set too high. Consistent long-term pacing may generally be effected by impulses of 2 to 5 mAmp, 2 to 6 volts, and 5 to 20 μjoules.

Important drugs that produce a rise in the stimulation threshold include the following: (1) insulin and glucose in the presence of hypopotassemia (3.9 mEq./L. or less); (2) 3 per cent NaCl; (3) mineralocorticoids (aldosterone and 9-alpha fluorohydrocortisone); (4) diphenylhydantoin; (5) procaine amide, which causes a slight (15 per cent) increase; (6) isoproterenol which, after an initial decrease immediately following its administration, causes a marked rise (56 per cent); and (7) propranolol (increase of 40 to 90 per cent). Propranolol in addition prevents the decrease in the stimulation threshold following exercise as a result of inhibition of catecholamine effects. Commonly used drugs that decrease the stimulation threshold include the following: (1) epinephrine; (2) ephedrine; (3) prednisone; (2) methylprednisone; and (5) dexamethasone. A number of cardioactive drugs have no significant effect on the stimulation threshold, despite their electrophysiologic actions, including: (1) quinidine; (2) digitalis; (3) lidocaine; (4) 10 per cent dextrose; (5) 0.9 per cent NaCl; (6) calcium gluconate; and (7) hydrocortisone (since it has both mineralocorticoid and glucocorticoid effects.

Moreover, various everyday physiologic alterations, such as eating, sleeping, and exercise, have an effect on the stimulation threshold. Minute-to-minute variations in the stimulation threshold as a result of these commonplace events may in borderline situations be significant in precipitating episodes of pacemaker malfunction or pacemaker-induced arrhythmias.

TEMPORARY PACING

Temporary pacing of the heart may be required as an emergency procedure and is also employed on an elective basis in certain situations. Because initiation of pacing without delay is often crucial and since temporary pacing, by definition, is employed for only a matter of days or weeks, the pacemakers used for this purpose are either completely external or only partially implanted. Partially implanted models consist of an external impulse generator with endocardial or myocardial electrodes in direct contact with the heart (Figs. 37–1, 37–2).

Indications. The most urgent indications for temporary pacing, which require the immediate initiation of stimulation, are: (1) Stokes-Adams attack (see Chapter 16) (Fig. 37–3); and (2) third degree A-V heart block occurring during cardiac surgery or acute myocardial infarction (see Chapters 10 and 28). Pacing is most rapidly instituted by use of an external pacemaker or by percutaneous insertion of electrodes into the right ventricle. This latter technique is rarely employed because of the serious complications it

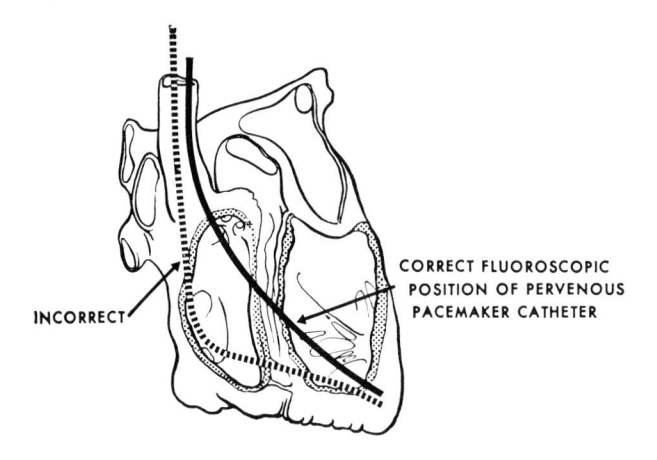

Figure 37-1. Correct and incorrect catheter angles in the right heart. (From Allen, P. R., and Rotem, C. E.: Ann. Thorac. Surg., 8:146, 1969.)

entails and because safer methods are available. In less urgent situations, when it is safe to delay the initiation of pacing for 15 minutes or longer, it is preferable to use an external impulse generator attached to electrodes that reach the ventricular endocardium by way of the antecubital vein. Situations in which this form of temporary pacing are indicated include the following: (1) preparation prior to insertion or replacement of a permanent pacemaker; (2) for prophylaxis in patients who have bradyarrhythmias of any type and are undergoing operation, including thoracotomy for insertion of myocardial electrodes; (3) for suppression of arrhythmias following open heart surgery, electrode wires may be attached to the atria or ventricles at surgery, enabling the pacing of these patients from either the atrial or the ventricular site; this provides optimal antiarrhythmic and hemodynamic benefits; (4) to suppress tachyarrhythmias, which are unresponsive to

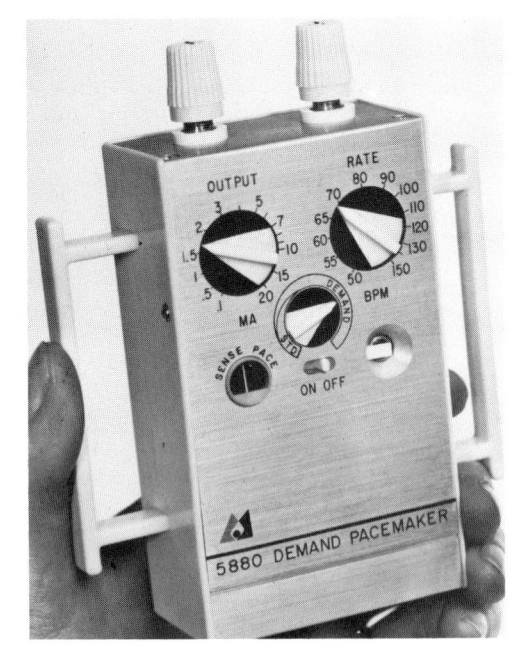

Figure 37-2. An external demand pacemaker for temporary use. The output and rate ranges are clearly indicated. The electrodes are placed in the heart pervenously or percutaneously and attached to the pulse generator. The handles provide for easy attachment to the patient's arm or waist. (Manufactured by Medtronic, Inc., Minneapolis, Minn.)

ARTIFICIAL PACEMAKERS

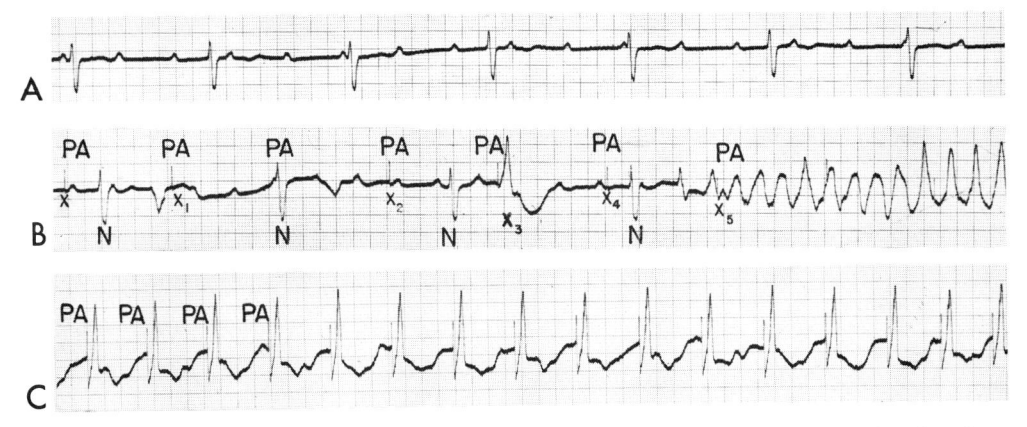

Figure 37-3. Shows the effect of artificial pacemaker in complete A-V heart block and Stokes-Adams syndrome.

(A) (Control) Complete A-V block (atrial rate 94 per minute, ventricular rate 36 per minute).

(B) Note failure of pacemaker to take over ventricular pacemaking at X, X_1, X_2; it produces a beat at X_3; it fails again at X_4. Note inception of ventricular flutter at X_5.

(C) Voltage of stimulation was increased and pacemaker (PA) takes over at 79 per minute.

drugs and countershock. If these are repetitive, a permanent pacemaker may be necessary.

Overdrive Suppression. When atrial tachyarrhythmias such as atrial flutter, paroxysmal atrial tachycardia, junctional and reciprocating tachycardias are refractory to drug therapy and electric countershock, cardiosuppression through rapid atrial or ventricular pacing is often successful. This is achieved by fixed-rate atrial pacing set in competition with the ectopic pacemaker. The tachyarrhythmia may be terminated by one of several mechanisms: (1) The atria may be captured by the artificial pacemaker firing at a rate higher than the spontaneous one. This may produce overdrive suppression of the ectopic pacemaker and establish normal sinus rhythm when the artificial pacemaker is turned off (Fig. 37-4). Similarly, ventricular tachyarrhythmias may be terminated with

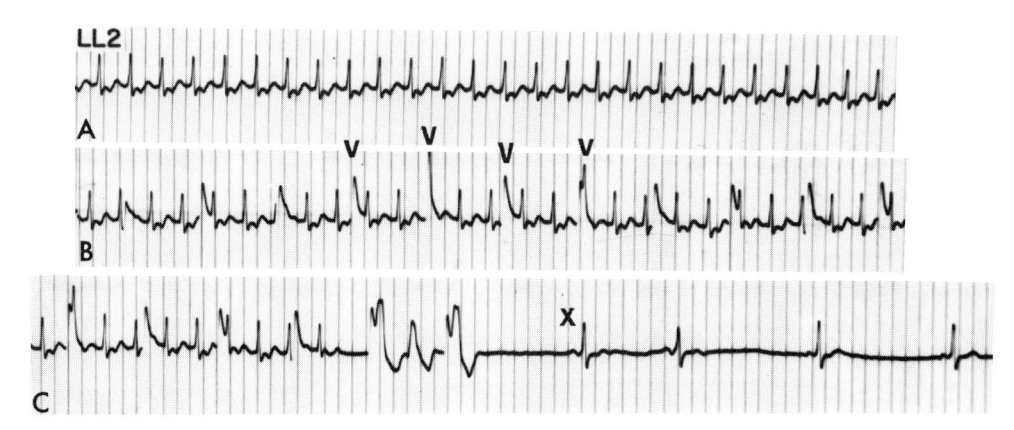

Figure 37-4. Overdrive pacing for atrial tachycardia occurring in association with the W-P-W syndrome.

(A) Supraventricular tachycardia with a rate of 144 per minute.

(B) Ventricular overdrive suppression (v) (rate 100 per minute).

(C) Note return to normal sinus rhythm at complexes marked X.

atrial or ventricular pacing by overdrive suppression of the ectopic focus. (2) Another mechanism of action of overdrive which may be operative is the release of acetylcholine. (3) Suppression of ectopic activity can be obtained by using pacemaker rates above the spontaneous sinus rate but below the rate of the ectopic tachycardia, by altering the rate of ventricular repolarization, duration of diastole, and length of the refractory period.

PERMANENT PACING

Long-term pacing may be achieved by several types of fully-implanted artificial pacemakers. The electrode placement in the patient depends upon the operative approach; systems using myocardial electrodes require thoracotomy and general anesthesia, while transvenous electrodes can be implanted under local anesthesia. The operative techniques have been described by Chardack (1969), Furman and Escher (1970), Siddons and Sowton (1967), Thalen et al. (1969), and others. A variety of pulse generators can be used in combination with the electrode systems, allowing the physician to choose the most beneficial site, schedule, and rate of stimulation for each patient.

Indications. The indications for permanent cardiac pacing are continually undergoing revision. The most common include: (1) prophylaxis against Stokes-Adams attacks, (2) symptomatic relief in complete A-V heart block, (3) persistent second degree A-V heart block following acute myocardial infarction, (4) persistent and symptomatic bradycardia, (5) certain cases of bifascicular block, (6) carotid sinus syncope, (7) atrial fibrillation with a slow ventricular rate to permit adequate digitalization, and (8) oversuppression for occasional cases of refractory tachyarrhythmias (Figs. 37–5, 37–6).

Sites of Electrode Placement. Pacemaker electrodes may be placed in the myocardium surgically by means of a thoracotomy; however, the most common type of electrode placement employed at present is the endocardial type, which is accomplished transvenously.

Endocardial Placement. An endocardial electrode is inserted through a peripheral vein and positioned in the right ventricle. This method has the great advantage of avoiding operative exposure of the heart; moreover, electrode replacement or correction of malposition, often necessary, can be easily performed without thoracotomy.

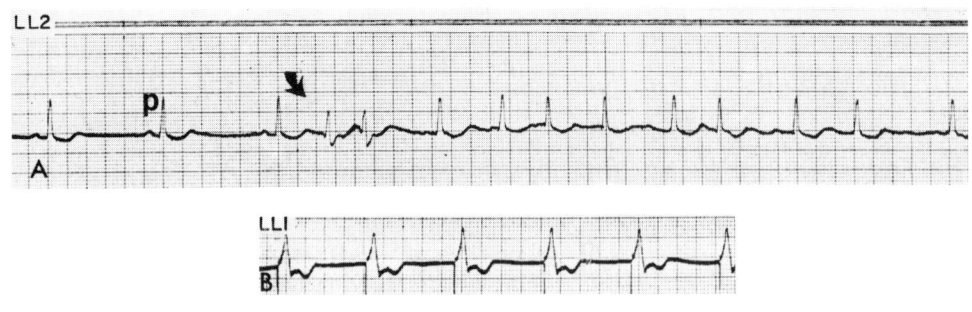

Figure 37–5. Artificial pacemaker for frequent episodes of paroxysmal atrial fibrillation. These produced intense discomfort and anxiety.
(A) Note the occurrence of sinus rhythm with episode of atrial fibrillation starting at arrow.
(B) Pacemaker inserted showing a regular rate which was maintained with loss of cardiac manifestations (palpitation and precordial discomfort).

ARTIFICIAL PACEMAKERS

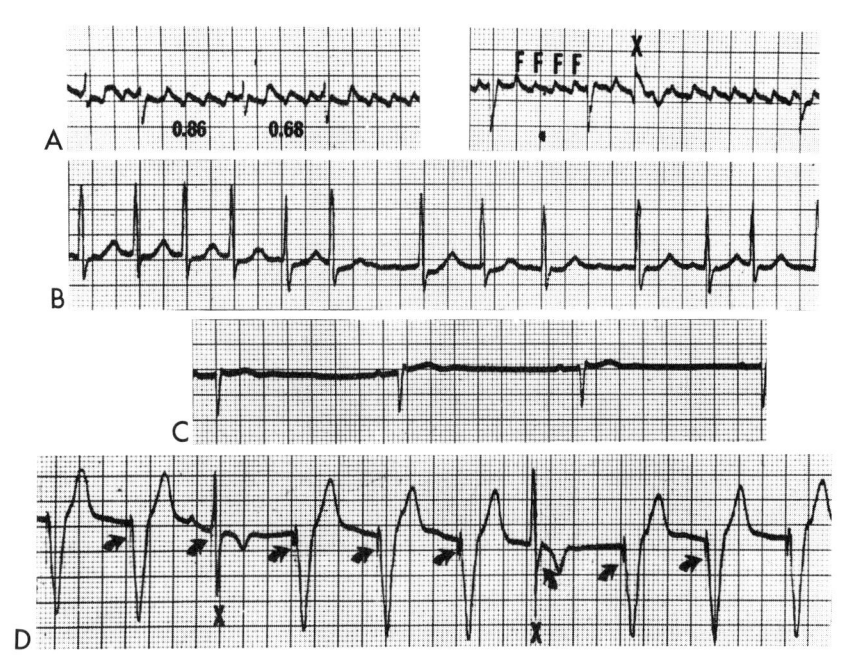

Figure 37-6. Use of pacemaker in treating brady-tachyarrhythmias. Tracing taken from a patient, 71 years of age, with episodes of coronary insufficiency that occurred at rapid ventricular rates and dizziness that occurred with slow heart rates.

(A) The first strip shows atrial flutter with varying degrees of A-V heart block (note cycle lengths). The second strip shows an aberrant beat at X.

(B) Atrial flutter-fibrillation. The initial five cycles show a rapid rate averaging 150 per minute. Thereafter, it becomes somewhat slower.

(C) Sinus bradycardia with normal sinus rhythm with a heart rate of 37 per minute.

(D) After insertion of a fixed-rate pacemaker (rate = 86 beats per minute), the dizzy spells disappeared; the patient was able to take digitalis, which improved the heart failure. At X is a normal beat. Remaining widened QRS complexes are the result of the pacemaker; note the stimulus artifact (arrows).

The electrode catheter is passed via the external or internal jugular vein and when positioned near the apex of the right ventricle (see Fig. 37-1) is fixed with sutures at the neck. The cephalic vein on either side may also be used. Very fine insulated wires with small electrode tips have recently been introduced and are positioned by a blind technique in which the electrode is placed in a peripheral vein and advances slowly so that the blood flow sweeps the tip through the right ventricle. Final positioning of the tip is accomplished by monitoring the electrocardiogram recorded from an intracavity lead in the same wire. The peripheral end of the electrode is then connected to the impulse generator, which is usually implanted beneath the breast. Because of the high risk of electrode displacement soon after insertion and the potentially serious consequences of unexpected cessation of pacing, the electrocardiogram should be monitored continuously for several days after electrode implantation.

Bipolar electrode stimulation, with both an anode and a cathode in the catheter tip in the heart, is most commonly employed, but unipolar stimulation, with the cathode placed at the heart and the anode placed in the subcutaneous tissue near the pulse generator, has also proven quite satisfactory.

Myocardial Electrode Placement. A

less commonly used method for long-term pacing is the implanted pacemaker with the electrodes positioned epicardially by thoracotomy (Fig. 37–7). The left ventricle is exposed by a limited anterior thoracotomy incision and the electrodes placed to just penetrate the myocardium. The electrodes may also be sewn into the left atrial appendage for atrial pacing or for sensing atrial activity in synchronous ("P" triggered) pacing. The electrodes may be bipolar or unipolar; unipolar types require an indifferent electrode that is usually placed close to the pacemaker implanted in the abdominal or chest wall.

Atrial Pacing. Atrial electrode placement has several hemodynamic and electrophysiologic advantages over ventricular pacing. First, experimental and clinical evidence indicates that atrial systole contributes significantly to ventricular filling by augmenting the stroke volume and cardiac output; this is of considerable help in subjects with myocardial derangement (see Chapter 3). Secondly, when the excitation process follows a normal sequence in the ventricles, a synchronized ventricular contraction results. Thirdly, if competitive rhythms occur between the pacemaker and an intrinsic atrial focus, ventricular fibrillation will be no more likely than when atrial premature beats occur (see Chapter 8).

The types of atrial electrodes vary with acute (or transient) and permanent placement. In transient atrial placement, a catheter electrode is passed pervenously into the atrium. This at present is not suitable for extended or permanent use because the electrode is not securely attached and can be dislodged relatively easily. It has been shown that transvenous pacemaker electrodes positioned in the atrium in this manner, however, are adequate for temporary pacing and produce the expected hemodynamic benefits for a short period of time. Permanent atrial pacing may be accomplished by a fish-hook electrode; however, this is not too satisfactory for long periods. The best procedure is

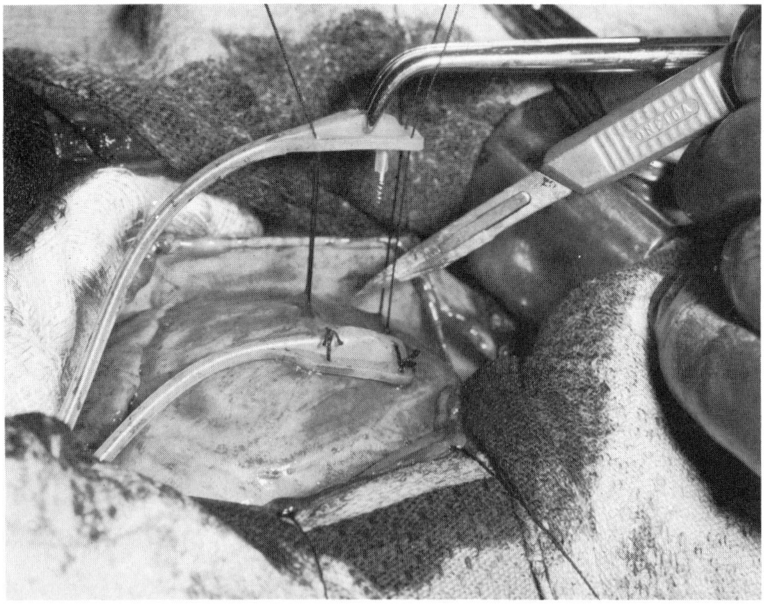

Figure 37–7. Insertion of a myocardial electrode. (From Chardack, W. M., and Greatbatch, W. *In* Gibbon, J. H., Jr., Sabiston, D. C., Jr., and Spencer, F. C., Surgery of the Chest, 2nd Ed. W. B. Saunders, 1969.)

affected by sewing the electrode to the left atrial appendage through a small thoracotomy incision.

Because of the difficulties in permanent atrial pacing, various methods have been devised. An interesting one consists in the *permanent pervenous atrial pacing from the coronary vein,* recently reported by Kramer and Moss (1970). This has been used in symptomatic bradycardia and in the bradycardia-tachycardia syndrome. There was no evidence of pacemaker perforation or coronary vein thrombosis.

Atrial pacing is indicated in the following situations: (1) marked sinus bradycardia; (2) passive A-V junctional bradyarrhythmias resulting from slow atrial rates incident to sluggish and sick sinus syndromes; (3) bradycardia following cardiac surgery including transplantation in which autonomic innervation to the S-A node is disrupted; (4) carotid sinus syncope; (5) sinoatrial heart block; (6) overdrive suppression; (7) termination of PAT, atrial flutter, and certain arrhythmias due to digitalis toxicity; and (8) augmentation of cardiac output in the presence of complete A-V heart block. Atrial pacing may *not* be advantageous in certain cases, especially in older patients with arteriosclerotic heart disease and the sick sinus syndrome, since a high percentage (70 per cent) of these patients manifest or tend to develop A-V junctional disturbances. It has been estimated that as many as two-thirds of patients in the older age group with sinoatrial or atrial disease have concomitant disease of the A-V junction. Therefore, if A-V conduction defects occur during artificial pacing at rates below 130 beats per minute, atrial pacing is contraindicated. In these cases, ventricular pacing is preferable; sequential pacing or bifocal demand pacing may be advantageous because atrial pacing continues as long as A-V junctional conduction is adequate, but when it is not, ventricular demand pacing is automatically initiated.

Types of Implanted Pulse Generators. Several types of pulse generators are available to meet the requirements for optimal pacing, namely: (1) a discharge rate suitable to the patient; (2) avoidance (within feasible limits) of competitive rhythms; and (3) capacity for rate change in patients who may benefit from it. The principal types of pulse generators that are used to accomplish these goals are: (1) fixed-rate (asynchronous) models, which ordinarily stimulate the ventricle but may also be used for atrial pacing; (2) atrial-triggered (synchronous) models, which follow the patient's own sinus rate by detecting atrial activity and discharging an impulse to the ventricles after an artificial P-R interval; and (3) ventricular-programmed pacemakers (comprising the "demand" and "standby" types), which detect the R wave and discharge their impulses on a schedule that avoids competition of rhythms.

Fixed-rate (Asynchronous) Pacemakers. These are the oldest and most stable type of artificial pacemaker; however, these are generally being supplanted by the demand types (see p. 413). Their great reliability results from simple circuitry and very low battery drain. The pulse generator discharges at a pre-set constant rate that is independent of and may compete with the intrinsic cardiac rhythm.

Atrial-triggered or "Synchronous" Pacemakers. As a result of the recently accumulated data on the important role of atrial contraction in increasing stroke volume and cardiac output and other advantages, a pacemaker was devised in which the pulse generator is triggered by the P wave; this is sensed by a separate electrode attached to the atrium (Benchimol and Liggett, 1966). After a delay of 0.12 second (artificial "P-R interval"), the pacemaker delivers a stimulating impulse to the ventricle (Fig. 37–8). The atrial-triggered pacemaker functions as an electronic A-V conduction sys-

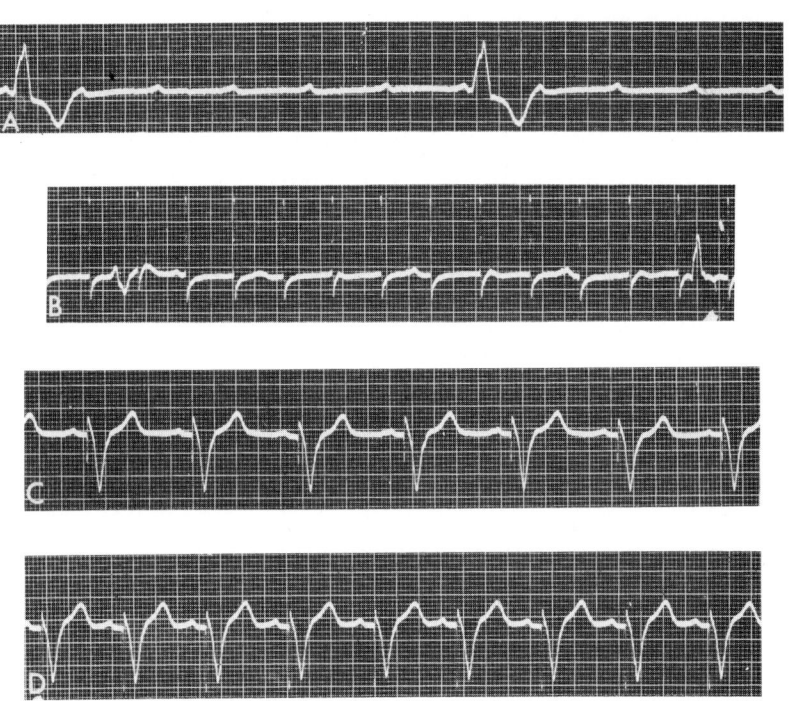

Figure 37-8. The use of the synchronized pacemaker (activation of the ventricles from the atria). Seventy-three-year-old man with arteriosclerotic heart disease, complete A-V heart block since 1959; pacer implanted 8/24/62.

(A) Complete A-V heart block. (B) Intracardiac electrocardiogram showing positive atrial potentials. (C) Synchronization, atrial and ventricular rate of 63 per minute. (D) Synchronization—after exercise, atrial and ventricular rate 80 per minute. (From Nathan, D. A., Center, S., Wu, C., and Keller, W.: Amer. J. Cardiol., *11*:362, 1963.)

tem with a pre-set P-R interval. Provisions have been made so that rapid supraventricular rates such as occur with PAT, atrial flutter or atrial fibrillation are not transmitted to the ventricles. Most synchronous pacemakers develop a 2:1 block when the atrial rate exceeds 110 to 120 beats per minute and a 3:1 block when the rate exceeds 180 beats per minute. Conversely, atrial-triggered pacemakers must be able to compensate for sinus bradycardia or sinus arrest if that situation should arise. Synchronous pacemakers therefore must be set for a critical rate at which to take over if no atrial impulse is detected; usually, they are pre-set to discharge at a fixed minimal rate of about 60 per minute if the atrial rate falls below this level (i.e., if the atrial cycle length exceeds 1.0 second).

Synchronous pacemakers offer the following advantages over the fixed-rate units: (a) the cardiac output may be varied according to demand by changes in rate as well as stroke volume; (b) they do not give rise to a parasystolic focus if A-V conduction should resume and therefore they tend to avoid one of the most serious complications ascribed to artificial pacing, namely, ventricular fibrillation and sudden death; and (c) they coordinate atrial systole with ventricular diastole, preserving the atrial contribution to ventricular filling.

Some of the disadvantages of this system include the more complicated mechanism which presents a greater possibility for malfunction and a shorter battery life and the fact that insertion of the atrial sensing electrode presently requires thoracotomy. A common finding is that, although synchrony is observed immediately following pacemaker implantation, the device later reverts intermittently to fixed-rate asynchronous firing in as many as 50 per cent of patients. In any case, the ability to increase the heart rate has little value in patients whose exercise tolerance is severely restricted by their underlying disease. Furthermore, the number of patients in whom this type may be used is limited because patients subject to attacks of supraventricular tachycardia, atrial flutter, or fibrillation are not ideally suitable for this type of pacemaker. In recent years, this type of pacemaker has been less popular, and it has generally been supplanted by the various demand types of pacemaker.

Ventricular-programmed ("Demand" and "Standby") Pacemakers. These types of pacemakers were devised to avoid the problem of competitive rhythms. All types of ventricular-programmed pacemakers employ a single ventricular electrode, which both senses the R wave and stimulates the ventricle. There are two basic varieties of ventricular-programmed pacemakers. The true "demand" pacemaker is inhibited by the intrinsic R wave and supplies impulses only when the intrinsic R-R interval (ventricular cycle length) exceeds a predetermined duration. The second variety of ventricular-programmed pacemaker is the "standby" pacemaker. The impulse generator is triggered by the R wave and immediately discharges an impulse, which falls into the naturally occurring QRS complex. If after a pre-set interval a QRS complex does not occur, the pacemaker initiates an impulse. Both the "demand" and the "standby" pacemaker are similar in that they avoid "competition" under most circumstances and they revert to fixed-rate firing in the presence of a slow intrinsic rate.

VENTRICULAR-INHIBITED ("DEMAND") PACEMAKER. The most commonly employed ventricular-programmed pacemaker is a fixed-rate asynchronous pacemaker which operates as any other fixed-rate unit when the inherent rate is slow. However, a sensor in the pacing electrode (which can be either epicardial or endocardial) detects and follows the QRS of the electrocardiogram. When the intrinsic ventricular rate becomes more rapid than the pre-set rate of the pacemaker, an inhibitory circuit is activated which blocks any further stimulus discharge until the ventricular rate once more falls below the critical level.

VENTRICULAR-TRIGGERED ("STANDBY") PACEMAKERS. The "standby" pacemaker employs a single electrode placed in the ventricle to detect spontaneous ventricular activity and to deliver the pacemaker impulses. If a spontaneous R wave is detected within a predetermined cycle length (R-R interval) after the preceding beat, the pacemaker discharges an impulse immediately. If the impulse falls in the absolute refractory period of the intrinsic ventricular complex or refractory period of the pacemaker, no beat occurs. If, however, no R wave is detected within the predetermined cycle length (R-R interval after the preceding beat), the pacemaker discharges an impulse immediately, thus assuring a minimal ventricular rate (Fig. 37–9).

Bifocal Demand Pacing. Although ventricular pacing remains the most popular method of increasing the heart rate in symptomatic patients with bradycardia, recent advances have been directed toward increasing the hemodynamic benefits of pacing while at the same time eliminating the various problems encountered in the other types of pulse generators. Bifocal (sequential A-V) demand pacing employs a pulse generator which combines a ventricular demand pacemaker with a QRS-inhibited atrial demand pacemaker, each having separate escape rates so that the unit may be dormant or may stimulate either the atria or the atria and ventricles. An endocardial ventricular electrode both monitors the ventricular electrical activity and delivers the ventricular stimulus while a transvenously positioned atrial electrode (with a special J-shaped end) serves to stimulate these chambers. If, as in a case of sinus bradycardia with normal A-V conduction, the sensing electrode does not detect a QRS complex within 600 msec. (atrial escape limit), an impulse is delivered to the atria. The ventricular escape rate is set at 72 beats per minute (R-R interval of 840 msec.), so that if the atrial impulse is conducted normally through the A-V junction (i.e., in less than 240 msec.), the artificial ventricular pacemaker impulse is inhibited; but if A-V junctional disease is present and the atrial impulse is blocked, a ventricular impulse is delivered at 840 msec. (Fig. 37–10). The hemodynamic benefit of sequential atrial contraction, which may be extremely important with severe myocardial disease (e.g.,

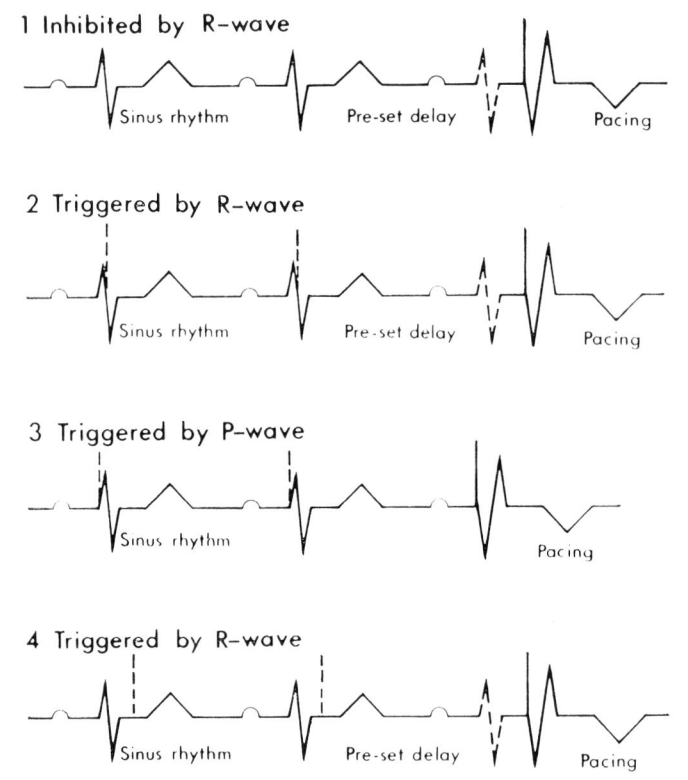

Figure 37–9. Diagrammatic representation of four types of pacing that avoid competing rhythms. (1) Pacemaker is inhibited by spontaneous QRS, but stimulates at a fixed rate if QRS does not occur. (2) Pacemaker is triggered by spontaneous QRS and delivers an ineffective stimulus; if no QRS appears the pacemaker stimulates the ventricle at a fixed rate. (3) Atrial-triggered pacemaker detecting spontaneous atrial activity and stimulating ventricle after a fixed delay equivalent to the P-R interval; in sinus rhythm the stimulus is ineffective. If no atrial potential is detected the pacemaker stimulates the ventricle at a fixed rate. (4) Atrial-triggered pacemaker arranged with the atrial pick-up electrode on the ventricle instead of the atrium. The pacemaker now functions as a ventricular-triggered pacemaker with a delay between detection of ventricular activity and delivery of the pacing stimulus. If no QRS appears the pacemaker stimulates at a fixed rate. (From Sowton, E.: Brit. Heart J., 30:363, 1968.)

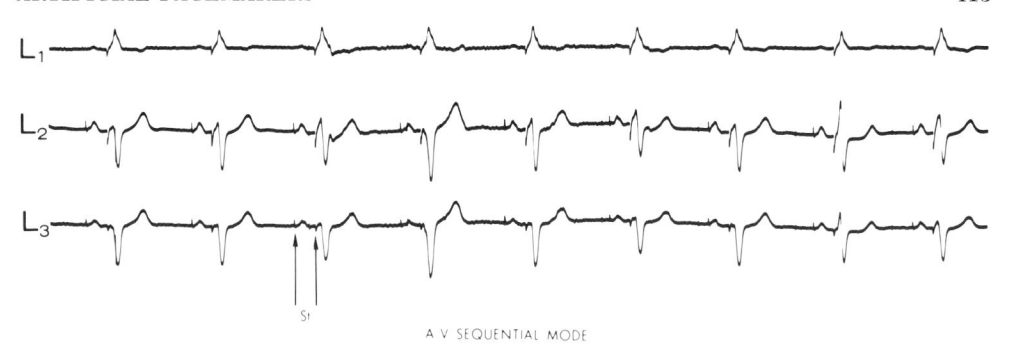

Figure 37-10. A bifocal demand pacemaker operating in the A-V sequential mode. Note the stimuli (ST) preceding both P waves and QRS complexes. The atrial stimuli occur at approximately 600 msec. following the preceding QRS complex. It is followed 240 msec. later by the ventricular stimulus. (Courtesy Dr. B. Berkovits, American Optical Corp.)

myocardial infarction), is maintained in all modes of bifocal demand pacing.

Bifocal pacing is indicated in the following instances: (1) intermittent sinoatrial or atrioventricular block; (2) patients with symptomatic bradycardia with borderline cardiac function in whom atrial transport provides substantial improvement; and (3) elderly patients with sinus bradycardia, sinoatrial block or atrial standstill in whom A-V heart block, although not present at the time of pacemaker implantation, may and often does ensue. This method is still experimental. More experience is required to evaluate its feasibility (Berkovits et al., 1969).

Atomic Power Supply. Several cardiac pacemakers derive their power from a self-contained electrical generator whose energy source is a capsule of plutonium. An alpha particle emitting isotope produces direct current electricity by heating a thermocouple; an electronics package contained in the unit modifies the current to produce the pacemaking impulse. It has been calculated that in 11 years the unit would lose only 8 per cent of its thermal energy. This long-life power supply has necessitated the development of a new pacemaker unit. The unit is 6.0 x 5.0 x 2.8 cm. and weighs 100 g. The materials employed in its construction were chosen on the basis of which would best resist corrosion and shield the radioactivity and which would be the most chemically inert. Two of the completely assembled units have been undergoing tests and have run for 6000 and 3300 hours without failure. Modifications and production of fixed-rate and demand models will permit clinical tests of new units. These pacemakers have been designed so that gradual depletion of the power supply will result in a progressive slowing of the impulse rate, which would be detectable long before the pulse generator fails.

Up to 1971, four patients were maintained on atomic powered pacemakers. These units have been functioning successfully for relatively short periods; thus, conclusions regarding efficacy and safety cannot yet be drawn from these studies. Certain problems confined to the atomic power unit are recognized (e.g., possible radiation of subject and the effect of traumatic disruption of the power supply); others await the result of larger clinical experience.

Hemodynamic Effects of Pacing. The common feature of all the conditions listed as indications for pacemakers is that excessive depression or elevation of the heart rate causes the cardiac output to be suboptimal or inadequate. Since the chief value of a pacemaker is to sustain an adequate cardiac output, the pacemaker should be chosen with an eye to its effects on the hemodynamic status in each individual case.

Hearts paced by a fixed-rate pacemaker are able to vary the cardiac output by change in stroke volume, but with any type of pacemaker, the hemodynamic limits of the heart's response depend upon the underlying condition of the myocardium. Therefore, in a heart with a severely damaged myocardium (Fig. 37–11A) in which cardiac output reaches a maximum (albeit still

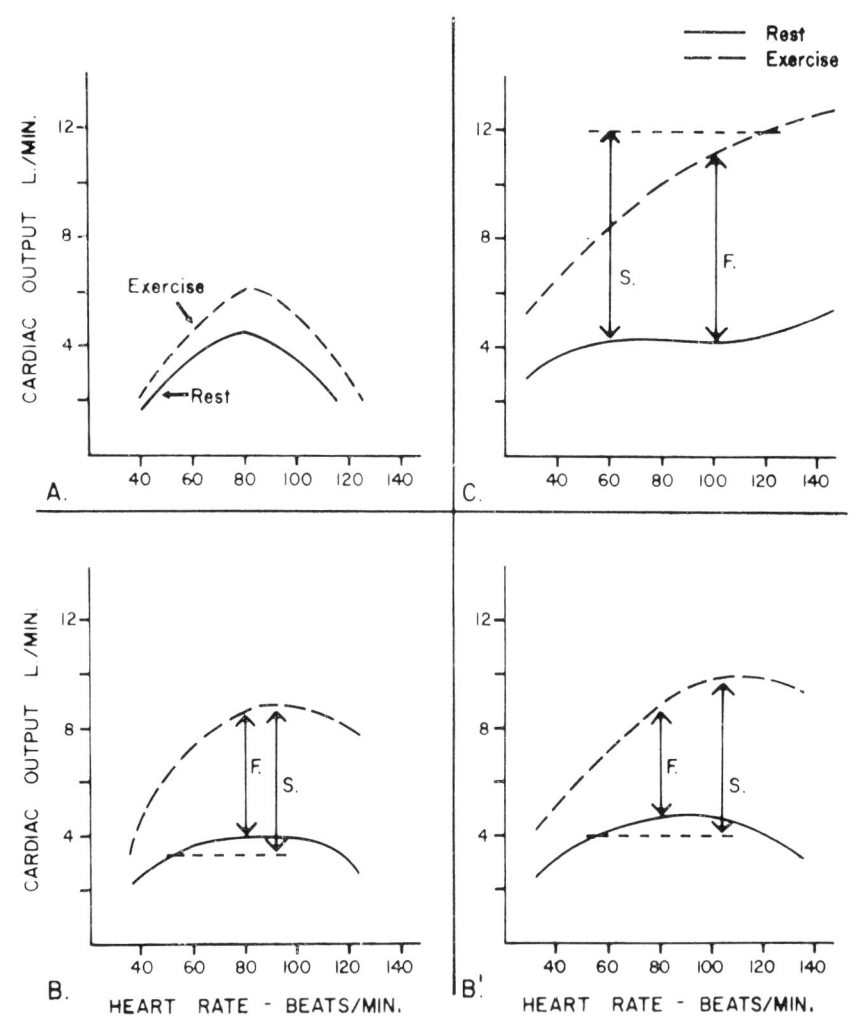

Figure 37–11. Resting and exercise rate-output (C.O.) curves in complete A-V heart block and the effects of cardiac pacing. F, fixed rate pacemaker; S, synchronous pacemaker. The arrows depict the range of C.O. available in each situation with the two types of units. The broken horizontal line represents the minimal or maximal cardiac output with a synchronous pacemaker with a range set at 60 to 120 beats per minute. (A) This patient shows a narrow range of rates in which cardiac output is maximal as a result of severe myocardial abnormality. (C) A nearly normal rate-output relationship. The majority of patients requiring pacemaker therapy fall between A and C and present situations such as (B) and B'. (B) A moderately damaged heart in which the maximal C.O. occurs at a rate of 90 beats per minute whereas in B' a less damaged heart in which the maximal C.O. is attained at a rate of 105 beats per minute. (From McNally, E. M., and Benchimol, A.: Amer. Heart J., 75:679, 1968.)

suboptimal) at a rate of 80 beats per minute, a synchronous pacemaker would clearly be a liability since it could potentially produce dangerously low cardiac outputs (e.g., 2.0 L./minute at 120 beats per minute). Thus, in this case a fixed-rate pacemaker set at 80 beats per minute would supply the maximal hemodynamic benefits. Conversely, in a heart with a healthy myocardium (see Fig. 37–11C), the synchronous pacemaker allows a wide and physiologic range of cardiac outputs and appears more beneficial.

When choosing the appropriate type of pacemaker one must remember that: (1) the optimal increase in cardiac output can usually be obtained at a pacing rate of 60 to 90 beats per minute; (2) patients with good myocardial reserve have the capacity to increase their cardiac output considerably in response to exercise and increased heart rate and may benefit from a pacemaker that gives them this capability; and (3) patients with severe myocardial disease have a narrow range of rates at which cardiac outputs are optimal and should be treated by a pacemaker that keeps the heart rate fixed or within this range.

Problem of Competitive Rhythms. If normal A-V conduction resumes in a patient with an implanted fixed-rate pacemaker, the ventricles will be stimulated by two competing pacemakers: the patient's own supraventricular pacemaker and the artificial pacemaker. This situation is referred to as competitive rhythms, which might result in the initiation of ventricular fibrillation or prefibrillatory arrhythmias. This subject is somewhat controversial; although the theoretical basis exists, the number of clearly documented cases in which this phenomenon has occurred are not numerous. In addition, sudden death in patients with pacemakers may be due to causes other than induced ventricular fibrillation, namely: (1) pacemaker failure, (2) increase in stimulation threshold, (3) circadian rhythms which may change the stimulation and fibrillation thresholds, and (4) the action of certain drugs. In fact, it would not be unexpected that pacemaker failure or causes totally unrelated to the pacemaker may result in sudden death in these patients, because the majority have severe cardiac derangement. Competitively produced ventricular fibrillation is rare and when it does occur, it is associated with one or more of the following conditions: (1) hypoxia, (2) electrolyte imbalance, (3) coronary occlusion, (4) acidosis or alkalosis, or (5) drug toxicity. Nevertheless, some unexplained deaths in paced patients whose pacemakers were functioning properly may be due to such "competition," and the present goal of ventricular programmed pacemaking is to avoid this possible complication (Furman and Escher, 1970; Chardack, 1969).

Cardioactive Drugs and Pacing. Many patients with pacemakers are also being treated with cardioactive drugs of various types. The hemodynamic and electrophysiologic effects of these agents in conjunction with artificial pacing may be different than their effects in the nonpaced patient; certain agents may be harmful and others particularly beneficial. Digitalis, quinidine, procaine amide, and lidocaine may be used for their ordinary indications and with normal precautions without significant effect on pacemaker function. Isoproterenol, while increasing the cardiac index and increased tissue-oxygen demand, has adverse effects upon the energy level required for pacing and should be used cautiously.

Clinical Results with Artificial Pacing. The reports of numerous investigators reviewing large series of patients have established the effectiveness of long-term artificial cardiac pacing in the treatment of the symptoms of complete A-V heart block and the Stokes-Adams syndrome. In addition, it is generally agreed that the artificial pacemaker also significantly increases survival (Fig. 37–12).

Recently, the reports of several groups (Edhag, 1969; Goldstein et al., 1970; Harthorne et al., 1969; Johansson, 1969; Torresani et al., 1969), comprising a total of 1200 patients with pacemakers who have been followed for at least 12 months, had a one-year mortality rate of 12.4 per cent. The five-year survival rate in this group was approximately 50 per cent. This latter survival rate must, however, be viewed in the context of the average mortality rate of 10 per cent per year (a five-year survival rate of 59 per cent) in the age group (>60 years) being considered. The life expectancy of patients in this age group is now within 10 per cent of that of a normal population of comparable age and sex. In contrast, the one-year mortality for patients with complete A-V heart block treated medically is 50 to 60 per cent (Friedberg et al., 1964; Johansson, 1966).

When pacemakers are employed in the therapy of arrhythmias associated with acute myocardial infarction, the severity and location of the infarction must be taken into account when considering the prognosis. Pacing does not appreciably affect the prognosis in anterior infarction complicated by complete A-V heart block. In one study, only three of 19 of the patients left the hospital and none survived one year, whereas 24 of 32 patients with inferior infarctions complicated by complete A-V heart block left the hospital and 22 survived at least one year (Julian et al., 1969).

The Prognosis of Triggered and Fixed-rate Pacemakers. It had been anticipated that noncompetitive pacemakers would prolong longevity and reduce patient mortality and rates compared to the asynchronous types.

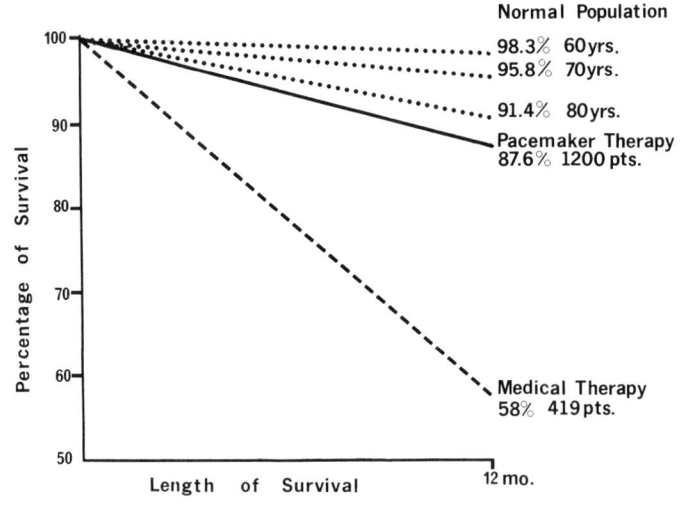

Figure 37–12. The effect of pacemaker therapy in complete A-V heart block. The graph depicts the one-year survival rates of patients with complete A-V heart block treated medically or with pacemakers compared with the survival rates for the healthy population at ages 60, 70, and 80. The data on medical therapy was compiled from Friedberg et al.: Ann. N.Y. Acad. Sci., *111*:85, 1964; and Johansson: Ann. N.Y. Acad. Sci., *167*:1031, 1969 and Acta Med. Scand., *180*, Supp. 451, 1966. The data on the pacemaker therapy was compiled from Johansson: Ann. N.Y. Acad. Sci., *167*, 1031, 1969; Edhag: Acta Med. Scand. (Supp.), 502, 1969; Torresani et al.: Ann. N.Y. Acad. Sci., *167*:995, 1969; Hawthorne et al.: Circulation, *40*:III–102, 1969; and Goldstein et al.: Brit. Heart J., *32*:35, 1970. The data on the normal population was compiled from the Society of Actuaries Basic Tables.

The ventricular inhibited (demand) pacemaker was also anticipated to have a greater longevity in the presence of A-V conduction since long periods might elapse when only the pacemaker-sensing circuit would be operative (Furman et al., 1971a). Recent data (Furman et al., 1971a) has shown that the mortality rates are equal to those of asynchronous pacemakers, and pacemaker longevity has been somewhat shorter. This is due to problems that exist uniquely to triggered pacemakers, namely, electromagnetic interference, pacemaker-induced arrhythmias, and inadequacies in sensing physiologic signals with bipolar electrodes (Furman et al., 1971a). These factors contribute to the complications observed with this type of pacemaker.

Complications of Pacing. The main problems of this type of therapy are: (1) pacemaker-induced arrhythmias (Fig. 37-13), (2) electrode disruption, (3) pacemaker failure, either electrical or mechanical, and (4) physical problems with the implanted pulse generator. Although the mortality from complete A-V heart block has been dramatically reduced by the use of pacemakers, the mortality and morbidity of pacemaker therapy may be itself decreased by an awareness of the complications and the means of correcting them. The incidence and seriousness of such occurrences may be reduced by: (1) the use of properly designed equipment; (2) adherence to careful technique during implantation; (3) periodic examination of the patient and pacemaker system; and (4) techniques for early detection of complications.

Arrhythmias with Specific Types of Pacemaker. Iatrogenically produced arrhythmias in paced patients may be due to interaction between intrinsic cardiac automatic tissue and a normally functioning pacemaker, or they may be a manifestation of abnormal pacemaker function that portends impending failure of the instrument. Persistent ectopic ventricular beats may result from irritation by the catheter electrode and may arise spontaneously. If they persist, they may be treated with quinidine, procaine amide, propranolol, or lidocaine. Right bundle branch block may be an early transient complication of transvenous pacemaking.

Asynchronous (fixed-rate) pacemakers may cause A-V dissociation phenomena with aberrant ventricular conduction when the pacemaker impulse is discharged at the end of the absolute refractory period, and isorhythmic dissociation when pacemaker and intrinsic rhythms are similar. The abnormal ventricular complexes may be similar to those seen with the W-P-W syndrome. Furthermore, when a patient's intrinsic rhythm returns following implantation of an artificial pacemaker, the rhythm produced will be parasystole.

Demand pacemakers may produce: "escape capture bigeminy," in which a pacemaker-induced escape beat is followed by a supraventricular beat; trigeminy, in which a supraventricular beat is followed by a fusion beat and a pacemaker beat or by two pacemaker beats; a "pacemaker induced ventriculophasic sinus arrhythmia," in which the P wave following a pacemaker beat occurs earlier than expected; "postextrasystolic pacemaker escape," wherein the compensatory pause that usually follows a premature beat does not occur in the presence of a pacemaker whose escape interval is shorter than the compensatory pause; and the "concertina effect," in which progressive changes in the QRS configuration manifest themselves as a gradual increase and decrease in the height and width of the QRS complex. This latter electrocardiographic pattern is due to progressively greater amounts of ventricular myocardium undergoing premature excitation.

When an unexpected irregularity

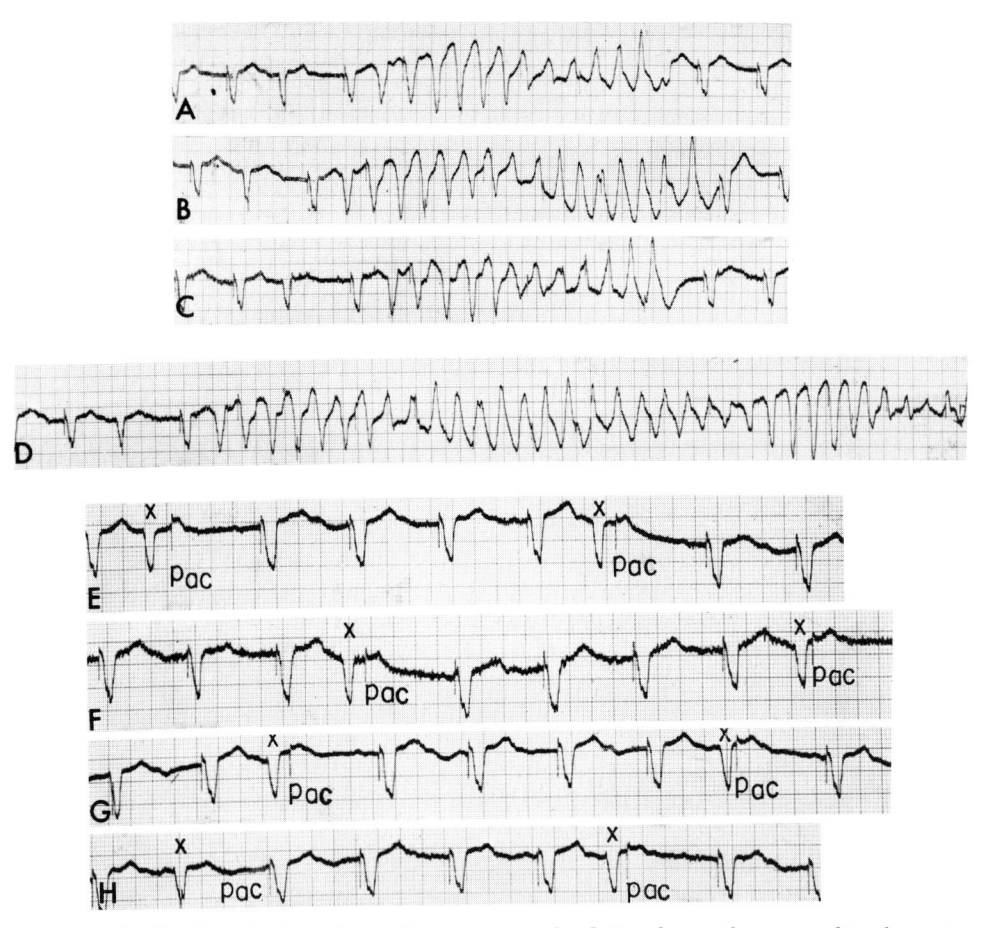

Figure 37–13. Ventricular tachycardia and ventricular flutter during the pacemaking by an implantable pacemaker. This patient, age 70, had many Stokes-Adams seizures with a complete A-V heart block; an implantable pacemaker was inserted two weeks prior to this tracing. The pacemaker produced ventricular impulses at 75 per minute. Ten days after the pacemaker had been implanted and had been working quite well, the patient developed episodes of ventricular tachycardia.

(A, B, C, and D) Show the beginning and ending of episodes of paroxysmal ventricular tachycardia. During the episodes the blood pressure fell to 60/40, and the patient appeared to be in a state of shock. She was given procaine amide (0.5 gm. q.i.d. intravenously), following which the ventricular tachycardia disappeared; however, occasional ventricular ectopic beats persisted.

(E) Shows the resumption of a slow ventricular rate and the occurrence of occasional premature ventricular beats; a single one occurs at a time.

(E, F, G, and H) Note that the pacemaker captures the ventricular beat except in the cycles marked X. When the stimulus occurs during the absolute refractory period (Pac), no ventricular beat results.

in rhythm occurs during pacing, one should determine whether this is due to pacemaker failure or to one of the variations of normal pacemaking function. The pauses that appear with normal pacemaking may be due to the escape interval (860 to 1000 msec.) or to failure of the demand pacemaker to sense an early premature beat. In order to avoid recycling of demand pacemakers by the QRS or T wave of the preceding beat, a refractory period is included in their mode of operation. A QRS occurring within the refractory period does not block the subsequent pacer impulse. The refractory period varies with the type of pacemaker. When the refractory period of the pacemaker is long (over 400 msec.), early spontaneous premature beats may fall in the refractory period and not be detected; bigeminy may thus result. When the refractory period is short (below 200 msec.), an early premature systole may be detected and considered as a beat by the pacemaker although it may be ineffective in producing a peripheral pulse.

Pacemaker-induced arrhythmias may produce few symptoms, but they make the patient's status more difficult to assess, and they may precipitate more serious arrhythmias.

Complications of Catheter Electrodes. The most common cause of pacing failure has been mechanical disruption of the stimulating electrode. Reports indicate that the use of more flexible wires now available are more favorable. Displacement of the electrode catheter has been reported in all large series and has an incidence of 10 to 15 per cent. The electrode catheter can perforate the myocardium during intracardiac manipulation. Such instances are usually asymptomatic, but cardiac tamponade has been reported and may require thoracotomy or pericardiocentesis. Late electrode displacement and late myocardial perforation by slow erosion of the ventricular wall have occurred but are relatively infrequent complications.

Pacing Failure. Failure of normal pacing may occur as a result of: (1) electrical failure of the pulse generator; (2) increase in the stimulation threshold above the capacities of the unit; and (3) electrical interference with synchronized units. Any type of pacing unit may fail or discharge at an excessively rapid rate (runaway pacemaker) (Figs. 37–14, 37–15); certain procedures have been developed to detect and correct these situations.

ELECTRICAL FAILURE OF PULSE GENERATORS. Failure of the pulse generator to produce an adequate energy level can be caused by a battery failure or mechanical failure to which all equipment is subject. Battery failure may result from a leak or simply from long use. Certain types of pulse generators (e.g., ventricular-triggered and fixed-rate) place an increased drain on the battery since they are continually active; battery failure is expected sooner in these models. Mechanical failure of the unit itself can be the result of various factors. These are discussed below.

DETECTION OF INCIPIENT PACEMAKER FAILURE (Figs. 37–16, 37–17). The postimplantation management of a patient with a permanent pacemaker should include regular examination of both the patient and the electronic unit and is best accomplished in a pacemaker clinic. An example of a routine system which has been employed to detect incipient pacemaker failure is as follows: (1) a monthly electrocardiogram is taken; (2) the pacemaker rate is measured to three significant decimal figures by an electronic counter; (3) the details of the pacemaker artifact are displayed on a wideband oscilloscope and photographed; and (4) the unit is examined radiologically. This data may be computerized to allow for rapid analysis and to produce a clear, concise, and readily retrieved record. This procedure, or one resembling it, should be followed at three- or four-month intervals immediately following implantation and with increasing regularity after a year. Comparison with previous records can alert one to imminent pacemaker failure so that correction can be instituted rapidly and prior to complete disruption of pacemaker function.

In such a program the patients are seen one week after implantation and at 1, 6, 12, and 15 months and thereafter at monthly intervals until an elective battery change at two years. The routine standard six-lead electrocardiogram is obtained with a long rhythm

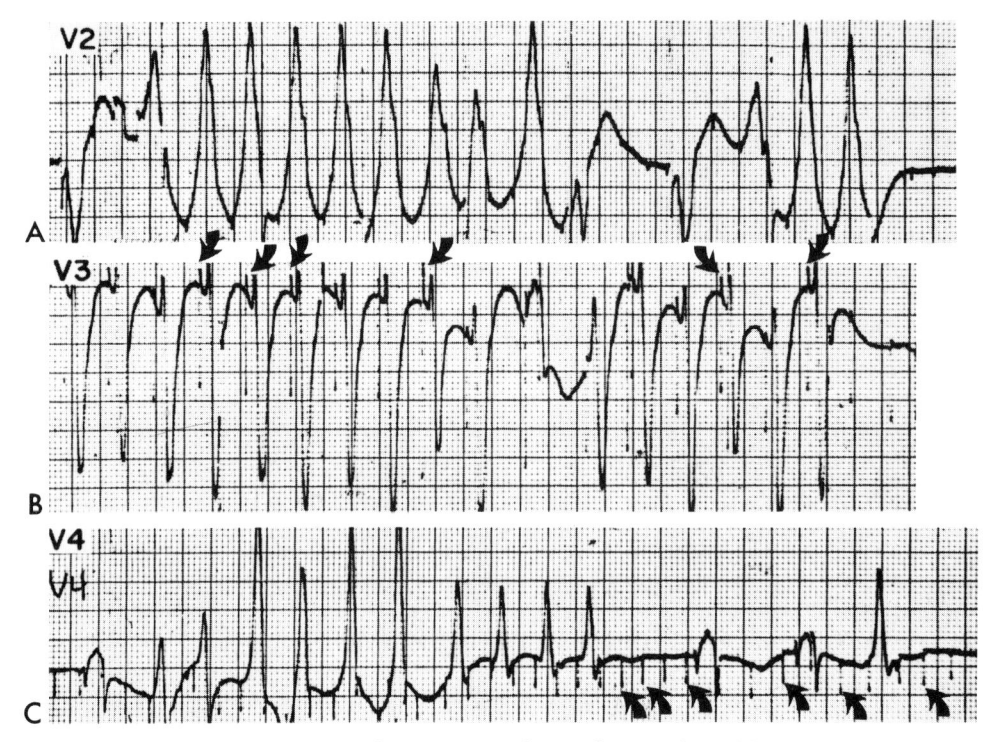

Figure 37-14. Runaway pacemaker; patient with complete A-V heart block on a fixed rate pacemaker. Pacemaker rate was 70 per minute.

(A) Note rapid ventricular complexes, rate 146 per minute.

(B) Note pacemaker artefact (at arrows), rate 187.5 per minute, followed by widened QRS. Note the occurrence of rapid rate in B (160 per minute).

(C) Note pacemaker artefacts (at arrows) most of which are not followed by a ventricular response (rate ranges from 250 to 375 per minute).

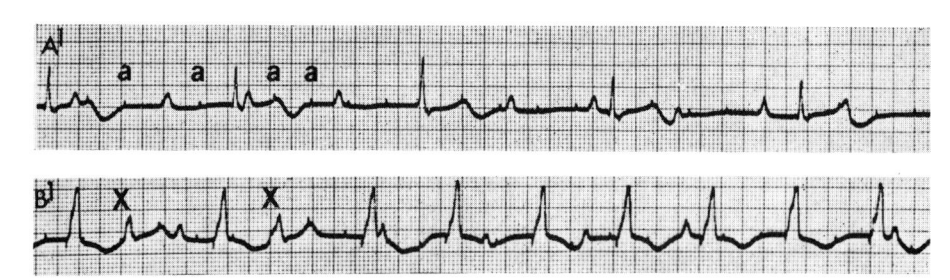

Figure 37-15. Runaway pacemaker in 75-year-old male patient with complete A-V heart block and arteriosclerotic heart disease. Because of battery exhaustion the current is inadequate to produce an effective contraction. A permanent demand pacemaker was implanted four years earlier and the pacing rate set at 72 per minute. Due to exhaustion of the battery, the pacemaker does not deliver adequate energy to stimulate the ventricle. In addition, the rate of the pacemaker was increased to 160 beats per minute (runaway pacemaker) and the demand system was not functioning. In (A¹), note pacemaker artefacts (a) (rate 160 per minute, which fails to activate the ventricle).

(B¹) A transvenous demand pacemaker was inserted in the same patient. It paced at the rate of 75 beats per minute. Note the difference in the ventricular complexes delivered by the new pacemaker which captures the ventricles at 75 per minute. Note that in this tracing stimuli delivered by the old implanted pacemaker at X now produce ventricular complexes when they occur 500 to 580 msec. after the stimulus of the newly inserted transvenous pacemaker. This may be due to supernormality resulting from the Wedensky effect.

ARTIFICIAL PACEMAKERS

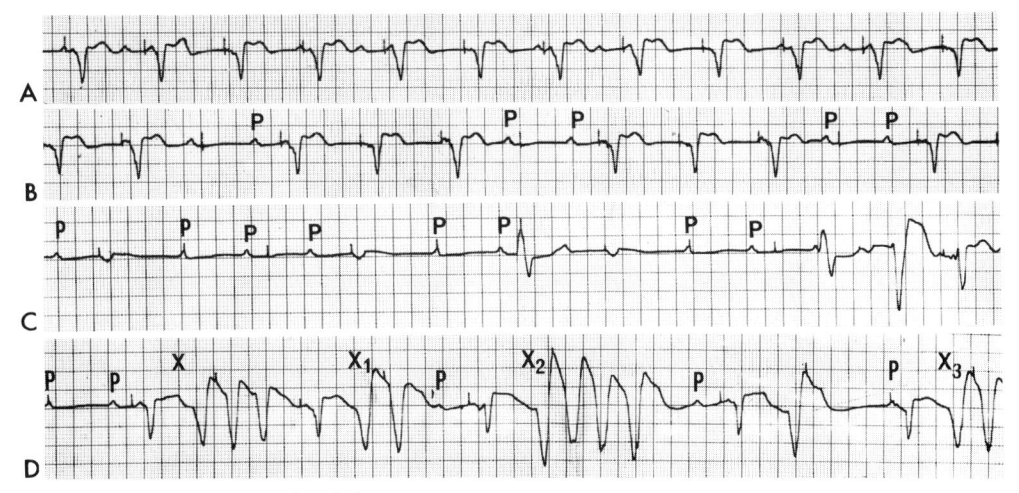

Figure 37–16. Pacemaker failure.
(A) Note the heart rate of 68 per minute with a normal pacemaker artefact.
(B) Shows intermittent failure of ventricular captures with three long cycles of asystole.
(C) Note even longer periods of asystole. The pacemaker fails to capture any of the complexes in this strip.
(D) With continuation of pacemaker failure, note the appearance of numerous ventricular premature beats occurring in groups at X, X_1, X_2, and X_3.

strip. This is compared with previous records for the presence of the pacer artifact and the myocardial response (Q, R, S, T) to each artifact falling in the nonrefractory phase of the cycle. Absence of an artifact confirmed in more than one lead may be due to failure of the pulse generator, a break in the electrode or demand (R wave suppression) response to spontaneous activity. Failure to respond may be a threshold problem due to a battery depletion, current loss from an insulation leak, malposition of an electrode, or increased resistance. Loss of sensor response in triggered pacemakers may be an early sign of battery depletion, malfunction of the pulse generator or malposition of the electrodes (Escher and Furman, 1971).

The electronic evaluation of the stimulus artifact is studied in Lead I; this refers to the shape, amplitude, duration, polarity, and repetition rate of the stimulus artifact. The artifact is visualized on an oscilloscope with a

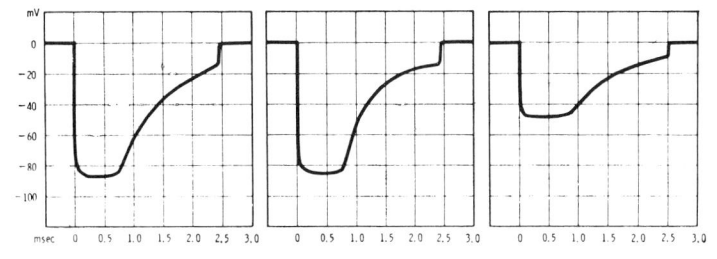

Figure 37–17. Monitoring pacemaker impulse to detect incipient failure. Data is derived at two-month intervals at pacemaker clinic. Note that the pulse generator showed progressive premonitory signs of failure over the four-month period. The rate has declined by approximately two beats and both the pulse duration and plateau time have become prolonged. Pulse generator replacement was indicated. (See text.) (From Furman, S., et al.: Surgery, 49:98, 1961.)

variable time base and a differential vertical amplifier and recorded on a Polaroid camera (Escher and Furman, 1971).

Loss of sensory response or questionable levels of pacing threshold are reasons to consider a change of the pulse generator. A follow-up program of this type can effect a sharp decrease in emergency replacements of the pulse generator due either to failure to pace or to marked changes in indexes implying immediately impending failure (Escher and Furman, 1971).

TRANS-TELEPHONIC PACEMAKER EVALUATION. This method is indicated particularly in patients who cannot come to the physician's office or to the clinic; it consists of the observation of the magnetic mode pacer rate by telephone transmission from the patient's home to a laboratory where facilities for evaluation are located (Furman et al., 1971b). A magnet in one electrode is applied over the pulse generator to convert pacing to the magnetic mode. This method involves electronic conversion of the pacemaker stimulus artifact into a sound tone which is transmitted over the telephone to the receiving station. This allows decimal point accuracy in counting even if the physician and patient are physically remote (Escher and Furman, 1971). This method serves to evaluate the pacemaker function and may lead to extension of the pacemaker's life.

References

Baratta, F. G., Meia, H., Furman, S., and Escher, D. J. W.: Maintenance of functional improvement during chronic cardiac pacing. Circulation, 39–40:III-39, 1969.

Benchimol, A., and Liggett, M.: Cardiac hemodynamics during stimulation of the right atrium, right ventricle and left ventricle in normal and abnormal hearts. Circulation, 33:933, 1966.

Benchimol, A., Wu, T. L., and Liggett, M. S.: Effect of exercise and isoproterenol on the cardiovascular dynamics in complete heart block at various heart rates. Amer. Heart J., 70:337, 1965.

Berkovits, B.: Bifocal demand pacing (In press).

Berkovits, B., Castellanos, A., Jr., and Lemberg, L.: Bifocal demand pacemaker. Circulation, 39–40:III-44, 1969.

Castellanos, A., Jr., and Lemberg, L.: Electrophysiology of Pacing and Cardioversion. New York, Appleton-Century-Crofts, 1969.

Castillo, C., Lemberg, L., Castellanos, A., Jr., and Berkovits, B.: Bifocal (sequential atrioventricular) and demand pacemaker for sinoatrial and atrioventricular conduction disturbances. Amer. J. Cardiol., 25:87, 1970.

Chardack, W. M.: Cardiac pacemakers and heart block. In Gibbon, J. H., Jr., Sabiston, D. C., Jr., and Spencer, F. C. (eds.): Surgery of the Chest, ed. 2. Philadelphia, W. B. Saunders, 1969.

Chardack, W. M., et al.: The long-term treatment of heart block. Prog. Cardiov. Dis., 9:105, 1966.

DeSanctis, R. W.: Diagnostic and therapeutic uses of atrial pacing. Circulation, 43:748, 1971.

DeSanctis, R. W., Kastor, J. A., Leinbach, R. C., and Harthorne, J. W.: Long-term pervenous atrial pacing. Circulation, 37–38:VI-65, 1968.

Donoso, E., et al.: Effects of digitalis in compensated and decompensated patients with internal cardiac pacemakers. Amer. Heart J., 73:590, 1967.

Durrer, D., et al.: The role of premature beats in the initiation and the termination of supraventricular tachycardia in the Wolff-Parkinson-White syndrome. Circulation, 36:644, 1967.

Edhag, O.: Long-term cardiac pacing. Experience of fixed rate pacing with an endocardial electrode in 260 patients. Acta Med. Scand. (Supp.), 502, 1969.

Editorial: Plutonium for pacemakers. Brit. Med. J., 2:447, 1969.

Escher, D. J. W.: The treatment of tachyarrhythmias by artificial cardiac pacing. Amer. Heart J., 78:829, 1969.

Escher, D. J. W., and Furman, S.: Modern methods of follow-up of the patient with an implanted cardiac pacemaker. Amer. J. Cardiol., 28:359, 1971.

Friedberg, C. K., Donoso, E., and Stein, W. G.: Non-surgical acquired heart block. Ann. N.Y. Acad. Sci., 111:85, 1964.

Furman, S., and Escher, D. J. W.: Choice of cardiac pacemaker. Ann. N.Y. Acad. Sci., 167:557, 1969.
cardiac pacemaker. N.Y. Acad. Sci., 167:557, 1969.

Furman, S., and Escher, D. J. W.: Temporary transvenous pacing. In: Principles and Techniques of Cardiac Pacing, New York, Harper & Row, 1970.

Furman, S., Escher, D. J. W., and Parker, B.: The failure of triggered pacemakers. Amer. Heart J., 82:28, 1971a.

Furman, S., Escher, D. J. W., Parker, B., and Solomon, N.: Electronic analysis for pacemaker failure. Ann. Thorac. Surg., 8:57, 1969.

Furman, S., Parker, B., and Escher, D. J. W.: Transtelephone pacemaker clinic. J. Thorac. & Cardiov. Surg., 61:827, 1971b.

Goldstein, S., Moss, A. J., Ribers, R. J., Jr., and Weiner, R. S.: Transthoracic and transvenous pacemakers: A comparative clinical experience with 131 implantable units. Brit. Heart J., 32:35, 1970.

Harthorne, J. W., Leinbach, R. C., and Sanders, C. A.: Late results of permanent endocardial pacing. Circulation, 39–40:III-102, 1969.

Johansson, B. W.: Complete heart block. Clinical, hemodynamic and pharmacological study in patients with and without an artificial pacemaker. Acta Med. Scand., 180: Suppl., 451, 1966.

Johansson, B. W.: Longevity in complete heart block. Ann. N.Y. Acad. Sci., 167:1031, 1969.

Judge, R. D., Preston, T. A., Lucchesi, B. R., and Bowers, D. L.: Myocardial threshold in patients with artificial pacemakers. Amer. J. Cardiol., 18:83, 1966.

Julian, D. G., Lassers, B. W., and Goodman, M. J.: Pacing for heart block in acute myocardial infarction. Ann. N.Y. Acad. Sci., 167:911, 1969.

Kramer, D. H., and Moss, A. J.: Permanent pervenous atrial pacing from the coronary vein. Circulation, 42:427, 1970.

Lagergren, H., and Johansson, L.: Intracardiac stimulation for complete heart block. Acta Clin. Scand., 125:562, 1963.

McNally, E. M., and Benchimol, A.: Medical and physiological considerations in the use of artificial cardiac pacing. Part II. Amer. Heart J., 75:679, 1968.

Massumi, R. A., Kiston, A. D., and Tawakkol, A. A.: Termination of reciprocating tachycardia by atrial stimulation. Circulation, 36:637, 1967.

Parsonnet, V., Myers, G. H., Zucker, I. R., and Gilbert, L.: Detection of incipient pacemaker failure. Circulation, 35–36:II-206, 1967.

Preston, T. A., Fletcher, R. D., Lucchesi, B. R., and Judge, R. D.: Changes in myocardial threshold. Physiologic and pharmacologic factors in patients with implanted pacemakers. Amer. Heart J., 74:235, 1967.

Siddons, H., and Sowton, E.: Cardiac Pacemakers, Springfield, Ill., Charles C Thomas, 1967.

Tavel, M. E., and Fisch, C.: Repetitive ventricular arrhythmias resulting from artificial internal pacemaker. Circulation, 30:493, 1964.

Thalen, H. J. Th., van den Berg, J. W., van der Heide, J. N. Homan, and Nieven, J.: The Artificial Cardiac Pacemaker. Springfield, Ill., Charles C Thomas, 1969.

Torresani, J., Bernard, Y., Monties, J. R., and Jouve, A.: Clinical experience in transvenous and myocardial pacing. Ann. N.Y. Acad. Sci., 167:995, 1969.

Zoll, P. M., and Frank, H. A.: Long-term cardiac pacemakers: Current controversies. Med. Counterpoint, 1:9, 1969.

Zuckerman, W., Matloff, J. M., Harken, D. E., and Berkovits, B. V.: Clinical application of demand pacing. Ann. N.Y. Acad. Sci., 167: 1055, 1969.

Chapter 38 Defibrillation and Electric Countershock

DEFIBRILLATION
  Shocks Initiating Ventricular Fibrillation
  Shocks Terminating Ventricular Fibrillation
  Optimal Conditions for Closed Chest Defibrillation
ELECTRIC COUNTERSHOCK
  Mechanism of Action
    Autonomic Effects
      Factors Favoring Simultaneous Depolarization
  Clinical Regimen for Cardioversion
    Analgesia
    Technique of Countershock
    Postcountershock Arrhythmias
      Drugs Employed to Prevent Postcountershock (PCS) Arrhythmias
      Clinical Results
      Immediate Results
      Long-term Results
  Hemodynamics Following Conversion of Atrial Fibrillation
  Hemodynamics Following Conversion of Other Rapid Arrhythmias
  Indications
  Contraindications
    Relative Contraindications
  Complications
  Place in Therapy

A *defibrillator* is an instrument that delivers an electric shock to the heart for the purpose of converting ventricular fibrillation to normal sinus rhythm. The current, which is applied directly to the heart or through the intact chest wall, may be AC or DC and is one of a variety of wave forms. *Countershock* or *cardioversion* employs direct current, usually applied to the heart through the closed chest to convert various tachyarrhythmias to normal sinus rhythm.

DEFIBRILLATION

The subject of defibrillation has assumed a great deal of practical importance in recent years because of: (a) the recognition of the many factors that induce ventricular fibrillation; (b) the frequent onset of ventricular fibrillation in patients in a hospital setting where immediate recognition and treatment are possible; (c) the presence of defibrillators in many areas of the hospital and especially in coronary care facilities, where medical and nursing personnel are thoroughly trained in their use; (d) the advent of the mobile coronary care unit, which brings the defibrillator to the patient's home for use in postmyocardial infarction emergencies; and (e) the experience gained during surgery and during emergency resuscitations elsewhere, especially in the coronary care unit which has shown that ventricular fibrillation is a completely reversible process in many instances.

Shocks Initiating Ventricular Fibrillation. Many investigators have shown that if shocks exceeding a threshold value are delivered during the ventricular vulnerable period, which is present late in the relative refractory period of the cardiac cycle, multiple extrasystoles or ventricular fibrillation result (Ferris et al., 1936; Lown et al.,

DEFIBRILLATION AND ELECTRIC COUNTERSHOCK

1963). Although the exact mechanism of this phenomenon is not known, it is generally accepted that stimuli delivered during the vulnerable period encounter persisting areas of refractory myocardium and wander slowly through the tissue around these areas, forming multiple re-entrant paths which result in self-perpetuating fibrillation (see Fig. 38-1).

Shocks Terminating Ventricular Fibrillation. The immediate recognition of ventricular fibrillation and the application of a defibrillating countershock is a lifesaving procedure. Monitoring equipment for the recognition of this arrhythmia and various types of defibrillators are usually available in the hospital environment, especially in the coronary care facility, and often can be brought to the patient's home by the mobile coronary care unit or specially equipped ambulance. Even though closed-chest compression can circulate sufficient blood to sustain the brain and heart, the quicker the heart is defibrillated, the better is the chance for successful resuscitation.

Optimal Conditions for Closed Chest Defibrillation. It is of the utmost importance that all possible cardiopulmonary resuscitative measures (e.g., artificial respiration, closed chest cardiac compression) be instituted as soon as possible, both before and concomitant with defibrillation (see emergency treatment of cardiac arrest, p. 217). While both AC and DC countershocks of sufficient strength will defibrillate a heart that is in fairly good condition, DC is quite effective in the severely hypoxic heart (see Fig. 38-2). Since fibrillating hearts in poor condition respond better to higher energy levels and since small currents are usually ineffective, discharges in the range of 100 to 400 watt-seconds should be employed in closed chest defibrillation. For terminating ventricular fibrillation, the use of unsynchronized DC precordial shock is the procedure usually employed.

ELECTRIC COUNTERSHOCK

Mechanism of Action. Electric countershock consists of the use of a synchronized direct current shock applied directly to the heart or through the chest wall to convert certain tachy-

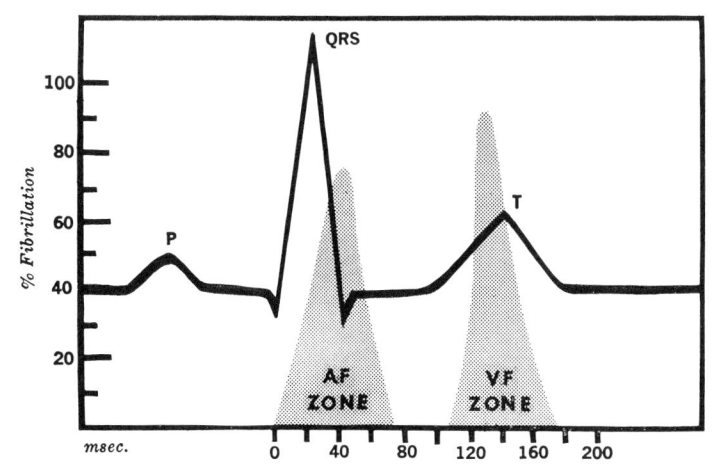

Figure 38-1. Fibrillation danger zones charted on the electrocardiogram. Shaded triangles represent zones where electroshock is most likely to produce atrial fibrillation (AF) or ventricular fibrillation (VF). (From Lown, B., Amarasingham, B., Neuman, J., and Berkovits, B. V.: J. Clin. Invest., 41:1381, 1962; courtesy of American Optical Corp.)

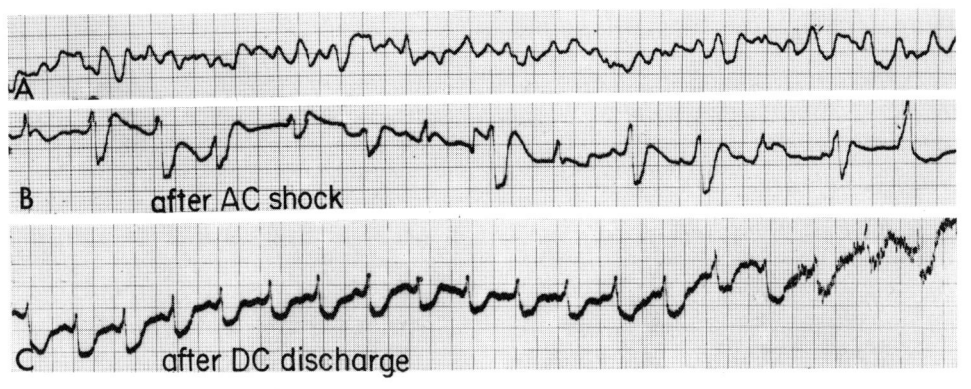

Figure 38–2. (A) Ventricular fibrillation.
(B) After AC shock, note the occurrence of occasional sinus beats; however, the rhythm is markedly abnormal due to varying types of aberration.
(C) After DC discharge, note the return to normal rhythm.

arrhythmias to normal sinus rhythm. The pulse discharge is synchronized with the R wave, thereby avoiding the ventricular vulnerable period at the peak of the T wave. The shock depolarizes all fibers that are excitable at the instant of stimulation, resulting in fusion of all wavelets and abolition of all available re-entry pathways. The restoration of normal sinus rhythm depends upon the ability of the sino-atrial node to function normally and initiate the first postshock impulse as well as the integrity of the atrial muscle or intra-atrial conduction pathways which allow normal conduction and contraction.

Autonomic Effects. In addition to the direct effects of electric countershock to depolarize cells, it also produces stimulation of the autonomic innervation of the heart. Excitation of the intracardiac sympathetic nerves by countershock and by other forces of electric stimulation has been shown to cause release of norepinephrine. In addition, countershock is frequently followed by bradycardia, suggestive of a parasympathetic effect.

FACTORS FAVORING SIMULTANEOUS DEPOLARIZATION. Simultaneous depolarization of the entire heart is necessary to terminate arrhythmias. Therefore, before cardioversion is attempted, the levels of serum potassium and arterial pO_2 and pH (if disturbed) should be restored to normal; this restitution in some cases may be sufficient to terminate the arrhythmia. Since postcountershock (PCS) arrhythmias are related to the degree of sympathetic activation and, hence, to the strength of the shock, one should employ the lowest possible energy to terminate the arrhythmia.

Clinical Regimen for Cardioversion. The regimen must provide appropriate analgesia, antiarrhythmic medication if indicated, and a plan for choosing the intensity and duration of shocks to be delivered. The following is a suggested routine for the conversion of atrial fibrillation and other arrhythmias.

Maintenance quinidine therapy is begun 48 to 72 hours prior to the procedure with quinidine sulfate, 300 mg., every 6 hours or long-acting quinidine gluconate (Quinaglute, Dura-Tabs), 500 mg., every 8 hours. The purpose of the quinidine administration is to establish an adequate plasma level in order to prevent prompt recurrence of the arrhythmia, to lower the incidence of conversion-induced arrhythmias, to facilitate conversion of atrial arrhythmias at a lower energy level, and to determine whether quinidine is well tolerated. In fact 10 to 20 per cent of patients with chronic atrial fibrillation revert to normal sinus rhythm on this dosage of quinidine alone. The usual precautions should be observed in administering this drug.

Digitalis intoxication may prevent successful conversion and precipitate postcountershock (PCS) arrhythmias including ventricular fibrillation (Fig. 38–3). Therefore, digitalis medication is suspended 24 to 48 hours prior to countershock and withheld for 24 hours following conversion. If digoxin is the glycoside used, withdrawal one day before the procedure is sufficient. Long-acting preparations (digitoxin or the powdered leaf) may be withheld as long as a week before the procedure. Whenever the preconversion electrocardiogram shows abnormalities suggestive of digitalis overdose, elective cardioversion should be postponed. In emergencies, in which immediate conversion is mandatory and the patient has received large doses of digitalis, cardioversion should be attempted at an initially low energy level or by intra-atrial stimulation by a catheter electrode. This method is employed for the control of digitalis-induced tachyarrhythmias without danger of precipitating ventricular fibrillation. This technique may in fact become the standard mode of treatment in this situation (Lister et al., 1968).

In patients with a previous history of embolic phenomena, with rheumatic valvular damage, or with other indications that there is significant risk of an embolic episode, prophylactic anticoagulation is indicated. This measure significantly reduces the occurrence of postcountershock embolization.

Analgesia. Mild anesthesia may be achieved by using one of the following agents: (1) sodium pentobarbital; (2) sodium thiopental; (3) sodium methohexital; (4) diazepam; or (5) methoxyflurane.

Technique of Countershock. One should be prepared for complications and have ready a defibrillator, a pacemaker, lidocaine, and other antiarrhythmic drugs. Before the procedure, the accuracy of the synchronized circuit should be checked several times. The electrode paddles should be liberally covered with conductive paste. The electrodes are placed, one in the second or third interspace to the right of the sternum and the other in the left fifth interspace in the midaxillary line. An alternate placement is one paddle placed anteriorly over the third and fourth interspaces centered in the parasternal area and the other placed below the left scapula.

The procedure should be initiated at low energy levels of 24 to 50 watt-sec. with further shocks administered in increasing strength until sinus rhythm is restored. Countershock at levels above 400 watt-sec. are generally not used, and it is seldom that more than four shocks are given in a series. Starting at a low level and increasing the energy of discharge in increments enables one to employ the minimal level necessary to restore normal sinus rhythm.

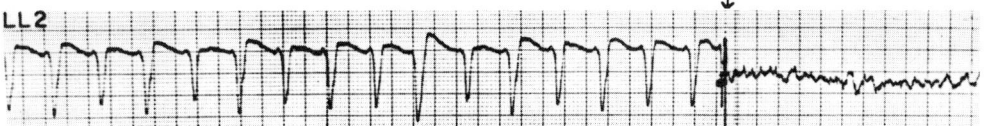

Figure 38–3. Ventricular fibrillation following countershock in the presence of digitalis toxicity. (Lead II), Control shows junctional paroxysmal tachycardia (rate, 150 per minute), probably the result of digitalis toxicity. Note occurrence of ventricular fibrillation following countershock at arrow.

For atrial fibrillation and other arrhythmias, quinidine maintenance is continued in the doses employed prior to countershock; the first dose is administered four hours after conversion, with further doses given every six hours thereafter. Long-acting preparations work very well for this purpose. Blood levels of quinidine should be determined frequently, particularly in patients with congestive heart failure or renal insufficiency.

Postcountershock Arrhythmias. The arrhythmias occurring immediately following cardioversion may be divided into the following categories: (1) The majority are atrial in origin and are usually of minor significance; they consist of single or multiple premature atrial beats which are usually transient. (2) Partial A-V heart block occurs frequently, usually indicating disease of the A-V junction or the effects of digitalis. (3) Delayed function or disease of the S-A node (i.e., sick sinus syndrome) may be manifested by a slow A-V junctional rhythm, sinus bradycardia, or A-V junctional escape. This is noted in 5 per cent of patients in whom atrial fibrillation was present for less than a year, and 45 per cent in whom atrial fibrillation was present over ten years. (4) Ventricular arrhythmias are less frequent but more serious (Figs. 38-4, 38-5).

DRUGS EMPLOYED TO PREVENT POSTCOUNTERSHOCK (PCS) ARRHYTHMIAS. Various drugs help maintain the patient in sinus rhythm after conversion. In general, they reduce excitability and prolong the refractory period. Quinidine, procaine amide,

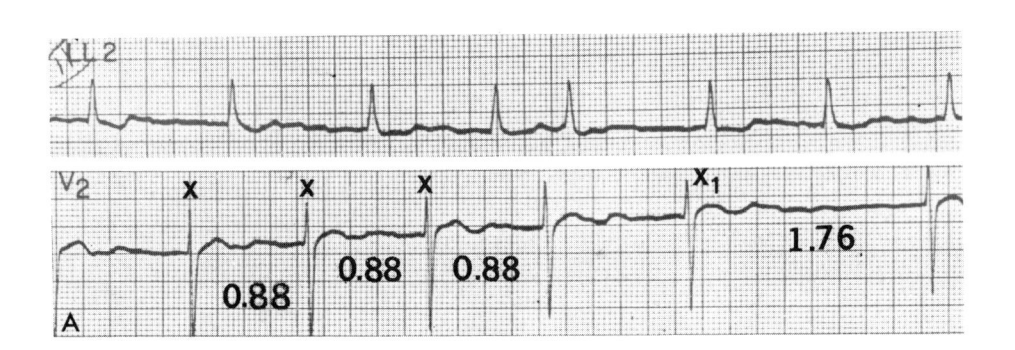

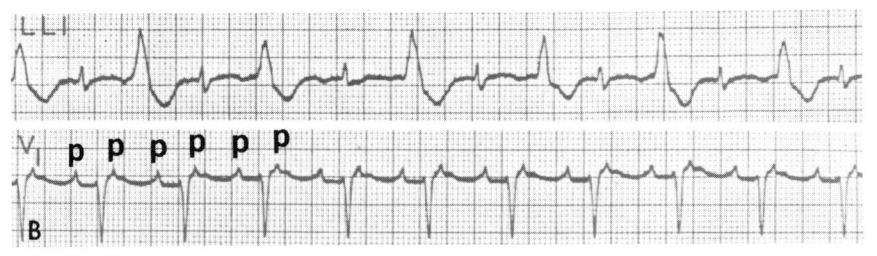

Figure 38-4. Countershock in atrial fibrillation; production of toxic digitalis effects in post-conversion period.

(A) Atrial fibrillation. Note that complexes at X have the same cycle length (0.88 sec.) (nodal rhythm). Cycle 4 is twice the regular cycle X. Exit block(?).

(B) After 200 watt-secs. countershock. Note upper strip (LI) with the occurrence of coupled ventricular premature beats. Lower strip (VI) shows an atrial tachycardia with a rate of 200 per minute. These arrhythmias are probably due to toxic digitalis effects.

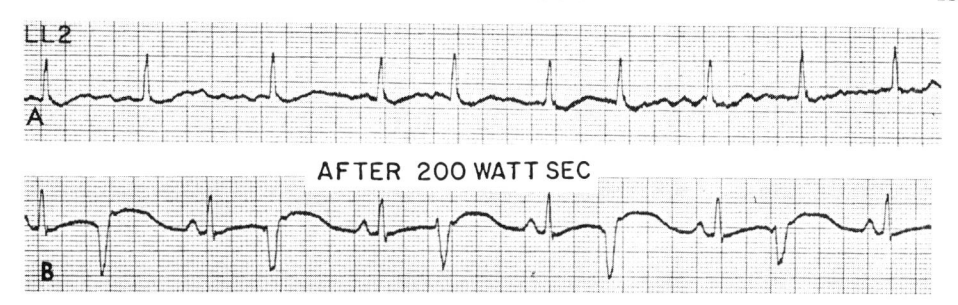

Figure 38-5. Conversion of atrial fibrillation to normal sinus rhythm. Note coupled premature ventricular beats.
(A) Atrial fibrillation with a ventricular rate averaging 75 per minute.
(B) Following cardioversion, note the presence of coupled premature ventricular beats.

and lidocaine are the drugs usually employed; diphenylhydantoin is occasionally effective for this purpose. These agents must be used with caution because in patients prone to PCS sinus bradycardia, these drugs may in certain cases prevent resumption of sinus rhythm by causing further depression of the sinus pacemaker.

Clinical Results. Electric countershock is an effective therapy for terminating many cardiac arrhythmias. The technique is simple and direct. Since it is applicable to ventricular as well as supraventricular arrhythmias, differentiation between the two is not critical to therapy with this procedure. Conductivity, contractility, and excitability of the heart are not depressed, and countershock does not commonly result in significant complications. The primary problem is maintenance of normal sinus rhythm once conversion has been effected.

Immediate Results. Of all patients receiving countershock, normal sinus rhythm is initially restored in approximately 90 per cent of patients. In a series of 1039 patients, 87 per cent (717 cases) of 820 episodes of atrial fibrillation were successfully converted to sinus rhythm (Figs. 38-6, 38-7), whereas 96 per cent (107) of 111 cases of atrial flutter were converted (Bellet, 1971). Supraventricular tachycardias (42 cases) were converted in 83 per cent (35) of cases and ventricular tachycardia was converted in 97 per cent (64) of 66 cases (Bellet, 1971) (Fig. 38-8).

Long-term Results. From 20 to 50 per cent of patients with atrial fibrillation treated by electric countershock remain in sinus rhythm for follow-up

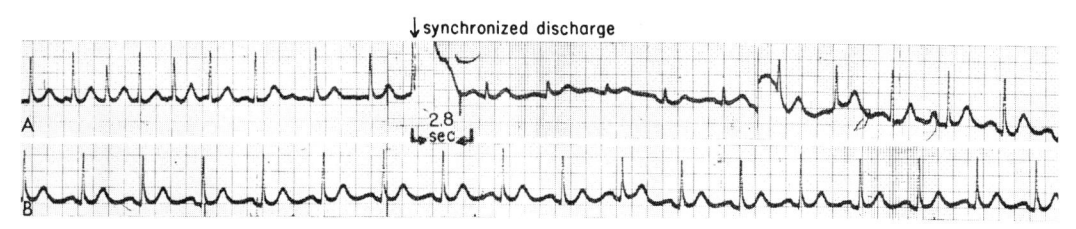

Figure 38-6. Reversion of atrial fibrillation to normal sinus rhythm. Male, 65 years old, with arteriosclerotic heart disease and atrial fibrillation of seven years' duration with borderline congestive heart failure.
(A) (Lead II) Shows atrial fibrillation. Synchronized discharge was applied at arrow and the resulting normal sinus rhythm is shown. The electrocardiogram was unreadable for 2.8 seconds, after which time normal sinus rhythm could be seen.
(B) Shows the tracing 10 minutes later with regular sinus rhythm.

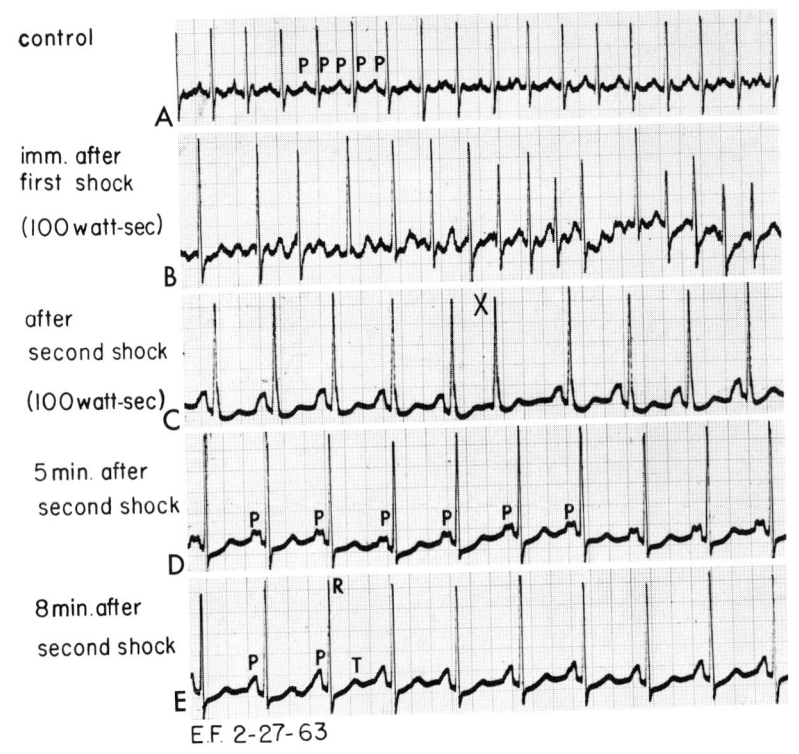

Figure 38-7. Steps in reversion of atrial flutter to normal sinus rhythm, 53-year-old male.
(A) Control. Shows 2:1 atrial flutter.
(B) After first synchronized discharge, atrial fibrillation with rapid ventricular response appears.
(C) After second synchronized discharge normal sinus rhythm is restored. Note the tall and broad P waves. A premature atrial beat is noted at X.
(D) Five minutes later the P waves become transiently notched.
(E) Eight minutes after the second shock the configuration of the P waves tends to become more normal.

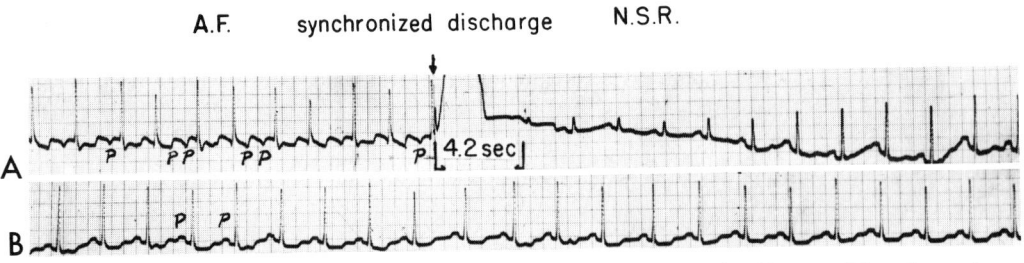

Figure 38-8. Reversion of atrial flutter to normal sinus rhythm. Male, 57 years old, with arteriosclerotic heart disease and mild congestive heart failure.
(A) (Lead II) Shows the reversion from atrial flutter to normal sinus rhythm. The electrocardiogram was unreadable for 4.2 seconds.
(B) Shows the tracing 10 minutes after reversion.

periods of 12 to 18 months. This variation is due to many factors: (a) the condition of the patient; (b) the type and extent of cardiac involvement; and (c) the method of administering quinidine. The degree of physical activity and of anxiety on the part of the patient also affects the duration of normal sinus rhythm. Quinidine is most effective when the doses are taken regularly by the patient, when frequent determinations of the plasma level are made in order to adjust dosages, and when long-acting preparations are used in appropriate cases.

In a typical series of 100 patients with atrial fibrillation restored to normal sinus rhythm by countershock, 16 reverted to atrial fibrillation in the first 24 hours, and by the end of the 12-month follow-up period, 60 were again in atrial fibrillation (Szekely et al., 1969). An inverse relationship exists between the duration of atrial fibrillation prior to cardioversion and the length of the maintenance of sinus rhythm afterwards. Those patients who have been in atrial fibrillation for less than one year have a much lower incidence (33 per cent) of return to the arrhythmia after 12 months than those who had been in atrial fibrillation for more than a year (89 per cent) (Szekely et al., 1969).

Normal sinus rhythm is maintained for long periods of time, chiefly in the group with only slight or moderate cardiac enlargement and those in whom normal physical activity is well-tolerated. It is also maintained in patients who have hemodynamically minor heart disease and in those patients who have undergone ameliorative surgery. Marked atrial dilatation, associated with severe underlying pathology, is associated with frequent recurrence of the arrhythmia. Recurrence is also more common in subjects over the age of 55. The value of electrical conversion appears to be limited in patients with chronic atrial fibrillation associated with stable or progressive heart failure.

Hemodynamics Following Conversion of Atrial Fibrillation. Conversion to normal sinus rhythm improves the hemodynamics in most patients with atrial fibrillation. Numerous studies show that there is a progressive return of cardiac output and ventricular rate to normal levels several days to several weeks following successful cardioversion. Although the mechanism is unknown, the improvement in myocardial function appears to be cumulative and involves the entire myocardium, both atrial and ventricular. This results in a progressive improvement in mechanical systole. Because of the absent atrial contribution, ventricular filling may be 30 per cent below normal (see Chapter 3), and as a result ventricular contraction is less effective. The irregular cycle lengths result in variable ventricular function and variable stroke volume (60.7 ± 18 ml.), blood pressure, and cardiac output.

As a result of conversion, the ventricular rate decreases and does not rise excessively in response to exercise. The stroke volume rises and remains at a fairly constant level and the cardiac output is significantly greater both at rest and during exercise. Additional details relative to this section are discussed in Chapter 7.

Hemodynamics Following Conversion of Other Rapid Arrhythmias. In tachyarrhythmias other than atrial fibrillation, the immediate postconversion benefits are derived primarily from the ability of countershock to decrease the heart rate. Since heart rates above 160, common in supraventricular tachyarrhythmias, cause significant decreases in cardiac output, the reduction of cardiac rate results in a significant return toward normal values. In patients with atrial flutter, atrial tachycardia, junctional tachycardia, and ventricular tachycardia of varying duration, significant improvement in cardiac output averaging 11 per cent and an increase in stroke output of almost 100 per cent has been observed by Wright et al. (1970). The magnitude of the increase in cardiac output is proportional to the heart rate prior to conversion so that the advantageous effects of countershock will be relatively greater in the patients with the more rapid tachyarrhythmia.

Indications. Countershock is generally indicated as the initial method of therapy in subjects with advanced forms of myocardial abnormality, in the presence of heart failure, hypotension or a shock-like state, and when drug therapy has been attempted and proved unsuccessful. It is also the method of choice in the more severe arrhythmias (e.g., atrial flutter and ventricular tachycardia).

Countershock is generally indicated for the following arrhythmias: (1) atrial fibrillation (Figs. 38–6, 38–7, 38–8), (2) atrial flutter, (3) paroxysmal atrial and junctional tachycardias, (4) other supraventricular tachycardias, (5) PAT with block, (6) supraventricular tachycardia associated with the W-P-W syndrome, and (7) ventricular tachycardia (Fig. 38–9).

Although other methods of therapy may be initially tried, countershock remains the method of choice where drug therapy has been unsuccessful and when the patient is severely ill.

Contraindications. Although the technique is simple and direct, there are several definite contraindications to its use: (1) Supraventricular arrhythmias with complete heart block. The existing hemodynamic changes cannot be reverted to sinus rhythm and little benefit can be achieved by countershock. (2) Digitalis toxicity. Countershock is not indicated for arrhythmias due to digitalis toxicity except when the toxicity is mild, inasmuch as countershock for digitalis-induced supraventricular arrhythmia is associated with a significant incidence of complications. Preferred therapy consists of withdrawal of digitalis and use of quinidine, propranolol, or diphenylhydantoin. If this is not successful and if a potentially fatal hemodynamic situation exists because of the arrhythmia, electrical conversion may be considered, employing small energy shocks (1 to 5 watt-sec.), or the use of right atrial stimulation. (3) Inability to tolerate quinidine in patients with a marked predisposition for the recurrence of atrial fibrillation. These circumstances make return of the arrhythmia a virtual certainty despite use of the other drugs employed for maintenance therapy. Propranolol may prove to be of some efficacy in this situation; however, administration of this drug alone is not dependable for maintenance. (4) In addition, when atrial fibrillation or other arrhythmias recur immediately after repeated countershock despite adequate quinidine therapy, subsequent countershock is contraindicated and other measures should be instituted for

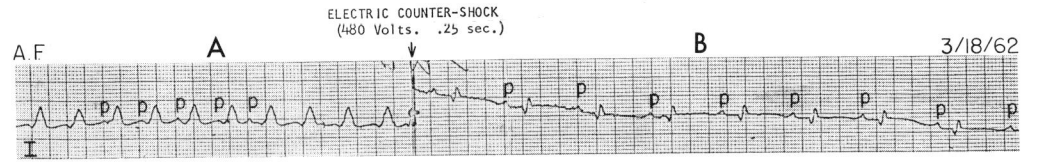

Figure 38–9. Effect of electric countershock in a patient with ventricular tachycardia refractory to drug therapy. (Lead I)

(A) Taken from a patient, age 75, with a ventricular tachycardia refractory to the usual methods of therapy. Note the ventricular rate of 145 per minute with markedly widened QRS complexes and P waves occurring at a slower rate independent of the ventricular complexes complete A-V dissociation).

(B) After the electric countershock (480 volts, 0.25 second). Note the restoration of a normal sinus rhythm with a P-R interval of 0.24 second. (From Medow and Dreifus: Amer. J. Cardiol.)

therapy. (5) There are also a small number of patients with angina pectoris whose symptoms are relieved during atrial fibrillation. Persistence of this arrhythmia in this group may be more desirable than a return to normal sinus rhythm.

Relative Contraindications. In some instances cardioversion is unlikely to be beneficial and the advisability of using this modality should be carefully considered for each patient in the following instances:

1. The recent onset of supraventricular arrhythmia is not an indication for immediate countershock, since other simpler measures are available in therapy. Electrical conversion should be deferred and drug therapy instituted.

2. Electric countershock is usually contraindicated and is of little efficacy for repetitive tachycardia.

3. In the presence of atrial fibrillation cardioversion should be used cautiously under the following conditions: (a) Candidates for cardiac surgery should be given the appropriate surgical treatment before conversion is considered. (b) Postoperative cardiac patients: There is a high rate of recurrence of atrial fibrillation when countershock is employed either at the time of surgery or immediately thereafter. Electrical conversion should be deferred for 8 to 12 weeks until postoperative convalescence is nearly complete. (c) A majority of patients with atrial fibrillation associated with hyperthyroidism will revert to sinus rhythm spontaneously when the euthyroid state is achieved. There is also a low success rate in maintaining normal rhythm in hypermetabolic patients. Electrical conversion should not be considered until after the hyperthyroid patient has been returned to the euthyroid state. (d) A patient who has suffered a recent systemic embolism should not be considered for countershock.

4. Cardioversion is not indicated for sinus tachycardia or normal sinus rhythm with atrial, junctional, or ventricular premature beats.

5. In general, countershock should not be employed when a critical evaluation of the factors argue against the probability of maintenance of sinus rhythm after conversion.

Complications. The major complications encountered include: (1) ventricular tachycardia and fibrillation, which occur in 1 to 2 per cent of patients treated; (2) pulmonary or systemic emboli, which occur in 1 to 2 per cent of patients who are not properly anticoagulated, but in less than 1 per cent of those who are; (3) pulmonary venous congestion with episodes of pulmonary edema (1 to 2 per cent); (4) elevation of serum glutamic-oxalacetic transaminase, lactic dehydrogenase, and creatine phosphokinase may occur in 20 per cent or more of patients, due to the skeletal muscle damage associated with countershock; and (5) various electrocardiographic changes may occur, especially transient S-T segment elevation in the precordial leads. Other less significant or very infrequent complications include: (1) hypoventilation, myocardial depression, and cardiac irritability associated with anesthesia; (2) drug reactions (potentiation of digitalis and quinidine toxicity); (3) A-V junctional rhythm; (4) occasionally, severe bradycardia; (5) multiple premature ventricular beats immediately following cardioversion; (6) rarely, cardiac arrest.

Place in Therapy. Electric countershock has been shown to occupy an important place in the treatment of rapid ectopic rhythms. It has the following advantages: (a) rapidity of conversion; (b) relative safety; and (c) avoidance of delay, uncertainty, and possible toxic effects of drugs. The use of electric countershock has been a notable advance in the therapy of certain arrhythmias.

Countershock is the method of choice

in the conversion of ventricular tachycardia, atrial flutter, and atrial fibrillation. However, the original enthusiasm for its use has been tempered somewhat by the fact that following conversion (e.g., in atrial fibrillation, the most common arrhythmia), reversion to the arrhythmia often occurs after a short period—three to six months in 50 to 70 per cent of patients. In the light of larger experience, this method has now undergone a somewhat more realistic evaluation than was originally considered. The problem at present is greater selectivity in the choice of patients and the maintenance of normal sinus rhythm following conversion by careful selection of therapeutic regimens for each individual patient. Concentration upon better methods of maintenance must be sought. Use of the longer acting quinidine preparations under adequate control in carefully adjusted dosage and judicious use of propranolol and other antiarrhythmic agents in selected cases may be of help in decreasing the incidence of recurrence.

References

Aberg, H., and Cullhed, I.: Direct-current countershock complications. Acta med. Scand., *183:*415, 1968.

Bell, H., Pugh, D., and Dunn, M.: Failure of cardioversion in mitral valve disease. Arch. Intern. Med., *119:*257, 1967.

Bellet, S.: Clinical Disorders of the Heart Beat, 3rd ed., Philadelphia, Lea & Febiger, 1971.

Bjerkelund, C., and Orning, O. M.: An evaluation of DC shock treatment of atrial arrhythmias. Acta med. Scand., *194:*481, 1968.

Cobb, F. R., Wallace, A. G., and Wagner, G. S.: Cardiac inotropic and coronary vascular responses to countershock. Circ. Res., *23:*731, 1968.

Ferris, L. P., Spence, P. W., King, B. G., and Williams, H. B.: Effect of electric shock on the heart. Electrical Engineering, *55:*498, 1936.

Gilbert, R., and Cuddy, R.: Digitalis intoxication following conversion to sinus rhythm. Circulation, *32:*58, 1965.

Kleiger, R., and Lown, B.: Cardioversion and digitalis. Part II. Clinical studies. Circulation, *33:*878, 1966.

Lister, J. W., Cohen, L. S., Bernstein, W. H., and Samet, P.: Treatment of supraventricular tachycardias by rapid atrial stimulation. Circulation, *38:*1044, 1968.

Lown, B., Bey, S. K., Perlroth, M., and Abe, T.: Comparative studies of ventricular vulnerability to fibrillation. J. Clin. Invest., *42:*953, 1963.

Lown, B., Kleiger, R., and Williams, J.: Cardioversion and digitalis drugs: Changed threshold to electric shock in digitalized animals. Circ. Res., *17:*519, 1965.

Peleska, B.: Srdecni defibrillator. Sbornik vynalezu a zlepsovacich navrhu ve zdrarotnictvi, *3:*33, 1955.

Radford, M. D., and Evans, D. W.: Long-term results of DC reversion of atrial fibrillation. Brit. Heart J., *30:*91, 1968.

Szekely, P., et al.: Direct current shock and digitalis. Brit. Heart J., *31:*91, 1969.

Wright, J. S., Fabian, J., and Epstein, E. J.: Immediate effect on cardiac output of reversion to sinus rhythm from rapid arrhythmias. Brit. Med. J., *3:*315, 1970.

Zoll, P. M., Linenthal, A. J., and Phelps, M. D., Jr.: Termination of refractory tachycardia by external electric countershock. Circulation, *24:*1078, 1961.

Zoll, P. M., Linenthal, A. J., and Zarsky, L. R. N.: Ventricular fibrillation: treatment and prevention by external electric currents. New Eng. J. Med., *262:*105, 1960.

Glossary

It is difficult in briefly defining a term to include all of its characteristics; these definitions are intended to convey the more important features. A more complete discussion is given in the text.

Aberration: Abnormal spread of the supraventricular impulse in the ventricle brought about by delayed activation of one of the branches of the bundle of His, with resultant widening of the ventricular complex. The right bundle branch is the branch most frequently involved. See also Gouaux-Ashman Phenomenon.

Accrochage: The transient synchronization of the inherently different rhythms of two contiguous cardiac elements (*e.g.*, when the atrial and ventricular rhythms become synchronous for a few beats during complete A-V heart block and other instances of slow ventricular rates).

All or None Law: A phenomenon characteristic of cardiac tissue whereby the weakest stimulus capable of causing a contraction at all (minimal stimulus) will produce the maximal contraction. On the other hand, a stimulus — no matter how powerful — will fail to produce a contraction during the absolute refractory period.

Alternation of the Heart: Refers to a regular variation in the electrical or mechanical activity of the heart in the presence of a regular rhythm. The term "pulsus alternans" has been replaced by the term "heart alternation." Two main types are observed: (*a*) *mechanical alternation* — a regular alternation in the presence of normal sinus rhythm. This may be reflected in the pressure curves of the individual chamber or in the peripheral vessels; in the case of the left ventricle and the pulmonary artery in the case of the right ventricle; (*b*) *electrical alternation* — the regular variation in amplitude of the various phases of the electrocardiogram: QRS, T, P-R interval or P waves in alternate beats.

Anomalous Beats or Complexes: These terms have been used to embrace all ventricular complexes that differ from the dominant pattern of the sinus beats. This includes both aberrant and ectopic beats.

Antegrade Conduction: Conduction in the usual manner from the S-A node to the atria to the A-V junction and bundle of His to the bundle branches (in contrast to retrograde conduction, in which the impulse is conducted in the reverse direction through some or all of the conducting system).

"As-Vs" Interval: (Analogous to the P-R interval, A-V conduction time.) The time interval elapsing between the beginning of atrial and ventricular systole.

Atrial: Refers to the main upper chamber of the heart. (In this book, the term "atrial" is used rather than "auricular" in describing premature beats, flutter, and fibrillation originating in this chamber of the heart.)

Atrial Complex: That portion of the electrocardiogram which is associated with atrial activity. The P wave represents depolarization and the T_p wave represents repolarization of atrial muscle.

Atrial Fibrillation: A rhythm of the atria manifested in the electrocardiogram by continuous and contiguous atrial oscillations, irregular in form, amplitude and cycle length and having in man an average rate of about 450 per minute. A high variable degree of A-V heart block is associated with a resultant irregular ventricular rhythm and a ventricular rate which, in the untreated case, usually ranges from 100 to 180 per minute.

Atrial Flutter: Rapid regular contractions of the atria occurring at an average rate of 300 per minute. Regular F (or P) waves representing each of these contractions are visible on the electrocardiogram. The ventricles usually respond to a fraction of these atrial impulses, rarely to all of them.

Atrial Fusion Beat: Simultaneous stimulation of the atria by a sinus or ectopic atrial impulse and a retrograde impulse from an A-V junction. The latter may be a premature ventricular systole or an escape beat. Fusion of two atrial excitation waves is rare.

Atrial Premature Beat: A premature beat arising in the atrium.

Atrial Tachycardia (Paroxysmal Atrial Tachycardia): A rapid regular beating of the atria, usually paroxysmal, with a rate ranging from 140 to 200 per minute.

Atrioventricular Bundle (Bundle of His): A bundle situated below the A-V junction at its bifurcation into the left bundle branch and right bundle branch systems, thus forming the stem of the neuromuscular system that unites the musculature of the atrium and ventricle anatomically and functionally.

Atrioventricular Junction: The structure over which the sinus impulse is transmitted to the ventricles. This consists of (1) the anatomic A-V node, which corresponds to the electrophysiologic N region, and (2) the atrial-nodal junction and the nodal-His junction, which correspond to the electrophysiologic A-N and N-H regions respectively.

Atrioventricular Node: See Atrioventricular Junction.

Atrium: (Left and right) Refers to the main upper (atrial) chamber of the heart.

Auricle: (Not a synonym for atrium) Anatomically, the term "auricle" refers to an atrial appendage and should not be used to indicate the main atrial chamber.

Automaticity: An inherent property of cardiac pacemaker cells by which they spontaneously depolarize and initiate action potentials independent of electrical or mechanical connections with other cells.

A-V Dissociation: Independent action of atria and ventricles, each beating in response to its own pacemaker. The ventricular rate is usually more rapid than the atrial: the atria respond to a pacemaker usually situated in the S-A node; the ventricles, to a pacemaker situated in the A-V junction or upper portion of the interventricular septum. This dissociation may be complete or, in the presence of ventricular captures, incomplete. A-V dissociation should not be considered an "arrhythmia" but only a result of an arrhythmia.

A-V Heart Block (First Degree): That type of heart block in which there is persistent P-R prolongation without dropped ventricular beats. The P-R interval is prolonged over the normal limit of 0.2 second because of an increase in duration of the refractory period of the A-V junction, which results in slowing of the impulse as it traverses the A-V junction; however, every sinus impulse, although slowed, reaches the ventricle. Therefore, a QRS complex is present after every P wave without exception.

A-V Heart Block (Second Degree): That type of heart block in which some of the atrial impulses fail to reach the ventricles, with the result that ventricular beats are not initiated at this time. The following types are observed: (*a*) Mobitz type I, with Wenckebach periodicity, and (*b*) Mobitz type II, without changes of P-R time in consecutive beats. In the latter type there is no periodicity; the A-V block occurs suddenly and is unpredictable.

A-V Heart Block (Complete or Third Degree): That type of A-V heart block in which all atrial impulses are prevented from reaching the ventricles, so that the heart is then controlled by two pacemakers—the atria by the sinus node or another supraventricular focus, and the ventricles by an A-V junctional or idioventricular focus. The atria usually beat regularly at a rate of 60 to 80 per minute, and the ventricles at a rate of 30 to 40 per minute. Should be differentiated from other types of A-V dissociation.

A-V Interval: See P-R Interval.

A-V Junctional: Referring to the A-V junction. This term is now commonly used instead of "nodal" or "A-V nodal."

A-V Junctional Escape: A single beat originating from the A-V junction which assumes control of the cardiac activity following a long sinus pause.

A-V Junctional Rhythm: A cardiac rhythm with the pacemaker originating in the A-V junction.

A-V Junctional Tachycardia: A rapid ectopic rhythm with the pacemaker focus located in the A-V junction. There are two forms: paroxysmal (rate 150 to 220) and nonparoxysmal (rate 70 to 100).

Bachman's Bundle: A bundle containing specialized and undifferentiated cardiac fibers, which connects the left and right atria.

Bidirectional Junctional Tachycardia: A type of tachycardia in which the QRS deflection is alternately positive and negative; these complexes arise from different portions of the A-V junction; they can be slowed by carotid sinus pressure and are usually due to toxic digitalis effects.

GLOSSARY

Bigeminy: A rhythm in which every other beat is premature so that each two beats appear coupled. See also Pseudobigeminy.

Bilateral Bundle Branch Block: Partial or complete block in both bundle branches; block may be complete in one and partial in the other.

Block: A phenomenon whereby an impulse is slowed or stopped at a time when it would be expected to arrive at a given point.

Bundle of His: See Atrioventricular Bundle.

Cardiac Arrest: Failure of the entire heart (both atria and ventricles) to contract.

Cardioversion: See Countershock.

Carotid Sinus Syndrome: (Carotid sinus syncope) A syndrome consisting of dizziness, convulsions, and/or unconsciousness caused by reflex vagal slowing of the heart (cardioinhibitory form most common), or by peripheral vasodilatation with hypotension (vasodepressor form) or a combination of both. These effects result from reflex stimulation of a hypersensitive carotid sinus.

Chaotic Heart Action: A phenomenon in which the heart shows a multiplicity of ectopic beats in the form of successive premature systoles having several points of origin and showing a bizarre configuration.

Circus Movement: A continuous movement of an ectopic excitation wave occurring in a circular fashion around a ring of muscle in various portions of the musculature of the heart or within the conduction system. See Re-entry. Compare Unifocal Theory.

Compensatory Pause: Following a premature beat, the pause is longer than the preceding cycle length — the pause compensates for the decreased cycle length preceding the premature beat. The R-R interval between the QRS complex preceding the premature beats and the QRS following it is equal to that of two normal cycle lengths. In certain instances the pause may be short (noncompensatory). With a fully compensatory pause, the premature beat does not prematurely discharge the S-A node; when the pause is not fully compensatory, the premature beat has discharged the S-A node.

Complexes (Electrical): Those portions of an electrogram or electrocardiogram which are associated with electrical activity in the areas from which the recording is made.

Concealed Conduction: An impairment of impulse propagation in which the impulse travels only part way through its pathways. It results from unequal depression of excitability in adjacent parts of the heart with cessation of the impulse propagation in the most depressed area. The degree of penetration of the impulse can be measured only indirectly by its effect on the subsequent impulse conduction or impulse formation.

Concordant Alternation: Alternation occurring in both systemic and pulmonary circuits. See Discordant Alternation.

Conduction Velocity: The rate at which excitation travels from its point of origin to other parts of a tissue. The excitation spreads through the Purkinje fibers at a rate of 4000 mm. per second, atrial muscle at a rate of 900 mm. per second, ventricular musculature at 200 mm. per second and nodal tissue at 200 mm. per second.

Coronary Care Unit: An area in a hospital for patients suffering from acute myocardial infarction. The coronary care unit is equipped with electronic monitoring equipment and drugs for the early detection and immediate treatment of arrhythmias. The emphasis is on prevention and immediate treatment of various arrhythmias, including ventricular fibrillation and cardiac arrest and the institution of resuscitative therapy with the early recognition and treatment of complications, especially congestive failure and shock.

Coronary Sinus Rhythm: A type of rhythm arising in the upper portion of the A-V junction that shows inverted P waves in leads II, III, and aVF of the electrocardiogram with a P-R interval ranging from 0.10 to 0.17 second. The focus of origin of the P wave is believed to be situated in the lower portion of the right atrium, probably in the coronary sinus area.

Countershock: The use of electrical current, usually D.C., preferably synchronized to the T wave of the electrocardiogram, which is applied to the heart directly or across the chest wall to convert various arrhythmias to normal sinus rhythm.

Coupling: A normal beat followed by a premature beat at a regular repeated sequence.

Decrement: A decrease in the conduction velocity due to a change of the properties of the conduction fiber at a particular point.

Default: Assumption of ventricular automaticity by a lower focus usually located in the A-V junction due to slowing of the higher pacemaker (the S-A node).

Defibrillator: An instrument that delivers an electric shock to the heart to convert ventricular fibrillation to normal sinus rhythm. The current, which is applied directly to the heart or through the intact chest wall, may be A.C. or D.C.

Delta Wave: The slow-rising, slurred, initial portion of the QRS deflection seen in the W-P-W syndrome caused by pre-excitation of a part of the ventricular myocardium. These waves may be observed occasionally in conditions other than W-P-W syndrome.

Depolarization, Diastolic: A slow decrease of the resting membrane potential which begins immediately after the end of repolarization, and continues until a more rapid depolarization action potential begins. It has been recorded from pacemaker areas and Purkinje fibers, but is not found in other portions of the heart muscle.

Discordant Alternation: Alternation in mechanical (blood pressure) or electrical units occurring either in the systemic or the pulmonary circulation, not in both systems.

Dissociation: Asynchronous and independent activity of two different pacemakers in the heart; the common type involves the S-A node and A-V junction, with the result that the P waves occur independently of the QRS complexes. The ventricular rate is usually more rapid than the atrial rate. However, other types of asynchronous activity may occur. See A-V Dissociation.

Double Pathway: Generally, a condition in which two pathways are available for the impulse to reach a certain destination (*e.g.*, in the W-P-W syndrome one impulse passes through the normal pathway—the A-V junction—the other by a more direct pathway through the bundle of Kent). See also Dual Transmission in the A-V Junction.

Dropped Beat: The occurrence of a nonconducted (blocked) beat in second degree A-V heart block.

Dual Transmission (in the A-V Junction): The presence of two separate transmission systems in the A-V junction, one of which conducts impulses slowly, the other more rapidly. This results in an early recovery and earlier responsiveness of one of these pathways.

Dysrhythmia: Used in preference to the term "arrhythmia" to indicate disturbances of cardiac pacemaker activity, but not necessarily an irregularity in rhythm.

Echo Beats: Beats produced by an excitation wave which spreads from one chamber of the heart to another, from which it returns to give rise to another beat (*e.g.*, "return extrasystoles" and "reciprocal beats").

Ectopic Beats or Rhythm: A beat or series of beats resulting from activity of a pacemaker other than the sinus node.

Electrical Alternans (Total): The type of alternation which involves the various deflections of the electrocardiogram—*P waves*, P-R interval, QRS complexes, and T waves.

Electrogram: A recording of the electrical activity of the heart taken with the recording electrode (unipolar or bipolar) placed directly on the surface of uninjured cardiac muscle.

Electrotonic: Referring to the cable or core-conductor properties of the cell membrane, *i.e.*, the excitable cell membrane responds to stimulus with conduction along a relatively long distance on the membrane rather than dissipating the impulse through internal (cytoplasmic) conduction.

Entrance Block: Unidirectional block caused by an area of refractory tissue surrounding a constantly active parasystolic focus, thus protecting it against capture by another cardiac pacemaker. See Protection Block; compare Exit Block.

Escape Beat: Beat from a lower and slower focus (passive beat) allowed to assume the role of pacemaker if the impulse of the higher focus is delayed or blocked (*e.g.*, A-V junctional escape).

Excitability: The property of muscle by virtue of which it responds to stimulation by propagation of the impulse.

Exit Block: A condition in which some or all impulses originating from an automatic focus are not conducted because of myocardial derangement (*e.g.*, fibrosis) or electrophysiologic alteration (*e.g.*, decremental conduction). The focus is effectively isolated from the remainder of the heart. Exit block may appear electrocardiographically as a sudden decrease in the heart rate to half or other fraction of the original rate. It involves particularly the A-V junction and less frequently the S-A node.

Extrasystoles: A term loosely applied to premature beats; strictly applied only to interpolated premature beats. According to the site of origin: atrial, A-V junctional, and ventricular extrasystoles.

f Waves: Represent the small irregular oscillations of the atria, characteristically found in atrial fibrillation.

F Waves: Characteristic undulating waves of atrial activity seen in atrial flutter (labeled F or P). These probably represent the manifestation of both atrial depolarization and repolarization occurring in rapid succession from an ectopic focus.

Fibrillation: See Atrial Fibrillation and Ventricular Fibrillation.

Fixed Coupling: Observed in premature beats when the interval between QRS of the basic rhythm and QRS of the premature beat is constant.

Fusion Beat: The complex that results from the collision and electrocardiographic summation of wave fronts within the ventricles or atria. The resulting (fusion) beat represents the sum-

GLOSSARY

mation of the two electrical forces. (Synonyms: combination beats, transitional beats.)

Gouaux-Ashman Phenomenon (Ashman phenomenon): Aberrant conduction of a supraventricular impulse when a beat with a short R-R interval follows one with a long R-R interval. The long preceding cycle length causes a long refractory period and the impulse of the short cycle is confronted with relatively refractory tissue, usually in the right bundle branch, causing aberration.

His Bundle Electrogram: A recording of A-V junctional electrical activity by a catheter electrode positioned in the right and occasionally the left ventricle. The various intervals observed include:

A-N Interval: The interval between the onset of the atrial deflection and the nodal potential (normal 40 to 100 msec.).

A-H Interval: Interval between the onset of the atrial deflection and the onset of His bundle potential (50 to 120 msec.).

N-H Interval: Interval between the nodal potential and the His bundle potential (10 to 20 msec.).

H-Q (H-V) Interval: Interval between the His potential and the Q wave of the QRS complex (36 to 44 msec.).

RB-Q Interval: The interval between the right bundle branch potential and the Q wave of the QRS complex (15 to 20 msec.).

Idioventricular Beat: Passive ventricular beat originating below the bifurcation of His bundle.

Idioventricular Rhythm: Passive ventricular rhythm consisting of a series of idioventricular beats, usually with a rate of 40 per minute or less. This is to be distinguished from *idioventricular rhythm associated with acute myocardial infarction* in which the rate may transiently range from 55 to 110 per minute.

Idioventricular Tachycardia: Idioventricular beats with a rate of 55 to 110 per minute observed in sequences of 30 beats or less. Also called (1) *accelerated idioventricular rhythm;* (2) *idioventricular rhythm;* (3) *slow ventricular tachycardia;* (2) *nonparoxysmal ventricular tachycardia.*

Indirect Leads: Leads in which both contacts are applied to the limbs or to other tissue at a distance from the heart.

Interference: (Most common connotation): In A-V dissociation, the rhythm is the result of two different pacemakers, *e.g.,* one in the atrium or A-V junction and the other in the ventricles. Interference is said to exist when the A-V dissociation is interrupted by conducted beats (captures). (Less common usage): Term used to indicate that there is a collision of the impulses from two different pacemakers.

Intermittent Parasystole: A parasystolic rhythm which is interrupted (discharged) and subsequently resumes.

Interpolated Premature Systoles: A true extrasystole that occurs as a premature ventricular contraction between two normal ventricular contractions. It is not followed by a compensatory pause.

Isoelectric Period: A period of the heart's cycle in which the galvanometric string stands at zero (*e.g.,* the T-P segment in the electrocardiogram).

Isorhythmic Dissociation: Atria and ventricles beat independently but at almost identical rates. P-R or R-P intervals are short and P wave often overrides QRS complexes. A theory to explain this phenomenon is that of accrochage or synchronization. See Accrochage.

"J" Point: Junction between QRS and ST.

Mobitz Type I A-V Block: The type of second degree A-V block showing Wenckebach periodicity. See Wenckebach Phenomenon.

Mobitz Type II A-V Block: The type of second degree A-V heart block (called also "type II" second degree A-V block) in which, following a fixed P-R interval, 2:1 or higher degrees of partial A-V heart block suddenly appear (in contrast to Wenckebach type).

Monophasic Action Potential: The measurement obtained from an electrode in contact with cardiac tissue during excitation. This is very similar to the true *transmembrane potential* as measured by an intracellular electrode. The *resting potential*, obtained when the cardiac cell is at rest, is approximately 80 to 90 mv. During excitation and repolarization of the cardiac cell, the monophasic action potential goes through five phases. *Phase 0* is the rapid upstroke of depolarization. *Phase 1* is the early rapid repolarization followed by *phase 2*, which is a plateau phase. *Phase 3* is again a more rapid (not as rapid as phase 1) repolarization phase. *Phase 4* is the diastolic phase when repolarization is complete. In automatic cells during this phase, the transmembrane potential gradually rises (diastolic depolarization) until threshold is reached and phase 0 is initiated; in undifferentiated myocardial cells, the phase 4 level is held constant.

Resting Potential: (Transmembrane resting potential) The potential obtained when a microelectrode is inserted into a resting cardiac cell. This usually is 80 to 90 mv. and is negative with respect to the external surface electrode.

Threshold Potential is that critical level to which the transmembrane potential must be reduced in order to produce a propagated response from an excitable tissue.

Nodal: See A-V Junctional.

Oculocardiac Reflex: A vagovagal reflex in which compression of the eyeball results in slowing or transient sinus pauses of the heart beat via vagal stimulation.

Orthograde Conduction: See Antegrade Conduction.

"P" Cell: The characteristic specialized cell of the S-A node and A-V junction. This cell appears to be the "pacemaker" cell.

P Wave: The initial deflection of the electrocardiogram, which represents the depolarization of the atria.

Pacemaker (Artificial): An electronic device that acts as an artificial automatic fiber to initiate and sustain a regular cardiac rhythm. There are several types of discharge schedules:

Types of Impulse Delivery:
(1) *Fixed-rate* — a unit which discharges impulses at a uniform and uninterrupted rate.
(2) *Atrial-triggered* — a unit which delivers a stimulus to the ventricle in response to the P wave which is detected by a sensor in the atrium.
(3) *Ventricular-programmed* (ventricular synchronous) — an electrode which is attached to the ventricle senses the QRS complex; the pacemaker either does or does not deliver an impulse depending on whether it is demand or standby.
  (a) *Demand* (ventricular-inhibited) — The sensed QRS inhibits the pacemaker discharge; thus, the pacemaker discharges when a QRS complex is not sensed within a pre-set interval (*e.g.*, 0.86 second).
  (b) *Standby* (ventricular-triggered) — The sensed QRS triggers the pacemaker discharge which occurs during the refractory period of the ventricle. If a QRS is not sensed within a pre-set interval, the pacemaker discharges at a fixed rate.
(4) *Sequential pacing* — an impulse is delivered to the atria and after a pre-set delay an impulse is delivered to the ventricles.
(5) *Bifocal demand pacing* — the combination of a QRS-inhibited ventricular pacemaker with a QRS-inhibited atrial pacemaker. This type may stimulate the atria, the atria and ventricles or may be inactive.

Parasystole: Condition in which at least one ectopic focus in addition to the normal pacemaker is firing at a regular and uninterrupted rate.

Parasystolic Rhythm: A rhythm originating in either the atria or ventricles (most commonly), which is the result of the activity of an ectopic pacemaker. The beats of the ectopic pacemaker occur regularly and manifest no relation to those of the dominant rhythm (see Entrance Block).

Paroxysmal Atrial Tachycardia with Block: Rapid ectopic atrial rhythm in the range of 140 to 220 per minute, associated with varying degrees of partial (usually 2:1) A-V heart block.

Paroxysmal Tachycardia: Regular tachycardia which begins and ends quite abruptly and which is presumably ectopic (atrial, nodal, or ventricular) in origin.

Postextrasystolic Potentiation: The occurrence of an increased inotropic effect (*i.e.*, increased systolic stroke output) in the beat following an extrasystole or artificially induced nonconducted premature beat.

P-R Interval: The interval between the beginning of P and QRS in the electrocardiogram; it represents the time interval between the beginning of atrial and ventricular depolarization (A-V conduction time).

Pre-excitation: The excitation of the ventricles by a supraventricular impulse which bypasses partially or completely the normal A-V conduction pathway. The pre-excitation syndromes include: (1) the W-P-W syndrome and its variations and (2) the Lown-Ganong-Levine syndrome.

Premature Beat: (Often used synonymously with "extrasystole.") Beats which in the course of basic rhythm of the heart (occasionally with an abnormal rhythm) arise prematurely, thus disturbing the rhythmic series of beats. This may or may not be followed by a compensatory pause.

Protection Block: An area of abnormal unidirectional block, associated with parasystole, which prevents the discharging of the ectopic pacemaker by an impulse originating in the sinus node or by another ectopic impulse. The normal impulse depolarizes the ventricles except in the area of the parasystolic focus, so that the latter's activity is not interrupted by the passage of the sinus or other impulse. (See Entrance Block.)

Pseudobigeminy: Term coined to distinguish "true bigeminy" (*i.e.*, extrasystolic bigeminy) from other bigeminal rhythms (pseudobigeminy), *e.g.*, in 3:2 A-V block, A-V alternans, alternating 2:1 and 4:1 A-V conduction in atrial flutter.

Pulse Deficit: Difference between the apical rate and the peripheral pulse rate. This condition, frequently encountered in atrial fibrillation, multiple premature beats and, less commonly, in other arrhythmias, is due to failure of a very early ventricular contraction to propel an adequate amount of blood to the periphery to produce a palpable pulse.

Purkinje Fibers: That part of the conduction system which is continuous with the bundle branches extending into the myocardium and lining the greater part of the interior of both ventricles.

QRS Group of Deflections: The initial deflections of the ventricular electrocardiogram; they correspond to the spread of the excitation wave in the ventricle (ventricular depolarization).

Reciprocal Beat or Rhythm: A beat or rhythm in which an impulse, arising in any automatic fiber, activates the atria or ventricles, and the same excitation front, after exciting these chambers, returns to activate the original chamber. Thus, an atrial or ventricular reciprocal beat, while traversing the A-V junction, initiates a retrograde impulse in another pathway which returns to activate the chamber of origin after the antegrade impulse has stimulated the other chambers.

Re-entry: A mechanism postulated to explain the production and maintenance of premature beats and other arrhythmias. An area of depressed excitability is present in the myocardium, which is capable of being activated after most of the myocardium has become refractory. Then, when the rest of the heart emerges from the refractory state, this now active focus propagates the impulse throughout the myocardium. This explains ventricular premature beats with fixed coupling and other arrhythmias. See Circus Movement.

Refractory Period: The period following the upstroke of the ventricular action potential during which the heart's excitability is depressed or absent. Several *periods* comprise the refractory state:

Absolute refractory period (*ARP*): The period following excitation when the myocardial fiber will not respond to even the highest intensity electrical impulse.

Effective refractory period (*ERP*): The period during which impulses may appear but are too weak to be conducted.

Relative refractory period (*RRP*): The period between the ERP and the end of the refractory period during which fibers respond only to stimuli greater than the diastolic stimulation threshold and the evoked impulses are conducted more slowly than normal.

Total refractory period (*TRP*): The sum of the ARP and RRP.

Repolarization: Immediately following depolarization of the cell, certain physiochemical processes take place which result in a gradual restoration of the positive and negative charges to their respective positions along the surface of the membrane. This constitutes the return of the stimulated muscle to the resting state. On the electrocardiogram this activity is represented by the S-T segment and T wave.

Retrograde Beat: A beat of the atria which starts in the ventricle or A-V junctional system and is propagated to the atrium (*i.e.*, in a direction the reverse of the normal).

Retrograde Conduction: Propagation of an impulse through the conduction system or cardiac muscle in a manner opposite to that of the normal impulse. See Antegrade Conduction.

S-A Block: A condition in which the sinus node apparently continues to discharge uninterruptedly; however, an exit block prevents the normal 1:1 response of the atria and ventricles. S-A block may be categorized as first, second, or third degree, as is A-V heart block.

Sick-Sinus Syndrome (SSS): A chronic ischemic, sclerotic or inflammatory disease of the S-A node and atria associated with sinus bradycardia, supraventricular tachycardia, chronic atrial fibrillation, and sinoatrial block.

Sinoatrial (S-A) Node: An interlacement of fine muscle fibers and nerve elements, buried in the mammalian heart near the cephalic end of the sulcus terminalis. In the normally beating heart this constitutes the cardiac pacemaker (primary focus).

Sinus Arrest: Long-lasting pause in sinus activity. Not distinguishable from complete S-A block.

Sinus Arrhythmia: An irregularity in which the whole heart, beating in response to impulses formed in the pacemaker, participates uniformly. When the varying rate of discharge is related to respiratory cycles, it is a respiratory sinus arrhythmia; when it occurs irregularly or unrelated to respiration, it is known as the nonrespiratory form of sinus arrhythmia.

Sinus Pause: Long-lasting absence of sinus P waves; may be caused by high degree of S-A block or sinus arrest.

Sluggish Sinus Node Syndrome: A syndrome of decreased S-A nodal automaticity. This is often antecedent to the development of the sick sinus syndrome.

Stokes-Adams Syndrome: A syndrome due to an abnormal cardiac mechanism associated with fainting or convulsive attacks; the basic cause is sudden cerebral hypoxia due to failure of the heart to supply blood to the vital centers. The cardiac mechanism may be one of the following —cardiac standstill, ventricular standstill with the maintenance of atrial beating, ventricular flutter, ventricular fibrillation, or any combination of these.

Supernormal Phase: A phase of hyperexcitability of the cardiac muscle immediately after the relative refractory phase in which the response is greater and the strength of stimulus required to produce the response is less than normally expected at this time.

Supraventricular Impulse: An impulse arising in any portion of the atrium including the S-A node, the A-V junction, or in the His bundle down to the point of its bifurcation.

T Wave: The chief end-deflection of the normal ventricular electrocardiogram; this represents the electrical repolarization of the ventricles.

Trigeminy: A condition in which two premature beats follow each normal beat, or two normal beats are followed by a premature beat.

U Wave: An inconstant and minor deflection of the normal electrocardiogram which occurs in early ventricular diastole. In electrolyte imbalance and certain abnormal states it may be quite prominent; this deflection may be superimposed upon the terminal portion of the T wave and may even exceed it in amplitude.

Unidirectional Block: Impaired conduction or absence of conductivity in one direction only (*e.g.*, complete A-V block with retrograde activation of atria; a unidirectional conduction is therefore present). Protection block and exit block in parasystole represent other examples of this phenomenon.

Unifocal Theory: Presumes that atrial tachycardia and flutter originate from and are perpetuated by a single rapidly discharging ectopic focus. Compare Circus Movement.

Usurpation: (Usually refers to a phenomenon observed with A-V dissociation.) Results from increased automaticity of the A-V node above that of the sinus node. This may occur when the nodal rate accelerates with or without slowing of the sinus rate, or when both pacemakers are slowed or accelerated to an unequal degree.

Ventricular Capture: In the presence of A-V dissociation, those atrial beats which occur during the nonrefractory period of both the A-V junction and the ventricles result in conducted sinus impulses, thus producing a ventricular response.

Ventricular Escape: A condition resulting from depression of the S-A nodal and A-V junctional pacemakers, allowing a focus in the ventricles, usually located in the upper portion of the interventricular septum, to assume the role of pacemaker. The resulting complexes are called "idioventricular beats."

Ventricular Extrasystole: An extrasystole (usually a premature beat) arising in the ventricle.

Ventricular Fibrillation: A condition of the ventricles yielding electrocardiographic deflections that are continuous, contiguous and varying greatly in form, amplitude, and incidence. The electrophysiologic background is chaotic and disorganized activity of the ventricular muscle resulting in totally ineffective pump action.

Ventricular Flutter: A condition bordering on chaotic heart action in which the ventricles contract weakly but regularly at a rate of about 200 per minute. In the electrocardiogram, the oscillations are represented by regular continuous waves of large amplitude and no distinction can be made between the QRS complex and T wave.

Ventricular Fusion Beat: Simultaneous stimulation of the ventricles by a supraventricular impulse having its origin in the sinus node, atrium or A-V junction and an impulse arising from a ventricular premature systole, a ventricular escape beat or a ventricular beat arising from a tachycardic ventricular pacemaker, or by two ventricular impulses from different foci.

Ventricular Standstill (Asystole): Absence of ventricular activity while atrial activity continues. See Stokes-Adams Syndrome.

Ventricular Tachycardia: A rapid ectopic rhythm with a rate of 130 to 180 per minute which originates in one of the ventricles or the conduction system below the bifurcation of the His bundle.

Ventriculophasic Sinus Arrhythmia: A type of sinus arrhythmia caused by ventricular activity as a consequence of vagal or mechanical influence upon the rhythmicity of sinus discharges. For example, in 2:1 or higher degrees of A-V heart block, the P-P intervals containing a QRS complex are shorter than those that do not.

Vulnerable Period: That interval during the relative refractory period of the heart cycle in which fibrillation is most easily produced by a single strong shock. The vulnerable period of the atrium is situated at the terminal portion of QRS complex; that of the ventricle coincides approximately with the peak of the T wave.

Wandering Pacemaker: A phenomenon in which the point of origin of the beat varies in successive cycles between different parts of the sinus node and A-V junction.

Wedensky Effect: A property of nervous and muscular tissue whereby subthreshold stimuli can, under certain circumstances, elicit a response. This is demonstrated in the following way: application of a subthreshold faradic current to the nerve of a nerve-muscle preparation may elicit no response; however, if during stimulation by this weak faradic current one strong induction shock is applied proximal to the area of faradization, the response will not be a single contraction but a brief tetanus. Thus, the conducted impulse temporarily alters the excitability of the nerve so that subthreshold stimuli can then elicit a response.

Wenckebach Phenomenon: Represents a periodicity or pattern of conduction that is observed in a single fiber, in the S-A node, A-V junction or ventricle. For example, in the A-V junction a progressive lengthening of the P-R interval occurs in successive cycles until a ventricular response fails to appear; this is followed by a cycle with a *short* P-R interval and the above events are repeated. In the S-A node a progressive lengthening of the S-A conduction time occurs until one of the sinus node impulses fails to be conducted to the atria.

Index

Aberration, 164–166
  definition of, 164
  differential diagnosis of, 165
  electrocardiogram in, 165
  therapy of, 166
Acid-base balance, maintenance of, 327. See also *Electrolytes.*
Acidosis, 392
Action potential, myocardial, normal, 11, 12, 13, 14
Addison's disease, arrhythmias in, 277
Adrenal glands, dysfunction of, arrhythmias and, 277
  hormones of, in cardiac regulation, 27
  therapeutic use of, 396, 405
Aldosterone, cardiac stimulation threshold and, 405
Alkalinizing agents, 336–338, 391–392. See also *Sodium lactate* and *Sodium bicarbonate.*
  for atrioventricular block, 123
  toxic effects of, 392
Allergic reaction, to procaine amide, 360, 361
Alprenolol, 364
Alternation of the heart, 222–228
  anatomic rotation hypothesis and, 224
  clinical features of, 224
  diagnosis of, 224–227
  etiology and clinical significance of, 222
  mechanisms involved in, 223–224
  prognosis in, 227
  therapy in, 227
  types of, 222–223
Aminophylline, therapeutic use of, 400
Amyloidosis, 321
Anatomic rotation hypothesis, 224
Anatomy, of heart, normal, 1–6
  pathologic changes in, 8–10
  of bundle branches, in atrioventricular block, 131
Anesthesia, and surgery, arrhythmias during, 279–283
  pathophysiology of, 280–281
  prior to cardioversion, 429
  proarrhythmic effects in, 401
  procaine amide and, 356
Angiocardiography, 286–288
  arrhythmias produced by, 287

Anomalies, cardiac, congenital, 261–265
Antazoline, 395–396
  dose and administration of, 396
Antihistaminic drugs, 395–396
Antistine, 395–396
Antithyroid drugs and isotopes, 394–395
  goitrogens, 394
  radioactive iodine, 395
Aorta, 4, 5
Aramine, therapeutic use of, 398–399
Arrhythmias. See also individual arrhythmias.
  cardiac physiology and, 21–24
  classification of, 38–39
  conditions simulating, 233–234
  definition of, 36
  diagnosis of, clinical, 40–41
    differential, 341
    electrocardiographic, 229–238
  during anesthesia and surgery, treatment of, 283
  during cardiac catheterization, 284–286
  endocrine disorders and, 275–278
  etiology of, 37–38
  factors leading to, 24–29
  familial occurrence of, 261–262
  hemodynamics in, 31–35. See also *Hemodynamics.*
  in fetus, 271
  in infancy and childhood, 267–270
  incidence of, 38
    in children, 266–267
  irregular, manifestations of, 39
  pathologic cardiac changes and, 8–10
  postcountershock, 430
  pregnancy and, 257–260
  respiratory maneuvers and, 322–324
  stress tests and, 248–256
  terminal, features of, 219
  therapy of, general methods in, 325–328. See also specific agents and techniques.
    in coronary care unit, 303
    prophylactic, 326
Arteriography, coronary, 288
Artifacts, electrocardiographic, 231
Asystole, partial, alternation of the heart and, 223
Atria, arrhythmias involving, 38
  beta-blocking effects on, 365

447

INDEX

Atria (Continued)
  hemodynamic roles of, 32
  impulse conduction and, 17
  normal anatomy of, 2
  relation of to arrhythmias, 43
Atrial capture, 169
Atrial fibrillation, 65–80
  arrhythmias associated with, 73
  conversion of, hemodynamics following, 433
  diagnosis of, 75
  electrocardiogram in, 70–75, 233
  electrophysiology of, 67
  etiology of, 65–66
  exercise and, 253
  hemodynamics in, 67–68
  in hyperthyroidism, 275
  in infants and children, 269
  in pregnancy, 259
  incidence of, 65
  paroxysmal, manifestations of, 70
    predisposing factors in, 65
    treatment of, 78
  pathology and pathophysiology of, 66–67
  precipitating factors in, 66
  premature beats initiating, 91
  prognosis in, 79
  symptoms and signs of, 69
  treatment of, 75–79
Atrial flutter, 55–64
  carotid sinus pressure for, 341
  complicating arrhythmias in, 61
  diagnosis of, 61–62
  electrocardiogram in, 233
  etiology of, 55–56
  hemodynamics in, 58
  impure, 59, 60
  in hyperthyroidism, 275
  in infancy and childhood, 269
  in pregnancy, 259
  mechanism of, 56
  prognosis in, 64
  symptoms and signs in, 56–58
  treatment of, 62–64
Atrial fusion beats, 98
Atrial pacing, 410
  indications for, 411
  uses of, 254–255
    in atrioventricular block, 118
    in digitalis toxicity, 385
Atrial parasystole, 95
Atrial premature beats, 91–95
  etiology of, 92
  hemodynamics in, 87
  prognosis in, 95
  treatment of, 95
Atrial standstill, 53–54
  diagnosis of, 53
Atrial tachycardia, during cardiac catheterization, 286
  multifocal, 106
  paroxysmal. See *Paroxysmal atrial tachycardia.*
  persistent, 107
  repetitive, 107
Atropine, effect of in arrhythmias, 335

Atropine (Continued)
  for atrioventricular block, complete, 139
    partial, 123
  for bradycardias, 336
  for cardioinhibitory syncope, 243
  indications for therapy with, 335
  mechanism of cardiac action of, 335
  toxic effects of, 336
Atrioventricular (A-V) heart block, 115–143
  atrial flutter with, 61
  atrial pacing and, 254
  complete (third degree), 116, 118, 124–139, 305
    acquired, 126
      clinical features of, 127–128
    alkalinizing agents for, 392
    arrhythmias associated with, 131
    congenital, 126
      clinical manifestations and diagnosis of, 262
      prognosis of, 263
    diagnosis of, 137–138
    electrocardiogram in, 128–131
    etiology of, 124–126
    hemodynamics in, 126–127
    patterns of, 131–137
    prognosis in, 139
    right bundle branch block, (RBBB), 132
    treatment of, 138–139
      ephedrine for, 398
      meperidine for, 401
      sodium lactate for, 390
      temporary pacemaker for, 405
    types of, 128
  definition of, 115
  fascicular blocks and, 132
  fetal, 272
  in infants and children, 269
    treatment of, 270
  in pregnancy, 259
    treatment of, 260
  Mobitz Type I. See *Atrioventricular (A-V) heart block, partial.*
  Mobitz Type II. See *Atrioventricular (A-V) heart block, partial.*
  paroxysmal atrial tachycardia (PAT) with, 110–113
    diagnosis of, 112
    incidence and etiology of, 111
    mechanism of, 111
    prognosis in, 113
    symptoms and signs of, 111
    treatment of, 112
      carotid sinus pressure for, 341
  partial, 119–123
    congenital, 264
    electrocardiogram in, 121–123
    etiology of, 119–120
    first degree, 116, 117, 305
      electrocardiogram in, 121
    pathology of, 120
    prognosis in, 123
    second degree, 116, 118, 305
      Mobitz Type I, electrocardiogram in, 121
      electrogram in, 118

INDEX

Atrioventricular (A–V) heart block, partial, second degree (*Continued*)
　　Mobitz Type II, electrocardiogram in, 122
　　　electrogram in, 118
　　　prognosis in, 123
　　　Wenckebach phenomenon, 116, 118, 121
　symptoms and signs in, 120–121
　treatment of, 123
　physiologic effects of, 120
　premature beats with, 91
　third degree. See *Atrioventricular (A-V) heart block, complete.*
　types of, 116–117
Atrioventricular (A–V) conduction, disturbances of, exercise and, 252
Atrioventricular (A–V) dissociation, 168–177
　auscultatory findings in, 175
　definition of terms in, 168–169
　diagnosis of, 175
　duration and fate of, 176
　electrocardiogram in, 175
　in A-V block, 128
　incidence and etiology of, 170–171
　mechanisms producing, 170
　potential, zone of, 169
　prognosis in, 177
　treatment of, 176–177
　types of, and modes of onset, 171–175
Atrioventricular (A–V) escape, 153–154
Atrioventricular (A–V) junction, anatomy of, 3
　arrhythmias involving, 38
　atrial fibrillation and, 73
　beta-blocking effects on, 365
　blood supply of, 6
　disturbances in region of, 144–167
　impulse conduction and, 18
　myocardial infarction and, 297
　premature beats and, 95–96
　procaine amide therapy and, 354
　reciprocal rhythm and, 155–156
　　diagnosis in, 156
Atrioventricular (A–V) junctional escape, electrocardiogram in, 153
　etiology of, 153
　treatment of, 154
Atrioventricular (A–V) junctional rhythm, 145–149
　diagnosis of, 149
　electrocardiogram in, 146
　incidence and etiology of, 145
　pathology of, 146
　prognosis in, 149
　symptoms and signs of, 146
Atrioventricular (A–V) junctional tachycardia, 151–153
　nonparoxysmal form, 153
　paroxysmal form, 151
Auscultatory findings, in atrial fibrillation, 69
　in atrial flutter, 58
　in atrioventricular (A-V) dissociation, 175
　in atrioventricular (A-V) heart block, partial, 121
　in flutter-fibrillation, 70
　in paroxysmal atrial tachycardia (PAT), 105
　in premature beats, 89, 90

Automaticity, cardiac, 12, 20
　agents to decrease, 339–374
　　sympathetic blocking agents, 364–368
　drugs to increase, 326, 329–338
Autonomic control, of cardiovascular function, 24

Bachmann's bundle, 4, 5
Bacterial infections, cardiac involvement in, 320–321
Banthine, dose and method of administration of, 336
　indications for therapy with, 336
Baroreceptors, and cardiovascular function, 27
Beta-adrenergic blocking agents, 364
　contraindications for, 367
　effects of, 365
　for atrial fibrillation, 77
　for digitalis toxicity, 385
　for ventricular premature beats, 100
Bidirectional tachycardia, 151
Block, heart, atrioventricular. See *Atrioventricular (A-V) heart block.*
　unidirectional, and re-entry, 22
Blood flow. See also *Circulation.*
　coronary, 6–8
　　premature beats and, 83
　phasic, measurement of in arrhythmias, 34
　regional, during premature beats, 88
　effects of arrhythmias on, 33–34
Blood pressure, postural syncope and, 243, 245
Bradycardias, fetal, 271, 272
　hemodynamics in, 31, 33
　sinus, 45–46
　treatment of, atropine for, 336
　　in coronary care unit, 305
　　temporary pacemaker for, 406
Brain, circulation in, arrhythmias and, 33
　damage to, cardiac arrest and, 218
　effects of on heart, 292
　relationships of with heart, 290–294
Breath-holding, arrhythmias and, 322
Bretylium, 370–372
　contraindications for, 372
　effects of, 371
　for ventricular tachycardia, 203
Bundle branch block, atrial pacing and, 254
　degrees of, 135
　right (RBBB), 132. See also *Right bundle branch block.*
　Wenckebach phenomena in, 137
Bundle branches, anatomy of, 3
　in atrioventricular (A-V) block, 131
　blood supply of, 7
Bundle of His, anatomy of, 3
　electrogram of, 16
　　clinical applications of, 17
　　in atrioventricular (A-V) block, 117
　　in Wolff-Parkinson-White syndrome, 183
　　value of, 118
　myocardial infarction and, 297
　procaine amide and, 354

INDEX

Bundle of Kent, accessory, 4
  pre-excitation syndromes and, 179
Butidrine, 364

Caffeine, premature beats and, 83
  proarrhythmic effects of, 400
Calcium, body balance of, 317–318
  therapeutic use of, 389
Cardiac arrest, 214–221
  complications of, 217–218
  diagnosis of, 215–217
  in infants and children, 270
  in pregnancy, 260
  incidence and etiology of, 214–215
  pathophysiology of, 215
  prognosis following, 219
  treatment of, 217
    alkalinizing therapy for, 392
  types of, 214
Cardiac catheterization, 284–286
  arrhythmias during, 285
  etiology of, 284
Cardiac impulse, artificial pacemaking and, 404–425
  formation of, 12
    disturbances of, 22, 23
    sinoatrial (S-A) node initiation of, 13
  propagation of, 15–19
Cardiac output, following conversion of tachyarrhythmias, 433
  in atrial fibrillation, 67, 68
  in exercise, 249
  in pregnancy, 257
Cardio-auditory syndrome, 241, 272–273
Cardiovascular system, collapse of, 303. See also *Cardiac arrest.*
  digitalis toxicity and, 380, 381
  propanolol effects on, 367
Cardioversion. See also *Countershock.*
  clinical regimen for, 428
  for Wolff-Parkinson-White (W-P-W) syndrome, 186
  in atrial fibrillation, 77
Carotid sinus pressure, 327, 340–345
  arrhythmia diagnosis using, 341
  complications of, 344
  contraindications for, 344
  failure in therapy using, causes for, 343
  indications for, 340–342
    in atrial flutter, 62, 63
    in paroxysmal atrial tachycardia, 108
    in QRS widening, 164
  response to, factors in, 340
  technique of applying, 342–344
Catecholamines, anesthesia and, 279
  postural syncope and, 244
Catheterization, cardiac, 284–286
  arrhythmias during, 285
  etiology of, 284
Cedilanid. See also *Digitalis.*
  dosage schedule for, 379
  for atrial fibrillation, 76

Cedilanid-D, dosage schedule for, 379
Central nervous system, etiology of arrhythmias and, 24, 37, 293
  digitalis toxicity and, 381
  procaine amide and, 360
Cerebral cortex, cardiovascular regulation and, 24, 25
  circulation to, arrhythmias and, 33
Chaotic atrial tachycardia, 106
Cheyne-Stokes respiration, arrhythmias and, 323
Children, arrhythmias in, 266–274
  etiology and incidence of, 266–267
  types of, 267–270
  digitalization of, dosage schedules for, 379
Chlorothiazide, therapeutic use of, 400
Chlorpromazine, 368
Cinchonism, 352
Cineangiography, 287
Circulation, cerebral, arrhythmias and, 33
  syncopal attacks and, 239
  coronary, 6–8
    arrhythmias and, 31, 34
    atrial fibrillation, 67
    premature beats, 83, 87
  in anesthesia, hypoxia and, 281
  regional, during premature beats, 88
  effects of arrhythmias on, 33–34
Circulatory arrest, in coronary care unit, 303
Circus movement, in atrial flutter, 56
  in paroxysmal atrial tachycardia, 103
Clinical diagnosis, of arrhythmia, 40–41
Closed-chest cardiac resuscitation, 217
Coffee, proarrhythmic effects of, 83
Computers, in electrocardiographic diagnosis, 236–238
Concealed conduction, of cardiac impulse, 18
  in atrial flutter, 59
  in Mobitz Type II block, 122
Conduction, atrioventricular, 15–19, 21
  beta-blocking effects on, 365
  concealed, 18
    in atrial flutter, 59
    in Mobitz Type II block, 122
  disturbances of, 22, 23
    with atrial flutter, 61
  inhomogeneous, 22
  potassium effects on, 388
  retrograde, in atrioventricular (A-V) block, 129
  ventricular, aberrant, 164–166
Congenital cardiac anomalies, 261–265
  atrioventricular block, complete, 126
Congestive heart failure, in atrial fibrillation, 69
Contourogram, 235, 236
Contractility, myocardial, 21
  quinidine and, 346
Convulsions, in Stokes-Adams disease, 140
Cor pulmonale, cardiac involvement in, 321–322
Coronary arteriography, 288
Coronary artery disease, arrhythmias and, 28, 308

INDEX

Coronary artery disease *(Continued)*
  myocardial infarction and, 295–311
Coronary care unit (CCU), 300–307
  cardiac arrest in, prognosis following, 219
  general considerations and history of, 300
  intermediate, 306
  mobile, 307
  personnel for, 301
  physical design and instrumentation of, 301
  prophylactic therapy in, 302–303, 304
Coronary sinus rhythm, 149–150
Corticoids, therapeutic use of, 396
Corticosteroids, therapeutic use of, 396
Countershock, 427–436
  clinical results with, 431
  complications of, 435
  contraindications for, 434
  indications for, 434
    in atrial fibrillation, 78
    in atrial flutter, 63
      in pregnancy, 259
    in digitalis toxicity, 38
    in paroxysmal ventricular tachycardia, 203
  mechanism of action of, 427
  place of in therapy, 435
  technique of, 429
Crista terminalis, 4
Cyclopropane, proarrhythmic effects of, 401

Deafness, congenital, cardiac syndrome involving, 272
Death, criteria of, 219
  sudden, 309–310
    predisposing factors in, 309
Decremental conduction, 22
Defibrillation, 426–427
  closed-chest, optimal conditions for, 427
Degenerative processes, atrioventricular (A-V) heart block due to, 124
"Demand" pacemaker, 413
  complications with, 419
Demerol, proarrhythmic effects of, 401
Desacetyl-lanatoside C. See also *Digitalis*.
  dosage schedule for, 379
Dexamethasone, cardiac stimulation threshold and, 405
Diagnosis, clinical, of arrhythmias, guidelines for, 40–41
Diaphragm, disturbances involving, electrocardiogram and, 234
Digitalis, 375–386, 400
  absorption and metabolism of, 375–377
  administration of, 378–380
  dosage schedules for, 378, 379
  duration of action of, 380
  indications for therapy with, 377
    in atrial fibrillation, 75
    in atrial flutter, 62
    in paroxysmal atrial tachycardia, 109
      in infancy and childhood, 268
    in ventricular premature beats, 100
  mechanism of cardiac effects of, 375
  toxicity of, 380–385

Digitalis, toxicity of *(Continued)*
    in therapy of atrial fibrillation, 76
  manifestations of, 381
    cardiac, 380
  treatment of, 383
    diphenylhydantoin in, 369
    procaine amide in, 356
Digitoxin. See also *Digitalis*.
  dosage schedules for, 379
  duration of action of, 380
  for atrial fibrillation, 76
Digoxin. See also *Digitalis*.
  dosage schedules for, 379
  duration of action of, 380
  for atrial fibrillation, 76
  toxic complications with, 382
Dilantin, for ventricular tachycardia, 203
Diphenylhydantoin (DPH), 368–370
  absorption and metabolism of, 369
  cardiac stimulation threshold and, 405
  contraindications for, 370
  dose and administration of, 369
  for digitalis toxicity, 385
  for ventricular premature beats, 100
  for ventricular tachycardia, 203
  pharmacologic effects of, 368
  toxic effects of, 370
Direct current countershock. See *Countershock*.
Disease states, cardiac involvement in, 320–324
  etiology of arrhythmias and, 37–38
Dissociation. See also *Atrioventricular (A-V) dissociation*.
  definition of, 168
  potential, zone of, 169
Diuretic agents, therapeutic use of, 400
Doppler ultrasonic telemetry, 87
DPH. See *Diphenylhydantoin*.
Drug therapy. See also *Drugs*.
  in aberration, 166
  in alternation of the heart, 227
  in atrioventricular (A-V) heart block, 138
    partial, 123
  in cardio-auditory syndrome, 273
  in fibrillation, atrial, 75
    ventricular, 212
  in premature beats, ventricular, 99
    in pregnancy, 258
  in tachycardia, paroxysmal, atrial, 108, 109
    in infancy and childhood, 268
    ventricular, 202
    in pregnancy, 258
  in Wolff-Parkinson-White (W-P-W) syndrome, 185
  to prevent postcountershock (PCS) arrhythmias, 430
Drugs. See also *Drug therapy*.
  antihistaminic, 395–396
  antithyroid, 394–395
  artificial pacemaking and, 417
  cardiac stimulation threshold and, 405
  causing atrioventricular (A-V) heart block, 119
  causing ventricular fibrillation, 208

Drugs (*Continued*)
  proarrhythmic, 327, 400–402
  sympathetic-blocking, 364–368
  to decrease cardiac automaticity, 327, 344–374
  to increase cardiac automaticity, 326, 329–338
  vasopressor, 327, 396–399
Dysrhythmia, 37

Ebstein's anomaly, 264
Ectopic beats, 81
Ectopic rhythm, definition of, 36
Edecrin, 400
Edrophonium, therapeutic use of, 346
  for paroxysmal atrial tachycardia, 109
Electrical countershock. See *Countershock.*
Electrical shock, initiating ventricular fibrillation, 208, 426
  terminating ventricular fibrillation, 427
Electrical stimulation, experimental, of brain, arrhythmias and, 290–291
  therapeutic, 328
Electrocardiogram, configuration of, 15
  diagnostic use of, 229–238
  in aberration, 165
  in alternation of the heart, 223
  in atrial fibrillation, 70–75
  in atrial flutter, 58–61, 62
  in atrioventricular (A-V) dissociation, 175
  in atrioventricular (A-V) junctional escape, 153
  in atrioventricular (A-V) junctional rhythm, 146
  in atrioventricular (A-V) junctional tachycardia, 151
  in beta-blocking drug therapy, 366
  in cardio-auditory syndrome, 273
  in exercise, 250
  in exit block, 86
  in idioventricular rhythm, 198
  in norepinephrine therapy, 332
  in paroxysmal atrial tachycardia, 105, 107
  in paroxysmal ventricular tachycardia, 193
  in premature beats, 90–91
    atrial, 92, 93
    ventricular, 96
  in quinidine therapy, 348
  in syncopal attacks, 242, 245
  in tachycardias, T wave changes and, 199–200
  in ventricular fibrillation, 210–211
  in Wolff-Parkinson-White (W-P-W) syndrome, 182
  normal, 42–43
  of fetus, 270–272
  terminal, 219–220
Electroencephalogram, in evaluating syncopal episode, 245
Electrogram, His bundle, 16
  clinical applications of, 17
  in atrioventricular (A-V) heart block, 117
  in Wolff-Parkinson-White (W-P-W) syndrome, 183

Electrolytes, balance of, disturbances of, 312–319
  calcium, 317–318
  flux of, quinidine and, 347
  magnesium, 318–319
  potassium, 312–317
  therapeutic uses of, 387–393
Electrophysiology, of heart, 11–15
  in atrial fibrillation, 67
  in atrioventricular (A-V) heart block, 117–119
  in paroxysmal atrial tachycardia, 103
Emotions, arrhythmias and, 253, 292
Endocrine disturbances, arrhythmias and, 37, 275–278
  treatment in, 394–395
"Entrance block," 84
Ephedrine, cardiac stimulation threshold and, 405
  therapeutic use of, 398
Epinephrine, acute myocardial infarction and, 296
  cardiac stimulation threshold and, 405
  dose and administration of, 331
  hemodynamic effects of, 331
  indications for therapy with, 331
    in complete atrioventricular (A-V) block, 139
    in ventricular premature beats, 100
  mechanism of action of, 330
  postural syncope and, 244
Ethacrynic acid, 400
Excitability, of normal heart muscle, 20
  supernormal, 85
Exercise, arrhythmias and, 248–253
  premature beats, 83
  beta-blocking effects and, 365
  electrocardiogram in, 250
  hemodynamic effects of, 249
  isometric, arrhythmias induced by, 253
"Exit block," 84, 86
Extrasystole, 81

Fainting. See *Syncopal attacks.*
Familial arrhythmias, 261–262
Fetus, arrhythmias in, 271
  electrocardiograms of, 270–272
Fibrillation, atrial, 65–80. See also *Atrial Fibrillation.*
  threshold of, artificial pacemaking and, 404
  ventricular, 207–213. See also *Ventricular fibrillation.*
First degree atrioventricular (A-V) block, 116, 117, 305
  electrocardiogram in, 121
First degree sinoatrial (S-A) block, 48
Fluoroalkane gases, proarrhythmic effects of, 402
Flutter, atrial, 55–64. See also *Atrial flutter.*
Frank-Starling principle, 24, 31
Furosemide, 400
Fusion beats, atrial, 98
  premature, 98
  ventricular, 98

INDEX

Gallop rhythms, in premature beats, 89
Gastrointestinal system, digitalis toxicity and, 381
   disturbances of, arrhythmias and, 37
   procaine amide and, 360
Gitalin. See also *Digitalis.*
   dosage schedule for, 379
Glossary, 437-445
Glucose, cardiac stimulation threshold and, 405
Glycosides. See also *Digitalis.*
   half-life of, 380
Goitrogens, 394

Halothane, proarrhythmic effects of, 401
Heart, alternation of. See *Alternation of the heart.*
   anatomy of, 1-6
      pathologic changes in, 8-10
      in atrial fibrillation, 69
      of bundle branches, in atrioventricular (A-V) block, 131
   inflammatory diseases of, 28
   orthostatic paroxysmal acceleration of, 324
   physiology of, 11-30
   stimulation threshold of, 404
Heart beat, irregular, manifestations of, 39
   supernormal, in alternation of the heart, 224
Heart block, atrioventricular. See *Atrioventricular (A-V) heart block.*
Heart failure, in atrial fibrillation, 69
Heart rate, acceleration of, in QRS widening, 158
   arrhythmia diagnosis and, 40
   atropine and, 335
   autonomic control of, 43
   normal, 13
      factors determining, 19-20
   rapid, symptoms and signs with, 39, 44
   slow, manifestations with, 39, 46
   with QRS widening, 161
Heart sounds. See *Auscultatory findings.*
Hemochromatosis, 277, 321
Hemodynamics, 31-35
   alterations in, cardiac regulation and, 27
   beta-blocking agents and, 365
   following conversion of tachyarrhythmias, 433
   general considerations of, 31-32
   in acute myocardial infarction, 299
   in aramine therapy, 398
   in artificial pacemaking, 415
   in atrial fibrillation, 67-68
      following conversion, 68, 433
   in atrial flutter, 58
   in diphenylhydantoin therapy, 369
   in epinephrine therapy, 331
   in exercise, 249
   in isoproterenol (Isuprel) therapy, 333
   in lidocaine therapy, 362
   in metaraminol therapy, 398
   in norepinephrine therapy, 332
   in paroxysmal atrial tachycardia, 103-104
   in premature beats, 86-88
   in procaine amide therapy, 355

Hemodynamics *(Continued)*
   in ventricular fibrillation, 209
   in Wolff-Parkinson-White (W-P-W) syndrome, 184
Heroin, proarrhythmic effects of, 401
His bundle. See *Bundle of His.*
Histology, of atrioventricular (A-V) junction, 6
Hormone(s), adrenal, in cardiac regulation, 27, 277
   corticoid, therapeutic use of, 396
   thyroid, proarrhythmic effects of, 400
Hydrochlorothiazide, therapeutic use of, 400
Hypercalcemia, 318, 389
Hypermagnesemia, 319
Hyperpotassemia, arrhythmias and, 314, 389, 390
   alkalinizing agents for, 392
   diagnosis of, 315
   electrocardiogram in, 315, 316, 390
   etiology and clinical manifestations of, 313
   treatment of, 317
Hyperthyroidism, arrhythmias in, 275
Hyperventilation, arrhythmias and, 322
Hypocalcemia, 317
Hypoglycemia, arrhythmias and, 276
Hypomagnesemia, 318
Hypopotassemia, electrophysiology in, 313
   etiology of, 312
   therapy of, 313
Hyposystole, alternation of the heart and, 224
Hypotension, in bretylium therapy, 371
   orthostatic, 244
   vasopressor drugs for, 397
Hypothalamus, cardiovascular regulation and, 24, 25
   stimulation of, arrhythmias and, 291
Hypothermia, ventricular fibrillation and, 208
Hypoxia, and atrioventricular (A-V) heart block, 119
   during anesthesia, arrhythmias and, 281

Idioventricular rhythm, 198-199, 305
Imipramine hydrochloride, proarrhythmic effects of, 401
Impulse, cardiac, artificial pacemaking and, 404-425
   formation of, 12
   sinoatrial (S-A) node initiation of, 13
Inderal, dose and administration of, 367
Infants, arrhythmias in, 266-274
Infectious diseases, cardiac involvement in, 320-321
   atrioventricular (A-V) heart block and, 119
Infiltrative diseases, cardiac involvement in, 321
Inflammatory diseases, of heart, 28
Inhomogeneous conduction, 22
Insulin, cardiac stimulation threshold and, 405
Interference, definition of, 168
Internodal pathways, myocardial infarction and, 297
Iodine, radioactive, 395
Isometric exercise, arrhythmias induced by, 253

Isoproterenol, cardiac stimulation threshold and, 405
  dose and administration of, 334
    with artificial pacemaker, 417
  hemodynamic effects of, 333
  indications for therapy with, 333
    for atrioventricular (A-V) block, 123
      complete, 139
  mechanism of action of, 333
  toxic effects of, 334
Isuprel, dose and method of administration of, 334
  hemodynamic effects of, 333
  indications for therapy with, 333
  mechanism of action of, 333
  toxic effects of, 334

Junctional tachycardia, bidirectional, carotid sinus pressure for, 341

Kent, bundle of. See *Bundle of Kent.*
Kidneys, blood flow to, in arrhythmias, 34

Lanatoside C. See also *Digitalis.*
  dosage schedule for, 379
  duration of action of, 380
  for atrial fibrillation, 76
Largactil, 368
Lasix, 400
Left anterior hemiblock (LAH), 133
Left atrial rhythm, 150–151
Lidocaine, 361–364
  contraindications for, 364
  dose and administration of, 362
  electrophysiologic effects of, 361
  hemodynamic effects of, 362
  indications for therapy with, 362
    in ventricular fibrillation, 212
    in ventricular premature beats, 100
    in ventricular tachycardia, 202
  toxicity of, 363
Lignocaine, 363
Limbic system, cardiovascular regulation and, 24
Lown-Ganong-Levine syndrome, 180–181
Lung disease, arrhythmias and, 37

Macro-reentry theory, of paroxysmal atrial tachycardia, 103
Magnesium, cardiac function and, 318–319
  therapeutic use of, 389–391
Mahaim fibers, 5
  pre-excitation syndromes and, 179
Medulla, cardiovascular regulation and, 24, 25
Mellaril, proarrhythmic effects of, 401
Meperidine, proarrhythmic effects of, 401

Mephentermine, therapeutic use of, 399
  for alternation of the heart, 227
Metabolism, cardiovascular regulation and, 26
  of digitalis, 375–377
  of diphenylhydantoin, 369
Metaraminol, therapeutic use of, 398–399
Methantheline, dose and administration of, 336
  indications for therapy with, 336
Methimazole, 394
Methoxamine, therapeutic use of, 397–398
Methylprednisone, cardiac stimulation threshold and, 405
Mineralocorticoids, cardiac stimulation threshold and, 405
Mitral valve, 5
Mobitz Type I heart block, 116
  electrogram in, 118
Mobitz Type II heart block, 116
  electrocardiogram in, 122
  electrogram in, 118
  prognosis in, 123
Monitoring, computer uses in, 236–238
  contourography in, 235, 236
  long-term, 234–236
Morphine, proarrhythmic effects of, 401
Mortality, from myocardial infarction, 306
Multifocal atrial tachycardia, 106
Murmurs, in premature beats, 89
Myocardial circulation, 6–8
Myocardial infarction, 295–311
  acute, arrhythmias following, 296
    electrocardiographic diagnosis and, 299–300
    incidence of, 301–302
    premonitory, 302
    prophylaxis of, 302–303
  electrophysiologic factors in, 298–299
  hemodynamics following, 299
  involvement of specialized tissues in, 297–298
  mortality from, 306
  pathophysiology of, 28, 296–297
  prehospital management of, 306
  ventricular fibrillation and, 208
  healed, arrhythmias in, 308
Myxedema, arrhythmias in, 276

Neostigmine, dose and administration of, 346
  mechanism of action of, 345
Neo-Synephrine, therapeutic use of, 397
  for supraventricular tachycardia, 110
Nervous system, digitalis toxicity and, 381
  etiology of arrhythmias and, 24, 37, 293
  procaine amide and, 360
Neuromuscular disease, cardiac involvement in, 321
Nicotine, proarrhythmic effects of, 401–402
Norepinephrine, dose and administration of, 332
  hemodynamic effects of, 332
  indications for use of, 332
  mechanism of action of, 332
  toxic effects of, 333

INDEX

Oculocardiac reflex, 344
Open-chest cardiac resuscitation, 218
Orthostatic hypotension, 244
Orthostatic paroxysmal acceleration of heart, 324
Oscillations, atrial, in atrial flutter, 58, 59
Ouabain. See also *Digitalis*.
  dosage schedule for, 379
Output of heart. See *Cardiac output*.
Overdrive suppression, with artificial pacemaker, indications for, 407

P cells, of sinoatrial (S-A) node, 2, 13
P waves, electrocardiographic diagnosis and, 229
  in normal electrocardiogram, 15
Pacemakers, artificial, 404–425
  asynchronous, 411
    prognosis of, 418
  atomic-powered, 415
  bifocal demand type, 413
    indications for, 415
  cardioactive drugs and, 417
  clinical results with, 417
  failure of, causes and detection of, 421
  for atrioventricular (A-V) block, 127
    complete, 139
  for cardioinhibitory syncope, 243
  for paroxysmal ventricular tachycardia, 203
  for Stokes-Adams disease, 141
  for Wolff-Parkinson-White (W-P-W) syndrome, 186
  general considerations with, 404–405
  hemodynamic effects of, 415
  permanent use of, 408–424
    indications for, 408
    problems in, 417, 419
    sites of electrode placement in, 408
    types of implanted pulse generators for, 411
  placement of, 406
  synchronous, 411
    prognosis of, 418
  temporary use of, 405–408
    indications for, 405
    overdrive suppression in, 407
  ventricular-programmed, 413
  "wandering," 47–48
Pacemaker (P) cells, of sinoatrial (S-A) node, 2, 13
Palpitation, evaluation of, 40
Papillary muscle, 4, 5
Parasitic diseases, cardiac involvement in, 321
Parasympathetic blocking agents, 334–336
Parasympathetic effects, and cardiovascular function, 26
Parasympathomimetic drugs, 345–346
Parasystole, 24
  atrial, 95
  with premature beats, 84
Parathyroids, disorders of, arrhythmias and, 276

Paroxysmal atrial tachycardia (PAT), 102–114
  atrial pacing and, 254
  diagnosis of, 107–108
  digitalis therapy and, 378
  etiology of, 103
  in infancy and childhood, 268
  mechanisms of, 103
  prognosis in, 110
  symptoms and signs of, 104–105
  treatment of, 108–110
    patient's role in, 108
  with atrioventricular heart block (PAT with block), 110–113
    carotid sinus pressure for, 341
    diagnosis of, 112
    incidence and etiology of, 111
    mechanism of, 111
    prognosis in, 113
    symptoms and signs of, 111
    treatment of, 112
Paroxysmal ventricular tachycardia, 189–206. See also *Ventricular tachycardia*.
  complications of, 205
  diagnostic features of, 191
  electrocardiogram in, 193
  hemodynamics in, 190–191
  incidence and etiology of, 189–190
  mechanism of, 190
  prognosis in, 205
  symptoms and signs of, 192
  treatment of, 201
Pathologic findings, in arrhythmias, 8–10
  in atrial flutter, 58
  in paroxysmal atrial tachycardia, 103
PCS (postcountershock) arrhythmias, 430
Persistent atrial tachycardia, 107
Phenylephrine, therapeutic use of, 397
  for supraventricular tachycardias, 110
Physiology, cardiac, 11–30
  disordered, in atrial fibrillation, 66–67
    in atrioventricular (A-V) heart block, 117–119
  of normal muscle, 20–21
Polyuria, with paroxysmal atrial tachycardia, 105
Postcountershock (PCS) arrhythmias, 430
Postoperative period, arrhythmias in, 282
Postural syncope, 243–244
  treatment of, 244
Posture, changes in, cardiac reactions to, 324
Potassium, body balance of, 313–317
  therapeutic use of, 387–389
    dose in, 388
    for digitalis toxicity, 384, 389
    for PAT with block, 113
  tolerance to, factors in, 315
  toxic effects of, 388
P-P interval, in atrioventricular (A-V) heart block, 130
P-R interval, 15
  in atrioventricular (A-V) heart block, 120
  electrocardiographic diagnosis and, 230
  exercise and, 252
  in hyperthyroidism, 275
  propanolol and, 366

Practolol, 364
Prednisone, cardiac stimulation threshold and, 405
Pre-excitation syndromes, 178–187
　anatomic and pathologic considerations in, 178–180
　exercise and, 253
　Lown-Ganong-Levine syndrome, 180–181
　Wolff-Parkinson-White (W-P-W) syndrome, 181–187
Pregnancy, arrhythmias in, 257–260
　　etiology of, 257
　　types of, 257–260
Premature beats, 81–101
　atrial, 91–95. See also *Atrial premature beats*.
　atrial fibrillation and, 91
　atrial pacing and, 254
　atrioventricular (A-V) junctional, 95–96
　carotid sinus pressure for, 341
　diagnosis of, 90
　during angiocardiography, 287
　electrocardiogram in, 90
　etiology of, 83–84
　exercise and, 250, 251
　frequency of, and hemodynamics, 87
　in infancy and childhood, 267
　incidence of, 82–83
　mechanisms producing, 84–86
　pregnancy and, 257
　symptoms and signs of, 88–90
　ventricular, 96–101. See also *Ventricular premature beats*.
　with atrioventricular (A-V) heart block, 91
Proarrhythmic drugs, 400–402
Procaine amide, 354–361
　absorption and metabolism of, 355
　cardiac stimulation threshold and, 405
　contraindications for, 361
　dose and administration of, 356
　electrophysiologic effects of, 354
　for tachycardia, paroxysmal atrial, 109
　　in infants and children, 269
　for ventricular premature beats, 100
　for ventricular tachycardia, 203
　for Wolff-Parkinson-White (W-P-W) syndrome, 185
　hemodynamic effects of, 355
　indications for therapy with, 355
　pharmacologic effects of, 354
　toxicitiy of, 358
　　alkalinizing agents for, 392
Propanolol, cardiac stimulation threshold and, 405
　contraindications for, 367
　dose and administration of, 367
　electrocardiographic effects of, 366
　indications for therapy with, 366
　　for atrial fibrillation, 77
　　for atrial flutter, 63
　pharmacologic actions of, 365
　physiologic effects of, 354
　toxicity of, 367
Propylthiouracil, 394

Prostigmin, 345
"Protection block," 84
Pseudoalternation, differential diagnosis of, 226
"Pseudobigeminy," 60
Psychosomatic disorders, arrhythmias and, 292–293
Pulse generators, types of, in artificial pacemaking, 411
Pulsus alternans. See also *Alternation of the heart*.
　atrial pacing and, 254
　supernormal strong beat and, 224
Purkinje fibers, 4, 5
　cardiac impulse conduction in, 19
　normal anatomy of, 3
　procaine amide and, 354

QRS complex, electrocardiographic diagnosis and, 230
　in A-V junctional rhythm, 148
　narrowing of, paradoxical, 162
　widening of, 157–164
　　carotid sinus pressure and, 164
　　etiology and clinical significance of, 161
　　types of, 158
　　with heart rate acceleration, mechanisms of, 160
Q-T interval, propanolol and, 366
Quinaglute, 350, 351
Quinidine, 346–354
　absorption and metabolism of, 347
　contraindications for, 354
　dose and administration of, 349
　electrocardiographic effects of, 348
　electrophysiologic effects of, 346
　pharmacologic effects of, 345
　indications for therapy with, 349
　　for atrial fibrillation, 77
　　for atrial flutter, 63
　　for tachycardias, in infants and children, 269
　　　supraventricular, 109
　　　ventricular, 203
　　for ventricular premature beats, 99
　　for Wolff-Parkinson-White (W-P-W) syndrome, 185
　　prior to countershock, 428
　toxicity of, 352
　　alkalinizing agents for, 392

Radioactive iodine, 395
Radioelectrocardiography, 236, 251
RBBB. See *Right bundle branch block*.
Reciprocal rhythm, 155–156
　diagnosis of, 156
Re-entry, premature beats and, 84
Reflex mechanisms, cardiovascular, 25, 27
　in syncopal attacks, 241
　oculocardiac, 344

INDEX

Renal circulation, in arrhythmias, 34
Repetitive atrial tachycardia, 107
Respiration, Cheyne-Stokes, arrhythmias and, 323
  propanolol effects on, 367
  sinus arrhythmia and, 46
Respiratory maneuvers, arrhythmias associated with, 253–254, 322–324
  therapeutic, 327
Resuscitation, closed-chest, 217
  open-chest, 218
Reticular formation, stimulation of, arrhythmias and, 291
Retrograde conduction, in atrioventricular (A-V) block, 129
Right bundle branch block (RBBB), 132
  and QRS widening, 160
  during cardiac catheterization, 286
  with left axis deviation (LAD), 134
  and QV_1 ($RBBBQV_1$), 135

S-A node. See *Sinoatrial node*.
Second degree sinoatrial block, 48
Seizures, Stokes-Adams, 140–141
Sick sinus syndrome (SSS), 52
  diagnosis of, atrial pacing and, 254
Sinoatrial (S-A) block, 48–53
  arrhythmias associated with, 52
  etiology of, 50
  first degree, 48
  prognosis in, 53
  second degree, 48
  symptoms and signs of, 50
  treatment of, 52
Sinoatrial (S-A) node, arrhythmias involving, 38, 43
  automaticity in, 20
  beta-blocking effects on, 365
  blood supply of, 6
  cardiac impulse conduction and, 13
  normal anatomy of, 1
Sinus arrhythmias, 42–54. See also *Sinus bradycardia* and *Sinus tachycardia*.
  etiology of, 47
  pauses, prolonged, in S-A block, 51
  symptoms and signs of, 47
  versus normal rhythms, 232
Sinus bradycardia, 45–46
  clinical features of, 45
  diagnosis of, 46
  etiology of, 45
  symptoms and signs with, 46
  treatment of, 46
Sinus tachycardia, 43–45
  electrocardiographic signs of, 44
  in hyperthyroidism, 275
  symptoms and signs of, 44
  treatment of, 44
Sinusoidal circulation, 8
Sluggish sinus node syndrome, 52
Smoking, proarrhythmic effects of, 402

Sodium bicarbonate, 391–392. See also *Sodium lactate*.
  indications for therapy with, 337
    in complete atrioventricular (A-V) block, 139
    in hyperpotassemia, 389, 390
  mechanism of cardiac effects of, 336
  toxic effects and contraindications for, 337
Sodium lactate. See also *Sodium bicarbonate*.
  indications for therapy with, 337
  mechanism of cardiac effects of, 336
  toxic effects and contraindications for, 337
Solatol, 364
Splanchnic circulation, arrhythmias and, 34
"Standby" pacemaker, 413
Stimulation threshold, cardiac, artificial pacemaking and, 404
  determination of, 405
  drugs affecting, 405
Stokes-Adams seizures, 140–141
  clinical features of, 140
  prognosis in, 141
  therapy of, ephedrine for, 398
  temporary pacemaker for, 405
Stomach, blood flow to, in arrhythmias, 34
Stress, arrhythmia-producing, 4, 248–256
Strophanthin, dosage schedule for, in children, 379
Sudden death, 309–310
"Supernormal excitability," 85
Supraventricular arrhythmias, therapy of, in coronary care unit, 303. See also specific arrhythmias.
Surdo-cardiac syndrome, 272
Surgery, 279–284
  cardiac, arrhythmias during, 282
    cardiac arrest during, 214, 215
    prognosis following, 219
    for arrhythmias, 328
      Wolff-Parkinson-White (W-P-W) syndrome, 186
  general, arrhythmias during, 281
    ventricular fibrillation, 208, 212
  thoracic, arrhythmias during, 282
  procaine amide therapy and, 356
Sympathetic blocking agents, 364–368
  mode of action of, 364
Sympathetic effects, and cardiovascular function, 26
Sympathectomy, 328
Sympathomimetic amines, 329–334
  classification of, 330
  for atrioventricular (A-V) heart block, 139
  proarrhythmic effects of, 401
Syncopal attacks, 239–247
  cardiac causes in, 240–243
  complications of, 246
  differential diagnosis of, 246
  etiologic factors in, 239–240
    determination of, 244–246
  in atrial fibrillation, 69
  postural type, 243
  prognosis in, 246
  in Stokes-Adams disease, 140–141
Syphilis, cardiac involvement in, 320

T waves, changes in, following paroxysmal tachycardia, 199–200
  electrocardiographic diagnosis and, 233
  propanolol therapy and, 366
Tachycardia, atrial, paroxysmal. See *Paroxysmal atrial tachycardia.*
  conversion of, hemodynamics following, 433
  hemodynamics in, 31, 33, 104
  in pregnancy, 258
    bidirectional, 151
    carotid sinus pressure for, 341
  paroxysmal in infancy and childhood, 267
    T wave changes following, 199–200
  simple, electrocardiographic signs of, 44
  sinus, in hyperthyroidism, 275
  supraventricular, in infancy and childhood, 268
    in pregnancy, 258
  ventricular, in atrial flutter, 61
    paroxysmal. See *Paroxysmal ventricular tachycardia.*
Tensilon, therapeutic use of, 346
  for paroxysmal atrial tachycardia, 109
THAM, therapeutic use of, 337
Therapy, of arrhythmias, approach to, 325–326
  general methods in, 325–328
Thioridazine, proarrhythmic effects of, 401
Third degree sinoatrial block, 49
Thorazine, 368
Thyroid heart disease, 275–276
  treatment of, 395
Thyroid hormone, cardiac regulation and, 27
  proarrhythmic effects of, 400
Tofranil, proarrhythmic effects of, 401
Trasicor, 364
Tromethamine, therapeutic use of, 337

Unidirectional block, and re-entry, 22

Vagal effects, carotid sinus pressure and, 344
  cardiovascular regulation and, 25, 26
Valsalva maneuver, arrhythmias and, 253, 254, 322, 323
  for paroxysmal atrial tachycardia, 109
Vasodepressor syncope, 243
Vasopressor drugs, 396–399
Vasoxyl, therapeutic use of, 397–398
Vectorcardiogram, in Wolff-Parkinson-White (W-P-W) syndrome, 184
Venous circulation, myocardial, 8
Ventricles, arrhythmias involving, 39. See also specific arrhythmias.
  treatment of, in coronary care unit, 304
  function of, in atrial fibrillation, 67, 69, 71, 73
    in atrial flutter, 56, 59
    in atrioventricular (A-V) block, 130
  in beta-blocking therapy, 365
  impulse conduction in, 19
    aberrant, 164–166
Ventricular capture, 169

Ventricular fibrillation, 207–213
  cardiac mechanisms preceding, 209
  clinical diagnosis of, 209–210
  during cardiac catheterization, 285
  electrical shock and, 426, 427
  electrocardiogram in, 210–211
  etiology of, 208
  hemodynamics in, 209
  incidence of, 207
  mechanisms underlying, 209
  prognosis in, 212–213
  threshold of, factors affecting, 208–209
  treatment of, 211–212
    bretylium in, 371
Ventricular flutter, 207–213
Ventricular fusion beats, 98
Ventricular pacing, in digitalis toxicity, 385
Ventricular premature beats, 96–101
  electrocardiogram in, 96
  hemodynamics in, 87
  in atrial fibrillation, 73
  prognosis in, 100
  treatment of, 99
Ventricular tachycardia, arrhythmias simulating, 200
  differential diagnosis of, 200–201
  during cardiac catheterization, 286
  in atrial flutter, 61
  in pregnancy, 259
  types of, 195
    paroxysmal, 189–206. See also *Paroxysmal ventricular tachycardia.*
Viral diseases, cardiac involvement in, 321
Vision, digitalis toxicity and, 381
Vomiting, induction of, in paroxysmal atrial tachycardia (PAT), 109

Wenckebach phenomenon, 48, 49
  in atrioventricular (A-V) block, 116
    bundle branch block, 137
    electrocardiogram of, 121
    electrogram of, 118
Wolff-Parkinson-White (W-P-W) syndrome, 181–187
  arrhythmias associated with, 184
  cardiac status and, 182
  congenital anomaly and, 264
  diagnosis of, 182
    atrial pacing and, 254
  electrocardiogram in, 182
  incidence and etiology of, 181
  prognosis in, 187
  treatment of, 185
Wyamine, therapeutic use of, 399
"Wandering pacemaker," 47–48

Xanthines, premature beats and, 83
  therapeutic use of, 400

Zone of potential dissociation, 169